Basic
Histology

a LANGE medical book

Basic
Histology

seventh edition

L. Carlos Junqueira, MD
Director Emeritus, Laboratory of Morphology
Ludwig Institute for Cancer Research
São Paulo, Brazil
Honorary Research Associate in Biology
Harvard College, Boston
Formerly Research Associate
Medical School, University of Chicago

José Carneiro, MD
Professor of Histology & Embryology
Institute of Biomedical Sciences, University of São Paulo, Brazil
Formerly Research Associate, Department of Anatomy
Medical School, McGill University, Montreal, Canada
Formerly Visiting Associate Professor, Department of Anatomy
Medical School, University of Virginia, Charlottesville, Virginia

Robert O. Kelley, PhD
Chairman, Department of Anatomy
The University of New Mexico, School of Medicine
Professor of Anatomy & Biology
The University of New Mexico
Albuquerque, New Mexico

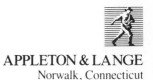

APPLETON & LANGE
Norwalk, Connecticut

0-8385-0576-7

Italian Edition: *Piccin Nuova Libraria, S.p.A., Via Altinate, 107, 35121 Padua, Italy*
Dutch Edition: *Kooyker Scientific Publications B.V., Postbus 24,*
2300 AA Leiden, The Netherlands
Indonesian Edition: *CV, E.G.C. Medical Publisher, P.O. Box 4276,*
10711 Jakarta, Indonesia
Japanese Edition: *Hirokawa Publishing Company, 27-14, Hongo 3, Bunkyo-ku,*
Tokyo 113, Japan
German Edition: *Springer-Verlag GmbH & Co. KG, Postfach 10 52 80,*
6900 Heidelberg 1, West Germany

Original title: *Histologia Basica,* 2nd ed. © 1971 by Editôra Guanabara Koogan S.A., Rio de Janeiro, Brazil

Many of the illustrations in this book were prepared with financial aid from the Fundação de Amparo à Pesquisa do Estado de São Paulo.

Prentice Hall International (UK) Limited, *London*
Prentice Hall of Australia Pty. Limited, *Sydney*
Prentice Hall Canada, Inc., *Toronto*
Prentice Hall Hispanoamericana, S.A., *Mexico*
Prentice Hall of India Private Limited, *New Delhi*
Prentice Hall of Japan, Inc., *Tokyo*
Simon & Schuster Asia Pte. Ltd., *Singapore*
Editora Prentice Hall do Brasil Ltda., *Rio de Janeiro*
Prentice Hall, *Englewood Cliffs, New Jersey*

ISBN: 0-8385-0576-7
ISSN: 0891-2106

Production Editor: Charles F. Evans
Cover Designer: Janice Barsevich

Table of Contents

Preface

The seventh edition of *Basic Histology* continues to be a concise, well-illustrated exposition of the basic facts and interpretation of microscopic anatomy. The information contained in this book is the foundation on which pathology and pathophysiology are built. Consequently, we continue to emphasize the relationships and concepts by which cell and tissue structure are inextricably linked with their function.

In revising *Basic Histology,* our intent is to provide our readers with the most contemporary and useful text possible. We do this in two ways: by describing the most important recent developments in the sciences basic to histology, and by recognizing that our readers are faced with the task of learning an ever-increasing number of facts in an ever-decreasing period of time. Because of this, every attempt has been made to shorten the text wherever possible and to organize information in a way that will facilitate learning.

INTENDED AUDIENCE

This text is designed for students in professional schools of medicine, veterinary medicine, dentistry, allied health, and nursing. It will also provide a useful, ready reference to both undergraduate students of microscopic anatomy and others in the structural biosciences.

ORGANIZATION

Because the study of histology requires a firm foundation in cell biology, *Basic Histology* begins with an accurate, up-to-date description of the structure and function of cells and their products and a brief introduction into the molecular biology of the cell.

This foundation is followed by a description of the 4 basic tissues of the body, emphasizing how cells become specialized to perform the specific functions of these tissues.

Finally, we devote a chapter to each of the organs and organ systems of the human body. Here, the emphasis on spatial arrangements of the basic tissues provides the key to understanding the functions of each organ. Again, we emphasize cell biology as the most fundamental approach to the study of structure and function.

As a further aid to learning, numerous photomicrographs and electron micrographs amplify the text and remind the reader of the laboratory basis of the study of histology. In addition, we place particular emphasis on diagrams, three-dimensional illustrations, and charts to summarize morphologic and functional features of cells, tissues, and organs.

NEW TO THIS EDITION

- All chapters have been revised to reflect new findings and interpretations, and the emphasis on human histology has been further strengthened.
- Basics of molecular biology related to the genomic contents of the cell nucleus have been included.
- The chapter on the immune system has been completely rewritten to include contemporary information and to organize that material into a readily assimilated body of knowledge.
- The chapter on hematopoiesis has been extensively reorganized and condensed.

- Existing diagrams have been revised and several new diagrams and figures have been added to enhance the usefulness of the text.
- Color has been added to highlight key points in illustrations and the principal issues in selected sections of the text.
- Clinical correlations in each chapter further illustrate the direct application of basic histologic information to the diagnosis, prognosis, pathobiology, and clinical aspects of disease. They are highlighted in color in each chapter.

ACKNOWLEDGMENTS

We wish to thank all the biomedical scientists and educators who provided information and micrographs that added to the usefulness of this edition. We also extend our appreciation to the staff of Appleton & Lange—Ruth Weinberg, Becky Hainz-Baxter, Alan Winick, Anne-Marie Zwierzyna and Muriel Solar—for their support and assistance.

We are pleased to announce that Italian, Dutch, Indonesian, Japanese, German, Serbo-Croatian, French, and Greek translations of *Basic Histology* are now available.

December 1991

L. Carlos Junqueira, MD
José Carneiro, MD
Robert O. Kelley, PhD

Methods of Study

Familiarity with the tools and methods of any branch of science is essential for a proper understanding of the subject. Some of the more common methods used to study cells and tissues and the principles involved in these methods will be reviewed here: units of measurement, preparation of tissues for examination, light microscopy, phase contrast microscopy, polarizing microscopy, electron microscopy, histochemistry, problems in interpretation of tissue sections, cryofracture, radioautography, examination of living cells and tissues, isolation and study in vitro of pure cell strains, and cell fractionation.

The most important units of measurement used in histology are given in Table 1–1. The **Ångström unit** (Å; 10^{-10} meter) is no longer recognized in the international system of units (Système International), and the **nanometer** (nm; 10^{-9} meter) is used in its stead (1 nm = 10 Å). The term **micrometer** (μm) has replaced the **micron** (μ) but has the same value (10^{-6} meter).

PREPARATION OF TISSUES FOR MICROSCOPIC EXAMINATION

The most common procedure used in the study of tissues is the preparation of histologic sections that can be studied with the aid of the light microscope. Under the light microscope, tissues are examined by transillumination. Since tissues and organs are usually too thick for transillumination, techniques have been developed for obtaining thin, translucent sections. In some cases, very thin layers of tissues or transparent membranes of living animals (eg, the mesentery, the tail of a tadpole, the wall of a hamster's cheek pouch) can be observed in the microscope without first sectioning the tissue. In such instances, it is possible to study these structures for long periods and under varying physiologic or experimental conditions. If a permanent preparation is desired, small fragments of these thin structures can be fixed, spread on a glass slide, stained, mounted with resin, and examined under the microscope. In most cases, however, tissues must be sliced into thin sections before they can be examined. These sections are cut by precision fine cutting instruments called **microtomes**

(Fig 1–1), and the organ or tissue is preserved and prepared for sectioning (see Table 1–2).

The ideal microscope tissue preparation would of course be preserved with suitable chemicals so that the tissue on the slide would have the same structure and molecular composition as it had in the body. This is sometimes possible but, as a practical matter, seldom feasible, and the artifacts resulting from the preparation process are almost always present.

Fixation

In order to avoid tissue digestion by enzymes (autolysis) or bacteria and to preserve physical structure, pieces of organs should be promptly and adequately treated prior to or as soon as possible following removal from the animal's body. This treatment—**fixation**—usually consists of submerging the tissues in stabilizing or cross-linking agents or perfusing them with these substances in order to preserve as much as possible of their morphologic and molecular characteristics.

The chemical substances used to preserve tissues are called **fixatives.** Some fixatives (eg, mercuric chloride, picric acid) promote the precipitation or clumping of proteins. Others (eg, formalin, glutaraldehyde) promote cross-linking but not course precipitation of proteins. All fixatives have both desirable and undesirable effects. The goal of combining the desirable effects and minimizing the undesirable ones has led to the development of several mixtures. The most commonly used mixtures are **Bouin's fluid,** composed of picric acid, formalin (a saturated solution—37% by weight of formaldehyde gas in water), acetic acid, and water; and **Zenker's formalin (Helly's fluid),** containing formalin, potassium dichromate, mercuric chloride, and water. The simple fixatives most commonly used are a 10% solution of formalin in saline and a 2% solution of buffered glutaraldehyde.

The chemistry of the process involved in fixation is complex and not well understood. However, formaldehyde and glutaraldehyde are known to react with the amine groups (NH_2) of tissue proteins. In the case of glutaraldehyde, the fixing action is reinforced by the fact that it is a dialdehyde and can cross-link.

In view of the high resolution afforded by the electron microscope, greater care in fixation is necessary

Table 1–1. Units of measurement used in light and electron microscopy.

Système International (SI) Unit	Symbol and Value
Micrometer	$\mu m = 0.001\ mm,\ 10^{-6}m$
Nanometer	$nm = 0.001\ \mu m,\ 10^{-9}m$

to preserve ultrastructural detail. Toward that end, a double fixation procedure, using a buffered glutaraldehyde solution followed by a second fixation in buffered osmium tetroxide, has become a standard procedure in preparations for fine structural studies. The glutaraldehyde cross-links proteins, while the effect of osmium tetroxide is to preserve and stain lipids and proteins.

Embedding:

In order to obtain thin sections with the microtome, tissues must be infiltrated after fixation with embedding substances that impart a rigid consistency to the tissue. Embedding materials include paraffin and plastic resins. Paraffin is used routinely for light microscopy; resins of the epoxy type are more commonly employed for electron microscopy.

The process of embedding or tissue impregnation is usually preceded by 2 main steps: **dehydration** and **clearing.** The water of the fragments to be embedded is first extracted by bathing successively in a graded series of mixtures of ethanol with water (usually from 70 to 100% ethanol). The ethanol is then replaced by a solvent miscible with the embedding medium. (In paraffin embedding, the solvent used is xylene.) As the tissues become infiltrated with the solvent, they

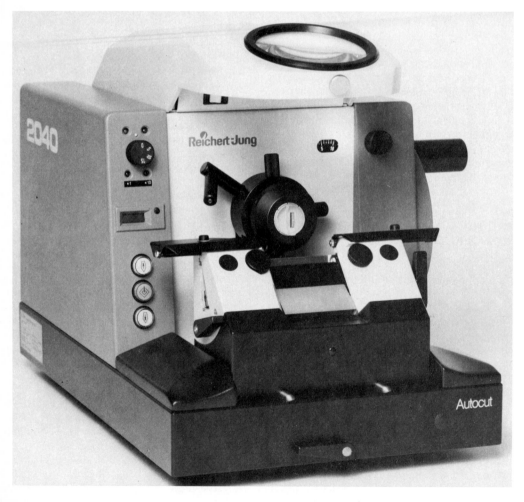

Figure 1–1. Microtome for sectioning resin- and paraffin-embedded tissues. Rotation of the drive wheel—seen with a handle on the right side of the instrument—moves the tissue-block holder up and down. Each turn of the drive wheel advances the specimen holder a controlled distance, generally 0.5, or 10 μm, and the embedded tissue passes over the knife edge, which cuts the sections. The sections adhere to each other, producing a ribbon of sections that is collected and affixed to a slide. (Courtesy of Cambridge Instruments.)

Table 1–2. Typical sequence of procedures in preparing tissues for observation under the light microscope. Following embedding in paraffin blocks, the tissues can be sectioned with a microtome (Fig 1–1).

Stage	Purpose	Duration
1. Fixation in simple or compound fixatives (Bouin's fluid, Zenker's formalin)	To preserve tissue morphology and molecular composition	About 12 h, according to the fixative and the size of the piece of tissue
2. Dehydration in graded concentrated ethyl alcohol (70% up to 100% alcohol)	To replace tissue water with organic solvents	6–24 h
3. Clearing in benzene, xylene, or toluene	To impregnate the tissues with a paraffin or a plastic resin solvent	1–6 h
4. Embedding in melted paraffin at 60 °C or plastic resin at room temperature	Paraffin or resin penetrates all intercellular spaces and even into the cells, making the tissues more resistant to sectioning	1–3 h

usually become transparent (this step is called **clearing**). Once the tissue is impregnated with the solvent, it is placed in plastic resin at room temperature or in melted paraffin in the oven, usually at 58–60 °C. The heat causes the solvent to evaporate, and the space becomes filled with paraffin. Tissues to be embedded with plastic resin are also dehydrated in ethanol and subsequently infiltrated with plastic solvents such as propylene oxide. These solvents are later replaced during the infiltration or embedding procedure by plastic solutions (eg, Epon, Araldite) that are hardened by means of cross-linking polymerizers and heat.

The small blocks containing the tissues are sectioned by the microtome's steel or glass blade to a thickness of 1–10 μm. The sections are floated on warm water and transferred to glass slides. Electron microscopy requires much thinner sections (0.02–0.1 μm); this is why embedding is performed with a hard epoxy plastic. The blocks thus obtained are so hard that glass or diamond knives are usually necessary to section them. Since the electron beam in the microscope cannot penetrate glass, the extremely thin plastic sections are collected on small metal (usually etched copper) grids. Those portions of the sections spanning the holes in the mesh of the grid can be examined in the microscope.

Immersion of tissues in solvents such as xylene dissolves the tissue lipids, which is an undesirable effect when these compounds are to be studied. To avoid loss of lipids, a **freezing microtome** has been devised in which the tissues are hardened at low temperatures to provide the rigidity necessary to permit sectioning. The freezing microtome—and its more elaborate and efficient successor, the **cryostat** (from Greek, *kryos*, cold, + *statos*, standing)— permit sections to be obtained quickly without going through the embedding procedure described above. Because they allow rapid study of pathologic specimens during surgical procedures, they are routinely used in hospitals. They are also effective in the histochemical study of very sensitive enzymes or small molecules, since freezing does not inactivate most enzymes and hinders the diffusion of small molecules.

Staining

With few exceptions, most tissues are colorless, so that observing them unstained in the light microscope is difficult. Methods of staining tissues have therefore been devised that not only make various tissue components conspicuous but also permit distinctions to be made between them. This is done by using mixtures of dyes that stain tissue components more or less selectively. Most dyes used in histologic studies behave like acidic or basic compounds and have a tendency to form electrostatic (salt) linkages with ionizable radicals of the tissues. Tissue components that stain more readily with basic dyes are termed **basophilic** (from Greek, *basis*, + *philein*, to love); those with an affinity for acid dyes are termed **acidophilic.**

Examples of basic dyes are toluidine blue and methylene blue. Hematoxylin behaves in the manner of a basic dye; ie, it stains the basophilic tissue components. The main tissue components that ionize and react with basic dyes do so because of acids in their composition (nucleoproteins and glycosaminoglycans). Acid dyes (eg, orange G, eosin, acid fuchsin) stain mostly the fundamental components present in cytoplasmic proteins.

Of all dyes, the combination of hematoxylin and eosin (H&E) is most commonly used. Hematoxylin stains the cell nucleus and other acidic structures (such as RNA-rich organelles) blue. In contrast, eosin stains the cytoplasm red and collagen pink. Many other dyes are used in different histologic procedures. Although they are useful in visualizing the different tissue components, they usually provide no insight into the chemical nature of the tissue being studied. Besides tissue staining with dyes, impregnation with such metals as silver and gold is commonly used, especially in studies of the nervous system.

LIGHT MICROSCOPY

Conventional light, phase contrast, and polarizing microscopy are all based on the interaction of photons and tissue components.

With the light microscope, stained preparations are usually examined by transillumination. The microscope is composed of both mechanical and optical parts. The mechanical components are illustrated in Fig 1–2. The optical components consist of 3 systems of lenses: condenser, objective, and ocular. The **condenser** collects and focuses the illumination to produce a cone of light that illuminates the object to be observed. The **objective** lens enlarges and projects the illuminated image of the object in the direction of the ocular lens. The **ocular** lens further magnifies this image and projects it onto the viewer's retina or a photographic plate. The total magnification is obtained by multiplying the magnifying power of the objective and ocular lenses.

Resolution

The critical factor in obtaining a crisp, detailed image with the microscope is **resolution,** the smallest distance between 2 particles at which the 2 particles can be seen as separate objects. For example, 2 particles will appear distinct if they are separated by a distance of 0.2 μm and the microscope has a resolving power of 0.2 μm. If the same particles are ex-

amined with a microscope that has a resolution of only 0.5 μm, they will appear as a single point. The highest resolution of the best light microscopes is approximately 0.2 μm; this permits good images magnified 1000 to 1500 times.

The quality of the image—its clarity and richness of detail—depends on the microscope's resolving power. The **magnification** is independent of its resolving power and is of value only when accompanied by high resolution. The resolving power of a microscope depends mainly on the quality of its objective lens. The ocular lens only enlarges the image obtained by the objective; it does not improve resolution.

PHASE CONTRAST MICROSCOPY

Unstained biologic specimens are usually transparent and difficult to view in detail, since all parts of the specimen have almost the same optical density. However, phase contrast microscopy employs a lens system that produces visible images from transparent objects (Fig 1–3).

The principle of phase contrast microscopy is based on the fact that light changes its speed and direction when passing through cellular and extracellular structures with different refractive indices. These changes cause the structures to appear lighter or darker relative to each other.

Differential interference (Nomarski) optics (as shown in Fig 1–3C produces an apparent 3-dimensional image of living cells and tissues.

POLARIZING MICROSCOPY

When normal light passes through a **Polaroid filter,** it exits vibrating in only one direction. If a second filter is placed in the microscope above the first one, with its main axis perpendicular to the first filter, no light passes through. In a polarizing microscope, the first filter is usually located below the condenser and is called the **polarizer.** A second filter **(analyzer)** is placed between the objective lens and the eyepiece. When polarizer and analyzer are disposed with their main axes perpendicular, no light passes, resulting in a darkfield effect. If, however, tissue structures containing oriented molecules (such as cellulose, collagen, microtubules, and microfilaments) are located between the polarizer and analyzer, their repetitive molecular structure allows them to rotate the axis of the light emerging from the polarizer. Consequently, they appear as bright structures against a dark background (Figs 5–10, 8–9, and 10–3). The ability to rotate the direction of vibration of polarized light is called **birefringence** and is present in crystalline substances or substances containing oriented molecules.

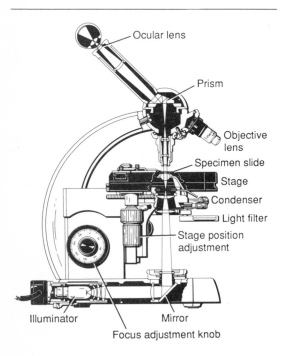

Figure 1–2. Schematic drawing of a light microscope showing its main components and the pathway of light from the source (substage lamp) to the eye of the observer. (Courtesy of Carl Zeiss Co.)

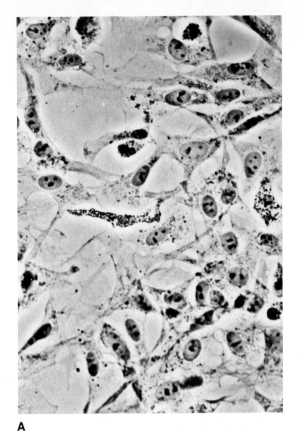

A

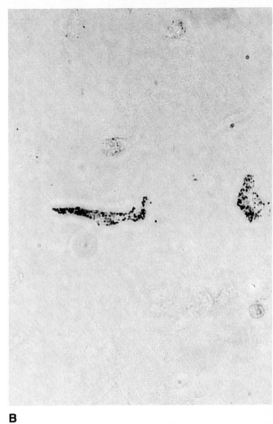

B

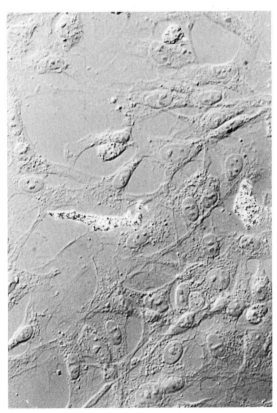

C

Figure 1–3. Cultured neural crest cells seen with different optical techniques. Unstained cells photographed with a phase contrast microscope **(A);** with a conventional light microscope **(B);** and using Nomarski differential interference microscopy **(C).** (Use the elongated pigmented cell for orientation in each image.) × 300. (Courtesy of S Rogers.)

ELECTRON MICROSCOPY

Both transmission and scanning electron microscopy are based on the interaction of electrons and tissue components.

The electron microscope is an imaging system that permits high resolution (0.1 nm). In practice, however, a resolution of 1 nm in tissue sections is considered satisfactory. This by itself permits enlargements to be obtained up to 400 times greater than those achieved with light microscopes.

The electron microscope functions on the principle that a beam of electrons can be deflected by electromagnetic fields in a manner similar to light deflection in glass lenses. Electrons are produced by high-temperature heating of a metallic filament (cathode) in a vacuum. The electrons emitted are then submitted to a potential difference of approximately 60–100 kV or more between the cathode and the anode (Fig 1–4). The anode is a metallic plate with a small hole in its center. Electrons are accelerated from the cathode to the anode. Some of these particles pass through the central opening in the anode, forming a constant stream (or **beam**) of electrons. The beam is deflected by electromagnetic lenses in a way roughly analogous to what occurs in the optical microscope. Thus, the condenser focuses the beam at the object plane and the objective lens forms an image of the object. The image obtained is further enlarged by 1–2 projecting lenses and is finally seen on a fluorescent screen or is projected onto photographic plates (Figs 1–4 and 1–5).

Differences Between Electron & Light Microscopes

Since electrons are easily scattered or absorbed by the specimen, very thin sections of tissue—usually 0.02–0.1 μm—must be used. Electrons are scattered or absorbed by portions of the specimen with high molecular weight, whereas in the light microscope light is absorbed by stained structures. Scattered electrons are absorbed by the aperture of the objective lens (usually a diameter of 25–100 μm). This aperture filters out the scattered electrons, which then do not contribute to image formation. The structures that scatter electrons thus appear in the fluorescent screen as dark bodies (electron-dense regions). The capacity to scatter electrons depends on the molecular weight and therefore the density of a given stain. Therefore, heavy metals (eg, uranium, lead) are used to stain tissue sections and thereby increase the contrast.

SCANNING ELECTRON MICROSCOPY

A variant of electron microscopy, scanning electron microscopy, permits pseudo-3-dimensional views

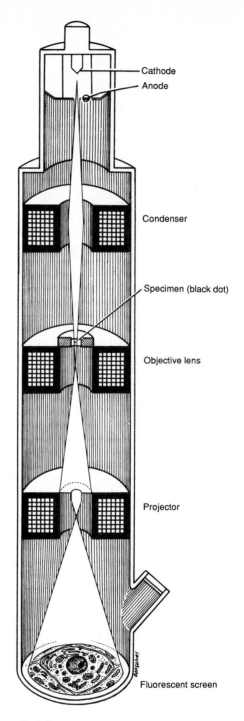

Figure 1–4 Pathway of the electron beam in the electron microscope. The ultrathin section is placed just over the objective electromagnetic lens. The image is projected onto a fluorescent screen and observed directly or through a 10× magnifying optical system.

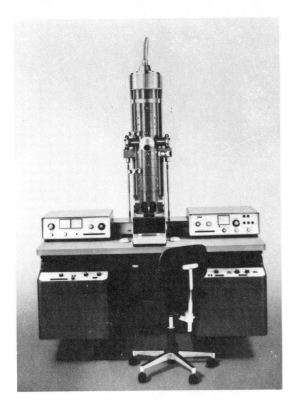

Figure 1–5. Photograph of the Zeiss model EM 10 electron microscope. (Courtesy of Carl Zeiss Co.)

PROBLEMS IN THE INTERPRETATION OF TISSUE SECTIONS

During the study and interpretation of stained tissue sections in microscope preparations, it should be remembered that the observed product is the end result of a series of processes that considerably distort the image observable in living tissue, mainly through shrinkage. This shrinkage is produced mainly by the heat (60 °C) needed for paraffin embedding; it is virtually eliminated when specimens are embedded in resin. As a consequence of these processes, the spaces frequently seen between cells and other tissue components are artifacts. Furthermore, there is a tendency to think in terms of only 2 dimensions when examining thin sections, when the structures from which the sections are made actually have 3 dimensions. In order to understand the architecture of an organ, it is therefore necessary to study sections made in different planes and to reason accordingly (Fig 1–6).

Another difficulty in the study of microscope preparations is the impossibility of differentially staining all tissue components on only one slide. It is therefore necessary to examine several preparations stained by different methods before a general idea of the composition and structure of any type of tissue can be obtained.

CRYOFRACTURE

Cryofracture permits the observation of tissue macromolecules with fewer artifacts than with other methods.

The technique of cryofracture (freeze fracture) is an important technical development in electron microscopy that permits examination of tissues without fixation and embedding. Although it is not free of artifacts, this technique is useful for verifying results obtained with other techniques in which ultrathin sections of fixed tissue are examined under the electron microscope. The cryofracture technique has furnished new information regarding the organization of the cell membrane and associated structures.

Fig 1–7 shows the replica of a freeze-fractured mouse intestinal epithelial cell in which most of the cell organelles can be seen, thus confirming their structure as shown by transmission electron microscopy (compare with Fig 15–34). An important feature of cryofracture is that cellular membranes are often split open, revealing details of their internal structure (see Chapter 3).

RADIOAUTOGRAPHY

Radioautography permits the localization of radioactive substances in cells or tissues by means of the

of surfaces of cells, tissues, and organs. The very narrow (10 nm) electron beam is moved sequentially from point to point across the surface to be examined. At each point, the primary electron beam interacts with atoms of the material being observed, giving rise to backscattered (reflected) electrons, x-rays characteristic of the irradiated atoms, and low-energy **secondary electrons.** Since elevations of the surface give rise to more secondary electrons, and depressions yield fewer secondary electrons, these secondary electrons are used to form an image of the topography of the surface. The fluctuation in electron signal is captured by a detector that modulates the brightness of a cathode ray tube whose electron beam is being moved (scanned) in synchrony with the primary electron beam of the microscope. The resulting photographs are easily understood, since they present a view that appears to be illuminated from above, just as our ordinary macroscopic world is filled with highlights and shadows caused by illumination from above.

Scanning electron micrographs illustrating the surface of the oocyte before and after fertilization and the initial stages of the formation of a morula are shown in Fig 23–15. Other scanning electron micrographs are shown in Figs 14–14, 16–14, 16–17, and 17–18.

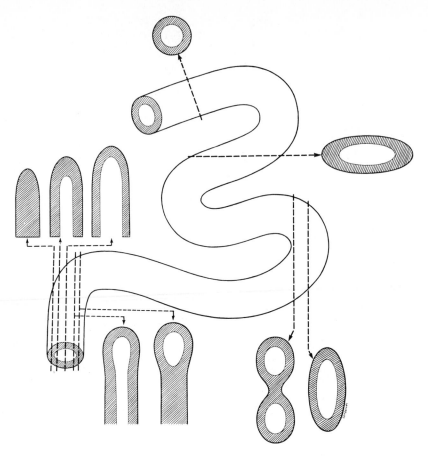

Figure 1–6. Some of the aspects a tube-shaped organ might exhibit when sectioned. The arrows indicate what is seen under the microscope in each particular section plane.

effect of emitted radiation on photographic emulsions. Silver bromide crystals present in the emulsion act as microdetectors of radioactivity. In radioautography, tissue sections obtained from animals previously treated with radioactive compounds are covered with photographic emulsion by dipping mounted sections in a glass container filled with a warmed mixture of gelatin and silver bromide. The slides, now covered with this thin layer of emulsion, are dried and stored in a lightproof box in a refrigerator. After various exposure times the slides are developed photographically and examined. All silver bromide crystals hit by radiation are reduced to small black granules of elemental silver, which reveal the existence of radioactivity in the structures in close proximity to these granules. The location and amount of radiation are thus determined; the quantity of silver granules is proportionate to the intensity of the radioactivity present. The tissue is then stained with regular stains, and the preparation is mounted in resin and covered with a coverslip. This procedure can be employed in electron microscopy by using thin sections of resin

embedded, radioactively labeled tissue. With the resolution provided by the electron microscope, silver granules usually appear as short, coiled filaments (Fig 1–8).

Radioautography is often used to study important dynamic biologic phenomena. As soon as it became possible to synthesize radioactive precursors of normal metabolites with the aid of carbon 14 and tritium, it was possible to study not only different metabolic pathways in tissue specimens but also the sequence and speed with which metabolic processes occurred. For example, the metabolism of proteins and nucleic acids can be studied by injecting labeled amino acids (eg, ^{14}C-leucine for studies of protein synthesis) and nucleotides (eg, ^{3}H-thymidine for studies of DNA synthesis) into animals. In both cases, precursors are incorporated into protein or nucleic acids within tissues and cells and can be localized and quantified with the aid of radioautography. If a fixed unit of time is used in the experiments, it is possible to estimate the speed of the metabolic process under study. The metabolism of proteins, carbohydrates, lipids, and

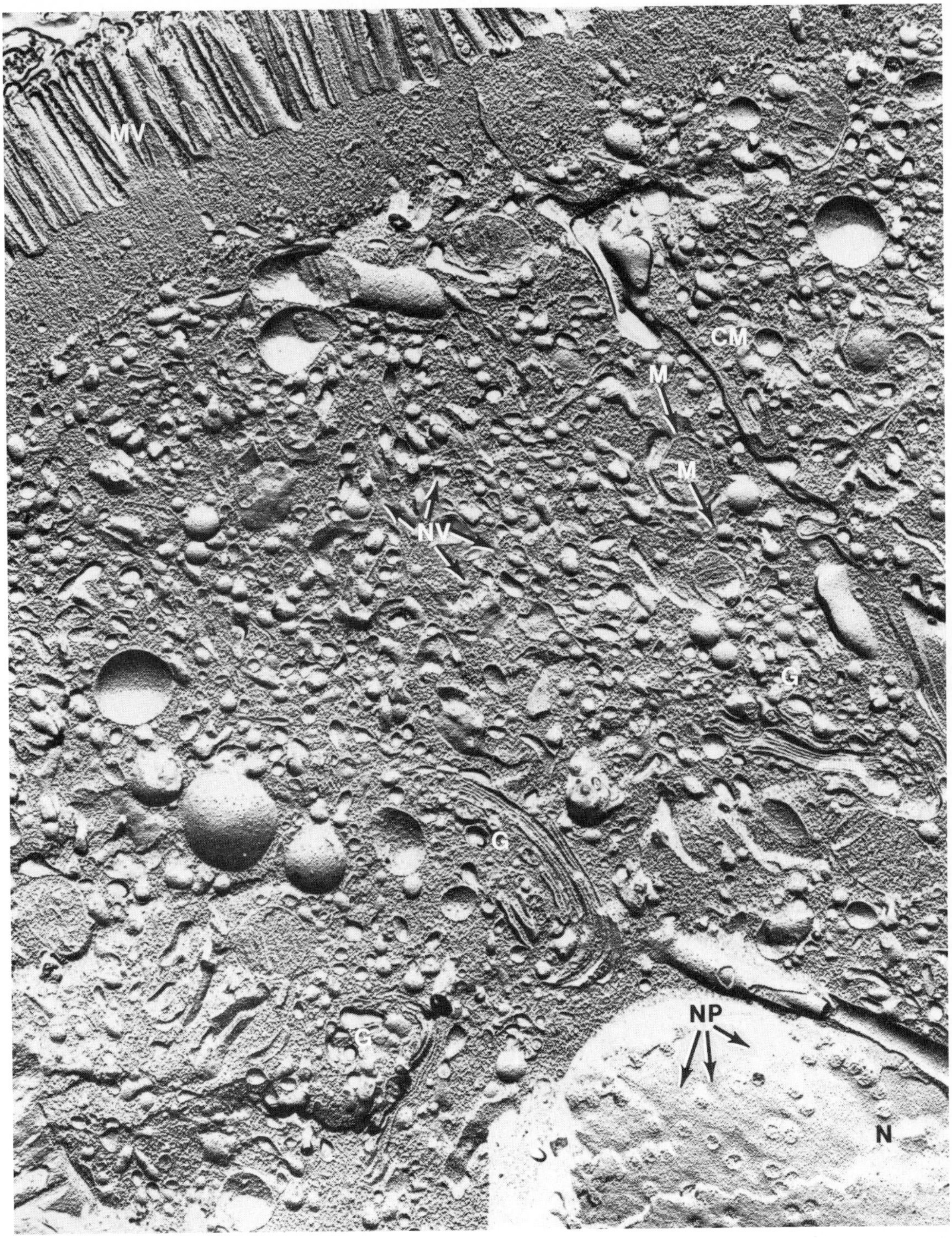

Figure 1–7. Electron micrograph of a mouse intestinal epithelial cell. The tissue was prepared by cryofracture. This process consists of freezing a fragment of tissue to very low temperatures and fracturing it with a sharpened metal blade. The fractured surface is kept at low temperature in a vacuum environment. A portion of the water in the surface sublimates, giving a bas-relief effect (etching). A replica of this surface is then obtained by coating it with a layer of platinum and carbon. In this picture, one can observe in material that has not been submitted to embedding and sectioning the presence of the various cell components described by classic transmission electron microscopy: microvilli (MV), cell membrane (CM), Golgi complex (G), nucleus (N), and nuclear pores (NP). × 24,000. (Courtesy of LS Staehelin.)

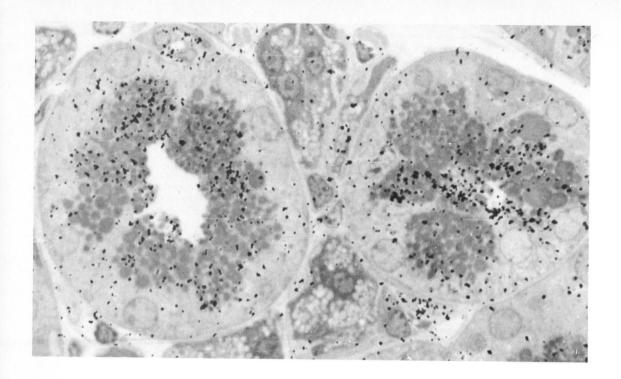

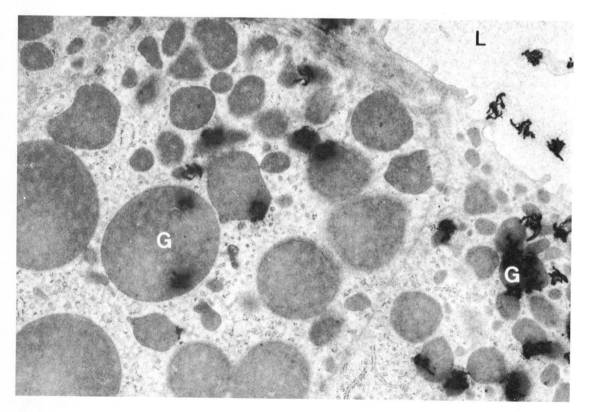

Figure 1–8. Radioautographs from the submandibular gland of a mouse injected 8 hours before sacrifice with ^{3}H fucose. **Top:** Photomicrograph showing black silver grains indicating radioactive regions in the cells. Most radioactivity is in the granules of the cells of the granular ducts of this gland. × 500. **Bottom:** The same cells in an electron micrograph. Observe the silver grains that, in this enlargement, appear as coiled structures localized mainly over the granules (G) and in the tubular lumen (L). × 9000. (Courtesy of TG Lima and A Haddad.)

nucleic acids has been localized and analyzed using this procedure. Specific examples include localization of the site and time of DNA synthesis in the nucleus and in mitochondria as well as the sulfation of glycoproteins in the Golgi complex of goblet cells and fibroblasts.

EXAMINATION OF LIVING CELLS & TISSUES

Cell- and tissue-culture techniques permit direct analysis of cell behavior. To accomplish this, cells and tissues are grown in chemically defined synthetic media to which growth factors, hormones, and serum components are frequently added.

In preparing cultures, cells can be dispersed mechanically or by prior treatment with enzymes such as trypsin or collagenase. Once isolated, the cells can be cultivated either in a suspension or spread out on a culture plate to which they can adhere as a single layer of cells (Fig 1–9).

Organs can also be cultured, starting from their embryonic rudiments. This technique permits study of the factors that influence the development of organs in conditions much simpler than those that exist inside the living organism. The term **organ culture** means primarily the culture of fragments of organs in conditions that keep the architecture of the organ intact. The term **in vitro** is applied to cells and tissue fragments isolated and maintained in a controlled cellular environment, as opposed to that which the cells experience **in vivo** as an integral part of their parent organism.

Cell culture has also been used for the study of the metabolism of normal and cancerous cells. In addition, this technique is useful in the study of parasites that grow only within cells, such as viruses, mycoplasma, and some protozoa. The use of extracellular matrix components such as collagens and laminin greatly increases the survival of cells in vitro. Thanks to these improvements in culture technology, most cell types can now be maintained in the laboratory, an important step in the study of normal cells. Most cells obtained from normal tissues have a finite, genetically programmed lifespan. Certain changes, however (mainly related to oncogenes; see Chapter 3), can promote cell "immortality," a process called **transformation**, which may be a first step in a normal cell becoming a cancer cell.

In cytogenetic research, tissue cultures permit the study of mitoses and of chromosomes in human cells. Determination of human karyotypes (the number and morphology of an individual's chromosomes) is accomplished by the short-term cultivation of blood lymphocytes or of skin fibroblasts.

In examining these cells during mitotic division in tissue cultures, one can detect anomalies in the

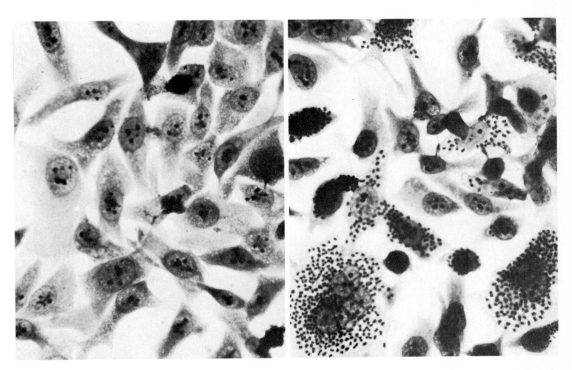

Figure 1–9. Photomicrographs of chicken fibroblasts grown in tissue culture. Giemsa stain. **Left:** Normal cells. **Right:** Fibroblasts infected by Trypanosoma cruzi. × 340. (Courtesy of S Yoneda.)

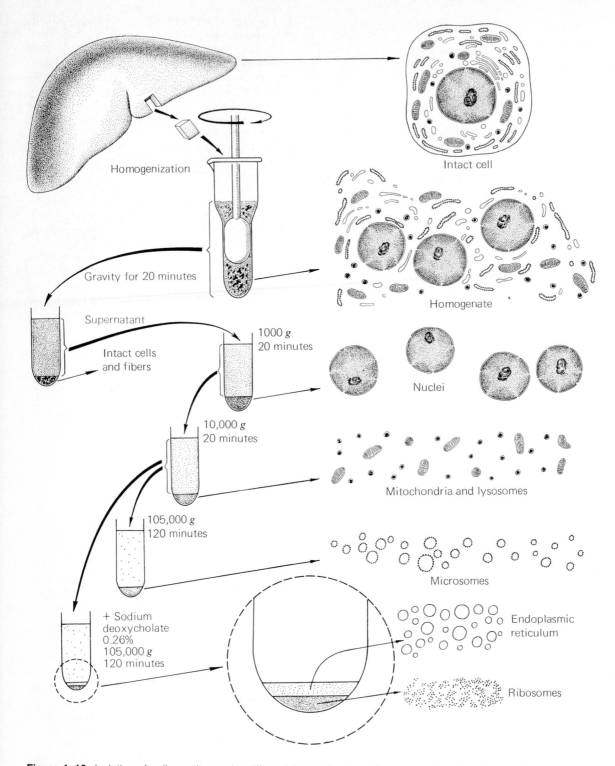

Homogenization

Intact cell

Homogenate

Gravity for 20 minutes

Supernatant

Intact cells
and fibers

1000 g
20 minutes

Nuclei

10,000 g
20 minutes

Mitochondria and lysosomes

105,000 g
120 minutes

Microsomes

+ Sodium
deoxycholate
0.26%
105,000 g
120 minutes

Endoplasmic
reticulum

Ribosomes

Figure 1–10. Isolation of cell constituents by differential centrifugation. The supernatant of each tube is centrifuged again at higher speeds. The drawings at right show the cellular organelles at the bottom of each tube after centrifugation. Centrifugal force is expressed by *g*, which is equivalent to the force of gravity. (Redrawn and reproduced, with permission, from Bloom W, Fawcett DW: *A Textbook of Histology,* 9th ed. Saunders, 1968.)

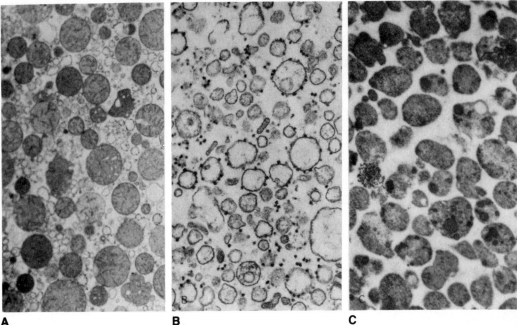

A   **B**   **C**

Figure 1–11. Electron migrographs of 3 cell fractions isolated by density gradient centrifugation. **A:** Mitochondrial fraction, contaminated with microsomes. × 13,000. **B:** Microsomal fraction. × 42,500. **C:** Lysosomal fraction. × 25,000. (Courtesy of P Baudhuin.)

number and morphology of the chromosomes. These anomalies have been shown to be related and are diagnostic of numerous diseases collectively called genetic disorders.

In addition, cell culture is central to contemporary techniques of molecular biology and recombinant DNA technology.

CELL FRACTIONATION

Cell fractionation is the physical process by which centrifugal force is used to separate organelles and cellular components as a function of their sedimentation coefficients. The sedimentation coefficient of a particle depends on its size, form, and density and on the viscosity of the medium. By means of differential centrifugation, certain cellular organelles can be isolated and their chemical composition and functions determined in vitro.

Differential centrifugation is achieved by subjecting a suspension of cellular components, obtained by disrupting the cells in a process called **homogenization,** to the action of different centrifugal forces (Fig 1–10). The organ or tissue from a recently killed animal is cut into very small fragments that are then immersed in an appropriate solution. Sucrose and inert soluble plastics of different compositions are often used to provide media with various densities and viscosities. The fragments of the organ in the inert so-

lution are placed in a homogenizer, often consisting of a glass cylinder containing a rod that turns with great velocity (Fig 1–10). The fragments of the tissues are crushed by the friction of the rod on the wall of the cylinder, breaking the cell membranes and liberating cell components into the solution.

After homogenization is complete, the suspension is allowed to rest for a few minutes so that the fibers of connective tissue, large cell remnants, and intact cells can settle out. The supernatant is then centrifuged, and the more dense particles separate first. The supernatant from each centrifugation is subjected again to greater centrifugal force, thus separating out the different cellular components, in decreasing order of their density, as shown in Fig 1–10.

An improvement in the technique of differential centrifugation is **centrifugation against a gradient, or density gradient centrifugation.** The gradient consists of solutions whose concentration (density) is maximal at the bottom of the tube and minimal at the top, with a gradual increase in concentration from top to bottom. The homogenate is placed on top of this stabilized gradient and centrifuged. The particles migrate centrifugally but stop at a level where an equilibrium exists between the action of the centrifugal force and the tendency of the particle to float (the buoyant density). This continuous gradient technique produces purer fractions of cell components.

It is also possible to use a discontinuous, or step, gradient, which is made up of superimposed zones whose density decreases from one zone to the other, starting from the bottom and proceeding to the top of the centrifuge tube.

All stages of the techniques described are carried out at a temperature slightly higher than the freezing point in order to inhibit the action of lytic enzymes that would disrupt the organelles during separation.

The homogeneity of the fractions thus obtained is examined with the light microscope (for nuclei, mitochondria, and secretory granules), with the electron microscope (for ribosomes, microsomes, etc [Fig 1–11]), or with biochemical methods. For example, the fraction containing lysosomes can be identified by the quantity of acid phosphatase, an enzyme usually found in these particles, and the fraction containing nuclei can be identified by the quantity of DNA it possesses.

Isolation of cellular components by differential centrifugation represented a great technical advance. It allows detailed study of cellular components obtained in a relatively pure state; eg, nuclei, nucleoli, mitochondria, rough endoplasmic reticulum, ribosomes, secretory granules, and pigment granules.

REFERENCES

Alberts B et al: *Molecular Biology of the Cell,* 2nd ed. Garland, 1989.

Bancroft JD, Stevens A: *Theory and Practice of Histological Techniques.* Churchill Livingstone, 1977.

Darnell J, Lodish H, Baltimore D: *Molecular Cell Biology,* 2nd ed. Sci Am Books, 1990.

Everhart TE, Hayes TL: The scanning electron microscope. *Sci Am* (Jan) 1972; **226**:54.

James J: *Light Microscopic Techniques in Biology and Medicine.* Martinus Nijhoff, 1976.

Rogers AW: *Techniques of Autoradiography,* 3rd ed. Elsevier, 1979.

Spencer M: *Fundamentals of Light Microscopy.* Cambridge Univ Press, 1982.

Stolinski C, Breathnack AS: *Freeze-Fracture Replication of Biological Tissues.* Academic Press, 1975.

Wischnitzer S: *Introduction to Electron Microscopy.* Pergamon, 1981.

Histochemistry & Cytochemistry

The chemistry of tissues and cells is studied by both microscopic and analytic methods. Chemical substances in tissues and cells can be identified and localized by chemical or high-affinity interactions that produce either insoluble colored compounds that can be observed with the light microscope or electron-scattering precipitates that can be observed with the electron microscope. In Perls's reaction, for example, potassium ferrocyanide reacts with ferric ions in tissues to produce an insoluble dark blue precipitate of ferric ferrocyanide.

BASIC HISTOCHEMICAL & CYTOCHEMICAL PRINCIPLES

Chemical reactions can be performed on cells and tissues, permitting identification and localization of chemical substances and enzymatic activities.

For a histochemical reaction to be recognized as valid and meaningful, it must fulfill the following basic requirements.

(1) The substances being analyzed must not diffuse out of their original sites.

(2) The product of the reaction should be insoluble and either colored or electron-scattering.

(3) The method used should be specific for the substance or chemical groups being studied.

(4) The procedure must not denature or block reactive groups.

In some histochemical reactions, the intensity of color produced is directly proportionate to the concentration of the substance being analyzed. Under these conditions, concentration of the substances under study can be determined by **microspectrophotometry.** This procedure is carried out by use of a microspectrophotometer, a combination microscope and spectrophotometer. By measuring the light absorbed by small areas of a cell or a tissue, it is possible to quantify chemical substances in this region. This method was improved by the introduction of scanning devices that analyze with great precision the optical density of the images produced by cytochemical methods and relay the information to a computer that processes the results.

EXAMPLES OF HISTOCHEMICAL METHODS

Ions

A. Iron: When sections of tissues containing ferric ions (Fe^{3+}) are incubated in a mixture of potassium ferrocyanide and hydrochloric acid, iron can be detected by the formation of a highly insoluble dark blue precipitate of ferric ferrocyanide (Perls's reaction). This method not only allows localization of cells that catabolize hemoglobin but also permits diagnosis of diseases in which deposits of iron occur in the tissues.

B. Phosphates: Phosphates are demonstrated by their reaction with silver nitrate. The silver phosphate formed is reduced by hydroquinone in the next phase of the reaction, producing a black precipitate of reduced silver (Fig 2–1). This reaction is frequently used to study bone and the ossification process, because the only insoluble phosphate found abundantly in the body is calcium phosphate, which is present in large amounts in bone tissue.

Lipids

Lipids are best revealed with dyes that are more soluble in the lipids than in the medium in which the dye is dissolved.

In this process, frozen sections are immersed in alcoholic solutions saturated with the appropriate dye. The stain then migrates from the alcohol to the cellular lipid droplets. The dyes most commonly used for this purpose are Sudan IV and Sudan black; they confer red and black colors, respectively, on the lipids.

Additional methods used for the localization of cholesterol and its esters, phospholipids, and glycolipids are useful in the diagnosis of metabolic diseases in which intracellular accumulations of different kinds of lipids occur.

Nucleic Acids

A. Deoxyribonucleic Acid (DNA): DNA is studied chiefly with Feulgen's reaction, a method that starts with the hydrolysis of DNA by hydrochloric acid. This process separates purine bases from sugar, promoting the formation of aldehyde groups in deoxyribose. The free aldehyde groups then react with the Schiff reagent (basic fuchsin bleached by sodium metabisulfite), producing an insoluble red substance. By using this staining procedure in conjunction with mi-

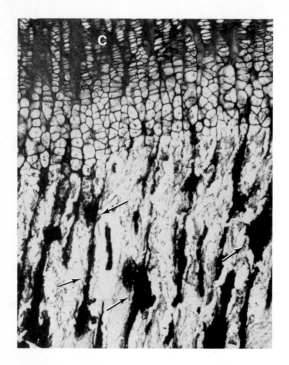

Figure 2–1. Photomicrograph of a section from the epiphysis of a bone treated with silver nitrate and subsequently reduced by hydroquinone. The black precipitate in the ossified tissue (arrows) indicates the presence of calcium phosphate. Nonreacting cartilage tissue (C) lies in the upper portion of the section. × 120.

crospectrophotometry, it is possible to quantitate the content of DNA in the nuclei of cells.

B. Ribonucleic Acid (RNA): RNA can be identified in tissues by virtue of its great affinity for basic stains (basophilia)—eg, it stains intensely with toluidine blue or methylene blue. Since RNA is not the only basophilic substance in the tissue, it is necessary to incubate a control slide with ribonuclease, an enzyme that removes RNA. Any structure that loses its basophilia as a result of pretreatment with ribonuclease is considered to contain RNA.

Proteins

Chemical methods do not permit localization of specific proteins in cells and tissues (Fig 2–2). This can be performed using the immunocytochemical methods presented later in this chapter, however. Specific enzymes such as RNase, DNase, collagenase, and elastase that digest cell and tissue components are used extensively to analyze the distribution of certain cell and tissue elements.

Polysaccharides & Oligosaccharides

Polysaccharides in the body occur either in a free state or combined with proteins. In the combined state, they constitute an extremely complex heterogeneous group. A ubiquitous polysaccharide in the body, not bound to protein, is **glycogen,** which can be demonstrated by the periodic acid-Schiff (PAS) reaction. The PAS reaction, based on the oxidative action of periodic acid (HIO_4) on 1, 2-glycol groups present in the glucose residues, gives rise to aldehyde groups, as shown in the equation below.

As in Feulgen's reaction, these aldehyde groups react with bleached fuchsin (Schiff's reagent), producing a new complex compound with a purple or magenta color. This can be seen in the light microscope, and we call such substances PAS-positive. Since other PAS-positive substances occur in cells, the specificity of this reaction depends on pretreatment with a glycogenolytic enzyme (eg, salivary amylase). Structures that stain intensely with the PAS reaction but fail to do so after pretreatment with amylase are considered to contain glycogen. Using this method, glycogen can be demonstrated in normal liver and striated muscle.

A variety of strongly anionic, unbranched long-chain polysaccharides containing aminated monosaccharides (amino sugars) constitute the **glycosaminoglycans** (known at one time as **mucopolysaccharides**). These substances contain chains of repeating disaccharide units containing an N-acetylated hexosamine coupled to uronic acid. Complexes of covalently bound glycosaminoglycans inserted at regular intervals along a protein core constitute the **proteoglycans.** In proteoglycans, which are significant constituents of connective tissue matrices (see Chapters 5 and 7), the carbohydrate moieties constitute the major component of the molecule.

Interest in the wide variety of sugar-containing macromolecules in the body gave rise to the general term **glycoconjugates** for these substances. This term

Glucose molecule from glycogen $+ HIO_4 \longrightarrow$ **Aldehyde groups resulting from action of periodic acid**

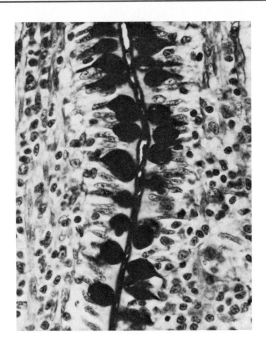

Figure 2–2. Photomicrograph of an intestinal villus stained by alcian blue. Staining is intense in the goblet cells because of their high content of acidic glycoproteins. × 400.

with a glycogenolytic enzyme. Using specific enzymes that digest proteoglycans and some glycoprotein components, one can distinguish these substances in tissue sections.

Glycolipids are characteristic constituents of most cell membranes and are significant components of the plasma membranes of nerve cells (eg, gangliosides, cerebrosides). The carbohydrate moieties of glycolipids are oligosaccharides similar to those of glycoproteins.

Many histochemical procedures are used frequently in laboratory diagnosis. Thus, the Perls's reaction for iron, the PAS-amylase and alcian blue reactions for glycogen and glycosaminoglycans, and the reactions for lipids are routinely used in biopsies of tissue taken from patients with diseases that store iron (eg. hemochromatosis, hemosiderosis), glycogen (glycogenosis), glycosaminoglycans (mucopolysaccharidosis), and sphingolipids (sphingolipidosis) in tissues.

Catecholamines

The fact that formaldehyde reacts with catecholamines to produce fluorescent compounds makes it

is applied to **glycoproteins** and **glycolipids** as well as proteoglycans. Glycoproteins differ in 4 major ways from proteoglycans: Glycoprotein molecules are generally smaller than proteoglycans; their carbohydrate moieties contain fewer sugar residues and are usually termed **oligosaccharides** rather than polysaccharides. The oligosaccharide chains of glycoproteins are often branched, whereas the polysaccharides of proteoglycans are more likely to be unbranched. In addition, the glycoprotein oligosaccharides are characterized by wide variability in the types and order of the individual sugars in the chain, while the polysaccharides of proteoglycans generally are much less diverse.

Glycoproteins such as thyroglobulin (present in the thyroid gland) and gonadotropins of the pituitary contain a high proportion of protein. Other glycoproteins with a low protein content, such as those produced by some epithelial cells, are identified as **mucous substances** that have a protective and lubricating function. Some glycoproteins (eg, neutral glycoproteins) contain no acidic groups; others (eg, acid mucous substances) have limited amounts of carboxyl or sulfate radicals. In contrast to glycoproteins, glycosaminoglycans are strongly anionic due to their high content of carboxyl and sulfate groups. For this reason, they react strongly with the alcian blue dye (Figs 2–2 and 2–3). Neutral glycoproteins can be identified in tissue sections by the fact that they react with the PAS method but are not digested by prior incubation

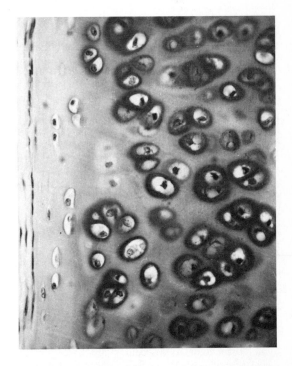

Figure 2–3. Photomicrograph of a section of hyaline cartilage stained with PAS and alcian blue. The region of the matrix close to the cartilage cells contains an abundance of acidic proteoglycans and stains blue with the alcian blue method. The rest of the matrix contains neutral glycoproteins that stain red using the PAS method. × 200.

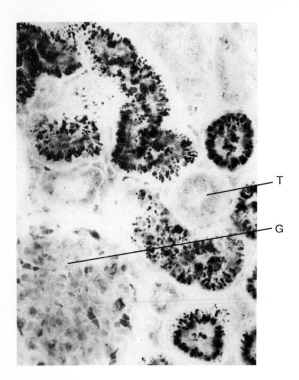

Figure 2–4. Photomicrograph of a rat kidney section treated by the lead acid phosphatase method. The lysosomes stain intensely as dark granules in the proximal convoluted tubule cells. The glomeruli (G) and other tubular cells (T) do not have enzymatic activity. × 400.

possible to localize epinephrine (adrenaline) and norepinephrine (noradrenaline) in tissue. This method is founded on the observation that ring hydroxylated phenylethylamines, indolealkylamines, and their corresponding amino acids are converted to fluorescent complexes in the presence of relatively dry formaldehyde vapor at 60–80 °C. This reaction has been helpful in studying the distribution of catecholamines and their precursors in neuronal pathways, cell bodies, and nerve endings.

Enzymes

Many histochemical methods are used to reveal and identify enzymes. When unstable enzymes are studied, sections of frozen, unfixed material must be used. Many enzymes, however, may retain a portion of their activity in tissues fixed with aldehyde fixatives such as formalin or glutaraldehyde. Most enzymatic histochemical procedures are based on the production of intensely stained or electron-dense precipitates at the site of enzymatic activity. Three examples of enzymes that can be shown by either the light or the electron microscope are described below.

A. Acid Phosphatase: The Gomori method of demonstrating acid phosphatase activity consists of incubating formalin-fixed tissue sections in a solution containing sodium glycerophosphate and lead nitrate buffered to pH 5.0. The enzyme hydrolyzes the glycerophosphate, liberating phosphate ions that react with lead nitrate to produce an insoluble, electron-dispersing colorless precipitate of lead phosphate at the site of the enzymatic activity. In a second step, the preparation is immersed in a solution of ammonium sulfide that reacts with the colorless lead phosphate to produce a black precipitate of lead sulfide. This method permits the localization of this enzyme's activity and is frequently used to demonstrate **lysosomes,** cytoplasmic organelles that contain acid phosphatase (Figs 2–4 and 2–5). The ammonium sulfide step is omitted when the tissue is to be examined in the electron microscope.

B. Dehydrogenases: These enzymes remove hydrogen from one substrate and transfer it to another. There are many different dehydrogenases in the body; they play an important role in several metabolic processes and can be distinguished by means of the substrate on which they act. The histochemical demonstration of dehydrogenases consists of incubating nonfixed tissue sections in a substrate solution containing **tetrazole,** a weakly colored soluble H^+ acceptor. The enzyme transports hydrogen from the substrate to tetrazole and reduces it to an intensely colored insoluble compound called **formazan,** which precipitates at the site of the enzymatic activity. By this method, succinate dehydrogenase—a key enzyme in the citric acid (Krebs) cycle—can be localized in mitochondria (Fig 2–6).

C. Peroxidase: This enzyme, which is present in several types of cells, promotes the oxidation of certain substrates with the transfer of hydrogen ions to hydrogen peroxide, forming molecules of water.

$$\begin{matrix} OH \\ | \\ | \\ OH \end{matrix} + \begin{matrix} OH \\ | \\ R \\ | \\ OH \end{matrix} \xrightarrow{\boxed{\text{PEROXIDASE}}} 2H_2O + \begin{matrix} O \\ \| \\ R \\ \| \\ O \end{matrix}$$

Hydrogen peroxide   Substrate   Insoluble and electron-dense precipitate

In this method, sections of adequately fixed tissue are incubated in a solution containing hydrogen peroxide and 3,3'-*diaminoazo*benzidine (DAB). The latter compound is oxidized in the presence of peroxidase, resulting in an insoluble, black, electron-dense precipitate that permits the localization of peroxidase activity in the optical and electron microscopes. Since the enzyme is extremely active, it produces an appreciable amount of insoluble precipitate in a short time, making this procedure a very sensitive histochemical assay. The DAB method is probably one of the most commonly used techniques of histochemistry, since it detects both the

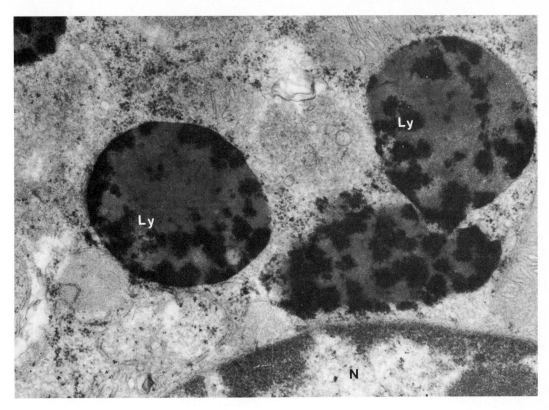

Figure 2–5. Electron micrograph of a rat kidney cell previously treated by the Gomori method for acid phosphatase. The 3 dark, rounded structures above the nucleus (N) are lysosomes (Ly). The dense heterogeneous precipitate within these structures is lead phosphate, which scatters the electrons. The information in this electron micrograph is equivalent to that in the light micrograph illustrated in Fig 2–4. × 25,000. (Courtesy of E Katchburian.)

peroxidase activity in blood cells (important in the diagnosis of leukemias) and the peroxidase used as a label in immunocytochemistry and in hybridization methods.

FLUORESCENT COMPOUNDS

This technique is based on the fact that when certain fluorescent substances are irradiated by light of a proper wavelength, they emit light with a longer wavelength. In fluorescence microscopy, tissue sections are usually irradiated with ultraviolet light so that the emission is in the visible portion of the spectrum. The fluorescent substances appear as brilliant, shiny particles on a dark background. A microscope with a strong ultraviolet light source is used, and special filters that eliminate ultraviolet light are used after the objective lens to protect the observer's eyes.

Some naturally fluorescent substances are normal constituents of cells, eg, vitamin A, vitamin B_2, and porphyrins. Other fluorescent compounds that have an affinity for tissues and cells are used as fluorescent stains. Acridine orange is most widely used, because it can combine with DNA and RNA. When observed in the fluorescence microscope, the DNA-acridine orange complex emits a yellowish-green light, and the RNA-acridine orange complex emits a reddish-orange light. It is thus possible to identify and localize nucleic acids in the cells (Fig 2–7).

Fluorescence spectroscopy is a method of analyzing the light emitted by a fluorescent compound in a microspectrophotometer. It can be used to characterize several compounds present in cells and is of particular importance in the study of catecholamines. The development of fluorescent probes (substances that react specifically with cell components) has permitted highly sensitive assays for various substances within cells.

IMMUNOCYTOCHEMISTRY

High-affinity interactions between macromolecules are the basis of such important techniques as

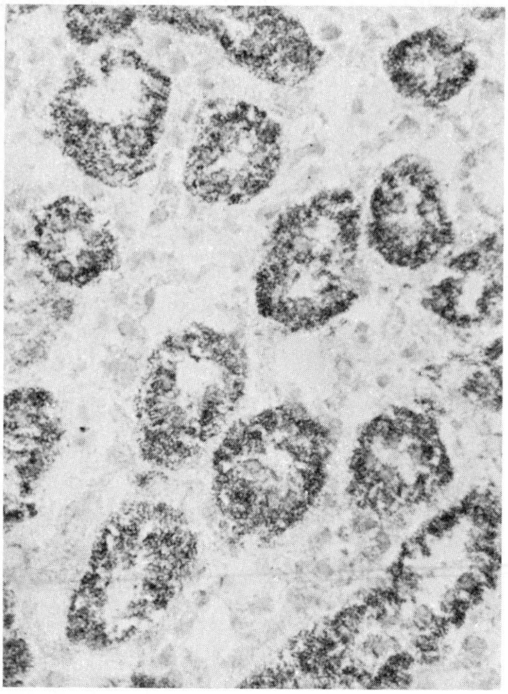

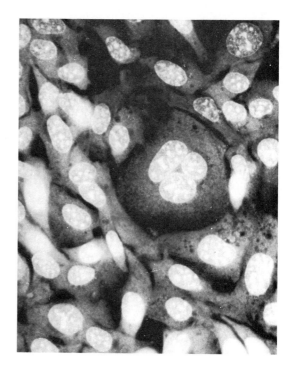

Figure 2–6. Photomicrograph of a frozen section of fresh, nonfixed kidney previously incubated in succinate plus monotetrazole. The dark precipitate seen in the tubules indicates the activity of succinate dehydrogenase. × 400. (Courtesy of AGE Pearse.)

immunocytochemistry, lectin histochemistry, and in situ hybridization. These methods permit the study of the presence and activity of specific macromolecules in cells and tissues. In addition, these interactions are reversible and do not depend on classical chemical bonds. The best studied example is the antigen-antibody interaction, the basis of immunology. High-affinity interactions are also used to locate segments of nucleic acids (hybridization) and specific carbohydrate moeities (lectin binding). Other high-affinity interactions provide molecular probes for macromolecules (eg, phalloidin interacts with actin in microfilaments).

Methods using labeled antibodies have proved most useful in localizing specific proteins and certain other macromolecules such as nucleic acids and polysaccharides. This test is based on the reaction of the body when exposed to foreign substances called **antigens** or **immunogens.** The body will respond by producing proteins called **antibodies** that react specifically and bind strongly to the antigen and result in neutralization of the foreign substance. Antibodies are proteins of the globulin group (immunoglobulins) that appear in plasma and tissue fluids after antigen injection. Their production enables the organism to oppose invasion by foreign microorganisms and to

eliminate certain proteins and other foreign matter not recognized as self. Immunocytochemistry is based on the coupling of immunoglobulins to substances that render them visible in the microscope without causing loss of the antibody's biologic activity. Since the labeled immunoglobulins bind specifically to their antigens, these compounds permit localization of specific antigens in tissue specimens. When a tissue section containing certain antigens is incubated in a solution containing labeled antibodies to these antigens, the antibodies bind specifically to the antigens, whose location can then be seen with either the light or the electron microscope.

Methods of Labeling Antibodies

Three methods of labeling antibodies are frequently used (Fig 2–8).

(1) Coupling with a fluorescent compound– This permits the identification of the site of specific antigens using a fluorescence microscope (Figs 2–8A and 2–9).

(2) Coupling with an enzyme– This permits detection of the labeled antibody by conventional enzyme cytochemistry. The enzyme most often used is

Figure 2–7. Photomicrograph of kidney cell culture transformed by infection with simian virus 40, stained with acridine orange, and photographed with the fluorescence microscope. A green fluorescence (shown as white in the photo) appears in the regions containing DNA (nucleus); a reddish-orange color (shown as gray) is characteristic of the RNA-rich cytoplasm. A giant cell is in the center. × 1000. (Courtesy of A Geraldes and JMV Costa.)

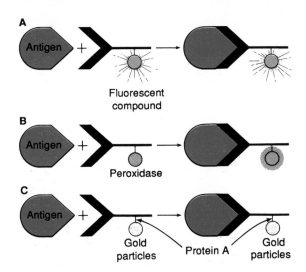

A

Antigen + ⟩ (Fluorescent compound) → Antigen⟩

Fluorescent
compound

B

Antigen + ⟩ (Peroxidase) → Antigen⟩

Peroxidase

C

Antigen + ⟩ (Gold particles / Protein A) → Antigen⟩ (Gold particles)

Gold
particles   Protein A   Gold
particles

Figure 2–8. Three current methods of labeling and identifying specific proteins by immunocytochemistry. **A:** The antibody is coupled with a fluorescent compound, such as fluorescein isothiocyanate or rhodamine. After incubation, the sections containing the antigen exposed to the labeled antibody solution are studied in the fluorescence microscope. **B:** The antibody is coupled with peroxidase. After the antigen-antibody reaction, the section is submitted to the histochemical method for peroxidase and studied with the light or the electron microscope (see text). **C:** The antibody is coupled with gold particles previously bound to protein A. This protein reacts with the antibody, labeling it. Preparations obtained by this method can also be studied by light and electron microscopy. The gold particle-protein A method is at present one of the most efficient and precise immunocytochemical methods.

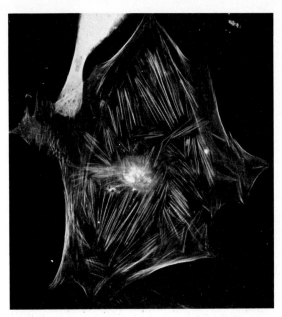

Figure 2–9. Actin fibrils composed of aggregates of actin filaments in the cytoplasm of a cultured human fibroblast preincubated in fluorescent actin antibody. × 1767. (Reproduced, with permission, from E Lazarides: *J Cell Biol* 1975; **65:**549.)

peroxidase, which can be detected by the method described above, using either the light or the electron microscope (Figs 2–8B and 2–10).

(3) Coupling with a colored electron-scattering compound that can be detected in light and electron microscopes–Gold particles that can be easily observed in both types of microscopy are at present the most commonly used label (Figs 2–8C, 2–12, and 21–15).

Methods of Localizing Antigens

There are both direct and indirect methods for antigen localization by immunocytochemistry.

(1) Direct method–Sections of a tissue suspected of containing an antigen (protein x) are incubated with a labeled antibody to x; the antibody will specifically combine with x. The excess antibody is washed off, and the tissue is processed according to the methods outlined above. The location of the antigen is then detected with the fluorescence microscope (Fig 2–11).

(2) Indirect method–Antibodies to protein x (the antigen) are produced in an animal, eg, a rabbit. Rabbit immunoglobulins are, in turn, capable of inducing

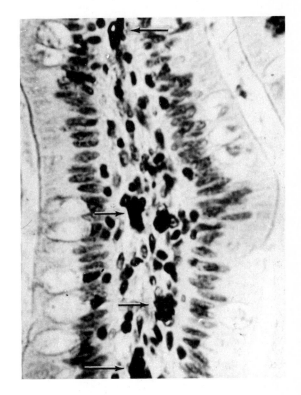

Figure 2–10. Photomicrograph of an intestinal villus showing macrophages stained by the immunoperoxidase method using antilysozyme antibodies (arrows). × 400.

A   B

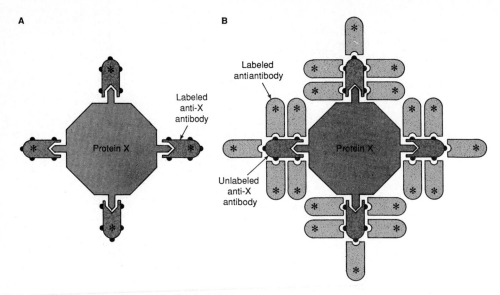

Figure 2–11. The direct **(A)** and indirect **(B)** techniques of immunocytochemistry. In the direct technique, a labeled anti-*x* antibody binds to an antigen present in the cells. In this case, each antigen molecule binds a few antibody molecules. In the first step of the indirect technique, nonlabeled anti-*x* antibody is bound to the antigen; in the second step, the labeled antiantibody then binds to the anti-*x* antibody. Because each anti-*x* antibody binds several molecules of labeled antiantibody, the indirect procedure is more sensitive than the direct method.

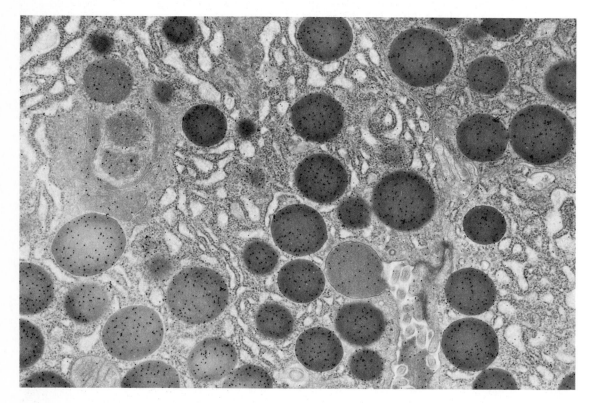

Figure 2–12. Section of a pancreatic acinar cell stained by the gold particle-protein A method after previous incubation with antiamylase antibody. The gold particles appear as very small black dots over the mature secretory granules and forming granules in the Golgi complex. (Courtesy of M Bendayan.)

Table 2–1. Partial list of the most commonly used proteins (antigens) important for the immunocytochemical diagnosis and subsequent treatment of disease.

Antigens	Diagnosis
Intermediate-filament proteins	
Cytokeratins	Undifferentiated tumors of epithelial origin, carcinomas, and adenocarcinomas
Glial fibrillary acid protein	Tumors of some glial cells
Vimentin	Tumors of connective tissue
Desmin	Muscle tumors
Other proteins	
Virtually all proteic or polypeptidic hormones	Protein or polypeptide hormone-producing tumors
Carcinoembryonic antigen (CEA)	Glandular tumors, mainly of the digestive tract and breast
Prostate-specific antigen	Prostate gland tumors
Steroid hormone receptors	Breast duct-cell tumors
Antigens produced by viruses	Specific virus infections

of all RNA transcripts expressed within a single cell type; and **Western analysis,** which detects a single protein species from among all other proteins expressed in a single cell or tissue.

Southern and Northern analyses are based on the high affinity observed between complementary sequences of nucleic acids (**hybridization**). Western analysis is based on the high affinity and specificity between antibodies and antigens.

Nucleic acid hybridization is the technique that allows the identification of specific sequences of DNA or RNA based on the ability of single-stranded segments of these nucleic acids to bind specifically to previously labeled known complementary single-stranded nucleic acid sequences. These known sequences, produced in the laboratory, are called **probes** and are usually labeled by the use of radioisotopes or by the coupling of their nucleotides with biotin. The isotope-labeled probe can then be detected by radioautography and the biotin-labeled probe by its high affinity to avidin (which was previously coupled with peroxidase; in a further step, peroxidase is

an antibody response in another animal, such as a sheep or goat, thus producing an antiantibody. A tissue section containing protein *x* is incubated with unlabeled rabbit anti-*x* antibodies. After washing, labeled rabbit antiantibodies are added, and the location of protein *x* can be seen by a microscopic technique appropriate for the label. This method has an advantage in that the technique is considerably more sensitive (Fig 2–11B) than the direct method (Fig 2–11A).

Several variations of immunocytochemical methods have been developed that permit both specificity and sensitivity. The gold particle-protein A method has been widely used and has contributed significantly to research in cell biology and to the improvement of medical diagnostic procedures (Fig 2–12). Table 2–1 shows some of the routine applications of immunocytochemical procedures in clinical practice.

IN SITU HYBRIDIZATION TECHNIQUES

The central challenge in modern cell biology is to understand the workings of the cell in molecular detail. This goal requires techniques that permit analysis of the molecules involved in the process of information flow from DNA to protein. These techniques include **Southern analysis,** which characterizes and quantitates the presence of DNA of a specific gene in the presence of all other genes in a eukaryotic organism; **Northern analysis,** which identifies and quantitates specific mRNA transcripts in the presence

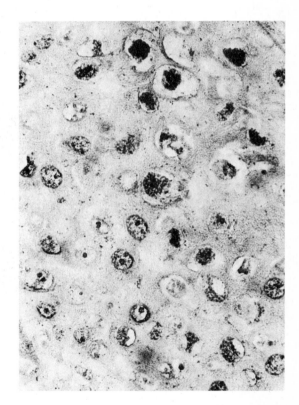

Figure 2–13. Photomicrograph of a section of human epithelial tumor (condyloma) in which in situ hybridization with the DNA of the human papilloma virus type II (HPVII) was performed. Observe dark staining in several nuclei, indicating the presence of the genome of this virus in this tumor, suggesting its possible participation in the genesis of the tumor. (Courtesy of JE Levi.)

detected by the DAB method currently used in immunohistochemistry). To localize specific DNA sequences (such as genes) or messenger RNAs in cells or cell components, in situ hybridization can be applied to tissue sections, smears, or chromosomes of squashed mitotic cells (Fig 2–13). This permits the localization of specific DNA (eg, cellular or viral genes) or gene expression, through the presence of messenger RNA (mRNA) in whole cells or cell components. The technique is highly specific and routinely used in research, clinical diagnosis, and forensic medicine.

REFERENCES

Bendayan M: Protein A-gold electron microscopic immunocytochemistry; Methods, applications and limitations. *J Electron Microsc Techn* 1984;**1**:243.

Cuello ACC: *Immunocytochemistry.* Wiley, 1983.

Hayat MA: *Electron Microscopy of Enzymes,* Vols 1–5. Van Nostrand-Reinhold, 1973–1977.

Murray RK et al: *Harper's Biochemistry,* 22nd ed. Appleton & Lange, 1990.

Pease AGE: *Histochemistry: Theoretical and Applied,* 4th ed. Churchill Livingstone, 1980.

Stoward PJ, Polak JM (eds): *Histochemistry: The Widening Horizons of its Applications in Biological Sciences.* Wiley, 1981.

The Cell

3

Cells are the structural units of all living organisms. It has been recognized for some time that there are, at least from the structural point of view, 2 fundamentally different types of cells. So many biochemical similarities exist between the 2 types that many investigators have postulated that one group evolved from the other.

The **prokaryotic** cell is found only in bacteria. These cells are small (1–5 μm long), may have a cell wall outside the limiting membrane (cell membrane, **plasmalemma**), and do not have a nuclear envelope separating the genetic material (DNA) from other cellular constituents. In addition, prokaryotes have no histones (specific basic proteins) bound to their DNA, and membranous organelles are usually not present.

In contrast, **eukaryotic** (from Greek, *eu*, good, + *karyon*, nucleus) cells are larger and have a distinct nucleus surrounded by a nuclear envelope (Fig 3–1). Histones are associated with the genetic material, and numerous membrane-limited organelles are found in the cytoplasm. This chapter is concerned almost exclusively with eukaryotic cells.

CELLULAR FUNCTIONS & DIFFERENTIATION

During the process of evolution, the cells of metazoa gradually became modified and specialized, resulting in increased efficiency of function. Through phylogenetic development, undifferentiated primitive cells exhibiting several functional activities, each with little efficiency, were transformed into a variety of differentiated cells that were collectively able to perform some specific functions with much greater efficiency. This process of cell specialization is known as **cell differentiation.**

During this differentiation, for example, the muscle cell elongates into a spindle-shaped cell that synthesizes and accumulates myofibrillar proteins. The resulting cell efficiently converts chemical energy into contractile energy. Another example is the pancreatic cell, which is specialized to synthesize and secrete digestive enzymes.

Morphologic modifications during differentiation are accompanied by chemical changes. The quantitative synthesis of specific proteins by each differenti-

ated cell type characterizes this process, for example, in the synthesis of the proteins actin and myosin by the muscle cell or of the several digestive enzymes by pancreatic acinar cells. The main cellular functions performed by specialized cells in the body are listed in Table 3–1.

Cells are not always restricted to a single, specialized function and frequently are capable of performing 2 or more functions. Thus, the cells of the proximal convoluted tubules of the kidney not only transport ions but also absorb metabolites and digest proteins. Similarly, the intestinal epithelial cells reabsorb metabolites and synthesize digestive enzymes (proteins) such as disaccharidases and peptidases (see Chapter 15).

It will be seen that the morphologic characteristics of a cell vary predictably according to its functions.

CELL COMPONENTS

The cell is composed of 2 basic parts: **cytoplasm** (from Greek, *kytos*, cell + *plasma*, thing formed) and **nucleus** (from Latin, *nux*, nut). Individual cytoplasmic components are usually not clearly distinguishable in common hematoxylin and eosin-stained preparations; the nucleus, however, appears intensely stained dark blue or black (Fig 4–1).

Cytoplasm

The outermost component of the cell, separating the cytoplasm from its extracellular environment, is the plasma membrane (plasmalemma). The cytoplasm itself is composed of a matrix in which are embedded several components, frequently called **organelles**, plus deposits of carbohydrates, lipids, and pigments.

Cell membranes divide the eukaryotic cells in discrete compartments that regulate intracellular traffic and interchanges between the cell and its environment.

Plasma Membrane

All eukaryotic cells are enveloped by a limiting membrane composed of lipids (phospholipids and cholesterol), protein, and oligosaccharides covalently linked to some of the lipids and proteins. The cell, or

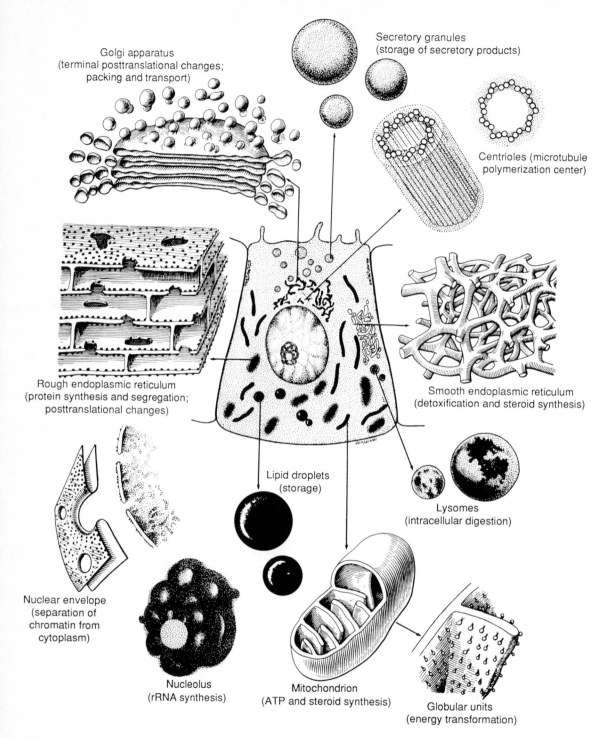

Figure 3–1. Diagram showing a hypothetical eukaryotic cell, in the center, as seen with the light microscope. It is surrounded by its various structures as seen with the electron microscope. (Redrawn and reproduced, with permission, from Bloom W, Fawcett DW: *A Textbook of Histology,* 9th ed. Saunders, 1968.)

Table 3–1. Cellular functions in some specialized cells.

Function	Specialized Cell(s)
Movement	Muscle cell
Conductivity	Nerve cell
Synthesis and secretion of enzymes	Pancreatic acinar cells
Synthesis and secretion of mucous substances	Mucous-gland cells
Synthesis and secretion of steroids	Some adrenal gland, testis, and ovary cells
Ion transport	Cells of the kidney and salivary gland ducts
Intracellular digestion	Macrophages and some white blood cells
Transformation of physical and chemical stimuli into nervous impulses	Sensory cells
Metabolite absorption	Cells of the intestine, kidney, etc.

plasma, membrane (plasmalemma) functions as a selective barrier that regulates the passage of certain materials into and out of the cell. In addition, membranes may facilitate the transport of specific materials through this limiting barrier. Membranes also carry out a number of specific recognition and regulatory functions (to be discussed later). For these reasons, the plasma membrane plays an important role in the way a cell interacts with its environment.

The membranes range from 7.5 to 10 nm in thickness and consequently are visible only in the electron microscope. Electron micrographs reveal that the plasmalemma—and, for that matter, almost all other organellar membranes—exhibit a trilaminar structure after fixation in osmium tetroxide (Fig 3–2). Because of the universality of this appearance, this 3-layered structure has been designated the **unit membrane** (Fig 3–3).

Membrane phospholipids, such as phosphatidyl-choline (lecithin) and phosphatidylethanolamine (cephalin) consist of 2 long, nonpolar (hydrophobic) hydrocarbon chains linked to a charged (hydrophilic) head group. Cholesterol is also a constituent of most membranes. Within the membrane, lipids are most stable when organized into a double layer with their hydrophobic (nonpolar) chains directed toward the center of the membrane and their charged (hydrophilic) heads directed outward (Fig 3–2). The lipid composition of each half of the bilayer is different. In the erythrocyte, phosphatidylcholine and sphingomyelin are more abundant in the outer half of the membrane, while phosphatidylserine and phosphatidylethanolamine are more concentrated in the inner half. Some of the lipids, known as glycolipids, possess oligosaccharide chains that extend outward from the surface of the cell membrane and thus contribute to the lipid asymmetry (Fig 3–4A). The trilaminar appearance of membranes in the electron microscope is apparently due to the deposition of reduced osmium on the hydrophilic groups present on each side of the lipid bilayer.

The proteins, which are a major molecular constituent of membranes ($> 50\%$ w/w), can be divided into 2 groups. **Integral proteins** represent a class of proteins that are directly incorporated within the lipid bilayer, while **peripheral proteins** exhibit a looser association with membrane surfaces. The loosely bound peripheral proteins can be easily extracted from cell membranes by use of salt solutions, while integral proteins can be extracted only by drastic methods involving the use of detergents.

From freeze-fracture electron microscopic studies, it appears that many integral proteins are distributed as globular molecules intercalated among the lipid molecules (Fig 3–4B). Some of these proteins are only partially embedded in the lipid bilayer, so that they may protrude from either the outer or inner surface. Other proteins are large enough to extend across the 2 lipid layers and protrude from both mem-

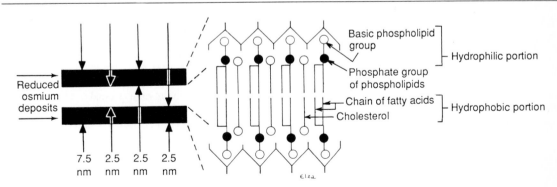

Figure 3–2. The ultrastructure and molecular structure (right) of the cell membrane. The dark lines at left represent the 2 dense layers observed in the electron microscope; these are caused by the deposit of osmium in the hydrophilic portions of the lipid molecules.

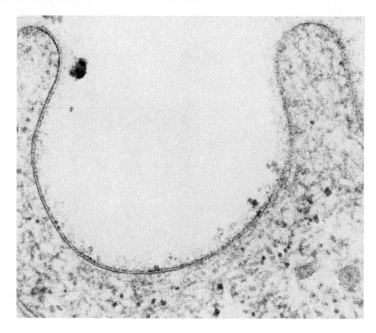

Figure 3–3. Electron micrograph of a section of the surface of an epithelial cell, showing the unit membrane with its 2 dark lines enclosing a clear band. On the surface of the membrane is a layer of granular material forming the cell coat. × 100,000.

brane surfaces. Some of the proteins that completely cross the membrane (transmembrane proteins) are believed to provide a channel through which water-soluble substances, such as ions, can pass back and forth between the extracellular and intracellular compartments. Other proteins, which may possess lipid (lipoproteins) or carbohydrate (glycoproteins and proteoglycans) side chains, are arranged as mosaics within the cell membrane (Fig 3–4). The carbohydrate moieties of glycoproteins and glycolipids project from the external surface of the plasma membrane and are important components of specific molecules called **receptors** that have been implicated as mediators of important interactions such as cell adhesion, recognition, and response to the action of protein hormones. As with lipids, the distribution of membrane proteins is different in the 2 surfaces of the cell membranes, and all cell membranes are therefore asymmetric (Fig 3–4).

Integration of the proteins within the lipid bilayer is the result of hydrophobic interactions between the lipids and nonpolar (hydrophobic) amino acids present on the outer shell of the integral membrane proteins (Fig 3–4A). The integral proteins are not bound rigidly in place, however, and are able to move by diffusing within the plane of the cell membrane. Under certain circumstances, these proteins can accumulate at one region of the plasma membrane, occasionally forming a localized aggregation of proteins. This process, called **capping,** has been ob-

served in several cell types and appears to be a general phenomenon. Experiments have also revealed that movement of some membrane proteins is not random but is probably controlled by intracellular mechanisms involving microfilaments. The association of actin-containing microfilaments with integral membrane proteins, via one to several peripheral membrane proteins, is becoming better understood, especially in the erythrocyte (red blood cell).

Fig 3–5 illustrates an experiment that demonstrates the fluidity of integral proteins within the cell membrane. The above-described "mosaic" disposition of membrane proteins, in conjunction with the fluid nature of the lipid bilayer, constitutes the basis of the **fluid mosaic model** for membrane structure shown in Figure 3–4A.

The plasma membrane is the site where materials are exchanged between the cell and its environment. Some ions, such as Na^+, K^+, and Ca^{2+}, are actively transported across the cell membrane using channels that are integral membrane proteins. Mass transfers of material also occur through the plasma membrane. The uptake of material is known generally as **endocytosis** (from Greek, *endon*, within, + *kytos*); the corresponding name for release of material is **exocytosis.** Several varieties of endocytosis are recognized.

A. Fluid-Phase Pinocytosis: Two examples of fluid incorporation into cells are recognized. First, small invaginations of the cell membrane form and entrap extracellular fluid and anything in solution in

A Carbohydrate chains bound to lipids and proteins

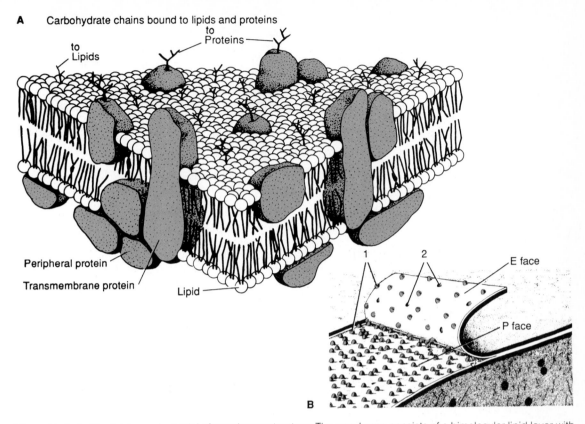

Figure 3–4. A. The fluid mosaic model of membrane structure. The membrane consists of a bimolecular lipid layer with proteins inserted in it or bound to the cytoplasmic surface. Integral membrane proteins are firmly embedded in the lipid layers. Some of these proteins completely span the bilayer and are called transmembrane proteins, while others are embedded in either the outer or inner leaflet of the lipid bilayer. The dotted line in the integral membrane protein is the region where hydrophobic amino acids interact with the hydrophobic portions of the membrane. Loosely bound to the inner surface of the membrane are the peripheral proteins. Many of the proteins and lipids have externally exposed oligosaccharide chains. **B.** Membrane cleavage occurs when a cell is frozen and fractured (cryofracture). Most of the membrane particles (1), generally thought to represent proteins or aggregates of proteins, remain attached to the half of the membrane adjacent to the cytoplasm (P, or protoplasmic, face of the membrane). Fewer particles are found attached to the outer half of the membrane (E, or extracellular, face). For every protein particle that bulges on one surface, a corresponding depression (2) appears in the opposite surface. Membrane splitting occurs along the line of weakness formed by the fatty acid tails of membrane phospholipids since only weak hydrophobic interactions serve to bind the 2 halves of the membrane together along this line. The study of these protein particles by cryofracture has contributed significantly to our knowledge of cell membranes. (Modified and reproduced, with permission, from Krstić RV: *Ultrastructure of the Mammalian Cell.* Springer-Verlag, 1979.)

the fluid. **Pinocytotic vesicles** (about 80 nm in diameter) pinch off from the cell surface (Fig 4–17), and most eventually fuse with lysosomes (see section on lysosomes later in this chapter). In the lining cells of capillaries (endothelial cells), however, pinocytotic vesicles may move to the surface opposite their origin. Here they fuse with the plasma membrane and release their contents onto the cell surface, thus accomplishing bulk transfer of material across the cell (see Fig 11–4). A second type of fluid-phase pinocytosis transports larger volumes of fluid and is performed by broad sheets of the cell membrane enfolding fluid into the cell interior (Fig 5–16).

B. Receptor-Mediated Endocytosis: Receptors for many substances, such as low-density lipoproteins and protein hormones, are located at the cell surface. The receptors are either originally widely dispersed over the surface or aggregated in special regions called **coated pits.** Binding of the ligand (a molecule with high affinity for a receptor) to its receptor causes widely dispersed receptors to accumulate in coated pits. The coating on the cytoplasmic surface of the membrane is composed of several polypeptides, the major one being **clathrin** (MW 180,000). These proteins form a lattice composed of pentagons and hexagons very similar in arrangement

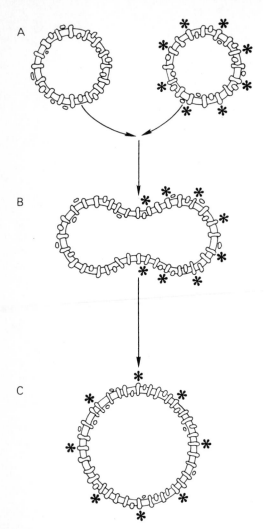

Figure 3–5. Experiment demonstrating the fluid nature of proteins within the cell membrane. The plasmalemma is shown as 2 parallel lines (representing the lipid portion) in which proteins are embedded. Some of these particles are characteristic of the cell at top right and are identified by asterisks. In this experiment, 2 types of cells derived from tissue cultures (one with a fluorescent marker [right] and one without) are fused (**A→B**) through the action of Sendai virus. Minutes after the fusion of the membranes, the fluorescent marker of the labeled cell spreads to the entire surface of the fused cells and finally covers it uniformly **(C)**.

cialized for taking up and disposing of invading bacteria, protozoa, fungi, damaged cells, and unneeded extracellular constituents. For example, after a bacterium becomes bound to the surface of a macrophage, cytoplasmic processes of the macrophage are extended and ultimately surround the bacterium. The edges of these processes fuse, enclosing the bacterium in an intracellular **phagocytic vacuole** (Fig 5–19). Lysosomes will then fuse with the vacuole, resulting in destruction of the bacterium (see also *Lysosomes* and Chapter 12).

Exocytosis is the term used to describe the fusion of a membrane-limited structure with the plasma membrane, resulting in the release of its contents into the extracellular space without compromising the integrity of the plasma membrane. A typical example is the release of stored products from secretory cells such as those of the exocrine pancreas and the mammary and salivary glands (Fig 4–19).

During endocytosis, portions of the cell membrane become an endocytotic vesicle; during exocytosis, the membrane is returned to the cell surface. This phenomenon is called **membrane trafficking.** Evidence is available that in several systems membranes are conserved and reused several times during repeated cycles of endocytosis. The significance of membrane trafficking for cell economy is self-evident.

The structures of other membranes (nuclear envelope, endoplasmic reticulum, Golgi complex, secretory granules, and lysosomes)—although not identical—are similar to those of the plasma membrane. The structural and functional differences observed are at present being actively investigated. Chemical differences have been noted, and structural differences have been associated with the presence of different structural proteins, lipids, enzymes, and receptors on them.

Cell Membranes Mediate Signal Reception

Cells in a multicellular organism need to communicate with one another in order to regulate their development into tissues, to control their growth and division, and to coordinate their functions. Cells communicate in 3 ways: They secrete chemicals that signal to cells some distance away; they display plasma-membrane-bound signaling molecules that influence other cells in direct physical contact; and they form communicating junctions that couple adjacent cells, allowing the exchange of small molecules (see Chapter 4).

Extracellular signaling molecules mediate 3 kinds of communication between cells. In **endocrine signaling,** hormones are carried in the blood to target cells throughout the body; in **paracrine signaling,** chemical mediators are rapidly metabolized so that they act on local cells only; and in **synaptic signaling,** neurotransmitters act only on adjacent nerve cells through special contact areas called synapses. Each

to the struts in a geodesic dome. It is believed that this arrangement produces a force that causes the coated pit to invaginate and pinch off, forming a **coated vesicle** that carries the ligand and its receptor into the cell (see Fig 3–16).

C. Phagocytosis: This term literally means *cell eating* and can be compared to pinocytosis, which means *cell drinking*. Certain cell types, such as macrophages and polymorphonuclear leukocytes, are spe-

cell type in the body contains a distinctive set of receptor proteins that enable it to respond to a complementary set of signaling molecules in a specific, preprogrammed way.

Signaling molecules can also be classified according to their solubility in water. Small **hydrophobic signaling molecules,** such as steroid and thyroid hormones, diffuse through the plasma membrane of the target cell and activate receptor proteins inside the cell. In contrast, **hydrophilic signaling molecules,** including neurotransmitters, most hormones, and local chemical mediators, activate receptor proteins on the surface of target cells. These, in turn, relay information to the cell interior.

Signaling Mediated by Intracellular Receptors

Steroid hormones are small hydrophobic molecules derived from cholesterol; they are transported in the blood by binding reversibly to carrier proteins in the plasma. Once released from their carrier proteins, they diffuse through the plasma membrane of the target cell and bind reversibly to specific steroid-hormone-receptor proteins in the cytoplasm or nucleus. The binding of hormone activates the receptor, enabling it to bind with high affinity to specific DNA sequences that act as transcriptional enhancers. Binding also increases the level of transcription from specific genes. The products of some of these activated genes may activate other genes in turn and produce a delayed secondary response, thereby extending the initial effect of the hormone. Each steroid hormone is recognized by a different member of a family of homologous receptor proteins. The same receptor protein regulates different genes in other target cells, presumably because the DNA-binding proteins required for specific gene transcription differ in these cells.

Mitochondria

Mitochondria (from Greek, *mitos,* thread, + *chondros,* granule) are spherical or filamentous organelles 0.5–1 μm wide that can attain a length of up to 10 μm. Their distribution in cells varies. They tend to accumulate in parts of the cytoplasm where metabolic activity is more intense, such as the apical ends of ciliated cells (Fig 17–2), in the middle piece of spermatozoa (Fig 22–4), or at the base of ion-transferring cells (Fig 4–17). In instances where they are not localized in specific regions of the cell, mitochondria have a tendency to be oriented along the long axis of long cells, or radially in round cells.

These highly efficient organelles, which are present in all eukaryotic cells, transform the chemical energy of the metabolites present in cytoplasm into energy that is easily accessible to the cell. This energy is partially stored as high-energy phosphate bonds in several compounds; approximately 50% of it is dissipated as heat. These compounds, the most important of which is adenosine triphosphate (ATP), promptly release energy when required by the cell to perform any type of work, whether it be of osmotic, mechanical, electrical, or chemical nature.

Cells contain great numbers of mitochondria—an estimated 800 in one liver cell—but always in a num-

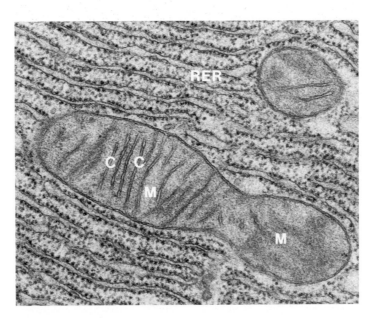

Figure 3–6. Electron micrograph of a section of rat pancreas. A mitochondrion with its membranes, cristae (C), and matrix (M) is seen in the center. Numerous flattened cisternae of rough endoplasmic reticulum (RER) with ribosomes on their cytoplasmic surfaces are also visible. × 50,000.

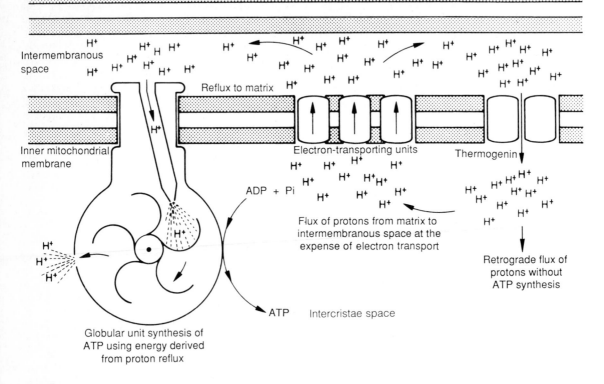

Figure 3–7. Drawing illustrating the chemiosmotic theory of mitochondrial energy transduction. **Middle:** the flux of protons is directed from the matrix to the intermembranous space promoted at the expense of energy derived from the electron transport system in the inner membrane. **Left:** half the energy derived from proton reflux produces ATP; the remaining energy produces heat. **Right:** the protein thermogenin, present in multilocular adipose tissue, forms a shunt for reflux of protons. This reflux, which dissipates energy as heat, does not produce ATP (see Chapter 6).

ber characteristic for that cell. Mitochondria are composed mainly of protein. Lipids are present to a lesser degree, along with small quantities of DNA and RNA. Like most cell components, mitochondria have a short life span, and their proteins are constantly being renewed. The average half-life of mitochondrial proteins in rat liver cells, for example, is 10 days.

Mitochondria generally have a characteristic structure under the electron microscope, with small variations according to the organ and species (Figs 3–1 and 3–6). They are composed of an **outer mitochondrial membrane** and an **inner mitochondrial membrane;** the latter projects folds, termed **cristae,** into the interior of the mitochondrion. These membranes enclose 2 spaces. The space located between the 2 membranes is termed the **intramembrane space** and is continuous with the **intracristal spaces** that penetrate the cristae. The other space, the **intercristal,** or **matrix, space,** is enclosed by the inner membrane and is in turn penetrated by the cristae. Filling the matrix space is a fine granular material of variable electron density. Most mitochondria have flat, shelf-

like cristae in their interiors (Figs 3–1 and 3–6), whereas cells that secrete steroids (eg, adrenal and gonadal cells; see Chapter 4) frequently contain tubular cristae (Fig 4–27). The cristae increase the internal surface area of mitochondria, and it is on these structures that enzymes and other compounds involved in the oxidative phosphorylation and electron transport systems are located. The adenosine diphosphate (ADP) to adenosine triphosphate (ATP) phosphorylating system is localized in globular structures connected to the membrane via cylindric stalks (Fig 3–1). The globular structures are a complex of proteins with ATP synthetase activity that, in the presence of ADP plus inorganic phosphate, form ATP. The most accepted theory (the chemiosmotic theory) suggests that ATP synthesis occurs at the expense of a flow of protons across this globular unit (Fig 3–7).

The number of mitochondria and the number of cristae in each mitochondrion are proportionate to the metabolic activity of the cells in which they reside. Thus, cells with a high rate of metabolism (eg, cardiac muscle, kidney tubule cells) have abundant mitochondria with a large number of closely packed cristae, whereas others with low metabolism have few mitochondria with short cristae.

Between the cristae is an amorphous **matrix** rich in protein and containing some DNA and RNA. In a great number of cell types, the mitochondrial matrix also exhibits rounded electron-dense granules rich in cations such as calcium and magnesium. Although their function is not completely understood, the granules are apparently related to the mitochondrion's ability to concentrate cations. Enzymes for the citric acid (Krebs) cycle and fatty acid β-oxidation are found to reside within the matrix space.

The DNA isolated from the mitochondrial matrix has been shown to be double-stranded and to have a circular structure. DNA strands are synthesized within the mitochondrion; their duplication is independent of nuclear DNA replication. Mitochondria are known to contain the 3 types of RNA (ribosomal RNA [rRNA], messenger RNA [mRNA], and transfer RNA [tRNA]). Particles resembling ribosomes are also present. Protein synthesis occurs in mitochondria, but because of the reduced amount of mitochondrial DNA, only a small proportion of the mitochondrial proteins are produced locally. Most of the mitochondrial proteins are coded by nuclear DNA and synthesized in polysomes. The proteins are then transported into mitochondria by mechanisms that are not fully understood but which require energy.

Metabolites are degraded within mitochondria by the catalytic activity of the enzymes of the citric acid cycle, and the energy liberated in this process is partially captured through oxidative phosphorylation. The end result of these reactions is the production of CO_2, water, and heat and the accumulation of energy in high-energy compounds such as ATP.

The initial degradation of proteins, carbohydrates, and fats is carried out in the cytoplasmic matrix. The metabolic end product of these extramitochondrial metabolic pathways is acetyl-CoA, which then enters the mitochondria. Within the mitochondria, acetyl-CoA combines with oxaloacetate to form citric acid. Within the citric acid cycle, there are several reactions of decarboxylation producing CO_2 and 4 pairs of hydrogen atoms are removed by specific reactions catalyzed by dehydrogenases. The H atoms ultimately react with oxygen to form H_2O. By virtue of the action of cytochromes a, b and c, coenzyme Q, and cytochrome oxidase, the **electron transport system,** located in the inner mitochondrial membrane, is capable of releasing energy that is captured at 3 points of this system through the formation of ATP from ADP and inorganic phosphate. Under aerobic conditions, the combined activity of extramitochondrial glycolysis and the citric acid cycle as well as the electron transport system gives rise to 36 molecules of ATP per mole of glucose. This is 18 times the energy obtainable under anaerobic circumstances, when only the glycolytic pathway can be utilized.

Origin & Evolution of Mitochondria

In the process of mitosis, each daughter cell receives approximately half the mitochondria originally present in the parent cell just before division. New mitochondria originate from preexisting mitochondria by accretion of material that leads to growth and subsequent division (fission) of the organelle itself.

The fact that mitochondria have some characteristics in common with bacteria has led to the hypothesis that mitochondria originated from an ancestral aerobic prokaryote that adapted to a symbiotic life within a eukaryotic host cell.

RIBOSOMES

Ribosomes are small electron-dense particles, about 20×30 nm in size. They are composed of 4 types of ribosomal RNA (rRNA) and almost 80 different proteins. Ribosomes are found in all cells, but each cell type has a characteristic number and distribution of these particles.

There are 2 classes of ribosomes: One class is found in prokaryotes, chloroplasts, and mitochondria; the other is found in eukaryotic cells. Both classes of ribosomes are composed of 2 different-sized subunits.

In eukaryotic cells, the RNAs of both subunits are synthesized within the nucleoli of the nucleus. Their numerous proteins are synthesized in the cytoplasm and then enter the nucleus and associate with rRNA. Subunits then leave the nucleus, via nuclear pores, to enter the cytoplasm and participate in protein synthesis.

Ribosomes, which are intensely basophilic because of the presence of numerous phosphate groups of the constituent rRNA that act as polyanions, react with such basic stains as methylene blue, toluidine blue, and hematoxylin. Thus, sites in the cytoplasm that are rich in ribosomes stain intensely with these dyes. These basophilic regions were described as early as the nineteenth century and were named according to the cell being studied. In glandular cells, they were know as **ergastoplasm** (from Greek, *ergaster,* workman, + *plasma*); in neurons, as **Nissl bodies;** and in other cells as **basophilic bodies** or **basophilic components.** Although ribosomes are below the resolution of the light microscope, they can be visualized indirectly because of their staining characteristics.

Ribosomes occur as individual granules or in clusters called **polyribosomes (polysomes).** The individual ribosomes of a polyribosome (Fig 3–8A) are held together by a strand of messenger RNA (mRNA). The message carried by mRNA is a code for the amino acid sequence of proteins being synthesized by the cell. Ribosomes play a crucial role in decoding, or translating, the message during protein synthesis. Proteins synthesized for use within the cell and destined to remain diffusely distributed in the cyto-

A. Free polyribosomes, whose proteins remain in the cytoplasm

B. Bound polyribosomes, showing protein synthesis and segregation into the rough endoplasmic reticulum

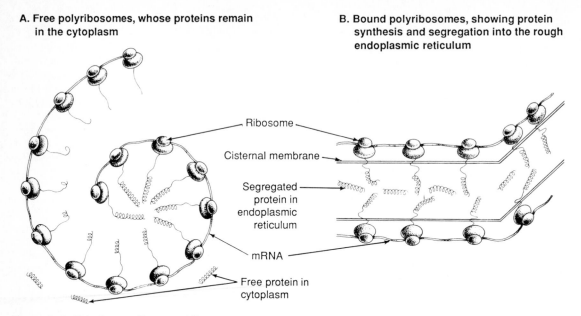

Ribosome

Cisternal membrane

Segregated protein in endoplasmic reticulum

mRNA

Free protein in cytoplasm

Figure 3–8. This diagram illustrates **(A)** the concept that cells synthesizing proteins (represented here by spirals) that are to remain within the cytoplasm possess (free) polyribosomes (ie, nonadherent to the endoplasmic reticulum). In **B,** where the proteins are segregated in the endoplasmic reticulum and may eventually be extruded from the cytoplasm (export proteins), not only do the polyribosomes adhere to the membranes of rough endoplasmic reticulum, but the proteins produced by them are injected into the interior of the organelle across its membrane. In this way, the proteins—especially enzymes such as ribonucleases and proteases, which could have undesirable effects on the cytoplasm—are separated from it.

plasm (eg, hemoglobin in immature red blood cells) are synthesized on free (or unattached) polyribosomes—polyribosomes existing as isolated clusters within the cytoplasm. Polyribosomes that are attached to the membranes of the endoplasmic reticulum (via their large subunits) translate mRNAs that code for proteins that are segregated into the cisternae of the reticulum (Fig 3–8B). These proteins can be secreted (eg, pancreatic and salivary enzymes) or stored in the cell (eg, enzymes of lysosomes and proteins within granules of white blood cells). In addition, most integral membrane proteins are synthesized on polyribosomes attached to membranes of the endoplasmic reticulum.

It should be emphasized that there are no intrinsic chemical differences between free and attached ribosomes. As seen below, it is the mRNA that possesses a signal which will cause ribosomes to attach to membranes of the endoplasmic reticulum.

Endoplasmic Reticulum

The endoplasmic reticulum (ER) is the site of lipid and carbohydrate synthesis, protein segregation from the cytoplasm, and the initial posttranslational modifications that prepare proteins for their specific function. This predominantly membranous organelle may appear as elongated, flattened, rounded, or tubular vesicles in electron micrographs. The endoplasmic

reticulum takes its name from the manner in which these structures anastomose with one another to form an intracellular network (reticulum). The disposition of endoplasmic reticulum membranes varies considerably from cell to cell and even from region to region within the same cell. Endoplasmic reticulum develops gradually during differentiation of embryonic cells and acquires a specialized appearance that varies with the size and functional state of different cell types. In fully differentiated cells, there are essentially 2 specialized types of endoplasmic reticulum: **rough** and **smooth.**

The 2 types of endoplasmic reticulum show differences in function as described below. These differences, however, are qualitative. The enzymes required for smooth endoplasmic reticulum function, for example, are synthesized in the rough endoplasmic reticulum, so there can be no absolute differences in the composition of these membranes. A probable exception to this statement, however, is the presence of ribophorins I and II only in rough endoplasmic reticulum (see below).

In general, the functions of the endoplasmic reticulum include segregation of newly synthesized proteins destined for export or intracellular utilization, limited proteolysis of the signal sequence of newly synthesized proteins, initial glycosylation of glycoproteins, posttranslational modifications of amino acids, assembly of multichain proteins, lipid synthesis, and chemical modification of endogenous and exogenous compounds. Note that some of these functions are more conspicuous in one type of reticulum than in the other.

Rough Endoplasmic Reticulum (RER): This form of endoplasmic reticulum is prominent in cells specialized for protein secretion, such as pancreatic acinar cells (digestive enzymes), fibroblasts (collagen), and plasma cells (immunoglobulins). The rough endoplasmic reticulum consists of tubules as well as parallel stacks of flattened cisternae (Figs 3–1 and 3–6), limited by membranes that are sometimes continuous with the outer membrane of the nuclear envelope (Fig 3–27). Although not obvious in a single thin section, the lumen of the rough endoplasmic reticulum is a single membrane-limited compartment within the cell. The name **rough endoplasmic reticulum** alludes to the presence of polyribosomes on the cytoplasmic surfaces of the endoplasmic reticulum membranes, giving them a rough or granular appearance (Figs 3–1 and 3–6). The presence of polyribosomes also confers basophilic staining properties on this organelle when viewed with the light microscope.

The principal function of the rough endoplasmic reticulum is to segregate proteins destined for export or intracellular utilization. Additional functions include the initial (core) glycosylation of glycoproteins having N-linked oligosaccharides, the synthesis of phospholipids, the assembly of multichain proteins, and certain posttranslational modifications of newly formed polypeptides.

All protein synthesis begins on polyribosomes that are not attached to the endoplasmic reticulum. Messenger RNAs of proteins destined to be segregated in the endoplasmic reticulum contain an additional sequence of bases at their 5′ end that code for approximately 20–25 mainly hydrophobic amino acids termed the **signal sequence.** Upon translation, the signal sequence interacts with a complex of 6 nonidentical polypeptides plus a 7S RNA molecule that is referred to as the **signal-recognition particle (SRP).** SRP acts to inhibit further polypeptide elongation until the SRP-polyribosome complex binds to a receptor in the membrane of the rough endoplasmic reticulum, the **docking protein**. Upon binding to the docking protein, SRP is released from polyribosomes, allowing the translation to continue (Fig 3–9). Also present in membranes of rough endoplasmic reticulum, but lacking in smooth endoplasmic reticulum, are 2 integral membrane proteins, **ribophorins I and II,** which may provide attachment sites for the large subunits of ribosomes. In addition, ribophorins may form hydrophilic channels through the hydrophobic core of rough endoplasmic reticulum membranes, allowing the pas-

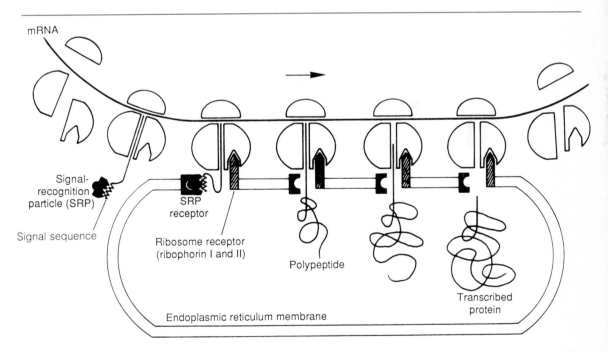

Figure 3–9. Diagram illustrating the transport of proteins across the membrane of the endoplasmic reticulum. The ribosomes bind to mRNA, and the signal peptide is initially bound to a signal-recognition particle (SRP). Ribosomes bind to the ER by interacting with the SRP and a ribosomal receptor. The signal peptide is then removed by a signal peptidase (not shown). These interactions cause the opening of a pore through which the protein is extruded into the endoplasmic reticulum.

sage of newly synthesized proteins into the lumen of the rough endoplasmic reticulum. This process is termed **vectorial discharge** to emphasize its unidirectional nature.

Once inside the lumen of the rough endoplasmic reticulum, the signal sequence is removed by a specific enzyme, **signal peptidase,** localized at the inner surface of the rough endoplasmic reticulum. Translation of the protein continues, accompanied by intracisternal secondary and tertiary structural changes as well as certain posttranslational modifications such as hydroxylation, glycosylation, sulfation, and phosphorylation.

The most important posttranslational modification is the initial (core) glycosylation, wherein high-mannose oligosaccharides are added to most proteins destined for export. Proteins synthesized in the rough endoplasmic reticulum can have several destinations: intracellular storage (eg, in lysosomes and specific granules of leukocytes), provisional intracellular storage of proteins for export (eg, in the pancreas, some endocrine cells), and as a component of other mem-

branes (eg, integral proteins). Proteins synthesized in cells may remain in the cytoplasm or be segregated from it and thus participate in a variety of cellular activities. These cells exhibit ultrastructures that correspond to their various activities (Fig 3–10).

Smooth Endoplasmic Reticulum (SER): This type of endoplasmic reticulum also takes the form of a membranous network within the cell; however, its ultrastructure differs from that of rough endoplasmic reticulum in 2 important ways. First, smooth endoplasmic reticulum lacks the associated ribosomes that characterize rough endoplasmic reticulum. Smooth endoplasmic reticulum membranes therefore appear smooth rather than granular. Second, its cisternae are more tubular and more likely to appear as a profusion of interconnected channels of variable shape and sizes than as stacks of flattened cisternae (Figs 3–1 and 4–27). Smooth endoplasmic reticulum membranes arise from rough endoplasmic reticulum, so that it is not surprising to see membrane continuity between the 2 forms.

Smooth endoplasmic reticulum not only exhibits a

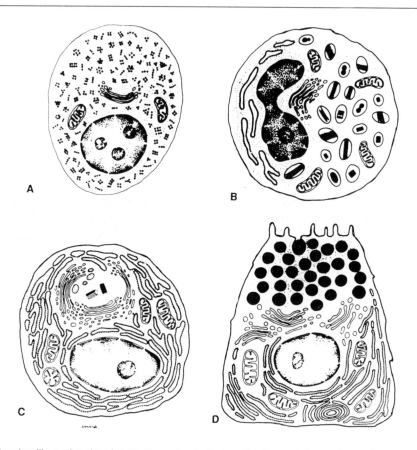

Figure 3–10. Drawing illustrating the ultrastructure of cells that synthesize proteins on free polyribosomes and remain in the cell (**A:** an erythroblast); cells that synthesize, segregate, and store proteins in organelles (**B:** an eosinophilic leucocyte); cells that synthesize, segregate, and directly export proteins (**C:** a plasma cell); and cells that synthesize, segregate, store, and export proteins (**D:** a pancreatic acinar cell).

diversity of morphologic appearances in different cell types but is also associated with a variety of specialized functional capabilities. For example, in cells that synthesize steroid hormones (eg, cells of the adrenal cortex), smooth endoplasmic reticulum occupies a large portion of the cytoplasm and contains some of the enzymes required for steroid synthesis (Figs 4–27 and 4–28). It is abundant in liver cells, where it is responsible for the oxidation, conjugation, and methylation processes employed by the liver to neutralize or detoxify certain hormones and noxious substances such as alcohol and insecticides. Smooth endoplasmic reticulum is also involved in the breakdown of glycogen in liver cells, where the enzyme glucose-6-phosphatase is a constituent of its membranes. This enzyme is also found in rough endoplasmic reticulum—an example of the lack of absolute partition of functions between these 2 organelles. Smooth endoplasmic reticulum participates in the contraction process in muscle cells, where it appears in a special-

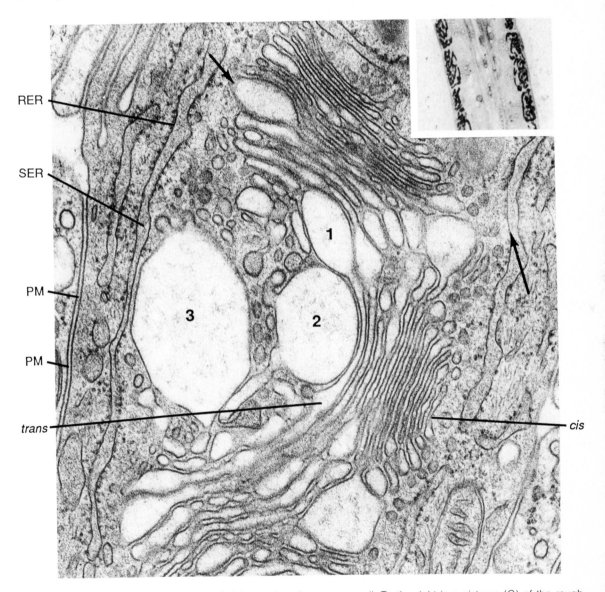

Figure 3–11. Electron micrograph of a Golgi complex of a mucous cell. To the right is a cisterna (C) of the rough endoplasmic reticulum containing granular material. Close to it are small vesicles containing this material. This is the *cis* face of the complex. In the center are flattened and stacked cisternae of the Golgi complex. Dilations can be observed extending from the ends of the cisternae. These dilations gradually detach themselves from the cisternae and fuse, forming the secretory granules (1, 2, and 3). This is the *trans* face. Near the plasma membrane of 2 neighboring cells (PM) is endoplasmic reticulum with a smooth section (SER) and a rough section (RER). × 30,000. Inset: The Golgi complex as seen in 1 μm sections of epididymis cells impregnated by silver. × 1200.

ized form called **sarcoplasmic reticulum** that is involved in the sequestration and release of the calcium ions that regulate muscular contraction (see Chapter 10).

The term **microsome,** as used in cytology and biochemistry, denotes vesicles generated by fragmentation of the endoplasmic reticulum during the process of homogenization that precedes differential or density-gradient centrifugation. This term should never be applied to intact cells. The broken ends of membrane fragments generated during homogenization fuse to produce small vesicles that may have ribosomes attached. These microsomes can then be isolated for biochemical analyses via centrifugation. The microsomes can be further fractionated and the attached polyribosomes separated from their membranes.

Golgi Complex (Golgi Apparatus)

The Golgi apparatus completes posttranslational modifications and packages and places an address on products that have been synthesized by the cell.

This organelle is composed of 3 distinct smooth-membrane-limited compartments (Figs 3–1, 3–11, and 3–12). The first and most obvious is a slightly curved stack of 3–10 flattened **cisternae.** The second is the numerous small **vesicles** seen around the periphery of the stack. Third, usually at one pole of the Golgi complex, are a few larger **vacuoles.** In highly polarized cells, such as columnar epithelial cells lining the intestine, the Golgi complex occupies a characteristic position in the cytoplasm between the nucleus and the apical plasma membrane. Because the Golgi complex is functionally an intermediary

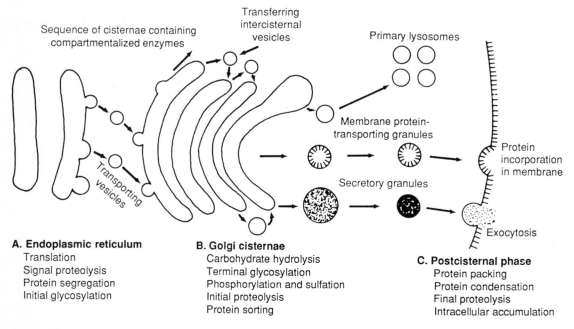

Figure 3–12. Main events occurring during trafficking and sorting of proteins through the Golgi complex. **A:** At the RER, proteins are synthesized and segregated into the RER, where they lose their signal sequence. Glycoproteins undergo their initial glycosylation, a process similar in all glycoproteins. Material from the RER undergoes one-way transport (via transporting vesicles) to the *cis* face of the Golgi cisternae. **B:** In the Golgi cisternae, glycoproteins undergo partial hydrolysis of their carbohydrate moiety and further glycosylation (terminal glycosylation) at various levels of the cisternae. This glycosylation is specific according to the fate of the glycoprotein. Phosphorylation and sulfation also occur at this level. The different proteins will be directed to different regions of a cell according to the type of glycosylation, phosphorylation, and probably also sulfation. Finally, material from the *trans* cisternae is aggregated in condensing vacuoles that bud from the cisternae. The transport of material from one cisterna to another probably occurs by budding and fusion of small vesicles. **C:** In the postcisternal phase, the material from condensing vacuoles is gradually concentrated (probably from the interaction of its component macromolecules) and stored in individual vesicles. Evidence shows that in this process, proteins combine with high-molecular-weight sulfated polyanions (eg, glycosaminoglycans) and thereby lose their osmotic activity. The consequent water loss from the vesicle produces local concentration of these materials. The proteolytic process that modifies some proteins within the cell is sometimes initiated in the cisternae and continues in these vesicles. The contents of the vesicles can then be distributed, according to cell type, to secretory granules, lysosomes, or the plasma membrane. The transformation of proinsulin to insulin is a good example of protein conversion occurring in the Golgi complex. A type of human diabetes has been described in which this transformation does not occur and there is a high blood level of proinsulin.

between the endoplasmic reticulum and the rest of the cell, it is sometimes difficult to demarcate its boundaries exactly.

In most cells, there is also polarity in Golgi structure and function. Near the Golgi complex, the rough endoplasmic reticulum can sometimes be seen budding off small vesicles (transport vesicles) that shuttle newly synthesized proteins to the Golgi for further processing. The Golgi cisterna nearest this point is called the forming, convex, or *cis,* face. On the opposite side of the Golgi complex—the maturing, concave, or *trans,* face—large Golgi vacuoles accumulate (see Fig 3–18). These are sometimes called **condensing vacuoles.**

These structures bud from the Golgi cisternae, generating vesicles that will transport proteins to various

sites. Cytochemical methods and the electron microscope have shown that the Golgi cisternae present different enzymes at different *cis-trans* levels and that the Golgi complex is important in the glycosylation, sulfation, phosphorylation, and limited proteolysis of proteins. Furthermore, it initiates packing, concentration, and storage of secretory products. Fig 3–12 gives an overall view of the currently accepted concepts regarding transit of material through the Golgi complex.

Lysosomes

Lysosomes are sites of intracellular digestion and turnover of cellular components.

Lysosomes are membrane-limited vesicles that contain a large variety of hydrolytic enzymes (more than

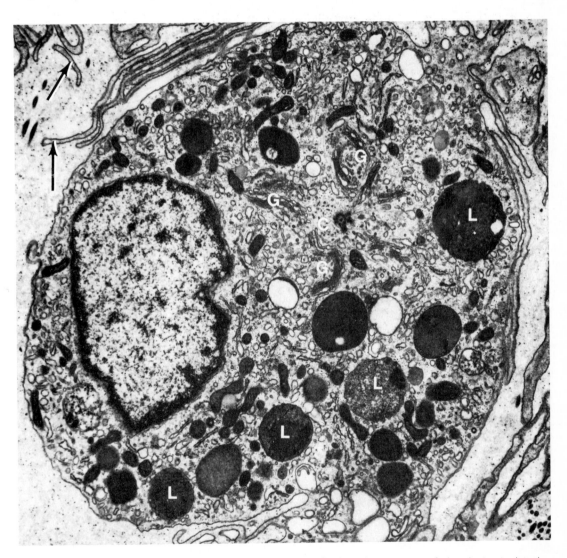

Figure 3–13. Electron micrograph of a mesenteric macrophage. Observe the presence of abundant cytoplasmic extensions (arrows). In the center is a centriole (C) surrounded by Golgi cisternae (G). Secondary lysosomes (L) are abundant. × 15,000.

40) whose main function is intracytoplasmic digestion (Figs 3–13, 3–14, 3–15, and 3–16). Lysosomes are present in almost all cells, but they are particularly abundant in cells exhibiting phagocytic activity (eg, macrophages, neutrophilic leukocytes). Although the nature and activity of lysosomal enzymes vary depending on the cell type being studied, the most common enzymes are acid phosphatase, ribonuclease, deoxyribonuclease, cathepsins (proteases), sulfatases, lipases, and β-glucuronidase. As can be seen from this list, lysosomal enzymes are capable of breaking down most biologic macromolecules. Generally, lysosomal enzymes are active at an acid pH.

Lysosomes are usually spherical, range in diameter from 0.05 to 0.5 μm, and present a uniformly granular electron-dense appearance in electron micrographs. The enveloping single unit membrane serves to separate the lytic enzymes from the cytoplasm, an important role in that it prevents the lysosomal enzymes from attacking and digesting cytoplasmic components (Fig 3–14).

Lysosomal enzymes are synthesized and segregated in the rough endoplasmic reticulum and subsequently transferred to the Golgi complex, where the enzymes are modified and packaged as lysosomes. These enzymes have oligosaccharides attached to them (as described earlier) but with an important modification. One or more of the mannose residues is phosphorylated at the 6' position. There are receptors for man-

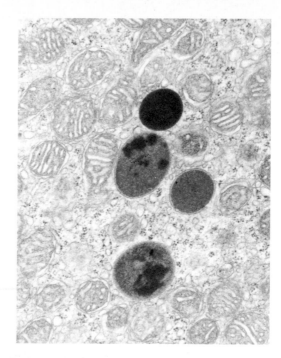

Figure 3–15. Electron micrograph showing 4 dark secondary lysosomes surrounded by numerous mitochondria.

nose 6-phosphate-containing proteins in the rough endoplasmic reticulum and Golgi complex that allow these proteins to be diverted from the main secretory pathway and segregated in lysosomes. This is the first indication of how the cell manages to sort out proteins going to different destinations (Fig 3–12).

Lysosomes that have not entered into a digestive event are identified as **primary lysosomes** (Fig 3–14). They can be very small (0.05 μm in diameter) membrane-limited vesicles, and they may be impossible to identify with certainty in the absence of a histochemical test of their content. This is the appearance of primary lysosomes in most cells. In a few cells, such as macrophages and neutrophilic leukocytes, primary lysosomes are larger, up to 0.5 μm in diameter, and thus just visible with the light microscope.

Lysosomes can digest materials taken into the cell from its environment, a process called **heterophagy.** The material is taken into a phagocytic vacuole (see p 30); primary lysosomes then fuse with the membrane of the phagosome and empty their hydrolytic enzymes into the vacuole. Digestion follows, and the composite structure is now termed a secondary lysosome.

Secondary lysosomes are those in which digestion occurs. They are generally 0.2–2 μm in diameter and present a heterogenous appearance in electron microscopes owing to the wide variety of materials they may be digesting (Fig 3–15). Again, the only sure

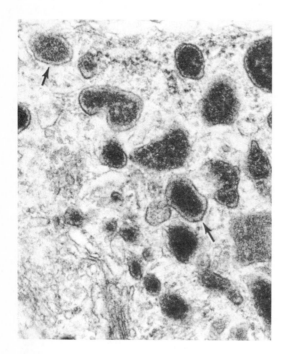

Figure 3–14. Electron micrograph of the cytoplasm of a macrophage showing primary lysosomes (arrows) characterized by uniform granular content and a limiting membrane. × 45,000.

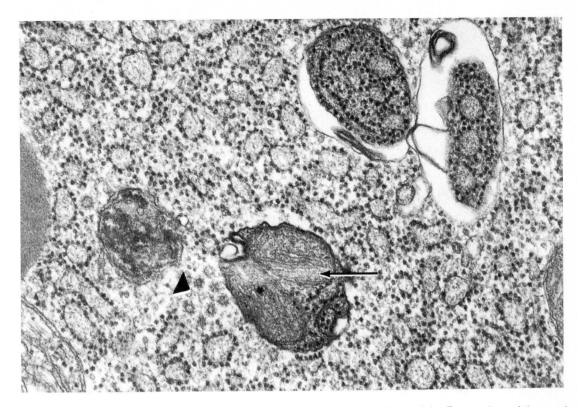

Figure 3–16. Section of a pancreatic acinar cell showing autophagosomes. **Upper right:** Two portions of the rough endoplasmic reticulum segregated by a membrane. **Below:** An autophagosome containing mitochondria (arrow) plus rough endoplasmic reticulum. **Left:** A secondary lysosome, or residual body, with undigestible material. Arrowhead shows a cluster of coated vesicles.

guide to their identification is histochemical methods to detect the presence of hydrolytic enzymes (eg, acid phosphatase) within these structures (Fig 2–5). Secondary lysosomes result from the fusion of endocytosed materials (from either phagocytosis or pinocytosis) with primary lysosomes to form a **phagosome.** The secondary lysosome is also known as a **phagolysosome.**

Following digestion of the contents of the secondary lysosome, nutrients diffuse through the lysosomal limiting membrane and enter the cytoplasm. Undigestible compounds are retained within the vacuoles, which are now called **residual bodies** (Figs 3–16 and 3–17). In some long-lived cells (eg, neurons, heart muscle, hepatocytes), large quantities of residual bodies accumulate and are referred to as **lipofuscin,** or **age pigment.**

Another function of lysosomes concerns the turnover of cytoplasmic organelles. Under certain conditions, organelles or portions of cytoplasm may become enclosed by a membrane. Primary lysosomes fuse with this structure and initiate the lysis of the enclosed cytoplasm (Figs 13–16 and 13–17). The resulting secondary lysosomes are known as **auto-**phagosomes (from Greek, *autos*, self, + *phagein*, to eat, + *soma,* body), indicating that their contents are of intracellular origin. The digested products of this hydrolysis are recycled by the cell to permit renewal, rearrangement, and reconstruction of the cytoplasmic contents. Cytoplasmic digestion by autophagosomes is enhanced in cells undergoing atrophy (as in prostatic epithelial cells after castration) and in secretory cells that have accumulated excess secretory product.

In some cases, primary lysosomes release their contents extracellularly, in which case their enzymes act in the extracellular milieu. An example is the destruction of bone matrix by the collagenases synthesized and released by osteoclasts. This type of reaction plays a significant role in the response to inflammation or injury. Several possible pathways relating to lysosome activities are schematically illustrated in Fig 3–17.

Lysosomes play an important role in the metabolism of several substances in the human body, and consequently many diseases have been ascribed to deficiencies of lysosomal enzymes. In **metachromatic leukodystrophy,** there is an in-

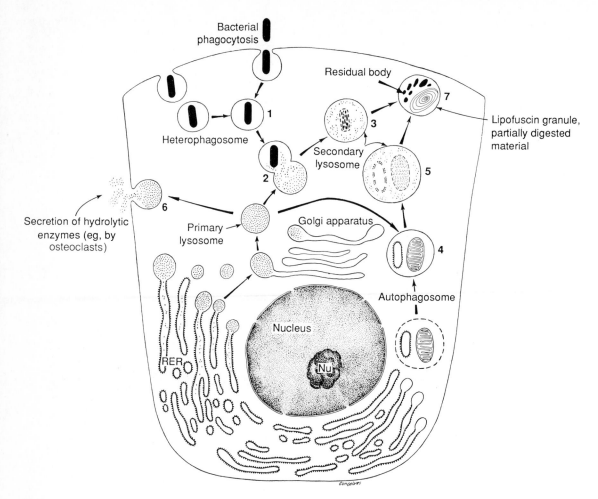

Figure 3–17. Present concepts of the functions of the lysosomes. Synthesis occurs in the rough endoplasmic reticulum (RER), and the enzymes are packaged in the Golgi complex. Numbers 1, 2, and 3 represent digestion of extracellular substance segregated into a heterophagosome; 4 and 5, digestion of segregated cytoplasmic material (autophagosome); 6, extrusion of lysosomal enzymes (eg, collagenase) that will act extracellularly; and 7, a residual body.

Table 3–2. Examples of diseases caused by lysosomal enzyme failure and accumulation of undigested material in different cell types.

Disease	Faulty Enzyme	Main Cell Type Affected	Main Organs Affected
Hurler	α L-iduronidase	Fibroblasts and osteoblasts accumulate dermatansulfate	Skeleton and nervous system
Sanfilippo Syndrome A	Heparan sulfate sulfamidase	Fibroblasts accumulate heparan sulfate	Skeleton and nervous system
Tay-Sachs	Hexosaminidase-A	Nerve cells accumulate glycolipids	Nervous system
Gaucher	β D-glycosidase	Macrophages accumulate glycolipids	Liver and spleen

tracellular accumulation of sulfated cerebrosides caused by lack of lysosomal sulfatase. In most of these diseases, a specific lysosomal enzyme is absent or inactive, and the digestion of certain substances (glycogen, cerebrosides, gangliosides, sphingomyelin, glycosaminoglycans, etc) does not occur. As a result, these substances accumulate in different cell types, interfering with their normal cell function. This diversity of affected cell types explains the variety of clinical symptoms observed in these diseases (Table 3–2).

Peroxisomes, or Microbodies

Peroxisomes (peroxide + *soma*) are spherical membrane-limited organelles whose diameter ranges from 0.5 to 1.2 μm (Fig 3–24). Their homogeneous matrix contains D- and L-amino oxidases and hy-

droxyacid oxidase. In some species, but not humans, a crystalline **nucleoid** is present that is composed of urate oxidase. All these enzymes oxidize their substrate and reduce O_2 and H_2O_2. Peroxisomes also contain catalase, an enzyme that decomposes hydrogen peroxide to water and oxygen ($2\ H_2O_2 \rightarrow 2\ H_2O + O_2$). Peroxisomes protect the cell from the effects of hydrogen peroxide, which could cause irreversible damage to many important cellular constituents.

There is evidence that peroxisomes contain enzymes involved in lipid metabolism. Thus the β-oxidation of long-chain fatty acids (18 carbons and longer) is preferentially accomplished by peroxisomal enzymes that differ from their mitochondrial counterparts. Certain hydroxylation reactions leading to the formation of the bile acids also have been localized in highly purified peroxisomal fractions.

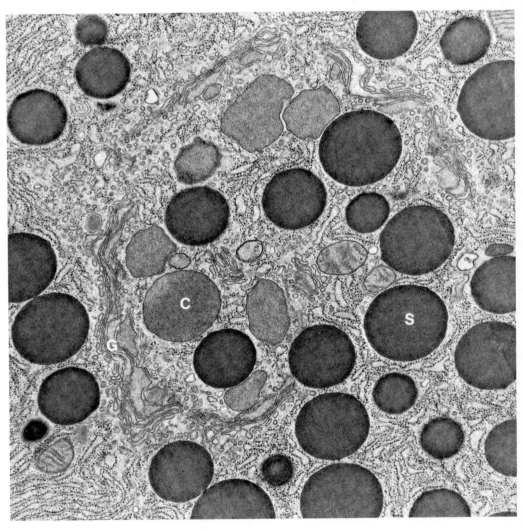

Figure 3–18. Electron micrograph of a pancreatic acinar cell from the rat. Numerous mature secretory granules (S) are seen in association with condensing vacuoles (C) and the Golgi complex (G). × 18,900.

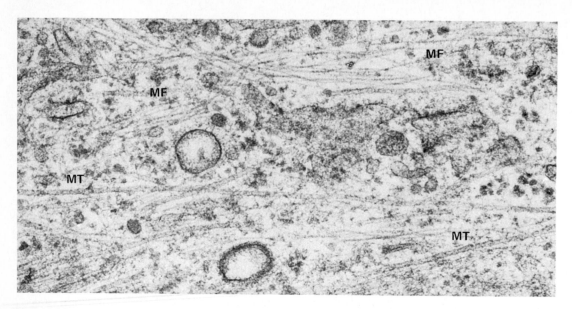

Figure 3–19. Electron micrograph of rat fibroblast cytoplasm. Observe the microfilaments (MF) and microtubules (MT). × 60,000. (Courtesy of E Katchburian.)

Regarding the biogenesis of peroxisomes, evidence has been presented that peroxisomal enzymes (catalase, enzymes of β-oxidation) are synthesized on free ribosomes and posttranslationally transferred to peroxisomes by an unknown mechanism. This is not consistent with the traditional view but is similar to the way in which certain proteins are incorporated into mitochondria.

Secretory Granules

Secretory granules are found in those cells that store a product until its release is signaled by a metabolic, hormonal, or neural message (regulated secretion). Secretory granules range in size from 0.2 to 2 μm in diameter. These granules are surrounded by a typical unit membrane and contain a concentrated form of the secretory product (Fig 3–18). The contents of some secretory granules may be up to 200 times more concentrated than in the rough endoplasmic reticulum. Binding proteins, nucleotides, or glycosaminoglycans may also be present. These constituents are thought to form complexes with the principal secretory product, thus rendering it less osmotically active. Secretory granules permit the storage of substances that could destroy the cell, such as digestive enzymes; in this case, the granules are usually referred to as **zymogen granules.**

THE CYTOSKELETON

In addition to the membrane-bound organelles, the cytoplasmic matrix contains a complex network of microtubules, microfilaments, and intermediate filaments (Fig 3–19). These structural proteins not only provide for the form and shaping of cells but also play an important role in cytoplasmic and cellular movement. Together, they are often called the **cytoskeleton** (*kytos* + Greek, *skeleton*, dried body), which is responsible for promoting movement and maintaining the shape and organization of the cell. The specific relationships of the cytoskeletal components to cellular functions are under active investigation.

Microtubules

Within the cytoplasmic matrix of eukaryotic cells are tubular structures known as microtubules. They have an outer diameter of 24 nm consisting of a dense wall 5 nm thick and a hollow core 14 nm wide. Microtubule lengths are variable, and individual tubules have often been observed to attain lengths of several micrometers (Fig 3–19). Occasionally, arms or bridges are found linking 2 or more tubules together (Figs 3–20 and 3–21).

The subunit of a microtubule is a heterodimer composed of α and β **tubulin** molecules of closely related amino acid composition, each with a molecular weight of about 50,000.

Under appropriate conditions (either in vivo or in vitro), tubulin subunits polymerize to form microtubules. Using special staining procedures, tubulin can be seen as heterodimers organized into a spiral. A total of 13 units are present in one complete turn of the spiral (Fig 3–21).

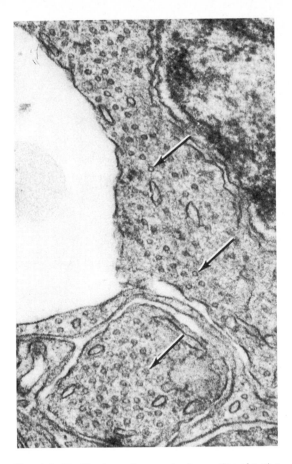

Figure 3–20. Electron micrograph of a section of a photosensitive retinal cell of a monkey. Observe the accumulation of transversely sectioned microtubules (arrows). Reduced slightly from × 80,000.

Polymerization of tubulins to form microtubules is believed to be directed by a variety of structures collectively known as microtubule organizing centers (MTOCs). These structures include basal bodies, centrioles, and the centromeres of chromosomes. Microtubule growth, via subunit polymerization, generally occurs more rapidly at the free end of existing tubules. This end is referred to as the fast-growing (+) end. If either colchicine or podophyllotoxin (antimitotic alkaloids that bind to tubulin heterodimers) is administered, the unavailability of heterodimers will block microtubule growth. Microtubules will eventually be broken down because the constant exchange of polymerized heterodimers with soluble heterodimers will proceed, but heterodimers with bound colchicine cannot polymerize. Another alkaloid, vinblastine, acts by depolymerizing the form of microtubules and, in a second step, aggregating to form paracrystalline arrays of tubulin heterodimers.

The antimitotic alkaloids are useful not only in cell biology (eg, colchicine is used to arrest chromosomes in prophase and to prepare karyotypes) but also in cancer chemotherapy (eg, vinblastine is used to arrest proliferation in tumors).

Within the cytoplasm, microtubules may exist in states ranging from an apparently random distribution to highly complex organized subcellular structures. Functions attributed to microtubules are usually based on 2 criteria: (1) the process must be sensitive to the pharmacologic agents, such as colchicine and vinblastine, known to interact with tubulin, and (2) morphologic data (numbers and orientation of tubules) must be sufficient to implicate tubules with a given cellular process.

Microtubules have been considered to play a significant role in the development and maintenance of cell forms based on the observation that tubules in intact cells or from cell-free preparations are normally quite straight and never exhibit oblique bends. These observations suggest that microtubules are rigid and lend support to the implication that they serve as a cytoskeletal element. Morphologic studies indicate a structural role, since microtubules are usually present in a proper orientation either to effect development of or to maintain a given cellular asymmetry. Procedures known to disrupt microtubules generally result in the loss of this cellular asymmetry.

Microtubules have also been implicated in the intracellular transport of other organelles. Timelapse cinematography of living cells reveals a significant movement and redistribution of cytoplasmic components (eg, mitochondria, vesicles). Examples include axoplasmic transport in neurons, melanin transport in pigment cells, chromosome movements along the mitotic spindle, and vesicle movements between the endoplasmic reticulum and Golgi complex and between the Golgi complex and the cell membrane. In each of these examples, movement is related to the presence of complex microtubule networks, and such activities are suspended if microtubules are disrupted.

Microtubules also provide the basis for several complex cytoplasmic components, including centrioles, basal bodies, cilia, and flagella. **Centrioles** are cylindric structures (0.15 μm in diameter and 0.3–0.5 μm in length) primarily composed of highly organized microtubules (Fig 3–22). Each centriole is composed of 9 sets of microtubule triplets arranged in the fashion of a pinwheel. The tubules are so close together that adjacent tubules of a triplet share a common wall. A single pair of centrioles is normally found in nondividing cells. In each pair, the long axes of the centrioles are at right angles to each other. Prior to cell division, more specifically during the S period of the interphase, each centriole duplicates itself. During mitosis, the resulting 2 pairs move to opposite poles of the cell and

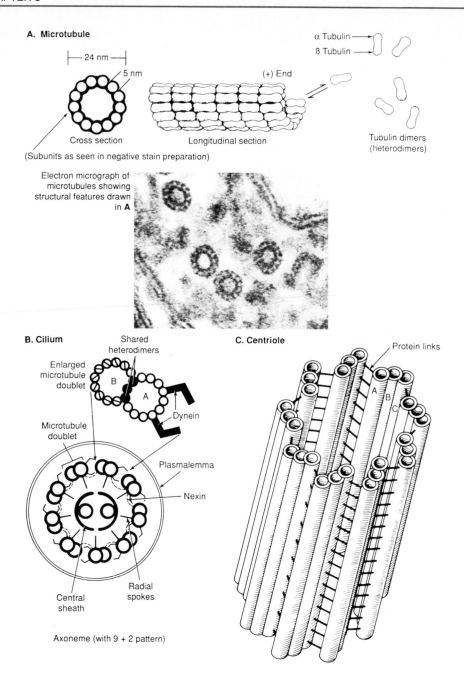

A. Microtubule

24 nm

5 nm

α Tubulin

ß Tubulin

(+) End

Cross section

Longitudinal section

Tubulin dimers
(heterodimers)

(Subunits as seen in negative stain preparation)

Electron micrograph of
microtubules showing
structural features drawn
in **A**

B. Cilium

Shared
heterodimers

Enlarged
microtubule
doublet

B

A

Dynein

Microtubule
doublet

Plasmalemma

Nexin

Central
sheath

Radial
spokes

Axoneme (with 9 + 2 pattern)

C. Centriole

Protein links

A

B

C

Figure 3–21. Schematic representation of microtubules, cilia, and centrioles. **A:** Drawing of microtubules as seen in the electron microscope following fixation with tannic acid in glutaraldehyde. The unstained tubulin subunits are delineated by the dense tannic acid. Cross sections of tubules reveal a ring of 13 subunits of dimers arranged in a spiral. Changes in microtubule length are due to the addition or loss of individual tubulin subunits. **B:** A cross section through a cilium reveals a core of microtubules called an axoneme. The axoneme consists of 2 central microtubules surrounded by 9 microtubule doublets. In the doublets, microtubule A is complete and consists of 13 subunits, while microtubule B shares 2–3 heterodimers with A. When activated by ATP, the dynein arms link adjacent tubules and provide for the sliding of doublets against each other. **C:** Centrioles consist of 9 microtubule triplets linked together in a pinwheel-like arrangement. In the triplets, microtubule A is complete and consists of 13 subunits, whereas tubules B and C share tubulin subunits. Under normal circumstances, these organelles are found in pairs with the centrioles disposed at right angles to one another.

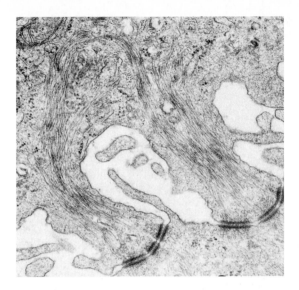

Figure 3–22. Electron micrograph of skin epithelial cell showing cytokeratin (intermediate) filaments associated with desmosomes.

become organizing centers for the developing mitotic spindles (Figs 3–36 and 3–38).

In nondividing cells, centriole pairs are usually found in a juxtanuclear position and in association with the Golgi complex. Associated with the centrioles are dense **pericentriolar bodies** from which microtubules seem to arise, suggesting that these bodies represent the organizing center for microtubule formation. This is confirmed by the observation that when isolated centrioles are added in vitro to depolymerized microtubular dimers, radial polymerization of microtubules occurs at these structures. The pair of centrioles, in conjunction with the Golgi complex, constitute the **cytocenter,** or cell center.

Cilia and **flagella** are motile processes with a highly organized microtubule core; they extend from the surface of many cell types. Ciliated cells usually possess a large number of cilia that range from 2 to 10 μm in length. Flagellated cells normally have only one flagellum, which ranges in length from 100 to 200 μm. Both cilia and flagella have a diameter of 0.3–0.5 μm and possess the same complexly organized core of microtubules.

This core consists of 9 pairs of microtubules surrounding 2 central tubules. This sheaf of tubules, possessing the characteristic 9 + 2 pattern, is called an **axoneme** (from Greek, *axon,* axis, + *nema,* thread). Each of the 9 peripheral pairs **(doublets)** shares a common wall of 2–3 heterodimers (Fig 3–21). The central pair of tubules are separated from each other and are enclosed within a **central sheath.** Adjacent doublets are linked to each other via protein bridges called **nexins** and are also linked to the cen-

tral sheath by **radial spokes.** The tubule units of each doublet are identified as subfibers A and B. Subfiber A is a complete microtubule with 13 heterodimers while subfiber B has only 10 or 11 heterodimers. Extending from the surface of subfiber A are pairs of arms formed by the protein **dynein,** which has ATPase activity (Fig 3–21).

At the base of each cilium or flagellum is a **basal body.** This body is essentially identical to a centriole except at its basal end, which has a complex central organization resembling a cartwheel. At the apical end of the basal body, the C tubule ends, while the A and B tubules are continuous with the corresponding tubules of the ciliary or flagellar axoneme. In developing cilia or flagella, the basal bodies act as a template to control the assembly of the axoneme subunits.

While basal bodies and centrioles have the same structure, they differ in the way in which they control the polymerization of tubulin monomers. Ciliary and flagellar axonemes are doublets that arise directly from the distal end of the basal body. In contrast, centrioles control the polymerization of single microtubules that characteristically radiate from the centriole and are not in direct contact with this organelle.

Recent experimental investigations show that the undulating motion exhibited by cilia and flagella is propagated by sliding of adjacent doublets within the axoneme. This sliding mechanism is mediated by two protein extensions from the A microtubule, formed mainly by the protein dynein (dynein arms). These arms exhibit ATPase activity (Fig 3–21B). It is currently thought that the dynein arms on microtubule A of one doublet binds to and "walks" along the surface of microtubule B of the adjacent doublet.

The sliding process occurring between adjacent pairs of microtubules does not occur freely and is constrained by the presence of nexin and the radial spokes. Thus, forces developed during the sliding process bend the cilia or flagella and account for their movements.

> Several mutations have been described in the proteins of the cilia and flagella. One of these is termed the **immotile cilia syndrome of Kartagener** and is characterized by the absence of dynein arms in these structures, leading to immotile sperm and male infertility and chronic respiratory infections caused by the lack of the cleansing action of cilia in the respiratory tract.

Microfilaments

Contractile activity in muscle cells results primarily from an interation between 2 proteins: **actin** and **myosin.** Actin is present in muscle as a thin (5–7 nm

Table 3–3. Examples of intermediate filaments found in eukaryotic cells

Filament Type	Cell Type	Examples
Cytokeratins	Epithelium	Both keratinizing and nonkeratinizing epithelia
Vimentin	Mesenchymal cells	Fibroblasts, chondroblasts, macrophages, endothelial cells, vascular smooth muscle
Desmin	Muscle	Striated and smooth muscle (except vascular smooth muscle)
Glial fibrillary acidic proteins	Glial cells	Astrocytes and Bergmann's glia
Neurofilaments	Neurons	Most, but probably not all, neurons

in diameter) filament composed of globular subunits organized into a double-stranded helix (Figs 10–6 and 10–8). Structural and biochemical studies reveal that actin may be an important component of the total protein of *all* cells. In non-muscle cells, actin is usually present as microfilaments.

Biochemical analyses reveal that non-muscle cells normally contain several species of actin, with some actins differing only by a single amino acid. The close similarities of actin within a given cell, as well as between cells of far-ranging species of the evolutionary scale, attest to the highly conserved nature of this protein. The differences in amino acid composition appear to be related to specific functional and stability characteristics of the various actins found within a cell. Within cells, microfilaments can be organized in many different forms: (1) In skeletal muscle, they assume a paracrystalline array integrated with thick (16-nm) myosin filaments. (2) In most cells, microfilaments are present as a thin sheath just beneath the plasmalemma. These filaments appear to be associated with membrane activities such as endocytosis, exocytosis, and cell migratory activity. Microfilaments are often found as an irregular lattice at the leading end of the cell in addition to constituting the primary structural component of migratory (pseudopodial and filopodial) processes. (3) Microfilaments are intimately associated with a number of cytoplasmic organelles, vesicles, and granules. The filaments are believed to play a role in moving and shifting cytoplasmic components (cytoplasmic streaming). (4) Microfilaments form a "purse-string" ring of filaments whose constriction results in the cleavage of mitotic cells. (5) In most cells, microfilaments are found

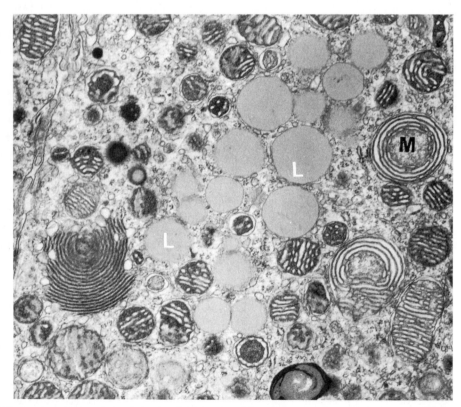

Figure 3–23. Section of adrenal gland showing lipid droplets (L) and abundant anomalous mitochondria (M). × 19,000.

scattered in what appears to be an unorganized fashion within the cytoplasm. It is currently thought that such actin networks provide part of the cytoskeleton or structural framework within the cell (Fig 3–19).

While actin filaments in muscle cells are structurally stable, microfilaments in non-muscle cells readily dissociate and reassemble. Microfilament polymerization appears to be under the direct control of minute changes in Ca^{2+} and cAMP levels. A large number of actin-binding proteins have been demonstrated in a wide variety of cells. Much current research is focused on how these proteins regulate the state of polymerization and lateral aggregation of microfilaments. Their importance can be deduced from the fact that only about half the cell's actin is in the form of microfilaments. In vitro, all cellular actin can be polymerized, demonstrating that other proteins (the actin-binding proteins) regulate the degree to which actin is polymerized to form microfilaments within the cell.

Presumably, most microfilament-related activities depend upon the interaction of **myosin** with actin. The structure and activity of the "thick" myosin filaments are described in the section on muscle tissues. Myosin is present in unpolymerized form in most motile non-muscle cells, polymerizing to form filaments only when participating in cell movement. Myosin-actin interactions are described in detail in the discussion of muscle tissue (see Chapter 10).

Intermediate Filaments

Ultrastructural and immunocytochemical investigations reveal that a third major filamentous structure is present in almost all eukaryotic cells. In addition to the thin (actin) and thick (myosin) filaments, cells contain a class of intermediate-sized filaments with an average diameter of 10–12 nm (Fig 3–22). The study of these **intermediate filaments** is a rapidly developing field (Table 3–3). Different proteins that form intermediate filaments

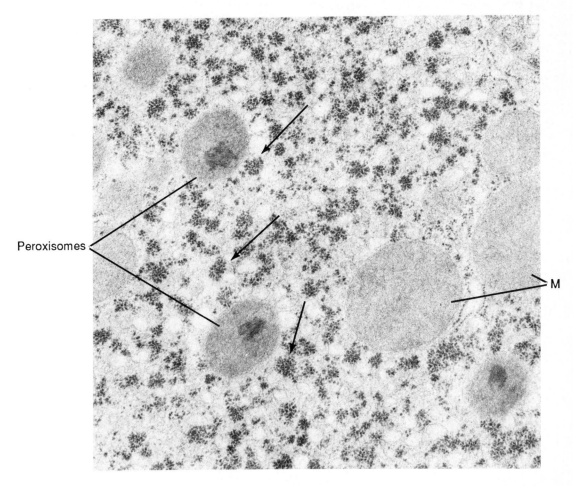

Peroxisomes

M

Figure 3–24. Electron micrograph of a section of a liver cell showing glycogen inclusions as accumulations of electron-dense particles (arrows). The dark structures with a dense core are peroxisomes. Mitochondria (M) are also shown. × 30,000.

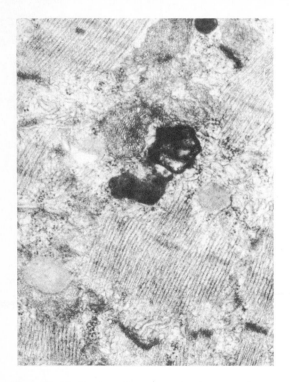

Figure 3–25. Section of heart muscle with a granule containing lipofuscin.

have been isolated and localized by immunocytochemical means.

Cytokeratins (*kytos* + Greek, *keras,* horn) are found in most epithelia and comprise a family of approximately 20 polypeptides (MW 40,000–68,000). They are coded by a family of genes and present different chemical and immunological properties. This diversity of keratin is not surprising and is probably related to the various roles these proteins play in the epidermis, nails, hooves, horns, feathers, scales, and the like in providing animals with defense against abrasion and loss of water and heat. They also supply them with camouflage, decoration, and physical protection.

Vimentin filaments are characteristic of cells of mesenchymal origin and of embryonic or undifferentiated cells. Vimentin is a single protein (MW 56,000–58,000) and may copolymerize with desmin or glial fibrillary acidic protein.

Desmin (skeletin) is found in smooth muscle and in the Z disks of skeletal and cardiac muscle (MW 53,000–55,000).

Glial filaments (glial fibrillary acidic protein [GFA]) are characteristic of astrocytes but are not found in neurons, muscle, mesenchymal cells, or epithelia (MW 51,000).

Neurofilaments consist of at least 3 high-molecular-weight polypeptides (MW 68,000, 140,000, and

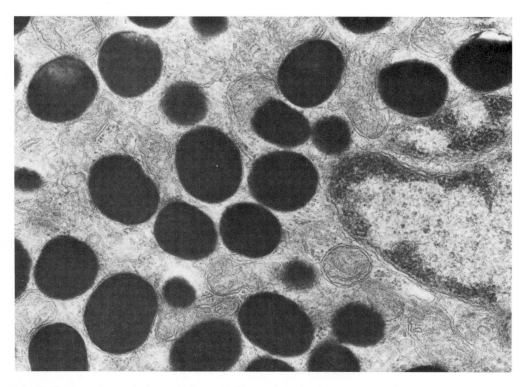

Figure 3–26. Section of a melanin-producing cell. The nucleus is shown at right. The cytoplasm is full of dense membrane-bound melanin granules. Mitochondria are also numerous. × 20,000.

210,000). These intermediate filament proteins have different chemical structures and different roles in cellular function.

> The presence of a specific type of intermediate filament in tumors is an important characteristic that can affect not only the diagnosis but also the treatment of tumors (see Table 2–1). Identification of intermediate filament protein is a routine procedure using immunocytochemical methods.

Cytoplasmic Deposits

These are usually transitory components of the cytoplasm, composed mainly of accumulated metabolites or deposits of varied nature. The accumulated metabolites occur in several forms, one of them being lipid droplets in adipose tissue, adrenal cortex cells, and liver cells (Fig 3–23). Carbohydrate accumulations are also visible in several cells in the form of glycogen. After impregnation with lead salts, this substance appears as collections of coarse, irregular electron-dense particles (Fig 3–24). Proteins are stored in glandular cells as **secretory granules** (Fig 3–18); these are periodically released into the extracellular medium.

Deposits of colored substances—**pigments**—are often found in cells. They may be synthesized by the cell (eg, in the skin melanocytes) or come from outside the body (eg, carotene). One of the most common pigments is **lipofuscin,** a yellowish-brown substance present mainly in permanent cells (eg, neurons, cardiac muscle) that increases in quantity with age. Its chemical constitution is complex. It is believed that granules of lipofuscin derive from secondary lysosomes and represent deposits of undigestible substances (Fig 3–25). Another widely distributed pigment, **melanin,** is abundant in the epidermis of the skin and in the pigment layer of the retina in the form of dense, intracellular, membrane-limited granules (Fig 3–26).

Cytomatrix

At one time, it was believed that the cytoplasm intervening between the discrete organelles and inclusions was unstructured and consisted of soluble enzymes, low-molecular-weight metabolites, ions, and water. This belief was reinforced by the widespread use of homogenization and centrifugation of the homogenates to yield fractions consisting of recognizable organelles. The final supernatant contains the soluble components of the cell and is called the **cytosol,** or soluble ground substance.

It now seems probable that homogenization of cells disrupts a delicate **microtrabecular lattice** that incorporates filaments, microtubules, and perhaps enzymes and other soluble constituents into a structured cytomatrix (*kytos* + Latin, *matrix,* mold).

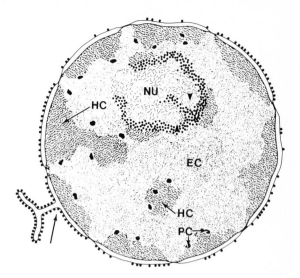

Figure 3–27. Structure of a nucleus. The nuclear envelope merges with the endoplasmic reticulum (arrow). Heterochromatin (HC) and euchromatin (EC) are shown. The large dark dots (PC) are perichromatin granules. Fibrillar and granular portions can be distinguished in the nucleolus (NU). The heterochromatin surrounding the nucleolus forms the **nucleolus-associated chromatin.** Portions of euchromatin appear interspersed with nucleolar material (arrowhead). This latter chromatin contains the genes that specify rRNAs.

This matrix may coordinate intracellular movements of organelles as well as provide an explanation for the viscosity of the cytoplasm. It has been suggested that soluble enzymes, such as those of the glycolytic pathway, might function more efficiently if they were organized in a sequence rather than relying on random collisions with their substrates. The cytomatrix may provide a framework for this organization.

THE NUCLEUS

In the nucleus, the DNA of the cell is so well organized that it can be partially or totally duplicated with few, if any, mistakes.

The nucleus of the cell appears as a rounded or elongated structure, usually in the center of the cell. In mammalian tissues, its diameter usually varies between 5 and 10 μm. The nucleus is composed of the **nuclear envelope, chromatin,** the **nucleolus,** and **nuclear matrix** (Fig 3–27). The size and morphologic features of nuclei in a specific tissue tend to be uniform, with rare exceptions.

> The presence of nuclei with irregular features (eg, variable size, atypical chromatin patterns),

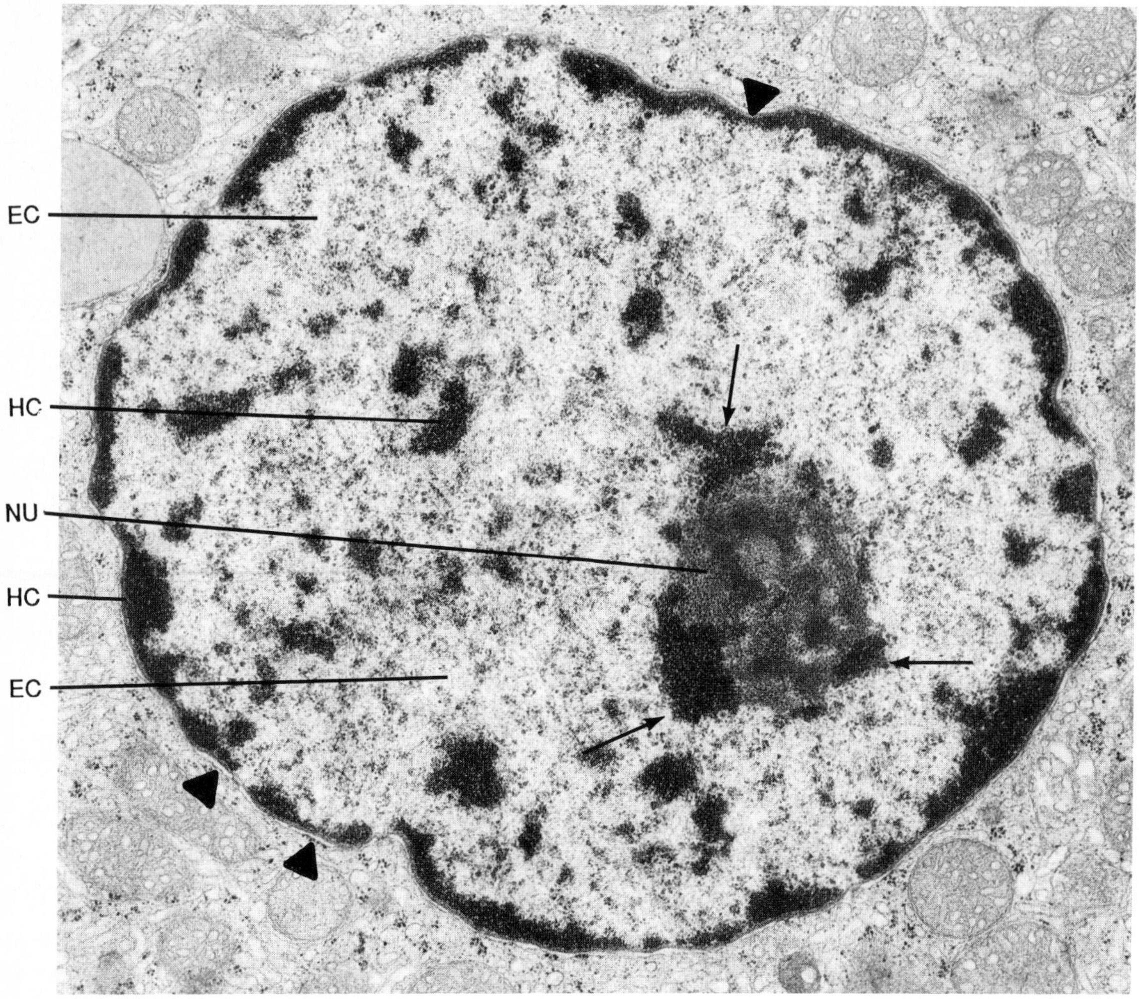

Figure 3–28. Electron micrograph of a nucleus, showing the heterochromatin (HC) and euchromatin (EC). Unlabeled arrows point to the nucleolus-associated chromatin around the nucleolus (NU). Arrowheads indicate the perinuclear cisterna. Underneath the cisterna is a layer of heterochromatin designated a **nuclear membrane** by optical microscopists. × 26,000.

plus the capacity to invade neighboring tissues, is the main morphologic characteristic used by pathologists to estimate the degree of malignancy of a tumor.

Nuclear Envelope

A "nuclear membrane" can be observed under the light microscope as a thin line surrounding the nucleus. Electron microscopy has revealed that the nucleus is actually surrounded by 2 parallel unit membranes separated by a narrow (40–70-nm) space called the **perinuclear cisterna.** Together, the paired membranes and the intervening space make up the nuclear envelope. What is seen in

the light microscope as the nuclear membrane is mainly a thin layer of heterochromatin that lines and binds to the internal surface of the nuclear envelope (Figs 3–28 and 3–29). Closely associated with the internal membrane of the nuclear envelope is a protein structure called the **fibrous lamina,** which varies in thickness from 80 to 300 nm depending on the cell examined. Nuclear pores are not blocked by this structure. The fibrous lamina is composed of 3 main polypeptides, called **lamins,** which form part of the nuclear matrix. During interphase, the chromatin adjacent to the centromeres of chromosomes is associated with the fibrous lamina. The pattern of association is very regular from cell to cell within a tissue. This finding has given rise to

Nucleus

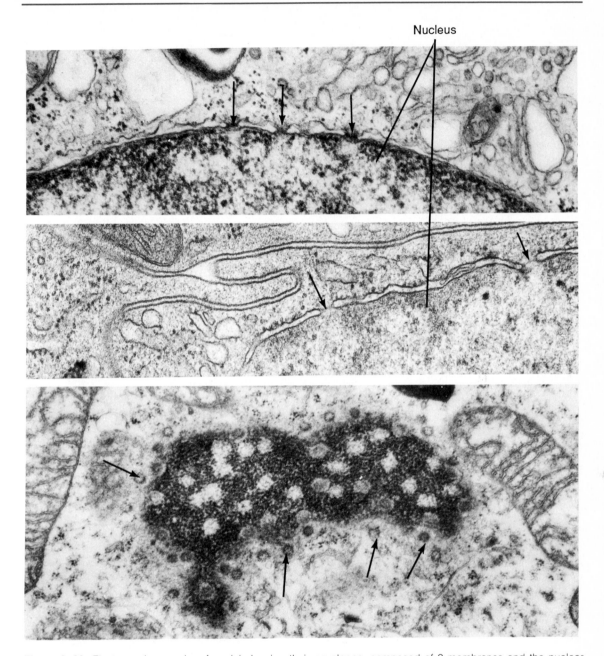

Figure 3–29. Electron micrographs of nuclei showing their envelopes, composed of 2 membranes and the nuclear pores (arrows). The 2 upper pictures are of transverse sections; the bottom is of a tangential section. Chromatin, frequently condensed below the nuclear envelope, is not usually seen in the pore regions. × 80,000.

the idea that chromatin has a definite organization within the nucleus. This organization could have an effect on the way in which genes are expressed. Polyribosomes are frequently attached to the outer membrane, and this portion of the nuclear envelope is sometimes continuous with the rough endoplasmic reticulum (Fig 3–27). When covered with polyribosomes, the nuclear envelope functions as

rough endoplasmic reticulum, synthesizing polypeptide chains and segregating them in the perinuclear cistern between its 2 membranes. Around the nuclear envelope, at sites where the inner and outer membranes fuse, there are circular gaps, the **nuclear pores** (Figs 3–29 and 3–30), that provide pathways between the nucleus and the cytoplasm. Nuclear pores have an average diameter of 70 nm

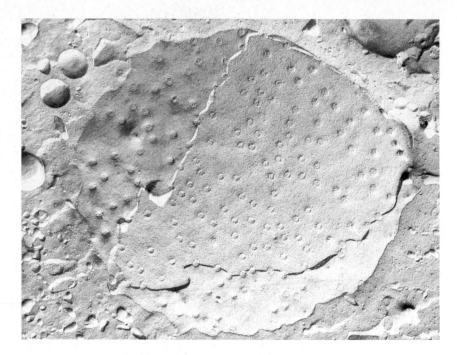

Figure 3–30. Electron micrograph of rat intestine preparation obtained by cryofracture, showing the 2 membranous components of the nuclear envelope and the nuclear pores. (Courtesy of P Pinto da Silva.)

and are composed of 8 subunits. The pores are not open but are bridged by an electron-dense membrane forming a single-layered diaphragm of protein. This structure is thinner than the membranes that constitute the nuclear envelope. The permeability of the nucleus to molecules is variable, but all pores are permeable to some macromolecules (eg, mRNA, cytoplasmic proteins).

Chromatin

Two types of chromatin can be distinguished with both the light and the electron microscopes (Figs 3–27 and 3–28). **Heterochromatin** (from Greek, *heteros*, other + *chroma*, color) which is electron-dense and appears as coarse granules in the electron microscope, is visible in the light microscope (after appropriate staining) as basophilic clumps of nucleoprotein. **Euchromatin** is visible as an organized structure only in the electron microscope. When viewed with the light microscope, however, lightly stained areas in the nucleus correspond to euchromatin recognized by electron microscopy. The proportion of heterochromatin to euchromatin accounts for the light-to-dark appearance of nuclei in tissue sections as seen in light and electron microscopes. The intensity of nuclear staining resulting from the chromatin is frequently used to distinguish and identify different tissues and cell types in the light

microscope. The morphologic characteristics of chromatin are therefore used throughout this book to aid in the study and identification of cells and tissues. It should be noted that these characteristics are important in the differential diagnosis between benign and malignant tumor cells.

Chromatin is composed mainly of coiled strands of DNA bound to basic proteins (histones); its structure is schematically presented in Fig 3–31. The basic structural unit of chromatin is the nucleosome. This consists of a core of 4 types of histones: 2 copies each of histones H2A, H2B, H3, and H4, around which are wrapped 166 DNA base pairs (Fig 3–31B). A further 48-base-pair segment forms a link between adjacent nucleosomes, and another type of histone (H1 or H5) is bound to this DNA. This organization of chromatin has been referred to as *beads-on-a-string* (Fig 3–31C). Non-histone proteins are also associated with chromatin, but their arrangement is less well understood.

The next higher order of organization of chromatin is the 30-nm fiber commonly referred to as a *solenoid*. In this structure, nucleosomes become coiled around an axis, with 6 nucleosomes per turn, to form the 30-nm chromatin fiber (Fig 3–31B). Higher orders of coiling must be necessary, especially in the condensation of chromatin into chromosomes during mitosis and meiosis.

Chromatin DNA represents the major form of DNA in the cell and consequently carries most of the genetic information. Within the chromatin, the precursors of the messenger, ribosomal, and transfer ribonucleic acids (mRNA, rRNA, and tRNA) are synthesized.

The nucleoprotein of chromatin is coiled, with the degree of coiling varying during cell activity. The chromatin pattern of a nucleus has been considered a guide to the cell's activity. In general, cells with light nuclei are more active than those with condensed, dark nuclei. In lightly staining nuclei (with few heterochromatin clumps), more DNA surface is available for the transcription of genetic information. In darkly staining nuclei, the coiling of DNA makes less surface available.

Careful study of the chromatin of mammalian cell nuclei has revealed the presence of a heterochromatin mass frequently observed in female cells but not in male cells. This chromatin clump is the **sex chromatin.** First observed in nerve cells obtained from female cats, it is present in cells of most mammals, including humans. This heterochromatin mass is one of the pair of X chromosomes that is visible in female cells during interphase. It remains tightly coiled and visible while the other X chromosome is uncoiled and not visible. Evidence suggests that the coiled X chromosome comprising the sex chromatin is genetically inactive. The male has one X chromosome and one Y chromosome as sex determinants; the X chromosome is uncoiled, and therefore no sex chromatin is visible. In human epithelial cells, sex chromatin appears as a small granule attached to the nuclear envelope. The cells lining the internal surface of the cheek are frequently used to study sex chromatin. Blood smears are also often used, in which case the sex chromatin appears as a drumsticklike appendage to the nuclei of the neutrophilic leukocytes (Fig 3–32).

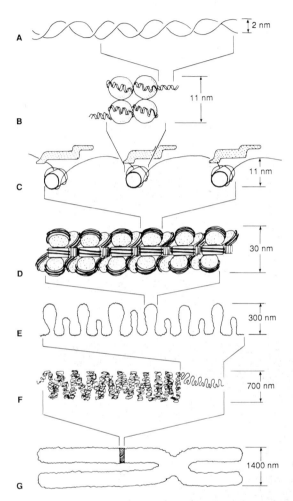

Figure 3–31. Drawing illustrating the orders of chromatin packing thought to exist in the metaphase chromosome. A short region of DNA double helix **(A)** coils twice around octamers of histones (4 dimers of H3, H4, H2A, and H2B) to form nucleosomes **(B).** Nucleosomes are linked by H1 histones **(C)** that aggregate further to form 30-nm fibers **(D).** These fibers form loops that spiral around a chromosomal protein core and form a section of the chromosome some 300 nm in diameter **(E).** Chromosomal loops may condense further to form a 700-nm coiled fiber **(F)** that can be seen as a visible band of the condensed metaphase chromosome **(G).** (Redrawn with permission, Alberts et al: *Molecular Biology of the Cell,* 2nd ed. Garland, 1989).

The study of sex chromatin has wide applicability to medicine, because it permits analysis of genetic sex in patients whose external sex organs do not permit diagnosis of gender, as in hermaphroditism and pseudohermaphroditism. It is essential for the study of other anomalies involving the sex chromosomes—eg, Klinefelter's syndrome, in which testicular abnormalities, azoospermia, and other symptoms are associated with the presence of XXY chromosomes in the cell.

The study of chromosomes of animals, and particularly of humans, made considerable progress after the development of methods of inducing cells to divide, arresting mitotic cells during metaphase, and subsequently causing cellular rupture. These techniques permit the separation, detailed observation, and analysis of chromosomes. Mitosis can be

Buccal epithelium

Polymorphonuclear
leukocyte

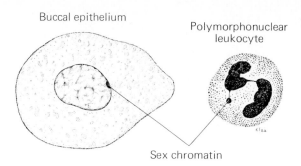

Sex chromatin

Figure 3–32. Morphologic features of sex chromatin in human female oral epithelium and in a polymorphonuclear leukocyte. In the epithelium, it appears as a small, dense granule adhering to the nuclear envelope. In the leukocyte, it has a drumstick shape.

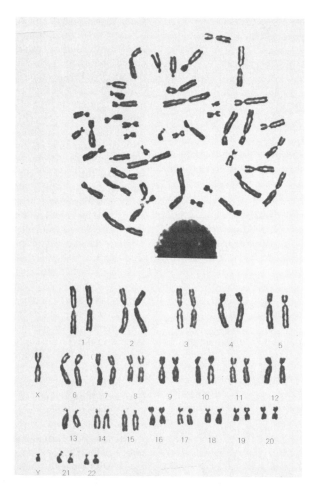

Figure 3–33. Top: Photomicrograph of chromosomes of a human cell obtained during metaphase. **Bottom:** Karyotype of a normal human male. The chromosomes are grouped according to their morphologic characteristics. (Courtesy of G Gimenez-Martin.)

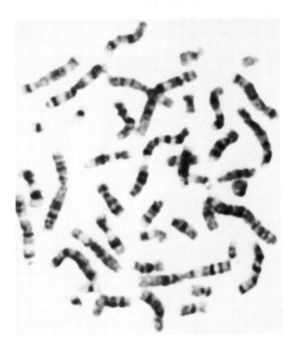

Figure 3–34. Human karyotype preparation using the GTG banding technique (G bands by Trypsin and Giemsa stain). Each chromosome has a particular pattern of banding, permitting identification of not only individual chromosomes but also the relationship of the banding pattern to genetic anomalies. × 2000. (Courtesy of A Wajntal.)

induced by phytohemagglutinin; it can be arrested in metaphase by colchicine. Rupture of cells is brought about by initial immersion in a hypotonic solution, causing swelling, after which cells are flattened and broken between a glass slide and a coverslip. The pattern of chromosomes obtained with a human cell after staining is illustrated in Fig 3–33. In addition to the 2 sex chromosomes X and Y, it is customary to group the remaining chromosomes, according to their morphologic characteristics, in 22 successively numbered pairs (Fig 3–33).

Until recently, recognition of individual chromosomes was not possible, because different chromosomes of the same karyotype often had the same general morphology. The development of techniques that reveal segmentation of chromosomes in transverse, differentially stained bands made possible not only the identification of individual chromosomes but also the detailed study of genetic deletion and translocation. These techniques are based mainly on the appearance of transverse bands in chromosomes previously treated with saline or enzyme solution and stained with fluorescent dies or Giemsa's blood staining technique (Fig 3–34; see also Chapter 12). In situ hybridization has also been used as a valuable proce-

dure to localize DNA sequences (genes) in chromosomes. These procedures have revolutionized the field of cytogenetics and made possible a series of important observations on human cytogenetics.

The number and characteristics of chromosomes encountered in an individual are known as the **karyotype** (Fig 3–34). Study of karyotypes has revealed chromosomal alterations associated with tumors, leukemias, and several types of genetic diseases.

Nucleolus

The nucleolus is a spherical structure, up to 1 μm in diameter, rich in rRNA and protein. It is usually basophilic when stained with hematoxylin and eosin. As seen with the electron microscope, the nucleolus consists of 3 distinct components. One to several pale-staining regions are composed of **nucleolar-organizer DNA**—sequences of bases that code for rRNAs (Fig 3–35). In the human genome, 5 pairs of chromosomes contain nucleolar organizers. Closely associated with the nucleolar organizers are densely packed 5–10-nm ribonucleoprotein fibers, the **pars fibrosa** (Fig 3–35), which is composed of primary transcripts of rRNA genes. The third component of the nucleolus is the **pars granulosa,** consisting of 15–20-nm granules (maturing ribosomes; see Fig 3–35). Proteins, synthesized in the cytoplasm, become associated with rRNAs in the nucleolus; ribosome subunits then migrate into the cytoplasm. Heterochromatin is often attached to the nucleolus **(nucleolus-associated chromatin),** but the functional significance of this association is not known (Figs 3–27 and 3–28).

Although each human cell has the potential of forming 10 separate nucleoli, only one or two are usually observed. This is because nucleoli tend to fuse during the interphase stage of the cell cycle. When nuclear chromatin becomes very condensed, as in lymphocytes, nucleoli become very difficult to visualize.

Large nucleoli are encountered in embryonic cells during their proliferation, in cells that are actively synthesizing proteins, and in rapidly growing malignant tumors. The nucleolus disperses during cell division but reappears in the telophase stage of mitosis.

Nuclear Matrix

The nuclear matrix is the component that fills the space between the chromatin and the nucleoli in the nucleus. It is composed mainly of proteins (some of which have enzymatic activity), metabolites, and ions. When its nucleic acids and other soluble components are removed, a continuous fibrillar structure remains, forming the **nucleoskeleton.** The fibrous lamina of the nuclear envelope is a part of the nuclear matrix. The functions of the nucleoskeleton are still

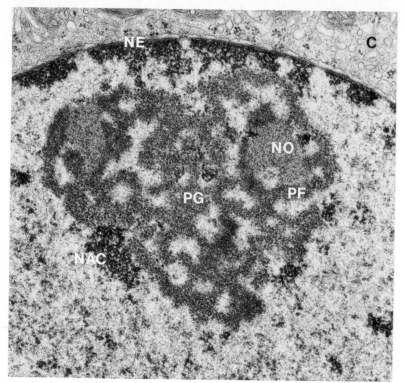

Figure 3–35. Nucleolus in a human adrenocortical cell showing the nucleolar-organizer DNA (NO), pars fibrosa (PF), pars granulosa (PG), nucleolus-associated chromatin (NAC), nuclear envelope (NE), and cytoplasm (C).

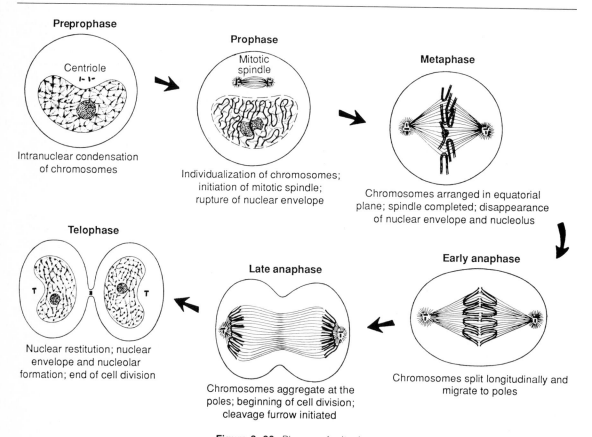

Preprophase

Centriole

Intranuclear condensation of chromosomes

Prophase

Mitotic spindle

Individualization of chromosomes; initiation of mitotic spindle; rupture of nuclear envelope

Metaphase

Chromosomes arranged in equatorial plane; spindle completed; disappearance of nuclear envelope and nucleolus

Early anaphase

Chromosomes split longitudinally and migrate to poles

Late anaphase

Chromosomes aggregate at the poles; beginning of cell division; cleavage furrow initiated

Telophase

Nuclear restitution; nuclear envelope and nucleolar formation; end of cell division

Figure 3–36. Phases of mitosis.

being studied, but the fact that it binds to hormone receptors and to recently synthesized DNA suggests an important role in nuclear functions.

CELL DIVISION

Cell division, or **mitosis,** can be observed with the light microscope. During this process, the parent cell divides, and each of the daughter cells receives a chromosomal karyotype identical to that of the parent cell. Essentially, a longitudinal duplication of the chromosomes takes place, and they are distributed to the daughter cells. The phase during which the cell does not undergo division is called **interphase,** and the nucleus appears as it is normally observed in microscope preparations. The process of mitosis is dynamic and continuous but is subdivided into phases to facilitate its study (Figs 3–36 and 3–37).

The **prophase** is characterized by the gradual coiling of nuclear chromatin, giving rise to several individualized rod- or hairpin-shaped bodies (**chromosomes**) that stain intensely. The nuclear envelope remains unaltered, and the chromosomes appear coiled in the nucleus. The centrioles separate, and a pair migrates to each pole of the cell. Simultaneously, the microtubules of the mitotic spindle appear between the 2 pairs of centrioles (Figs 3–36 and 3–37).

During **metaphase,** the nuclear envelope and the nucleolus disappear. The chromosomes migrate to the equatorial plane of the cell, where each divides longitudinally to form 2 chromatids. These attach to the microtubules of the mitotic spindle at a plaquelike, electron-dense region, the **centromere** (from Greek, *kentron,* center, + *meros,* part), or **kinetochore** (from Greek, *kinetos,* moving, + *chora,* central region); (see Figs 3–38 and 3–39.)

In **anaphase,** the sister chromatids separate from each other and migrate toward the opposite poles of the cell, following the direction of the spindle microtubules. Throughout this process, the centromeres move from the center, pulling along the remainder of the chromosome (Fig 3–36). It has been shown by immunofluorescence that microtubular protein (tubulin), actin, and myosin occur in the spindle region. It is possible that these proteins participate with microtubules in the process of chromosome migration to the cell poles, although the mechanism of this process is still a subject for discussion.

Telophase is characterized by the reappearance of nuclei in the daughter cells. The chromosomes revert to their semidispersed state, and the nucleoli, chromatin, and nuclear envelope reappear. While these nuclear alterations are taking place, a constriction develops at the equatorial plane of the parent cell and progresses until it divides the cytoplasm and its organelles in half (Figs 3–36 and 3–40). A beltlike accumulation of microfilaments containing both actin and myosin occurs beneath the cell membrane in the region of mitotic constriction.

Most tissues undergo a constant turnover because of continuous cell division and the ongoing death of cells. Nerve tissue and cardiac muscle cells are an exception, since they do not multiply postnatally and consequently cannot regenerate. The turnover rate of the cells varies greatly from one tissue to another—rapid in the epithelium of the alimentary canal and the epidermis, slow in the pancreas and thyroid.

THE CELL CYCLE

Mitosis is the visible manifestation of cell division, but there are other processes, not so easily observed with the light microscope, that play a fundamental role in cell multiplication. Principal among these is the phase in which DNA, the main chromosomal component, replicates. This process can be analyzed by the introduction of labeled, radioactive DNA precursors (eg, ^{3}H-thymidine), which are then traced by biochemical and radioautographic methods. DNA replication has been shown to occur during **interphase,** when no visible phenomena of cell division are observable with the microscope. This alternation between mitosis and interphase in all tissues with cellular turnover is known as the cell cycle. A careful study of the cell cycle reveals that it can be divided into 2 stages: mitosis, consisting of the 4 phases already described (prophase, metaphase, anaphase, and telophase), and interphase.

Interphase is itself divided into 3 phases: G_1 (presynthesis), S (DNA synthesis), and G_2 (post-DNA duplication) (Fig 3–41). Synthesis and replication of DNA and centrioles take place in the S phase. The sequence of these phases and the time involved are illustrated in Figure 3–41. It is during the G_1 (for gap) phase that RNA and protein synthesis occur and the cell volume, previously reduced to one-half by mitosis, is restored to its normal size. In cells that are not continuously dividing, the cell cycle activities may be temporarily or permanently suspended. Cells in such a stage of development are referred to as being in G_0 (eg, muscle, nerve).

Processes that occur during the G_2 phase are the production and accumulation of energy to be utilized during mitosis and the synthesis of tubulin to be assembled in microtubules during mitosis.

Rapidly growing tissues (eg, intestinal epithelium) frequently demonstrate cells in mitosis; the opposite is seen in slowly growing tissues. The increased number of mitotic figures and abnormal mitoses in tumors is an important characteristic distinguishing malignant from benign tumors. It is known that the organism has elaborate regulatory systems that control cell repro-

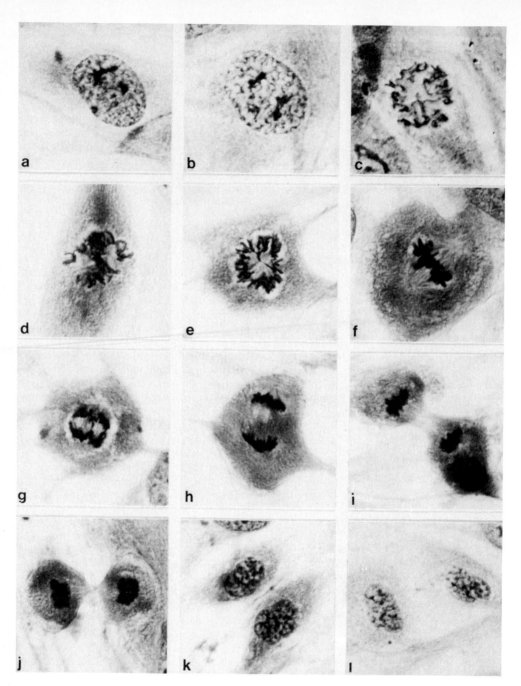

Figure 3–37. Stages of mitosis in cultured human fibroblasts. Feulgen stain with acrolein-thionine counterstain. × 1400.
A: Interphase. Note the structure of the chromatin and the large, somewhat branched nucleoli; at the lower left is a mass of heterochromatin representing the sex chromatin (arrow). **B:** Early prophase with the first manifestation of chromosomes as tortuous threads. Nucleoli are still present. **C:** Late prophase/early prometaphase. Nucleoli have disappeared; note the progressive condensation of chromosomes and the disappearance of the nuclear envelope. **D:** Late prometaphase. **E:** Metaphase in bottom view. Typical arrangement of chromosomes that have now reached their maximal degree of contraction. **F:** Metaphase seen in lateral view. The entire spindle figure is shown. **G:** Early anaphase. The sister chromosomes have just moved apart, following their centromeres. **H:** Late anaphase. Maximal diversion of the chromosome packages; note the interzonal connections. Constriction in the midzonal region of cytokinesis is about to start. **I:** Late anaphase with advanced cytokinesis. The chromosome packages do not seem to round up yet. **J:** Early telophase with completed cytokinesis. Remnants of interzonal connections unite both cells, with a thickening in the middle. **K:** Telophase. Rearrangement of nuclear material shown in both daughter cells. **L:** Late telophase with interphase arrangement of chromatin. Cells are moving apart. (Courtesy of J James.)

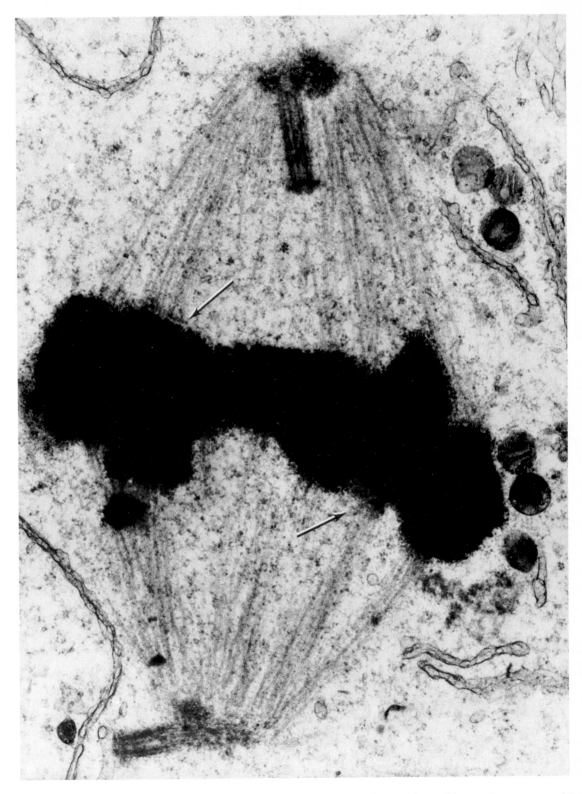

Figure 3–38. Electron micrograph of a section of a rooster spermatocyte in metaphase. Observe the presence of 2 centrioles in each pole, the mitotic spindle formed by microtubules, and the chromosomes in the equatorial plate. The arrows show the insertion of microtubules in the centromeres. Reduced from × 19,000. (Courtesy of R McIntosh.)

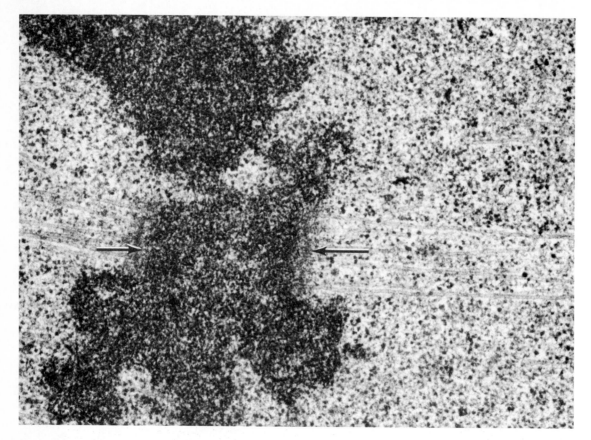

Figure 3–39. Electron micrograph of the metaphase of a human lung cell in tissue culture. Note the insertion of microtubules in the centromeres (arrows) of the densely stained chromosomes. Reduced from × 50,000. (Courtesy of R McIntosh.)

duction, either stimulating or inhibiting mitosis. It has been shown that normal cell proliferation and differentiation are controlled by a group of genes called **proto-oncogenes.** It has been further shown that altering the structure or expression of these genes promotes the production of tumors. Altered proto-oncogenes are present in tumor-producing viruses and are probably derived from cells. Altered oncogene activity can be induced by a change in the DNA sequence **(mutation),** an increase in the number of genes **(gene amplification),** or by gene rearrangement, in which genes are located close to an active promoter site. Altered oncogenes have been related to several tumors and hematologic neoplasia. Several proteins have been isolated that stimulate mitotic activity in different cell types, such as nerve growth factor, epithelial growth factor, fibroblast growth factor, and precursors of red blood cell growth factor (erythropoietin). The list of **growth factors** is extensive and is growing rapidly (see Chapter 13). Several

factors that inhibit cell reproduction have also been described and are collectively called **chalones** (see Chapter 4). Cell proliferation is usually regulated by precise mechanisms that can, when necessary, stimulate or retard mitosis according to the needs of the organism. Several factors (eg, chemical substances, certain types of radiation, viral infections) can induce abnormal cell proliferation that bypasses normal regulation mechanisms for controlled growth and forms tumors.

The term **tumor,** used initially to denote any localized swelling in the body caused by inflammation or abnormal cell proliferation, is now usually employed as a synonym for **neoplasm** (from Greek, *neos,* new, + *plasma*), which can be defined as an abnormal mass of tissue formed by uncoordinated cell proliferation. Neoplasms, or tumors, are either benign or malignant according to their characteristics of slow growth and no invasiveness (benign) or rapid growth and great capacity to invade other tissues and

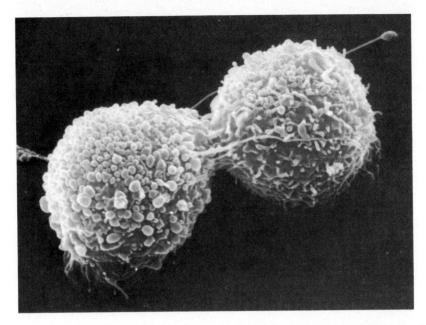

Figure 3–40. Scanning electron micrograph of cell division (telophase) in a Chinese hamster ovary cell in cell culture. The numerous blebs are characteristic of this stage of mitosis. × 5000. (Courtesy of J Aggelar.)

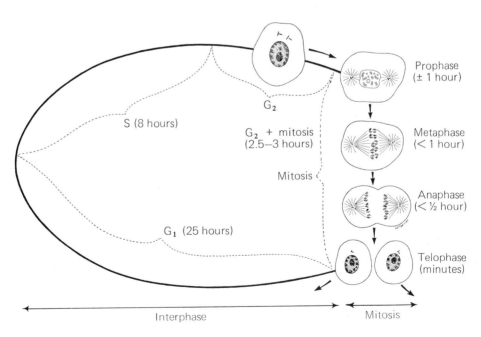

Figure 3–41. Phases of the cell cycle. The G_1 phase (presynthesis) is variable and depends on many factors, including the rate of cell division in the tissue. In this particular case of bone tissue, it lasts 25 hours. The S phase (DNA synthesis) lasts about 8 hours. The G_2-plus-mitosis phase lasts 2.5–3 hours. The times are from Young RW in *J Cell Biol* 1962; **14:**357.

organs (malignant). Between these 2 extremes exist many tumors with intermediate properties. **Cancer** is the common term for all malignant tumors. Cancers are of great importance in medicine and are responsible for 20–30% of all deaths. For this reason, this book presents basic information regarding the origin of the most frequently encountered human tumors.

CELL DYNAMICS

Study of the cell by means of the light or electron microscope gives the false impression that the cell is static. However, cinematography at accelerated rates (5–30 times normal) shows considerable activity in cells. Mitochondria, for example, demonstrate active wriggling movements in the cytoplasm. In only a few minutes, they can be seen to become fragmented and to fuse together again.

Profound cellular changes are also observed during cell differentiation. Depending upon the function of the cell, some organelles develop more than others and become major features of the cytoplasm. Cytoplasm in striated muscle cells is composed mainly of contractile fibrils, the myofibrils. Cells of the acinar pancreas that synthesize and secrete protein contain cytoplasm almost completely filled with rough endoplasmic reticulum and zymogen granules. Furthermore, in an already differentiated cell, modification of the organelles can be observed according to the phase of cell activity (this depends on whether the cell is hypoactive or hyperactive).

In addition to these morphologic aspects of the cell's continuous activity as reflected in its organelles, it should also be realized that with few exceptions, the cell's chemical components are continually being turned over.

Many diseases have been discovered that are caused by molecular alterations in a specific cell component. Several of these diseases present morphologic characteristics that can be detected by light or electron microscopy or histochemistry. Table 3–4 lists some of these diseases and emphasizes the importance of understanding the many different cell components in pathobiology and disease.

Table 3–4. Some human and animal diseases related to altered cellular components.

Cell Component Involved	Disease	Molecular Defect	Morphologic Change	Clinical Consequence
Mitochondrion	Mitochondrial cytopathy	Defect of oxidative phosphorylation	Increase in size and number of muscle mitochondria	High basal metabolism without hyperthyroidism
Microtubule	Kartagener's syndrome	Lack of dynein in cilia and flagella	Lack of arms of the doublet microtubules	Immotile cilia and flagella with male sterility and chronic respiratory infection
	Mouse (*Acomys*) diabetes	Reduction of tubulin in pancreatic β cells	Reduction of microtubules in β cells	High blood sugar content (diabetes)
Lysosome	Metachromatic leukodystrophy	Lack of lysosomal sulfatase	Accumulation of lipid (cerebroside) in tissues	Motor and mental impairment
	Hurler's disease	Lack of lysosomal α-L-iduronidase	Accumulation of dermatan sulfate in tissues	Growth and mental retardation
Secretory granule	Proinsulin diabetes	Defect of proinsulin-cleaving enzyme	None	High blood proinsulin content (diabetes)
Golgi complex	T-cell disease	Phosphotransferase deficiency	Inclusion-particle storage in fibroblasts	Psychomotor retardation, bone abnormalities

REFERENCES

Afzelius BA, Eliasson R: Flagellar mutants in man: On the heterogeneity of the immotile-cilia syndrome. *J Ultrastruct Res* 1979;**69**:43.

Alberts B et al: *Molecular Biology of the Cell*, 2nd ed. Garland, 1989.

Bittar EW (editor): *Membrane Structure and Function*. 4 Vols. Wiley, 1980–1981.

Bostock CJ, Sumner AT: *The Eucaryotic Chromosome.* North-Holland, 1978.

Bretscher MS: The molecules of the cell membrane. *Sci Am* (Oct) 1985;**253**:100.

Brinkley BR: Microtubule organizing centers. *Annu Rev Cell Biol* 1985;**1**:145.

Brown MS, Anderson RGW, Goldstein JL: Recycling receptors: The round-trip itinerary of migrant membrane proteins. *Cell* 1983;**32**:663.

Darnell J, Lodish H, Baltimore D: *Molecular Cell Biology,* 2nd ed. Scientific American Books, 1990.

DeDuve C: *A Guided Tour of the Living Cell.* Freeman, 1984.

DeDuve C: Microbodies in the living cell. *Sci Am* (May) 1983;**248**:74.

Dingle JT (editor): *Lysosomes in Biology and Pathology,* 6 vols. Elsevier/North-Holland, 1969–1979.

Dustin P: *Microtubules,* 2nd ed. Springer-Verlag, 1984.

Farquhar MG: Progress in unraveling pathways of Golgi traffic. *Annu Rev Cell Biol* 1985:**1**:447.

Fawcett D: *The Cell,* 2nd ed. Saunders, 1981.

Jordan EG, Cullis CA (editors): *The Nucleolus.* Cambridge Univ. Press, 1982.

Kornberg RD, Klug A: The nucleosome. *Sci Am* (Feb) 1981;**244**:52.

Krstić RV: *Ultrastructure of the Mammalian Cell.* Springer-Verlag, 1979.

Lloyd D, Poole PK, Edwards SW: *The Cell Division Cycle.* Academic Press, 1982.

Osborn M, Weber K: Intermediate filaments: Cell-type-specific markers in differentiation and pathology. *Cell* 1982;**31**:303.

Palade GE: Intracellular aspects of the process of protein synthesis. *Science* 1975;**189**:347.

Pfeffer SR, Rothman JE: Biosynthetic protein transport and sorting in the endoplasmic reticulum. *Annu Rev Biochem* 1987;**56**:829.

Rothman J: The compartmental organization of the Golgi apparatus. *Sci Am* (Sept) 1985;**253**:74.

Singer SJ, Nicholson GL: The fluid mosaic model of the structure of cell membranes. *Science* 1972;**175**:720.

Tzagoloff A: *Mitochondria.* Plenum, 1982.

Weber K, Osborn M: The molecules of the cell matrix. *Sci Am* (Oct) 1985;**253**:110.

Weissman G, Claiborne R (editors): *Cell Membranes: Biochemistry, Cell Biology, and Pathology.* HP Publishing Co. 1975.

Epithelial Tissue

Despite its complexity, the human body is composed of only **4 basic types of tissue:** epithelial, connective, muscular, and nervous. These tissues do not exist as isolated units but rather in association with one another and in variable proportions, forming different organs and systems of the body.

Each of these tissues is composed of several cell types. Approximately 200 types of cells are recognized in the human body. Almost all cell types can undergo abnormal changes in their growth that can generate tumors (neoplasms). Tumors can be derived from virtually every stage of differentiation for each cell type, accounting for the enormous diversity (several hundred types) of recognized tumors. Since each type of tumor has its own biological characteristics, this diversity explains the difficulty associated with diagnosis and clinical and surgical treatment.

An interesting observation regarding the tissue origin of cancer is worth noting. In children up to age 10, most tumors develop (in decreasing order) from hematopoietic organs, nerve tissues, connective tissues, and epithelial tissues. This proportion gradually changes with age, so that after 45 years of age, more than 90% of all tumors are of epithelial origin.

Connective tissue is characterized by the abundance of intercellular material produced by its cells: muscular tissue is composed of elongated cells that have the specialized function of contraction; and nervous tissue is composed of cells with elongated processes extending from the cell body that have the specialized functions of receiving, generating, and transmitting nerve impulses.

Epithelial tissues are composed of closely aggregated polyhedral cells with very little intercellular substance. Adhesion between these cells is strong. Thus, cellular sheets are formed that cover the surface of the body and line its cavities.

The principal functions of epithelial (from Greek, *epi,* upon, + *thele,* nipple) tissues are covering and lining surfaces (eg, skin), absorption (eg, the intestines), secretion (eg, the epithelial cells of glands), sensation (eg, neuroepithelium), and contractility (eg, myoepithelial cells).

Epithelia are derived from all 3 embryonic germ layers. Most of the epithelium lining the skin, mouth, nose, and anus has an ectodermal origin. The lining of the respiratory system, the digestive tract, and the glands of the digestive tract (eg, the pancreas and the liver) is derived from the endoderm. Other epithelia (eg, the endothelial lining of blood vessels) originate from mesoderm.

THE FORMS & CHARACTERISTICS OF EPITHELIAL CELLS

The forms and dimensions of epithelial cells are varied, ranging from high **columnar** to **cuboidal** to low **squamous** cells and including all intermediate forms (Fig 4–1). Their common polyhedral form is ac-

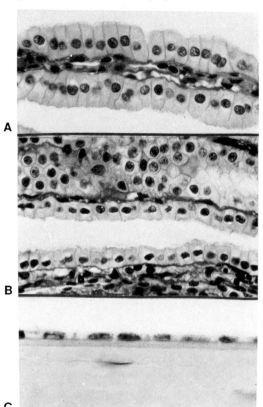

Figure 4–1. Examples of simple epithelia. **A:** Simple columnar type from the intestine. **B:** Simple cuboidal epithelium from the kidney. **C:** Simple squamous epithelium from the cornea. × 300.

counted for by their juxtaposition in cellular layers or masses. A similar phenomenon might be observed if a large number of inflated rubber balloons were compressed into a limited space. Epithelial cell nuclei have a distinctive appearance, varying from spherical to elongated or elliptic in shape. The nuclear form often corresponds roughly to the cell shape; thus, cuboidal cells have spherical nuclei and squamous cells have flattened, elliptic nuclei. The long axis of the nucleus is always parallel to the main axis of the cell.

Since the boundaries between cells are frequently indistinguishable at the light-microscope level, obser-

vation of the form of the cell nucleus is of great importance because it is an indirect clue to the shape and number of cells. This is also of value in determining whether they are arranged in layers, which is a primary morphologic criterion for classifying epithelia (Figs 4–1 and 4–2).

Basal Laminae & Basement Membranes

All epithelial cells in contact with subjacent connective tissue present, at their basal surfaces, a sheet-like extracellular structure called the **basal lamina.**

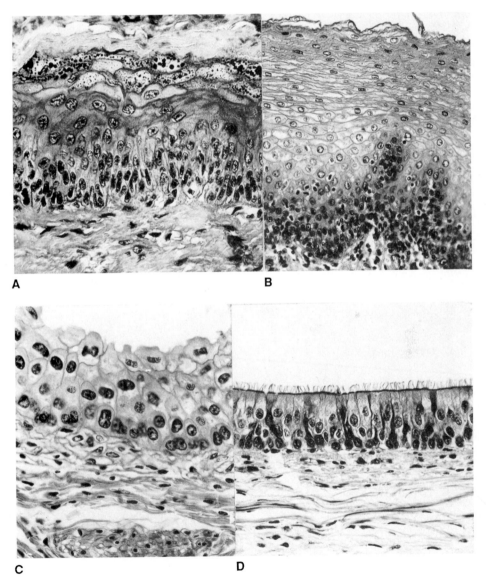

Figure 4–2. Photomicrographs of more complex types of epithelial tissue using H&E stain. **A:** Stratified squamous keratinized epithelium. **B:** Stratified squamous nonkeratinized epithelium. **C:** Transitional epithelium. **D:** Ciliated pseudostratified columnar epithelium. × 500.

A

Podocyte

Laminin

Proteoglycan
(heparan sulfate)

Endothelium

B

Hemi-
desmosome

Lamina densa

Basal
lamina

Anchoring
fibril

Lamina
lucida

Microfibrils

Reticular lamina

Figure 4–3. Two types of basement membranes. **A:** This type of basement membrane is thick because it is the result of fusion of two basal laminae produced by an epithelial and an endothelial cell layer, as found in the kidney glomerulus (shown here) and in the alveoli of the lung. It consists of a thick central **lamina densa** (darker colored zone) with a **lamina lucida** (**lamina rara;** lighter colored zone) on either side. **B:** The more common type of basement membrane that separates and binds epithelia to connective tissue is formed by assocation of the **basal** and **reticular laminae.** Observe the presence of the anchoring fibrils formed by type VII collagen, which binds the basal lamina to the subjacent collagen. Observe also microfibrils grouped in a bundle that perforate the basal lamina binding this structure to the elastic fiber system (see Fig 4–4).

This structure is visible only with the electron microscope. where it appears as a dense layer, 20–100 nm thick, consisting of a delicate network of fine fibrils (**lamina densa**). In addition to the lamina densa, basal laminae may have electron-lucent layers on one or both sides of the dense layer; these are called **laminae rarae** or **laminae lucidae.** Basal laminae are composed mainly of **type IV collagen,** a glycoprotein called **laminin,** and **proteoglycan** (heparan sulfate). Basal laminae are attached to the underlying connective tissues by anchoring structures (fibrils) formed by a special type of collagen (type VII) and by bundles of microfibrils that are part of the elastic elements of the superficial dermis (Figs 4–3 and 4–4).

A basal lamina is found not only in epithelial tissues; it is also present where other cell types come

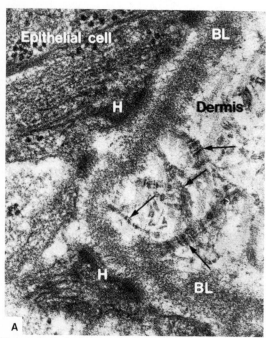

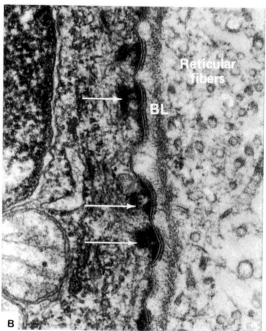

Figure 4–4. A: Section of human skin showing the zone of the epithelial-connective tissue junction. Observe the anchoring structures (arrows) that apparently insert into the basal lamina (BL). The characteristically irregular spacing of these fibrils distinguishes them from collagen fibrils. × 54,000. (Courtesy of FM Guerra Rodrigo.) **B:** Section of skin showing the basal lamina (BL) and hemidesmosomes (arrows). This is a typical example of a basement membrane formed by a basal lamina and a reticular lamina (to the right of the basal lamina in this micrograph). × 80,000.

into contact with connective tissue. It is therefore present around the endothelium of capillaries as well as around muscle, adipose, and Schwann cells (Fig 4–3B). These basal laminae provide a barrier limiting or regulating exchanges of macromolecules between connective tissue and the other tissues. A basal lamina is also found between adjacent epithelial layers, as in lung alveoli and the renal glomerulus (Fig 4–3A). In these cases, the basal lamina is thicker as a result of fusion of the basal laminae of each epithelial cell layer.

The components of the basal lamina are secreted by epithelial, muscle, adipose, and Schwann cells. In some instances, reticular fibers are closely associated with the basal lamina, forming a layer termed the **reticular lamina** (Figs 4–3B and 4–4). The reticular fibers are produced by connective tissue cells.

In addition to providing a selective barrier between connective tissue and other cells, the basal lamina seems to contain the information necessary for certain cell-cell interactions. An example is the reinnervation of denervated muscle cells. Presence of the basal lamina around a muscle cell is necessary for the establishment of new neuromuscular junctions. Another function of the basal lamina is to orient epithelial cell location and movement.

The passage of tumor cells across a basal lamina indicates the invasive quality of these cells and is an important clue to the pathologist in evaluating the degree of malignancy of certain tumors.

The term **basement membrane** is used to specify a PAS-positive layer, visible with the light microscope, beneath epithelia and in the kidney glomerulus and lung alveoli. The basement membrane is therefore thicker and is usually formed by the fusion of either 2

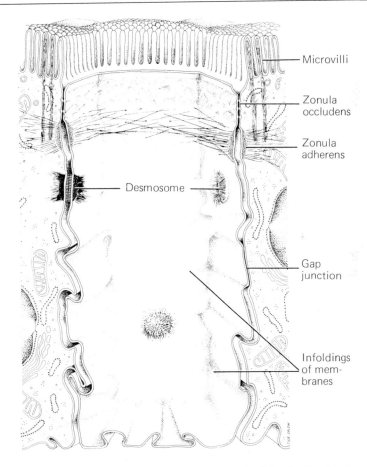

Figure 4–5. The main structures that participate in cohesion among epithelial cells. The drawing shows 3 cells from the intestinal epithelium. The cell in the middle was emptied of its contents to show the inner surface of its membrane. Observe that the zonulae occludens and adherens form a continuous ribbon around the cell apex, while the desmosomes and gap junctions make spot-like plaques. The zonula occludens is formed by multiple ridges where the membranes' outer laminae fuse. (Redrawn and reproduced, with permission, from Krstić RV: *Ultrastructure of the Mammalian Cell.* Springer-Verlag, 1979.)

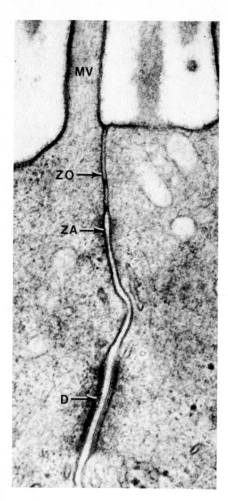

Figure 4–6. Electron micrograph of a section of epithelial cells in the large intestine showing a junctional complex with its zonula occludens (ZO), zonula adherens (ZA), and desmosome (D). Also shown is a microvillus (MV). × 80,000.

basal laminae (Fig 4–3A) or a basal lamina and a reticular lamina (Fig 4–3B). The use of these terms is not agreed upon by all authors; they are frequently used indiscriminately, causing confusion. In this book, the term **basal lamina** is used to denote the lamina densa and the variable presence of laminae rarae, structures seen with the electron microscope. When referring to the thicker structures seen with the light microscope, the term **basement membrane** is used.

Intercellular Junctions

Several membrane-associated structures promote cell aggregation and contribute to cohesion and communication between cells.

Epithelial cells are extremely cohesive, and relatively strong mechanical forces are necessary to separate them. This quality of intercellular adhesion is especially marked in those epithelial tissues usually subjected to traction and pressure (eg, the skin). This is due in part to the binding action of the glycoproteins, which are integral membrane proteins of the plasma membrane, and of a small amount of intercellular proteoglycan. Some glycoproteins lose their adhesiveness in the absence of calcium. The chelating agent EDTA, which complexes with calcium, is known to decrease cell adhesion and is therefore widely used in cell biology to separate epithelial cells, a necessary step in obtaining a suspension of isolated cells.

In addition to the cohesion effects of intercellular macromolecules and ions, the lateral membranes of epithelial cells exhibit several specializations that form **intercellular junctions.** These junctions serve not only as sites of **adhesion** but also as **seals** to prevent the flow of materials through the intercellular space (paracellular pathway) and to provide a mechanism for communication between adjacent cells. The various junctions are usually present in a definite order from the apex toward the base of the cell.

Tight junctions, or **zonulae occludentes** (singular, **zonula occludens**), are the most apical of the junctions. The Latin terminology gives important information about the geometry of the junction. *Zonula* refers to the fact that the junction forms a band completely encircling the cell, while *occludens* alludes to the membrane fusions that close off the intercellular space. In properly stained thin sections viewed in the electron microscope, the outer leaflets of adjacent unit membranes are seen to fuse, giving rise to a local pentalaminar appearance. One to several of these fusion sites may be observed, depending on the epithelium under observation (Figs 4–5 and 4–6). After cryofracture (Fig 4–7), the replicas show anastomosing ridges and grooves that form a netlike structure corresponding to the fusion sites observed in conventional thin sections. The number of ridges and grooves, or fusion sites, has a high correlation with the "leakiness" of the epithelium. Epithelia with one or very few fusion sites (eg, proximal renal tubule) are more permeable to water and solutes than are epithelia with numerous (12–15) fusion sites (eg, urinary bladder). Thus, the principal function of the tight junction is to form a more or less tight seal that prevents the flow of materials between epithelial cells (paracellular pathway) in either direction (from apex to base or base to apex) (Fig 4–18). In some epithelia, electrical potentials are set up across the epithelium that influence the ability of the epithelium to transport molecules. In these cases, more fusion sites are usually found, but some little-understood exceptions do occur.

In many epithelia, the next junctional type encountered is the **zonula adherens** (Figs 4–5 and 4–6). This junction encircles the cell and is thought to provide for the adhesion of one cell to its neighbor. A noteworthy feature of this junction is the insertion of numerous actin-containing microfilaments into dense plaques of material on the cytoplasmic surfaces of the junctional membranes. The plaques contain myosin,

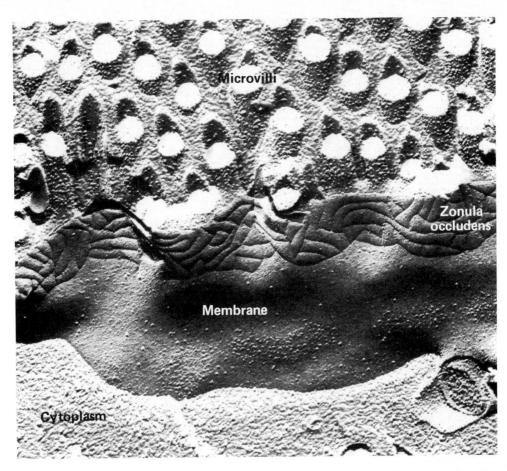

Figure 4–7. Electron micrograph of a freeze-fractured small-intestine epithelial cell. In the upper portion, the microvilli are fractured transversely; in the lower portion, the fracture crosses through the cytoplasm of the intestinal epithelial cell. The grooves, which actually lie in the lipid (middle) layer of each plasmalemma, reveal that the membranes of adjoining cells were fused in the zonula occludens. × 100,000. (Courtesy of P Pinto da Silva.)

tropomyosin, α-actinin, and vinculin. The microfilaments arise from the **terminal web**, a web of several types of filaments in the apical cytoplasm. In this region, most cytoplasmic organelles are excluded, and the terminal web is thought to provide a certain rigidity to the apex of the cell (see Fig 4–9).

Both of the above-described junctions are responsible for a structure long known to light microscopists as the **terminal bar** (Figs 4–12 and 4–13).

A **gap junction,** or nexus, can occur almost anywhere along the lateral membranes of most epithelial cells. Gap junctions are characterized, in conventional electron-micrographs, by the close (2 nm) apposition of adjacent cell membranes (Fig 4–8). After cryofracture, aggregates of intramembrane particles are found in circular patches in the plasma membrane (Fig 4–8B). Gap junctions have been isolated from liver, lens, and cardiac muscle. The major protein constituent is a polypeptide (MW 26,000–30,000).

Gap junction proteins form hexamers with a hydro-philic pore, about 1.5 nm in diameter in the center. This unit is called **connexon,** and connexons in adjacent cell membranes are aligned to form a hydrophilic channel between the 2 cells (Fig 4–8A). It has been shown that gap junctions permit the interchange between cells of molecules with a molecular weight below 1500. Thus, informational substances such as some hormones, cyclic AMP and GMP, and ions can spread information along cells of a tissue and integrate their behavior, causing the cells in many tissues to act in a coordinated manner rather than as independent units. A typical example is heart muscle cells, where gap junctions are greatly responsible for the heart's coordinated beat.

Cellular communication appears during embryogenesis and is probably important in the coordination of embryonic development.

Gap junctions can be rapidly formed between previously isolated cells. Metabolic inhibitors—especially those blocking oxidative phosphorylation

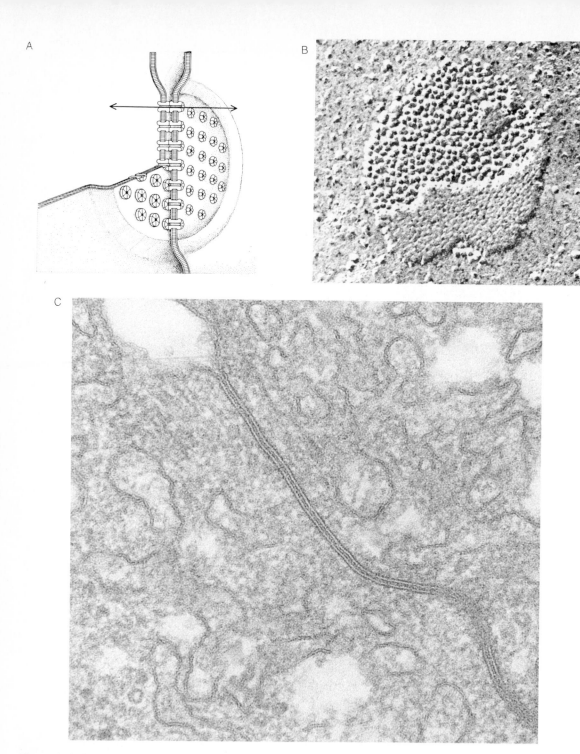

Figure 4–8. A: Model of a gap junction (oblique view) depicting the structural elements that allow the exchange of nutrients and signal molecules between cells without loss of material into the intercellular space. The communicating pipes are formed by pairs of abutting particles, which are in turn composed of 6 dumbbell-shaped protein subunits that span the lipid bilayer of each cell membrane. The channel passing through the cylindrical bridges is about 1.5 nm in diameter, limiting the size of the molecules that can pass through it. Fluids and tracers in the intercellular space can permeate the gap junction by flowing around the protein bridges. (Reproduced, with permission, from Staehelin LA, Hull BE: Junctions between living cells. *Sci Am* [May] 1978;**238**:41. Copyright © 1978 by Scientific American, Inc. All rights reserved.) **B:** Gap junction as seen on cryofracture preparation. It appears as a plaquelike agglomeration of intramembrane protein particles. × 45,000. (Courtesy of P Pinto da Silva). **C:** Gap junction between 2 rat liver cells. At the junction, 2 apposed membranes are separated by a 2-nm-wide electron-dense space, or gap. × 193,000. (Courtesy of MC Williams.)

—can inhibit the formation of junctions or undo junctions already present between cells. New junctions can be formed in the absence of protein synthesis, however. In this case, connexons may form from subunits diffusely scattered in the plasma membrane.

The final junctional type to be considered is the **desmosome,** or **macula adherens** (Figs 4–5 and 4–6). The desmosome is a complex disk-shaped structure at the surface of one cell that is matched with an identical structure at the surface of the adjacent cell. The cell membranes are very straight in this region and are usually somewhat farther apart (> 30 nm) than the usual 20 nm. In addition, some desmosomes possess a line of dense material in the intercellular space. Inside the membrane of each cell and separated from it by a short distance is a circular plaque of material called an **attachment plaque.** At least 12 proteins make up the plaque. Groups of intermediate filaments of the cytokeratin variety are inserted in the attachment plaque or make hairpin turns and return to the cytoplasm. Desmosomes are distributed in patches along the lateral membranes of most epithelial cells and are the only type of junction present in the stratified squamous epithelium of the skin. Their only function appears to be that of providing an especially firm adhesion of one cell to the next. The above description refers to the more complex desmosomes. Many cells, however, have a simpler structure with similar results.

In the contact zone between certain epithelial cells and the basal lamina, **hemidesmosomes** (from Greek, *hemi,* half, + *desmos,* band, + *soma*) can often be observed. Morphologically, these structures take the form of half a desmosome on the epithelial cell plasmalemma. They probably serve to bind the epithelial cell to the subjacent basal lamina (Fig 4–4B).

From the functional point of view, junctions between cells can be classified as **adhering junctions** (zonulae adherentes, hemidesmosomes, and desmosomes), **impermeable junctions** (zonulae occludentes), and **communicating junctions** (gap junctions).

The importance of these types of cell junctions will be discussed again in the chapters on muscle and nervous tissue.

SPECIALIZATIONS OF THE CELL SURFACE

Structural specializations reflect specific activities at the various cell surfaces and are an important part of cell polarity.

Terminal web   Microvilli   Cell coat

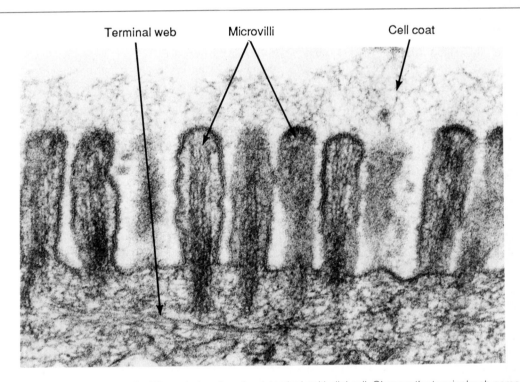

Figure 4–9. Electron micrograph of the apical region of an intestinal epithelial cell. Observe the terminal web composed of a horizontal network that contains mainly actin microfilaments. The vertical microfilaments that constitute the core of the microvilli are clearly seen. An extracellular cell coat (glycocalyx) is bound to the plasmalemma of the microvilli. × 45,000.

Microvilli

When viewed in the electron microscope, most cells are seen to have projections arising from the surface. These projections may be short or long fingerlike extensions or folds that pursue a sinuous course, and they range in number from a few to many. In absorptive cells, such as the lining epithelium of the small intestine and the cells of the proximal renal tubule, orderly arrays of many hundreds of microvilli (Latin, *microvillus*, a tuft of hair) are encountered (Figs 4–9 and 4–10). Each microvillus is about 1 μm high and 0.08 μm wide. Covering the microvillus is a filamentous coat of variable thickness, the **glycocalyx**, which contains glycoproteins and is thus PAS-positive. The complex of microvilli and glycocalyx is easily seen in the light microscope and is called the **brush** (or **striated**) **border** (see Fig 15–21).

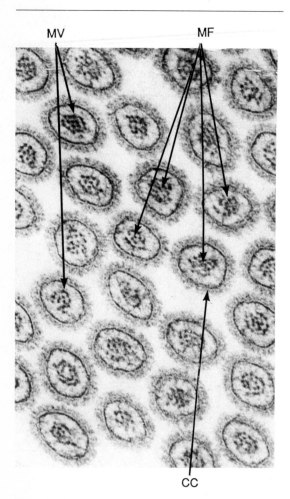

MV   MF

CC

Figure 4–10. Electron micrograph of a section from the apical region of a cell from the intestinal lining showing cross-sectioned microvilli (MV). In their interiors, note the microfilaments (MF) in a cross section. The surrounding unit membrane can be clearly discerned and is covered by a layer of glycocalyx, or cell coat (CC). × 100,000.

Each microvillus is an extension of the cytoplasm of the cell and is covered by plasma membrane, thus greatly increasing the surface area of the apex of the cell; there is a consequent increase in the absorptive efficiency of the cell. In their interiors, microvilli contain a cluster of 20–30 actin-containing microfilaments that are cross-linked to each other and to the surrounding plasma membrane by several other proteins. The basal ends of these microfilaments intermingle with microfilaments of the terminal web found just beneath the microvilli.

Stereocilia

Stereocilia are long, nonmotile processes of cells of the epididymis that are actually longer branched microvilli and should not be confused with true cilia.

Cilia & Flagella

Cilia are elongated, motile structures on the surface of epithelial cells, 5–10 μm long and 0.2 μm in diameter—much longer than and different in structure from the microvilli. Under the electron microscope in cross section, they are observed to be surrounded by the cell membrane and to contain a central pair of microtubules. At the periphery inside the membrane, arranged in a circle, are 9 more pairs of microtubules, all of which run in the direction of the long axis (Figs 3–21 and 4–11).

Cilia are inserted into **basal bodies,** which are electron-dense structures present at the apical pole just below the cell membrane (Fig 4–11). Basal bodies have a structure analogous to that of the centrioles (see Chapter 3).

In living organisms, rapid back-and-forth movement can be observed in cilia. Ciliary movement is frequently coordinated to permit a current of fluid or particulate matter to be propelled in one direction over the ciliated epithelium. ATP is the source of energy for ciliary motion.

It is estimated that a ciliated cell of the trachea can have about 250 cilia. Flagella, present in the human body only in spermatozoa, are similar in structure to cilia but are much longer and are limited in most cases to one per cell.

TYPES OF EPITHELIA

Epithelia are customarily classified according to their structure and function into 2 main groups: covering epithelia and glandular epithelia. This is an arbitrary division, for there are covering epithelia in which all cells secrete mucus (eg, the surface epithelium of the stomach) or in which glandular cells are very sparse (eg, mucous cells in the small intestine or trachea).

Covering Epithelia

Covering epithelia are tissues whose cells are organized in layers that cover the external surface or line the cavities of the body. They can be classified mor-

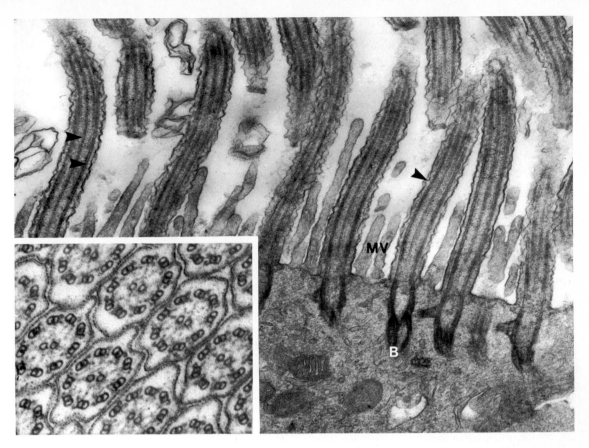

Figure 4–11. Electron micrograph of the apical portion of a ciliated epithelial cell. Cilia are seen in longitudinal section. At the left, arrowheads point to the central and peripheral microtubules of the axoneme. The arrowhead at right indicates the plasma membrane surrounding the cilium. Each cilium has a basal body (B) from which it grows. Microvilli are shown (MV). × 59,000. The inset shows cilia in cross section. The 9 + 2 array of microtubules in each cilium is evident. × 80,000. (Reproduced, with permission, from Junqueira LCU, Salles LMM: *Ultra-Estrutura e Função Celular.* Edgard Blücher, 1975.)

Table 4–1. Common types of covering epithelia in the human body.

Number of Cell Layers	Cell Form	Examples of Distribution	Function
Simple (one layer)	Squamous	Lining of vessels (endothelium). Serous lining of cavities: pericardium, pleura, peritoneum (mesothelium).	Facilitates the movement of the viscera (mesothelium), active transport by pinocytosis (mesothelium and endothelium).
	Cuboidal	Covering the ovary, thyroid.	Covering, secretion.
	Columnar	Lining of intestine, gallbladder.	Protection, lubrication, absorption, secretion.
Pseudostratified (layers of cells with nuclei at different levels; not all cells reach surface but all adhere to basal lamina)		Lining of trachea, bronchi, nasal cavity.	Protection, secretion; cilia-mediated transport of particles trapped in mucus out of the air passages.
Stratified (2 or more layers)	Squamous keratinized (dry)	Epidermis.	Protection; prevents water loss.
	Squamous nonkeratinized (moist)	Mouth, esophagus, larynx, vagina, anal canal.	Protection, secretion; prevents water loss.
	Cuboidal	Sweat glands, developing ovarian follicles.	Protection, secretion.
	Transitional	Bladder, ureters, renal calyces.	Protection, distensibility.
	Columnar	Conjunctiva.	Protection.

phologically according to the number of cell layers and the morphology of the cells in the surface layer (Table 4–1). **Simple** epithelium contains only one layer of cells, and **stratified** epithelium contains more than one layer (Figs 4–1, 4–2, 4–12, and 4–13).

Simple epithelium can, according to cell shape, be **squamous, cuboidal,** or **columnar.** The endothelium lining blood vessels and the mesothelium lining certain body cavities are examples of simple squamous epithelium (Fig 4–12A).

> Although endothelial and mesothelial cells present the same appearance in the light microscope, they should not be considered as one cell type differently localized. It is known that they differ not only in their embryologic origin and ultrastructural morphologic characteristics but also in their pathologic responses. Thus, they react differently to several types of insults and even produce different types of tumors.

An example of cuboidal epithelium is the surface epithelium of the ovary (Fig 4–12B), and an example of columnar epithelium is the lining of the small intestine (Figs 15–21 and 15–24).

Stratified epithelium is classified according to the cell shape of its superficial layer. These include **squamous, cuboidal, columnar,** and **transitional** epithelia. Pseudostratified epithelium forms a separate group, discussed below.

Stratified squamous keratinized epithelium is found mainly in the skin. Its cells form many layers; the cells closer to the underlying tissue are usually cuboidal or columnar. The cells become irregular in shape and flatten progressively as they get closer to the surface, where they are thin and squamous (Fig 4–13A; see Chapter 18 for details).

Stratified squamous nonkeratinized epithelium lines wet cavities (eg, mouth, esophagus, vagina), in contrast to the skin, whose surface is dry. Stratified squamous nonkeratinized epithelium is characterized by a flattened layer of living cells at the surface that retain their nuclei. This is not the case with the keratinized variety of this epithelium, where the surface cells are dead and their nuclei are not discernible (compare Fig 4–2A and 4–2B).

Stratified columnar epithelium is rare; it is present in the human body only in small areas such as the ocular conjunctiva and the ducts of large glands.

Transitional epithelium, which lines the urinary bladder, the ureter, and the upper part of the urethra, is characterized by the presence on its surface of domelike facet cells that are neither squamous nor columnar (Figs 4–2C and 4–13B). The form of these cells changes according to the degree of distention of the bladder. It is not unusual for these cells to be binucleate. This type of epithelium is discussed in detail in Chapter 19.

Pseudostratified epithelium is so called because the nuclei appear to lie in various layers. Although all

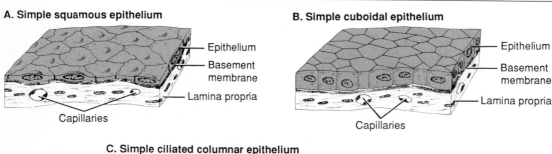

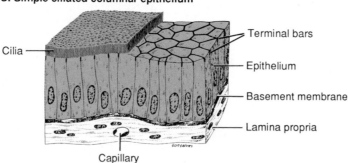

Figure 4–12. Diagrams of epithelial tissue. **A:** Simple squamous epithelium. **B:** Simple cuboidal epithelium. **C:** Simple ciliated columnar epithelium. All are separated from the subjacent connective tissue by a basement membrane. Note in **C** the terminal bars, which correspond in light microscopy to the zonula occludens and zonula adherens of the junctional complex.

A. Stratified squamous epithelium

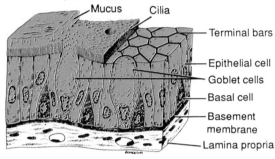

- Epithelium

- Basement membrane

- Lamina propria

B. Transitional epithelium

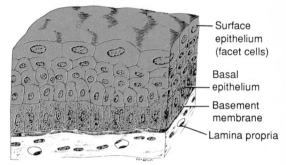

- Surface epithelium (facet cells)

- Basal epithelium

- Basement membrane

- Lamina propria

C. Ciliated pseudostratified epithelium

Mucus   Cilia

- Terminal bars

- Epithelial cell

- Goblet cells

- Basal cell

- Basement membrane

- Lamina propria

Figure 4–13. Diagrams of epithelial tissue. **A:** Startified squamous epithelium; **B:** Transitional epithelium; **C:** Ciliated pseudostratified epithelium. The goblet cells secrete mucus that forms a continuous mucous layer over the ciliary layer.

cells are attached to the basal lamina, some do not reach the surface. The best-known example of this tissue is ciliated pseudostratified columnar epithelium present in the respiratory passages (Figs 4–2D and 4–13C).

Two other types of epithelium warrant brief mention. **Neuroepithelial cells** are cells of epithelial origin with specialized sensory functions (eg, cells of taste buds). **Myoepithelial cells** are branched cells with a large number of actin microfilaments. They are specialized for contraction, mainly of the acini of the mammary, sweat, and salivary glands.

Glandular Epithelia

Glandular epithelia tissues are those formed by cells specialized to produce a fluid secretion that differs in composition from blood or intercellular fluid. This process is usually accompanied by the intracellular synthesis of macromolecules. These compounds are generally stored in the cells in small membrane-bound vesicles called **secretory granules.**

The chemical nature of these macromolecules is variable. Glandular epithelial cells may synthesize, store, and secrete proteins (eg, pancreas), lipids (eg, adrenal, sebaceous glands), or complexes of carbohydrate and proteins (eg, salivary glands). The mammary glands secrete all 3 substances—proteins, lipids, and carbohydrates. Less common are the cells of

glands that have low synthetic activity (eg, sweat glands) and in which secretion is mostly composed of substances transferred from the blood to the lumen of the gland.

In some cases, a gland may contain active synthesizing cells in association with cells specializing in ion transport. This occurs in most major mammalian salivary glands where secretory acini coexist with ion-transporting structures called **striated ducts** (see Chapter 16).

All gland cells produce and expel to an extracellular compartment products that are not used by the cell itself but are of importance to other parts of the organism.

Types of Glandular Epithelia

The epithelia that form the glands of the body can be classified according to various criteria; eg, unicellular glands consist of isolated glandular cells, and multicellular glands are composed of clusters of cells. An example of a unicellular gland is the **goblet cell** of the lining of the small intestine or of the respiratory tract (Fig 4–13C). The term *gland*, however, is usually used to designate large, complex aggregates of glandular epithelial cells, as in the salivary glands and pancreas.

Glands always arise from covering epithelia by means of cell proliferation and invasion of subjacent connective tissue, followed by further differentiation. Fig 4–14 shows how this occurs. **Exocrine glands** are glands that retain their connection with the surface epithelium from which they originated. This connection takes the form of tubular ducts lined with epithelial cells through which the glandular secretions pass to reach the surface. **Endocrine glands** are those whose connection with the surface from which they originated was obliterated during development. These glands are therefore ductless, and their secretions are picked up and transported to their site of action by the bloodstream rather than by a duct system.

Two types of endocrine glands can be differentiated according to cell grouping. In the first type, the agglomerated cells form anastomosing cords interspersed between dilated blood capillaries (eg, adrenal gland, parathyroid, anterior lobe of the pituitary) (Fig 4–14). In the second type, the cells line a vesicle or follicle filled with noncellular material (eg, the thyroid gland) (Fig 4–14).

Exocrine glands have a **secretory portion,** which contains the cells responsible for the secretory process; and the **ducts,** which transport the secretion to the exterior of the gland (Fig 4–14). **Simple glands** have only one unbranched duct, while **compound glands** have ducts that branch repeatedly (ramified ducts). The cellular organization within the secretory portion of the gland further classifies the glands. The simple glands can be tubular, coiled tubular, branched tubular, or acinar. Compound glands can be tubular, acinar, or tubuloacinar. Fig 4–15 illustrates these types of glands schematically. Some organs have both endocrine and exocrine functions, and one cell type may function both ways—eg, in the liver, where cells

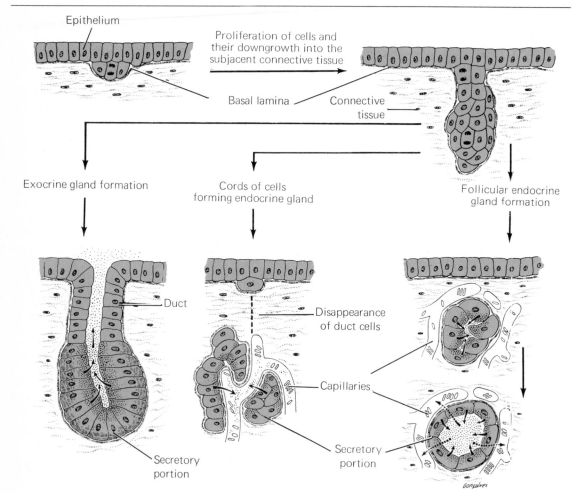

Figure 4–14. Formation of glands from covering epithelia. Epithelial cells proliferate and penetrate connective tissue. They may—or may not—maintain contact with the surface. When contact is maintained, exocrine glands are formed; without contact, endocrine glands are formed. The cells of these glands can be arranged in cords or follicles. The lumens of the follicles accumulate large quantities of secretion; cells of the cords store only small quantities in their cytoplasm. (Redrawn and reproduced, with permission, from Ham AW: *Histology,* 6th ed. Lippincott, 1969.)

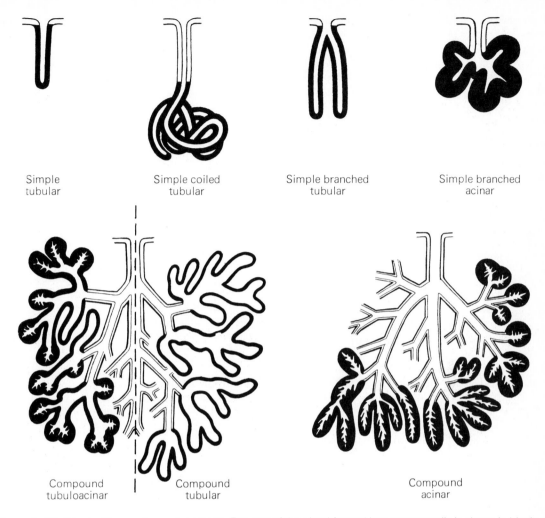

Simple
tubular

Simple coiled
tubular

Simple branched
tubular

Simple branched
acinar

Compound
tubuloacinar

Compound
tubular

Compound
acinar

Figure 4–15. Principal types of exocrine glands. The part of the gland formed by secretory cells is shown in black; the remainder shows the ducts. The compound glands have ramified ducts.

that secrete bile into the duct system also secrete some of their products into the bloodstream. In other organs, some cells are specialized in exocrine secretion and others are concerned exclusively with endocrine secretion; eg, in the pancreas, the acinar cells secrete digestive enzymes into the intestinal lumen while the islet cells secrete insulin and glucagon into the blood.

According to the way the secretory products leave the cell, glands may be classified as **merocrine** (*meros,* + Greek, *krinein,* to separate) or **holocrine** (from Greek, *holos,* whole, + *krinein*). In merocrine glands (eg, the pancreas), the secretory granules leave the cell by exocytosis with no loss of other cellular material. In holocrine glands (eg, sebaceous glands), the product of secretion is shed with the whole cell—a process that involves destruction of the secretion-filled cells. In an intermediate type—the **apocrine** (from Greek, *apo,* away from, + *krinein*)

gland—the secretory product is discharged together with parts of the apical cytoplasm.

Multicellular glands are not merely collections of cells but complete organs with a definite and orderly architecture. They usually have a surrounding capsule of connective tissue and septa that divide the gland into lobules. These lobules then subdivide, and in this way the connective tissue separates and binds together the glandular components. Blood vessels and nerves also penetrate and subdivide in the gland.

GENERAL BIOLOGY OF EPITHELIAL TISSUES

Underlying the covering epithelial tissues that line body cavities is a layer of connective tissue, the **lamina propria,** which is bound to the epithelium by the basal lamina. The lamina propria not only serves to support the epithelium but also binds it to neighboring structures. The contact between epithelium and lamina propria is increased by irregularities in the surface in the form of evaginations called **papillae** (Latin, diminutive of *papula,* nipple). These occur most frequently in epithelial tissues subject to stress, such as the skin and the tongue.

Polarity

An important feature of epithelia is their polarity; ie, they have a free, or apical, surface and a basal surface resting on a basal lamina. Since blood vessels do not normally penetrate an epithelium, all nutrients must pass out of the capillaries present in the underlying lamina propria. These nutrients and precursors of products of the epithelial cells then diffuse across the basal lamina and are taken up through the basolateral surface of the epithelial cell, usually by an energy-dependent process. Receptors for chemical messengers that influence the activity of epithelial cells (eg, hormones, neurotransmitters) are localized in the basolateral membranes. In absorptive epithelial cells, the apical cell membrane contains, as integral membrane proteins, enzymes such as disaccharidases and peptidases, which complete the digestion of molecules to be absorbed. It is thought that tight junctions help prevent the intermingling of the integral membrane proteins of the various cell membrane regions. Based on a simplified view of the fluid mosaic model of membrane structure, such intermingling might be expected.

Nutrition

Normally, blood vessels do not penetrate the epithelium, so there is no direct contact between these cells and blood vessels. Epithelial nutrition depends, therefore, on the diffusion of metabolites through the basal lamina and, frequently, through parts of the lamina propria as well. The diffusion process is probably enhanced by the papillae, which increase the area of contact between epithelium and lamina propria. Reduced diffusion probably limits the thickness of the epithelium.

Innervation

Most epithelial tissues receive a rich supply of sensory nerve endings from nerve plexuses in the lamina propria. Everyone is aware of the exquisite sensitivity of the cornea, the epithelium covering the anterior surface of the eye. This sensitivity is due to the great number of sensory nerve fibers that ramify between corneal epithelial cells.

Renewal of Epithelial Cells

Epithelial tissues are labile structures whose cells are renewed continuously by means of mitotic activity. This renewal rate is variable. It can be fast in such tissues as the intestinal epithelium, which is replaced every 2–5 days; or slow, as in the pancreas, where tissue renewal takes about 50 days. In stratified and pseudostratified epithelial tissues, mitosis occurs within the germinal layer, those cells closest to the basal lamina.

Metaplasia

Under certain physiologic or pathologic conditions, one type of epithelial tissue may undergo transformation into another epithelial type. This process is called **metaplasia** (Greek, *metaplasis,* transformation).

> The following examples illustrate this process. (1) In heavy cigarette smokers, the ciliated pseudostratified epithelium lining the bronchi can be transformed into stratified squamous epithelium. (2) In individuals with chronic vitamin A deficiency, epithelial tissues of the type found in the bronchi and urinary bladder are gradually replaced by stratified squamous epithelium. Metaplasia, which is not restricted to epithelial tissue, may also occur in connective tissue. The process, however, is reversible.

Control of Glandular Activity

The activity of a gland depends on 2 types of mechanisms: The first is genetic and depends on the expression of one or more genes that provide for the synthesis and secretion of specific compounds or products. The selection and expression of the genes that control secretion are determined during the differentiation of a glandular cell.

The second type of mechanism is related to exogenous or environmental controls. The nervous and endocrine systems are the main participants in its control. Most glands are sensitive to both nervous and endocrine control, but one is frequently more important than the other. Thus, exocrine secretion in the pancreas depends mainly on stimulation by the hormones secretin and cholecystokinin (from Greek, *chole,* bile, + *kystis,* bladder, + *kinein,* to move). The salivary glands, on the other hand, are essentially under nervous control.

The nervous and endocrine control of glands occurs through the action of chemical substances called **chemical messengers.** Neurotransmitters are the messengers produced by nerve cells, while hormones are the controlling factors produced by endocrine glands.

Chemical messengers may act by either of 2 mechanisms. In the first case, the messenger enters the cell, reacts with intracellular receptors, and activates one or more genes, initiating the production of specific proteins. Some steroid hormones, whose lipid structure makes them capable of easily crossing the cell membrane, exhibit this type of action. The antibiotic dactinomycin blocks the synthesis of messenger RNA and is known to inhibit this type of messenger activity.

A second mechanism is related to the interaction of a chemical messenger with a receptor located in the outer surface of the cell membrane. This chemical substance, referred to as the **first messenger,** acts by inducing the synthesis of yet another messenger, the **intracellular (second) messenger,** that initiates a series of events which ultimately promote a specific cell activity. Fig 4–16 summarizes this concept. Protein or polypeptide hormones and neurotransmitters that do not readily cross the cell membrane are known to act via this second-messenger mechanism.

BIOLOGY OF EPITHELIAL CELLS

As cells differentiate, they gradually acquire morphologic and physiologic characteristics related to the

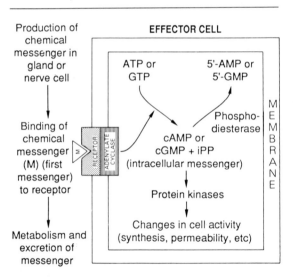

Figure 4–16. cAMP or cGMP is produced from ATP or GTP, respectively, owing to the activation of adenylate cyclase by the first messenger. Adenylate cyclase is located in the cell membrane, and a specific first-messenger receptor binds with this enzyme. The resulting intracellular (second) messengers are produced inside the cell, while the first messenger remains outside. The actions of many neurotransmitters and hormones are mediated by cAMP or cGMP. The action of the first messengers on different cell types depends on the presence of specific receptors associated with adenylate cyclase. Although cGMP is usually found in lower concentrations than is cAMP, it mediates a variety of cellular activities. In some cells, both cAMP and cGMP are known to interact, one stimulating and other inhibiting a specific cellular activity. (Based on Sutherland EW: Studies on the mechanism of hormone action. *Science* 1972;**177:**401. Copyright © 1972 by the American Association for the Advancement of Science.)

various functions they assume. Since these differentiated cells frequently have the same functions in different tissues and organs, descriptions of the basic epithelial cell types will be given.

Cells that Transport Ions

All cells have the ability to transport certain ions against a concentration and electrical-potential gradient, using ATP as an energy source. This is called **active transport** to distinguish it from passive diffusion down a concentration gradient. In mammals, the sodium ion (Na^+) concentration in the extracellular fluid is 140 mmol/L, while the intracellular concentration is 5–15 mmol/L. In addition, the interior of the cells is electrically negative with respect to the extracellular environment. Under these conditions, the positively charged sodium ion would tend to diffuse down both an electrical and a concentration gradient. The cell uses the energy stored in ATP to actively extrude Na^+ by means of an Mg^{2+}-activated Na^+/K^+-ATPase ("sodium pump"), thereby maintaining the required low intracellular sodium concentration.

Some epithelial cells (eg, proximal and distal renal tubules, striated ducts of salivary glands) exploit this mechanism to transfer sodium across the epithelium, from its apex to its base—**transcellular transport.** The apical surface of the proximal renal tubule cell is freely permeable to Na^+. To maintain electrical and osmotic balance, equimolar amounts of Cl^- and water follow the Na^+ ion into the cell. The basal surfaces of these cells are elaborately folded; many long invaginations of the basal plasma membrane are seen in electron micrographs (Figs 4–17 and 19–17). In addition, there is elaborate interdigitation of basal processes between adjacent cells. It has been shown that Mg^{2+}-activated Na^+/K^+-ATPase is localized in these invaginations of the basal plasma membrane but is also present in the lateral membranes. Located between the invaginations are vertically oriented mitochondria that supply the energy (ATP) for the active extrusion of Na^+ from the base of the cell. Chloride and water again follow passively. Thus, sodium is returned to the circulation and not lost in massive amounts in the urine.

Tight junctions play an important role in this process. Because of their relative impermeability to ions, water, and larger molecules, they prevent back-diffusion of materials already transported across the epithelium. Otherwise, a great deal of energy would be wasted.

Ion transport and the consequent flow of fluid may occur in opposite directions (ie, apical → basal, basal → apical) in different epithelial tissues. In the intestine, proximal convoluted tubules of the kidney, striated ducts of the salivary glands, gallbladder, etc, the flow is from the apex of the cell to its basal region. Flow is in the opposite direction in other epithelial sheets such as in the choroid plexus and ciliary body (Fig 4–18). In both cases, the tight

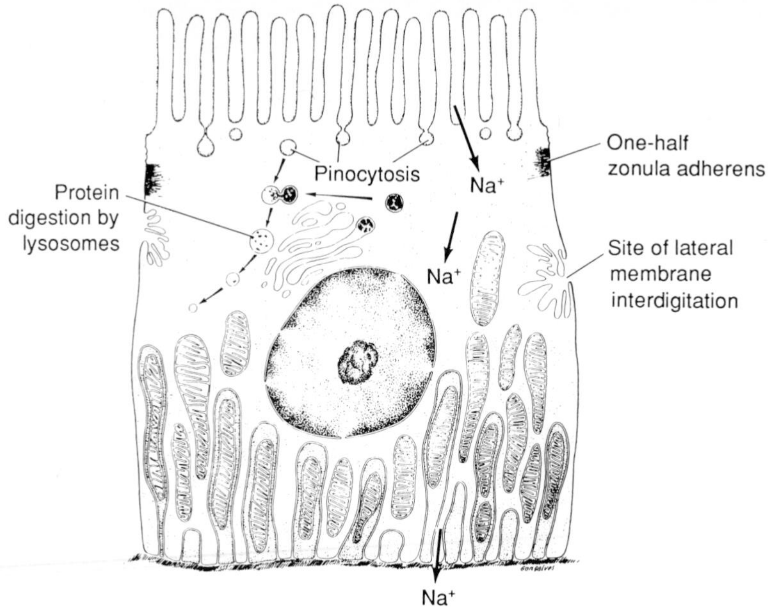

Figure 4–17. Ultrastructure of a proximal convoluted tubule cell of the kidney. Invaginations of the basal cell membrane outline regions filled with elongated mitochondria. This typical disposition is present in ion-transporting cells. Interdigitations from neighboring cells interlock with those of this cell. Protein being absorbed by pinocytosis and digested by lysosomes is shown in the upper left portion of the diagram. Sodium ions diffuse passively through the apical membranes of renal epithelial cells. These ions are then actively transported out of the cells by Na^+/K^+-ATPase located in the basolaterial membranes of the cells. Energy for this "sodium pump" is supplied by nearby mitochondria. This is an example of a cell with more than one function; it transports ions in addition to providing for protein digestion.

junctions seal the apical portions of the cells and provide for inner and outer tissue compartments.

Cells that Transport by Pinocytosis

In various cells of the body, pinocytotic vesicles that form abundantly on plasmalemma surfaces permit the transport of macromolecules across the plasma membrane. This activity is clearly observed in the simple squamous epithelial lining the blood vessels (endothelia) or the body cavities (mesothelia). These cells have few organelles other than the abundant pinocytotic vesicles found on the cell surfaces and in the cytoplasma. These observations, in conjunction with results obtained by injection of electron-dense colloidal particles (eg, ferritin, colloidal gold, thorium) followed by observation with the electron microscope, indicate that the vesicles transporting the injected materials flow in both directions through the cells.

Calculations based on these studies suggest that a pinocytotic vesicle can cross these cells in 2–3 minutes.

Chemical-Messenger– Producing Cells

The vertebrate body has many cell types whose main function is the production of messenger sub-

stances of a varied chemical nature that may influence the activities of other cells. These cells can be classified in 3 groups, according to the mode of delivery of the messenger:

Neurocrine (from Greek, *neuron,* nerve, + *krinein*) cells release chemical messages at interfaces where cytoplasmic extensions of the messenger cell approach the surface of the target cells. Neurons are an example of this type of messenger-producing cell, and the site where its extension makes contact with the effector cell is called a **synapse** (see Chapter 9).

Paracrine (from Greek, *parere,* to bring forth, + *krinein*) cells secrete a message that diffuses into the surrounding extracellular fluid and acts upon neighboring target cells. The mast cell, an example of this type of messenger-producing cell, secretes histamine that acts upon nearby capillary endothelial cells (see Chapter 5).

Endocrine (*endon* + *krinein*) cells secrete their messenger substances into the blood, which carries them directly to the target cells. Most endocrine cells produce steroid or protein messenger compounds. Some endocrine cells, however, produce biologically active amines.

Chemical-messenger–producing cells are derived from each of the 3 embryologic germ layers and subsequently reside in a variety of tissues within the

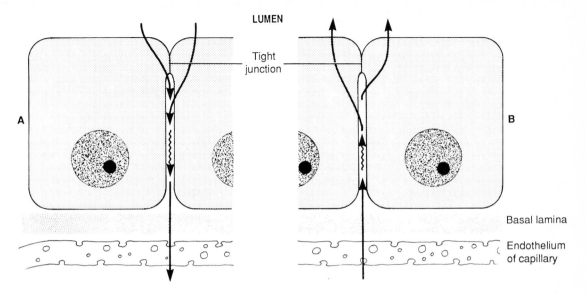

Figure 4–18. Ion and fluid transport can occur in different directions depending on which tissue is involved. **A:** The direction of transport is from the lumen to the blood vessel, as occurs in the gallbladder and intestine. This process is called absorption. **B:** Transport is in the opposite direction, as occurs in the choroid plexus, ciliary body, and sweat gland. This process is called secretion. Note the use of the intercellular space in the transport process and that the presence of occluding junctions is necessary to maintain compartmentalization and consequent control over ion distribution.

body. For example, neurocrine cells derive from ectoderm; mast cells derive from mesoderm; and thyroid follicular cells, which produce thyroid hormone, derive from endoderm.

Protein-Synthesizing Cells

All cells continuously synthesize small amounts of protein in order to replace cytoplasmic subunits utilized or lost through the normal turnover of cellular components. Some cells, however, synthesize large amounts of protein as a consequence of their differentiated function. These cells can be divided into 2 classes, based on the final distribution of their protein products. In one group, where the protein remains free within the cytoplasm, protein synthesis occurs primarily on free or unbound polyribosomes. Within this group are erythroblasts (Fig 13–7), rapidly dividing cells such as malignant tumor cells, and embryonic cells that must replace their cytoplasmic proteins rapidly after each cell division. These cells are characterized by their high content of polyribosomes that are not bound to the endoplasmic reticulum.

In the second group, synthesized proteins are segregated from other cytoplasmic components as a result of their injection into the rough endoplasmic reticulum. This group can be further subdivided in regard to whether the synthesized proteins are accumulated within or exported from the cell. Some leukocytes (eg, neutrophils, eosinophils) and macrophages synthesize lytic enzymes stored in membrane-bound granules that are usually retained within the cytoplasm and subsequently utilized for intracellular digestion (see Chapter 5 and Fig 5–17). Many protein synthesizers segregate their protein products, however, and eventually export them into the extracellular space in a process called **secretion.** Examples of protein secretors include fibroblasts, plasma cells, and pancreatic acinar cells. Within these cells, proteins are synthesized on membrane-bound polyribosomes, and the newly synthesized polypeptides are injected directly into cisternae of the rough endoplasmic reticulum.

Some cells **synthesize, segregate,** and **export** proteins without first accumulating them within the cytoplasm. In such cells (eg, the **plasma cell, fibroblasts** [Fig 5–24]), proteins are transferred from the endoplasmic reticulum to the Golgi complex. Small vesicles bud from the Golgi complex, migrate to the cell surface, and release their contents by exocytosis.

In other cell types, proteins are **synthesized, segregated,** and **accumulated** in the apex of the cell; they are then exported in response to specific stimuli. The acinar cells of the pancreas and parotid glands are typical examples of this cell type. They are polyhedral or pyramidal, with central, rounded nuclei and well-defined polarity. In the basal infranuclear region, these cells exhibit an intense basophilia, which results from local accumulation of rough endoplasmic reticulum in the form of parallel arrays of cisternae studded with abundant polyribosomes (Fig 4–19).

Mitochondria are frequently interspersed among endoplasmic reticulum cisternae. The position of the

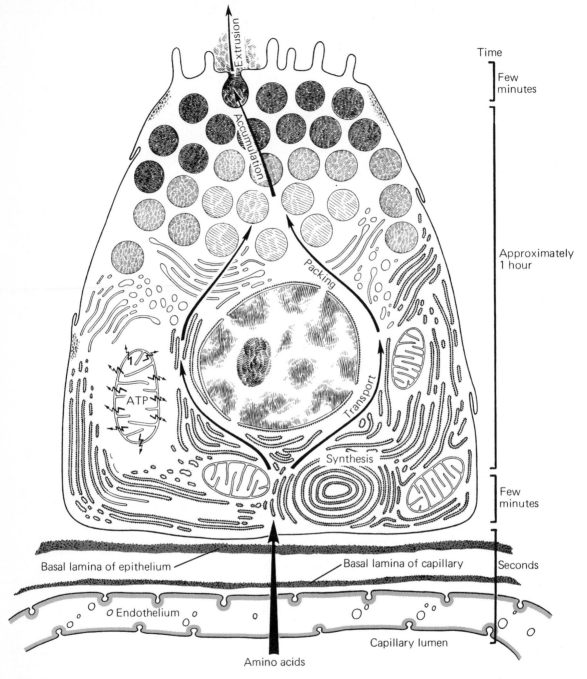

Figure 4–19. Diagram of a serous (pancreatic acinar) cell. Observe its evident polarity, with abundant basal rough endoplasmic reticulum. The Golgi complex and zymogen granules are in the supranuclear region. The secretory process is described in the text. To the right is a scale indicating the approximate amount of time necessary for each step. The darker color marks the epithelial and endothelial basal laminae; the lighter color highlights the endothelial cell membrane.

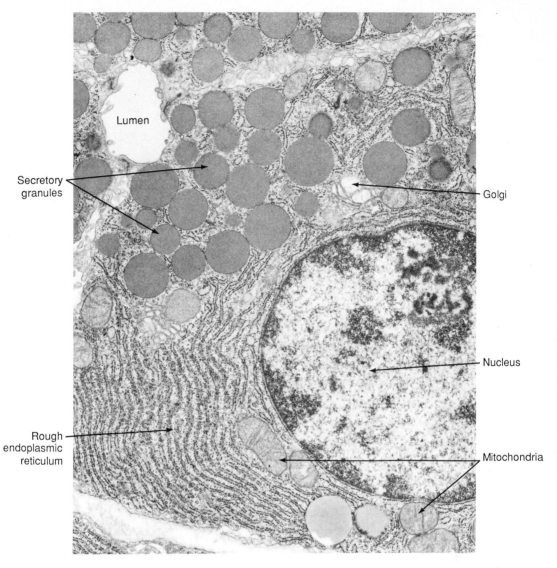

Figure 4–20. Electron micrograph of 2 frog pancreatic cells. Observe the nucleus, mitochondria, Golgi complex, secretory (zymogen) granules in various stages of condensation, and rough endoplasmic reticulum. × 13,000. (Courtesy of KR Porter.)

nucleus and the presence of an evident basal basophilic region in these cells and characteristics of protein-synthesizing cells and are used to distinguish them from mucus-secreting cells.

In the apical region just above the nucleus lies a well-developed Golgi complex. The rest of the cytoplasm is filled with rounded, protein-rich, membrane-bound **secretory granules.** In cells that produce digestive enzymes (eg, pancreatic acinar cells), these structures containing enzymes are called **zymogen granules** (Figs 4–19 and 4–20).

Enough evidence has been presented from biochemical and cytologic studies to define the secretory process in these cells as follows (see also Chapter 3):

(1) Amino acids from the bloodstream pass through the capillary walls and their basal lamina, through the secretory-cell basal lamina and plasma membrane, and into the cytoplasm. The entry of amino acids through the membrane is greatly accelerated by an active transport mechanism.

(2) Within the cell, the amino acids become associated with transfer RNA (tRNA). Polyribosomes initiate protein synthesis by utilizing the tRNA-associated amino acids to translate the message encoded in the mRNA. The mRNA code for segregated proteins includes a code for an initial

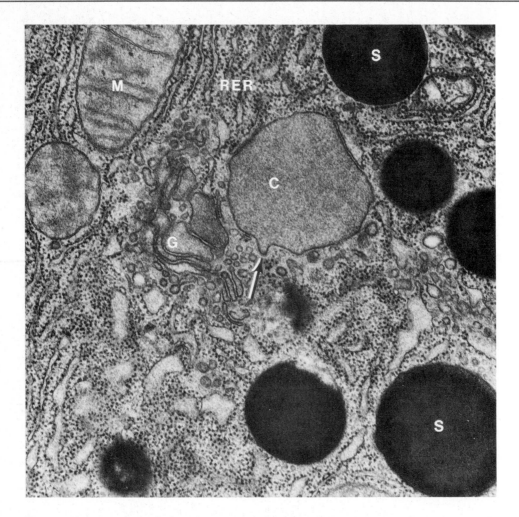

Figure 4–21. Electron micrograph of a part of a rat pancreatic acinar cell showing a condensing vacuole (C), which is presumed to be receiving a small quantity of secretory product (arrow) from the Golgi complex (G). M, mitochondrion; RER, rough endoplasmic reticulum; S, mature secretory (zymogen) granule. × 40,000.

N-terminal sequence of hydrophobic amino acids called a **signal peptide.** As the newly assembled peptide extends from the central core of the ribosome (Fig 3–9), the hydrophobic signal peptide penetrates the endoplasmic reticulum membrane. As the protein chain is assembled and injected into the endoplasmic reticulum cisterna, additional ribosomes are simultaneously attached to both the mRNA and the endoplasmic reticulum membrane, resulting in the formation of a membrane-bound polyribosome. The polypeptide thus formed is termed a **proprotein.** The hydrophobic signal peptide is enzymatically clipped off after the assembled protein enters the endoplasmic reticulum cisterna, resulting in a preproprotein. At this stage, the proteins are segregated within an extracytoplasmic space—the interior of the rough endoplasmic reticulum cisterna. This separation is significant in that it

avoids direct contact of the secretory product, often digestive enzymes (eg, ribonuclease, protease), with cytoplasmic components.

(3) The proteins thus segregated are transported from the endoplasmic reticulum to the Golgi complex. This occurs by formation of small, protein-containing **transfer,** or **shuttle, vesicles** that bud from the endoplasmic reticulum, migrating to and fusing with the convex surface of Golgi cisternae.

(4) This material is then accumulated in the Golgi cisternae. On the mature (concave) face of the Golgi, bulges form along the surface and lateral margins of the innermost cisternae. These bulges pinch off to form large membrane-bound **condensing vacuoles** or immature secretory granules (Fig 4–21). Frequently, proteins are synthesized as inactive proproteins that become functional, mature proteins only after limited proteolysis, which occurs in

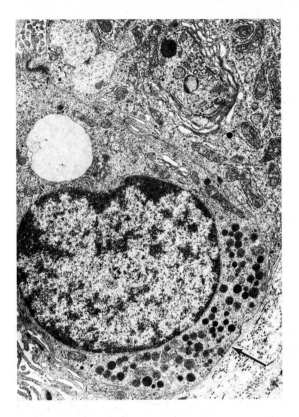

Figure 4–22. Electron micrograph of a somatostatin D cell from a human gastrointestinal tract. Note the accumulation of secretory granules in the basal region of the cell. The arrow indicates the basal lamina. × 13,500. (Courtesy of AGE Pearse.)

the Golgi complex, in the secretory granules, or after secretion.

(5) The newly formed granules in turn migrate to the cell apex and in doing so become more dense as water is removed from the protein. These have been designated **mature granules,** in contrast to the less dense, recently formed granules. Granules accumulate until they are mobilized. Accumulation occurs for periods of time that vary with the type of gland and its activity.

(6) When the cells release their secretory products, the membranes of the secretory granules fuse to the cell membrane and the granule contents spill out of the cell in a process called exocytosis. The energy for these processes is known to be furnished by oxidative phosphorylation at the mitochondrial level.

The Diffuse Neuroendocrine System (DNES)

Studies initially performed in the digestive system revealed the presence of endocrine cells interspersed among nonendocrine cells. The cytoplasm of these endocrine cells contains either polypeptide hormones or the biogenic amines epinephrine, norepinephrine, or 5-hydroxytryptamine (serotonin). In some cases, more than one of these compounds is present in the same cell. Many but not all of these cells are able to take up amine precursors and to exhibit amino acid decarboxylase activity. These characteristics explain the acronym APUD (amine precursor uptake and decarboxylation) by which they are known. Because

Table 4–2. Some of the better-known polypeptide-producing cells present in humans.

Hormone Produced	Major Action	Mechanism of Action			Location
		Neurocrine	Endocrine	Paracrine	
Gastrin	Secretes gastic acid and pepsin		+		Gastric antrum, duodenum (G cell)
Cholecystokinin (CCK)	Secretes pancreatic amylase	+	+		Duodenum, jejunum (I cell)
Secretin	Secretes pancreatic bicarbonate		+		Duodenum, jejunum (S cell)
Gastric inhibitory polypeptide (GIP)	Enhances insulin release, inhibits gastric-acid secretion		+		Small intestine
Vasoactive intestinal polypeptide (VIP)	Causes smooth-muscle relaxation; stimulates pancreatic-bicarbonate secretion	+			Pancreas (D1 cell)
Motilin	Causes intestinal motility		+		Small intestine (EC2 cell)
Somatostatin	Has numerous inhibitory effects	+		+	Stomach, duodenum, pancreas (D cell)
Calcitonin	Regulates calcium metabolism		+		Thyroid gland (C cell)
Insulin	Regulates glucose metabolism		+		Pancreas (B cell)

some of these cells stain with silver salts, they are also called **argentaffin** and **argyrophil** cells. It was initially thought that these cells derived from the nervous system, but their embryologic origin is currently being questioned.

Recent studies have shown that not all of these cells concentrate amine precursors. Therefore, the APUD designation is being gradually replaced by DNES (diffuse neuroendocrine system). DNES cells can be identified and localized by immunocytochemical methods or other cytochemical techniques for specific amines. DNES cells are widespread throughout the organism and constitute about 35 types of cells located in the respiratory and gastrointestinal systems, thyroid, hypophysis, and prostate. Some DNES cells are **paracrine cells** because they produce some of the chemical signals that diffuse into the surrounding extracellular fluid to regulate the function of neighboring cells without passing through the vascular system. Many of the polypeptide hormones and amines produced by DNES cells also act as chemical mediators in the nervous system. Amine-producing cells are described in Chapter 9. Polypeptide-secreting cells generally have distinctive dense granules about 100–400 nm in diameter located at the basal pole of these cells (Fig 4–22). They have a relatively small amount of rough endoplasmic reticulum, since they secrete at a slower rate than protein-secreting exocrine cells (eg, the pancreatic acinar cells) do.

Table 4–2 presents a series of the best-characterized polypeptide hormone-producing cells.

Several tumors derived from polypeptide-secreting cells of the DNES have been described; these are called **apudomas.** Clinical symptoms result from hypersecretion of the specific hormone involved. The diagnosis is usually confirmed using immunocytochemical methods on sections of these tumor biopsies.

Mucus-Secreting Cells

The most thoroughly studied example of a mucus-secreting cell is the **goblet cell** of the intestines. This cell is characterized by the presence of numerous large, lightly staining granules containing strongly hydrophilic glycoproteins called **mucins.** Secretory granules fill the extensive apical pole of the cell. The nucleus is usually located in the cell base. This region is rich in rough endoplasmic reticulum (Figs 4–23 and 4–24). The Golgi complex, located just above the nucleus, is exceptionally well developed, indicative of its important function in this cell. Data obtained by radioautography suggest that, in this cell, proteins are synthesized from amino acids at the level of the rough endoplasmic reticulum in the cell base. Monosaccharides are added to the core protein by enzymes termed **glycosyltransferases** located in the endoplasmic reticulum and Golgi membranes. In cells that produce sul-

fated glycoproteins, sulfation of sugars also occurs in the Golgi complex. When mucins are released from the cell, they become highly hydrated and form mucus, a viscous, elastic, protecting and lubricating gel.

The goblet cell of the intestines is only one of several types of cells that synthesize mucin glycoproteins. Others are found in the stomach, salivary glands, respiratory tract, and genital tract. These show great variability in the chemistry of their secretions and have somewhat different morphologic characteristics, described elsewhere in the text.

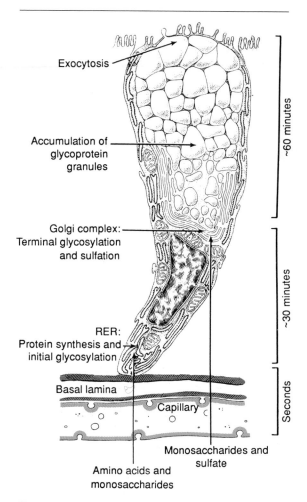

Figure 4–23. Diagram of a mucus-secreting intestinal goblet cell showing a typical constricted base, where the mitochondria and rough endoplasmic reticulum (RER) are located. Synthesis of the protein part of the glycoprotein complex occurs in the endoplasmic reticulum. A well-developed Golgi complex is present in the supranuclear region. In cells that secrete sulfated polysaccharides, the process of sulfation occurs in the Golgi complex. Darker color highlights the epithelial and endothelial basal laminae. (Redrawn after Gordon and reproduced, with permission, from Ham AW: *Histology,* 6th ed. Lippincott, 1969.)

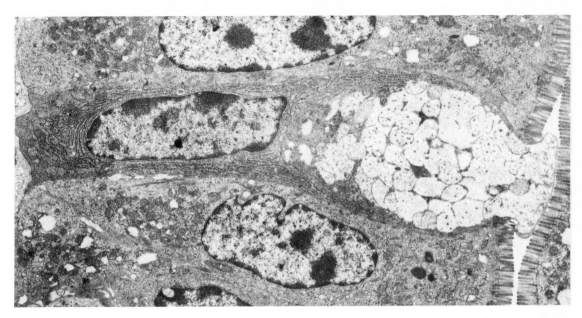

Figure 4–24. Electron micrograph of a typical goblet cell from the small intestine. The rough endoplasmic reticulum is present mainly in the basal portion of the cell (R), while the cell apex is filled with light secretory granules (SG). The Golgi complex (G) lies just above the nucleus. Typical columnar absorptive cells with microvillar borders (M) lie adjacent to the goblet cell. × 7000. (Reproduced, with permission, from Junqueira LCU, Salles LMM: *Ultra-Estrutura e Função Celular*. Edgard Blücher, 1975.)

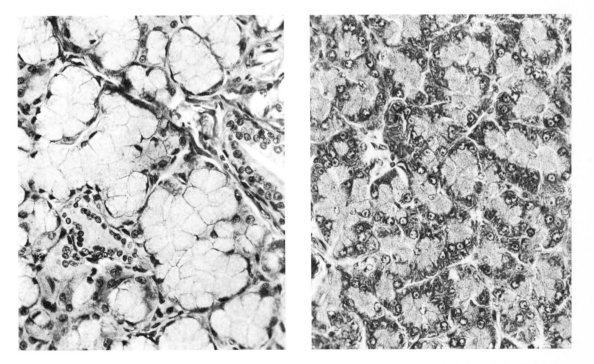

Figure 4–25. Two photomicrographs illustrating the differences between mucous cells (sublingual gland) **left,** and serous cells (pancreas), **right.** × 300.

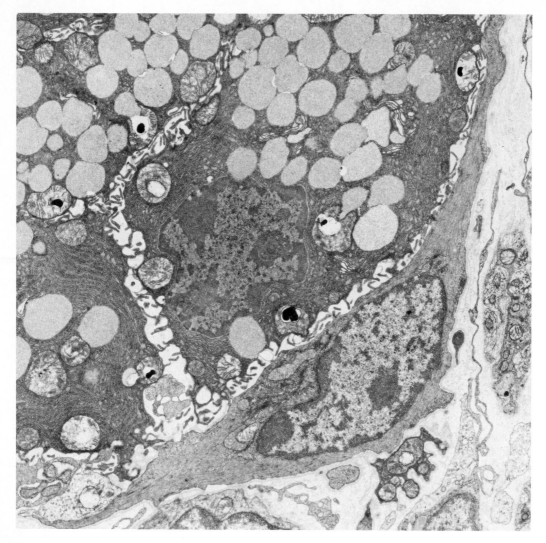

Figure 4–26. Electron micrograph of salivary gland showing secretory cells in the upper left; in the lower right of the image is a myoepithelial cell that embraces the secretory acinus. Contraction of the myoepithelial cell compresses the acinus and aids in the expulsion of secretory products.

Serous & Mucous Cells

Pancreatic acinar cells and goblet cells are typical examples of cells called serous and mucous cells, respectively, because of the molecular nature and consistency of their products of secretion. Mucous cells are characterized by the presence of large, translucent secretory granules that occupy most of the cell; there is also a nucleus containing condensed chromatin located at the cell base. Serous cells present a rounded euchromatic nucleus surrounded by rough endoplasmic reticulum in the basal third of the cell, in addition to clearly visible and easily stained secretory granules at the cell apex (Figs 4–25 and 16–1).

Myoepithelial Cells

Several glands (eg, sweat, lacrimal, salivary, mammary) contain stellate or spindle-shaped myoepithelial cells. These cells embrace gland acini as an octopus might embrace a rounded boulder. They are more longitudinally arranged along ducts. Myoepithelial cells are located between the basal lamina and the basal pole of secretory or ductal cells. In addition, they are connected to each other and to the epithelial cells by gap junctions and desmosomes. The cytoplasm contains numerous microfilaments (actin), as well as tropomyosin and myosin. Myoepithelial cells also contain intermediate filaments (10–12 nm in diameter) belonging to the cytokeratin family, con-

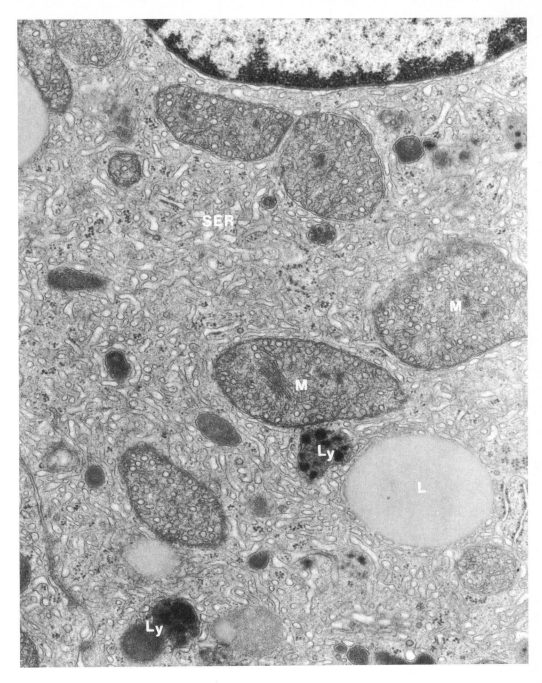

Figure 4–27. Electron micrograph of a steroid-producing cell from the human adrenal cortex. Note the mitochondria (M) with tubular cristae, the lipid droplets (L), the abundant smooth endoplasmic reticulum (SER), and the lysosomes (Ly). × 25,400.

firming their epithelial origin. The function of myo-epithelial cells is to contract around the secretory or conducting portion of the gland and thus help propel secretory products toward the exterior (Fig 4–26).

Steroid-Secreting Cells

Cells secreting steroids are found in various organs of the body (eg, testes, ovaries, adrenals.) They are endocrine cells specialized for synthesizing and secreting steroids with hormonal activity. They have the following characteristics (Figs 4–27 and 4–28):

(1) They are polyhedral or rounded acidophilic cells with a central nucleus and a cytoplasm that is usually but not invariably rich in lipid droplets.

(2) The cytoplasm of steroid-secreting cells contains an exceptionally rich, smooth endoplasmic reticulum, which takes the form of anastomosing tubules. Smooth endoplasmic reticulum contains the necessary enzymes to synthesize cholesterol from ac-

etate and other substrates and to transform the pregnenolone produced in the mitochondria into androgens, estrogens, and progestogens.

(3) The spherical or elongated mitochondria that are present usually contain tubular rather than the lamellar or shelflike cristae that are common in mitochondria of other epithelial cells. Besides being the main site of energy production for cell function, these organelles have the necessary enzymatic equipment not only to cleave the cholesterol side chain and produce pregnenolone but also to participate in subsequent reactions that result in steroid hormones. The process of steroid synthesis results, therefore, from close collaboration between smooth endoplasmic reticulum and mitochondria, a striking example of cooperation between intracellular organelles (Fig 22–11). It also explains the close proximity observed between these 2 organelles in steroid-secreting cells.

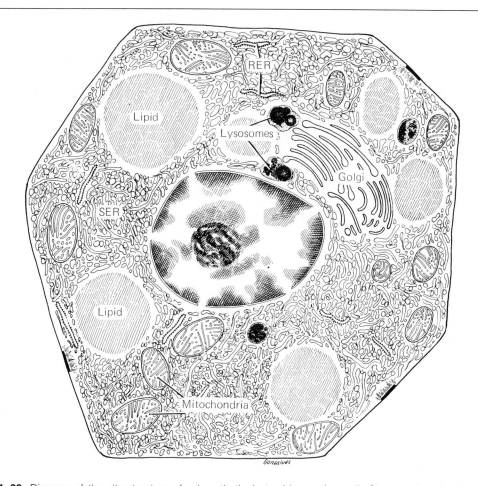

Figure 4–28. Diagram of the ultrastructure of a hypothetical steroid-secreting cell. Observe the abundance of the smooth endoplasmic reticulum (SER), lipid droplets, Golgi complex, and lysosomes. The numerous mitochondria have tubular cristae. They not only produce the energy necessary for activity of the cell but are also involved in a steroid hormone synthesis. Rough endoplasmic reticulum (RER) is also shown.

Epithelial-Cell–Derived Tumors

Both benign and malignant tumors can arise from most types of epithelial cells. A **carcinoma** (Greek, *karkinos,* cancer) is a malignant tumor of epithelial cell origin. Malignant tumors derived from glandular epithelial tissue are usually called **adenocarcinomas** (from Greek, *adenos,* gland, + *karkinos*); these are by far the most common tumors in adults.

Carcinomas composed of differentiated cells reflect cell-specific morphologic features and behavior (eg, the production of specific cytokeratins, mucins, and hormones). Undifferentiated carcinomas are often difficult to diagnose by morphologic methods alone. Since these carcinomas usually contain cytokeratins, the detection of these proteins by immunocytochemistry often helps determine not only the diagnosis but the treatment of these tumors as well (see Table 2–1).

REFERENCES

Alberts B, et al: *Molecular Biology of the Cell,* 2nd ed. Garland, 1989.

Berridge MJ, Oschman JL: *Transporting Epithelia.* Academic Press, 1972.

Darnell J, Lodish H, Baltimore D: *Molecular Cell Biology,* 2nd ed. Scientific American Books, 1990.

Farquhar MG, Palade GE: Junctional complexes in various epithelia. *J Cell Biol* 1963;**17:**375.

Fawcett D: *The Cell,* 2nd ed. Saunders, 1981.

Hall PF: Cellular organization for steroidogenesis. *Int Rev Cytol* 1984;**86:**53.

Hertzberg EL, Lawrence TS, Gilula NB: Gap junctional communication. *Annu Rev Physiol* 1981;**43:**479.

Hull BE, Staehelin LA: The terminal web: A reevaluation of its structure and function. *J Cell Biol* 1979;**81:**67.

Jamieson JD, Palade, GE: Intracellular transport of secretory protein in the pancreatic exocrine cell. 4 Metabolic requirements. *J Cell Biol* 1968;**39:**589.

Kefalides NA: *Biology and Chemistry of Basement Membranes.* Academic Press, 1978.

Krstić RV: *Illustrated Encyclopedia of Human Histology.* Springer-Verlag, 1984.

Krstić RV: *Ultrastructure of the Mammalian Cell.* Springer-Verlag, 1979.

Mooseker MS: Organization, chemistry, and assembly of the cytoskeletal apparatus of the intestinal brush border. *Annu Rev Cell Biol* 1985;**1:**209.

Simons K, Fuller SD: Cell surface polarity in epithelia. *Annu Rev Cell Biol* 1985;**1:**243.

Staehelin LA, Hull B: Junctions between living cells. *Sci Am* (May) 1978;**238:**141.

5

Connective Tissue

The connective tissues are responsible for providing and maintaining form in the body. Functioning in a mechanical role, they provide a matrix that serves to connect and bind the cells and organs and ultimately give support to the body. Unlike the other tissue types (epithelium, muscle, and nerve) that are formed mainly by cells, the major constituent of connective tissue is its **extracellular matrix,** composed of **protein fibers,** an amorphous **ground substance,** and **tissue fluid,** the latter consisting primarily of bound water of solvation. Embedded within the extracellular matrix are the **connective tissue cells.**

In terms of structural composition, connective tissue can be subdivided into 3 classes of components: **cells, fibers,** and **ground substance.** The wide variety of connective tissue types in the body represents variations in the composition and amount of these 3 components.

Connective tissue serves a variety of functions, the most conspicuous being structural. The capsules that surround the organs of the body and the internal architecture that supports their cells are composed of connective tissue. This tissue also makes up tendons, ligaments, and the areolar tissue that fills the spaces between organs. Bone, adipose tissue, and cartilage are specialized types of connective tissue that function to support the soft tissues of the body and to store fat.

The role of connective tissue in defending the organism is related to its content of phagocytic and immunocompetent cells as well as cells that produce pharmacologically active substances that are important in modulating inflammation. Phagocytic cells engulf inert particles and microorganisms that enter the body. Specific proteins called **antibodies** are produced by plasma cells in the connective tissue. The antibodies combine with foreign proteins of bacteria and viruses—or with the toxins produced by bacteria—and combat the biologic activity of these harmful agents. In addition, connective tissue matrix components provide a physical barrier, preventing the dispersion of microorganisms that pass through the epithelia.

The role of connective tissue in nutrition is a result of its close association with blood vessels. The connective tissue matrix serves as the medium through which nutrients and metabolic wastes are exchanged between cells and their blood supply.

Most connective tissues develop from the middle layer of the embryo, the **mesoderm.** Some of the connective tissues of the head, however, derive from the neural crest, a derivative of the ectoderm. Mesodermal cells migrate from their site of origin, surrounding and penetrating developing organs. These are the **mesenchymal cells,** and the tissue they form is called **mesenchyme.** Mesenchymal cells are characterized by an oval nucleus with prominent nucleoli and fine chromatin. They have relatively little cytoplasm, which extends as multiple thin processes away from the nucleus. The space between mesenchymal cells is occupied by a viscous ground substance containing few fibers. In addition to being the point of origin of all types of connective tissue cells, mesenchyme develops into other types of structures such as blood cells and blood vessels.

GROUND SUBSTANCE

The amorphous intercellular ground substance, a complex mixture of glycoproteins and proteoglycans (see Chapter 7) that participate in binding cells to the fibers of connective tissues, is colorless, transparent, and homogeneous. It fills the space between cells and fibers of the connective tissue; it is viscous and acts as a lubricant and also as a barrier to the penetration of the tissues by foreign particles. Because of its high water content and its amorphous appearance, it is difficult to study in both fresh and fixed material. When fixed, its components aggregate and appear as a granular material in the electron microscope (Fig 5–1). The ground substance is formed mainly by 2 classes of components: **glycosaminoglycans** and **structural glycoproteins.**

Glycosaminoglycans are linear polysaccharides formed by characteristic repeating disaccharide units usually composed of a uronic acid and a hexosamine. The term **acid mucopolysaccharides** was used originally to designate these macromolecules. In recent years, the term **glycosaminoglycans** has gained greater acceptance and is now used in place of **mucopolysaccharides.** The hexosamine can be **glucosamine** or **galactosamine,** and the uronic acid can

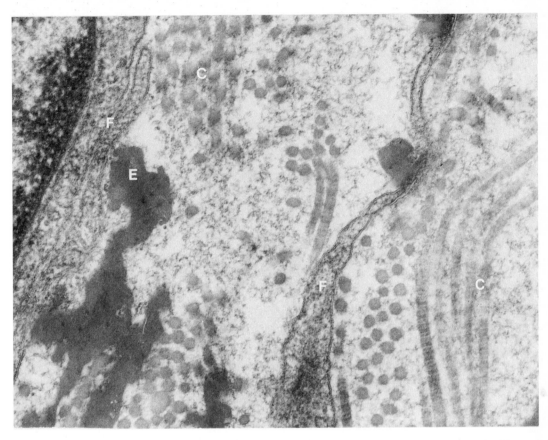

Figure 5–1. Electron micrograph showing the structural organization of the connective tissue matrix. The ground substance constitutes a fine granular material that fills the spaces between the collagen (C) and elastic (E) fibers, as well as surrounding fibroblast cells and processes (F). Ground substance granularity is an artifactual consequence of the glutaraldehyde-tannic acid fixation procedure. × 100,000.

be **glucuronic** or **iduronic acid.** With the exception of hyaluronic acid, these linear chains are bound covalently to a protein core (Fig 7–4), forming a **proteoglycan molecule.** This is a 3-dimensional structure that can be pictured as a test tube brush, with the wire stem representing the protein core and the bristles representing the glycosaminoglycans. In cartilage, the proteoglycan molecules have been shown to be bound to a hyaluronic acid chain, forming larger molecules—proteoglycan aggregates. Because of the abundance of hydroxyl, carboxyl, and sulfate groups in the carbohydrate moiety of most proteoglycans, they are intensely hydrophilic and act as polyanions. With the exception of hyaluronic acid, all other glycosaminoglycans are sulfated to some degree in the adult state. The carbohydrate portion is preponderant in proteoglycans and constitutes 80–90% of the weight of this macromolecule. Because of these characteristics, proteoglycans can bind to a great number of cations (usually sodium) by electrostatic (ionic) bonds; they are intensely hydrated structures with a thick layer of solvation water surrounding the molecule. When fully hydrated, these molecules fill a much larger volume (domain) than in their anhydrous state.

The main proteoglycans are composed of a core protein associated with the 4 main glycosaminoglycans: **dermatan sulfate, chondroitin sulfate, keratan sulfate,** and **heparan sulfate.** Table 5–1 shows the chemical composition and distribution of the glycosaminoglycans, as well as hyaluronic acid, in the tissues.

Dermatan sulfate is found mainly in dermis, tendons, ligaments, and fibrous cartilage, all structures that contain **collagen** (from Greek, *kolla*, glue, + *genin*, to produce) **fibers** (collagen type 1). Chondroitin sulfate predominates in hyaline and elastic cartilages, which are rich in collagen type II. Heparan sulfate seems to be associated mainly with **reticular fibers,** which contain collagen type III, and with basal laminae. The various collagen types are discussed below. The electrostatic interaction between their acidic groups and the basic amino acid residues of collagen causes proteoglycans to bind to collagen. (Fig 7–4).

Table 5–1. Composition and distribution of glycosaminoglycans in connective tissue and their interactions with collagen fibers.

| Glycosaminoglycan | Repeating Disaccharides | | Distribution | Electrostatic Interaction with Collagen |
	Hexuronic Acid	Hexosamine		
Hyaluronic acid	D-Glucuronic acid	D-Glucosamine	Umbilical cord, synovial fluid, vitreous humor, cartilage	. . .
Chondroitin 4-sulfate	D-Glucuronic acid	D-Galactosamine	Cartilage, bone, cornea, skin, notochord, aorta	High levels of interaction, mainly with collagen type II
Chondroitin 6-sulfate	D-Glucuronic acid	D-Galactosamine	Cartilage, umbilical cord, skin, aorta (media)	High levels of interaction, mainly with collagen type II
Dermatan sulfate	L-iduronic acid or D-glucoronic acid	D-Galactosamine	Skin, tendon, aorta (adventitia)	Low levels of interaction, mainly with collagen type I
Heparan sulfate	D-Glucuronic acid or L-iduronic acid	D-Galactosamine	Aorta, lung, liver, basal laminae	Intermediate levels of interaction, mainly with collagen types III and IV
Keratan sulfate (cornea)	D-Galactose	D-Galactosamine	Cornea	. . .
Keratan sulfate (skeleton)	D-Galactose	D-Glucosamine	Cartilage, nucleus pulposus, annulus fibrosus	. . .

The synthesis of proteoglycans begins in the rough endoplasmic reticulum with the synthesis of its protein moiety. Its glycosylation is initiated in the rough endoplasmic reticulum and completed in the Golgi complex where sulfation also occurs (see Chapter 3).

The degradation of proteoglycans is carried out by several cell types and depends on the presence of several lysosomal enzymes. The turnover of these compounds is rapid—2–4 days for hyaluronic acid and 7–10 days for sulfated proteoglycans. Several disorders have been described in which a deficiency in lysosomal enzymes causes glycosaminoglycan degradation to be blocked, with a consequent accumulation of these compounds in tissues. The lack of specific hydrolases in the lysosomes has been found as the cause of several disorders in humans, including Hurler's syndrome, Hunter's syndrome, Sanfilippo syndrome, and Morquio's syndrome.

Because of their high viscosity, intercellular substances act as a barrier to the penetration of bacteria and foreign particles. Bacteria that produce **hyaluronidase,** an enzyme that hydrolyzes hyaluronic acid and other glycosaminoglycans, have great invasive power since they reduce the viscosity of the connective tissue.

Structural glycoproteins are compounds containing a protein moiety to which carbohydrates are attached. In contrast to proteoglycans, the protein moiety usually predominates, and these molecules do not contain the linear polysaccharides formed by disaccharides containing hexosamines. Instead, the carbohydrate moiety of glycoproteins is frequently a branched structure.

Several glycoproteins have been isolated from connective tissue, and evidence shows that they play an important role not only in the interaction between neighboring adult and embryonic cells but also in the adhesion of cells to their substrate. **Fibronectin** (from Latin, *fibra,* fiber, + *nexus,* interconnection) is a glycoprotein synthesized by fibroblasts and some epithelial cells. This molecule, with a molecular weight of 222,000 to 240,000, has binding sites for cells, collagen, and glycosaminoglycans. These interactions help mediate normal cell adhesion and migration. **Laminin** is a large glycoprotein detected in basal laminae that is partially responsible for the adhesion of epithelial cells to these structures.

Participation of both fibronectin and laminin has been postulated in the increased ability of cancer cells to invade other tissues. **Chondronectin** is present in cartilage, where it mediates the adhesion of chondrocytes to type II collagen.

In connective tissue, in addition to the amorphous substance, there is a very small quantity of fluid—called **tissue fluid**—that is similar to blood plasma in its content of ions and diffusible substances. Tissue fluid contains a small percentage of plasma proteins of low molecular weight that pass through the capillary walls as a consequence of the hydrostatic pressure of the blood. Under normal conditions, the quantity of tissue fluid is insignificant.

Edema

Water in the intercellular substance of connective tissue comes from the blood, passing through the capillary walls into the intercellular regions of the tissue. The capillary wall is only slightly permeable to macromolecules but per-

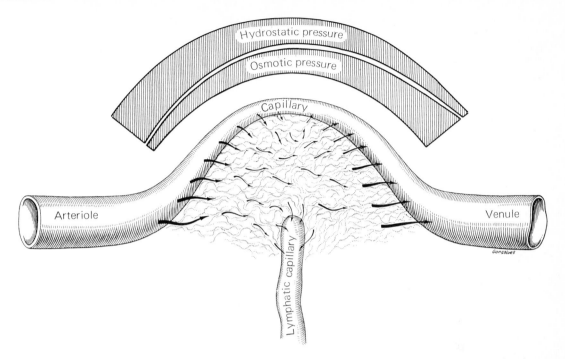

Figure 5–2. Movement of fluid through connective tissue. There is a decrease in hydrostatic pressure and an increase in osmotic pressure from the arterial to the venous ends of blood capillaries (upper part of drawing). Fluid leaves the capillary through its arterial end and repenetrates the blood at the venous end of the capillaries. Some fluid is drained by the lymphatic capillaries.

mits the passage of water and small molecules, including low-molecular-weight proteins.

Blood brings to connective tissue the different nutrients required by the cells and carries metabolic waste products away to the detoxifying and excretory organs (liver, kidney, etc).

There are 2 forces acting on the water contained in the capillaries: the hydrostatic pressure of the blood, a consequence of the pumping action of the heart, which forces water to pass through the capillary walls; and the colloid osmotic pressure of the blood plasma, which draws water back into the capillaries (Fig 5–2). Osmotic pressure is due mainly to plasma proteins. Because the ions and low-molecular-weight compounds that pass easily through the capillary walls have approximately the same concentration inside and outside these blood vessels, the osmotic pressures they exert are approximately equal on either side of the capillaries and cancel each other. The colloid osmotic pressure exerted by the blood protein macromolecules—which are unable to pass through the capillary walls—is not counterbalanced by outside pressure, however, and tends to bring water back into the blood vessel.

Normally, water passes through capillary walls to the surrounding tissues at the arterial end of a capillary. This occurs because the hydrostatic pressure here is greater than the colloid osmotic pressure; the hydrostatic pressure, however, decreases along the length of the capillary toward the venous end. As this hydrostatic pressure falls, osmotic pressure rises because of the progressive increase in the concentration of proteins, which is caused by the passage of water from the capillaries. As a result of this increase in protein concentration and fall in hydrostatic pressure, osmotic pressure becomes greater than hydrostatic pressure at the venous end of the capillary, and water is drawn back into the capillary (Fig 5–2).

The quantity of water drawn back is less than that which passes out through the capillaries. The water that remains in the connective tissue returns to the blood through the lymphatic vessels. The smallest lymphatic vessels are the lymphatic capillaries, which originate in connective tissue with blind ends. Lymphatic vessels drain into veins at the base of the neck (see Chapter 11).

Therefore, because of the equilibrium that exists between the water entering and the water leaving the intercellular substance of connective tissue, there is little free water in the tissue.

In several pathologic conditions, the quantity of tissue fluid may increase considerably, causing **edema.** Histologically, this condition is characterized by enlarged spaces between the components of the connective tissue caused by the increase in liquid. Macroscopically, edema is characterized by an increase in volume that yields easily to localized pressure, causing a depression that slowly disappears ("pitting" edema).

Edema may result from venous obstruction or a decrease in venous blood flow (eg, congestive heart failure). It may also be caused by chronic starvation; the consequent protein deficiency results in a lack of plasma proteins and a fall in colloid osmotic pressure. Water therefore accumulates in the connective tissue and is not drawn back into the capillaries.

Another possible cause of edema is increased permeability of the blood capillary endothelium resulting from chemical or mechanical injury or the release of certain substances produced in the body (eg, histamine). Edema may also be caused by the obstruction of lymphatic vessels, eg, by plugs of parasites or tumor cells.

FIBERS

Connective tissue fibers are long, slender protein polymers that are present in variable proportions in the different types of connective tissue.

There are 3 main types of connective tissue fibers: **collagen, reticular,** and **elastic.** Collagen and reticular fibers are known to be formed by the protein **collagen,** and the elastic fibers are composed mainly of the protein **elastin.** These fibers are distributed unequally among the different connective tissues. In many cases, the predominant fiber type is responsible for conferring specific properties on the tissue.

Evolution & Types of Collagen

During the process of evolution, a group of structural proteins developed that were modified by environmental influences and the functional requirements of the animal organism to varying degrees of rigidity, elasticity, and strength. These proteins are known collectively as **collagen,** and the chief examples among its various types are from the skin, bone, cartilage, smooth muscle, and basal lamina.

Collagen is the most abundant protein of the human body, representing 30% of its dry weight. The colla-

Table 5–2. Main characteristics of the different collagen types.

Collagen Type	Tissue Distribution	Optical Microscopy	Ultrastructure	Site of Synthesis	Interaction with Glycosamino-glycans	Function
I	Dermis, bone, tendon, dentin, fascias, sclera, organ capsules, fibrous cartilage.	Closely packed, thick, nonargyrophilic, strongly birefringent yellow or red fibers. Collagen fibers.	Densely packed, thick fibrils with marked variation in diameter.	Fibroblast, osteoblast, odontoblast, chondroblast.	Low level of interaction, mainly with dermatan sulfate.	Resistance to tension.
II	Hyaline and elastic cartilages.	Loose, collagenous network visible only with picro-Sirius stain and polarization microscopy.	No fibers: very thin fibrils embedded in abundant ground substance.	Chondroblast.	High level of interaction, mainly with chondroitin sulfates.	Resistance to intermittent pressure.
III	Smooth muscle, endoneurium, arteries, uterus, liver, spleen, kidney, lung.	Loose network of thin, argyrophilic, weakly birefringent greenish fibers. Reticular fibers.	Loosely packed thin fibrils with more uniform diameters.	Smooth muscle, fibroblast, reticular cells, Schwann cells, hepatocyte.	Intermediate level of interaction, mainly with heparan sulfate.	Structural maintenance in expansible organs.
IV	Epithelial and endothelial basal laminae and basement membranes.	Thin, amorphous, weakly birefringent membrane.	Neither fibers nor fibrils are detected.	Endothelial and epithelial cells, muscle cells, and Schwann cells.	Interacts with heparan sulfate.	Support and filtration.
V	Placental basement membranes.	Insufficient data.	Insufficient data.	Insufficient data.	Insufficient data.	Insufficient data.

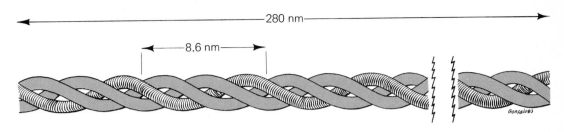

Figure 5–3. In the most abundant form of collagen, type I, each molecule (tropocollagen) is composed of two α1 (shown in color) and one α2 (shaded) peptide chains, each with a molecular weight of approximately 100,000, intertwined in a right-handed helix and held together by hydrogen bonds and hydrophobic interactions. Each complete turn of the helix spans a distance of 8.6 nm. The length of each tropocollagen molecule is 280 nm, and its width is 1.5 nm.

gens of vertebrates are a family of proteins, produced by several cell types, that are distinguishable by their differing chemical compositions, morphologic characteristics, distribution, functions, and pathologies (Table 5–2). Although more than a dozen types of collagen have been described, the most common, most important, and best studied are types I, II, III, IV, and V.

Collagen type I is the most abundant and has a widespread distribution. It occurs in tissues as struc-tures that are classically designated as **collagen fibers** and that form bones, dentin, tendons, organ capsules, dermis, etc.

Collagen type II is present mainly in hyaline and elastic cartilage. Only very thin fibrils are formed.

Collagen type III is usually associated with col-lagen type I in the tissues and is probably the major collagenous component of **reticular fibers.** Colla-gen type III can copolymerize with other types of collagen.

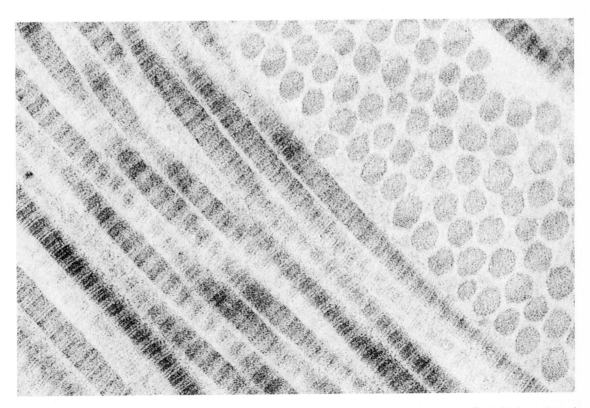

Figure 5–4. Electron micrograph of human collagen fibrils in cross and longitudinal sections. Each fibril consists of regular alternating dark and light bands that are further divided by cross-striations. Amorphous ground substance completely surrounds the fibrils. × 100,000.

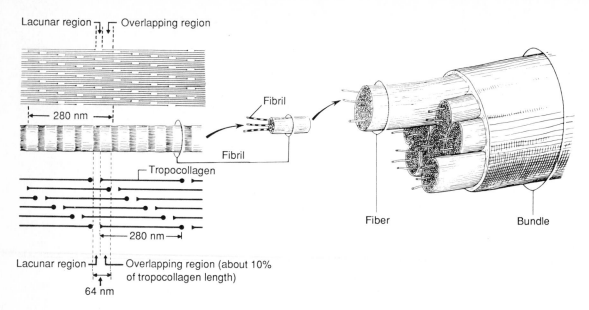

Figure 5–5. Schematic drawing of collagen molecules (tropocollagen), fibrils, fibers, and bundles. Under the electron microscope, the fibrils show a 64 nm periodicity of dark and light bands. This periodicity is explained by the stepwise overlapping arrangement of rodlike tropocollagen subunits, each measuring 280 nm. This arrangement results in the production of alternating lacunar and overlapping regions that cause the cross-striations characteristic of collagen fibrils.

Collagen type IV is present in the basal lamina (see Chapter 4). This type of collagen does not form fibrils or fibers.

Collagen type V is present in fetal membranes, in blood vessels, and in small amounts in other tissues.

Collagen synthesis, an activity thought originally to be restricted to fibroblasts, chondroblasts, osteoblasts, and odontoblasts, has been shown by studies in collagen biology to actually be very widespread, and many cell types produce this protein (Table 5–2). The principal amino acids that make up collagen are glycine (33.5%), proline (12%), and hydroxyproline (10%). Collagen contains 2 amino acids that are characteristic of this protein: **hydroxyproline** and **hydroxylysine.** These amino acids are not incorporated as such in the protein molecule but result from the hydroxylation of proline and lysine of nascent collagen polypeptides in the rough endoplasmic reticulum during collagen synthesis. The amount of collagen in a tissue can thus be determined by measurement of its hydroxyproline content.

The protein unit that polymerizes to form collagen fibrils is the elongated molecule called **tropocollagen,** which measures 280 nm in length and 1.5 nm in width. Tropocollagen consists of 3 subunit polypeptide chains intertwined in a triple helix (Fig 5–3). Differences in the chemical structure of these polypeptide chains are responsible for the different types of collagen.

In collagen types I, II, and III, tropocollagen molecules aggregate into microfibrillar subunits that are packed together to form **fibrils.** Hydrogen bonds and hydrophobic interactions are important in the aggregation and packing of these units. In a subsequent step, this structure is reinforced by the formation of covalent cross-links, a process catalyzed by the activity of the enzyme lysyl oxidase.

Collagen fibrils are thin, elongated structures with a variable diameter (ranging from 20 to 90 nm); they have transverse striation with a characteristic periodicity of 64 nm (Fig 5–4). The transverse striations of the collagen fibrils are determined by the overlapping arrangement of the subunit tropocollagen molecules (Fig 5–5). The dark bands retain more of the lead-based stain used in electron-microscope studies because their more numerous free chemical groups react more intensely with the lead solution than do the light bands. In collagen types I and III, these fibrils associate to form fibers. In collagen type I, the fibers can associate to form bundles (Figs 5–5 and 5–6). Collagen type II (present in cartilage) occurs as fibrils but does not form fibers (Fig 5–7). Collagen type IV, present in basal laminae, does not form either fibrils or fibers and probably occurs as unpolymerized or scarcely polymerized procollagen molecules. Collagen types I, II, and III, which form fibrils, are often referred to as **interstitial** collagens to distinguish them, as a group, from the other types of collagen that do not.

Collagen fiber

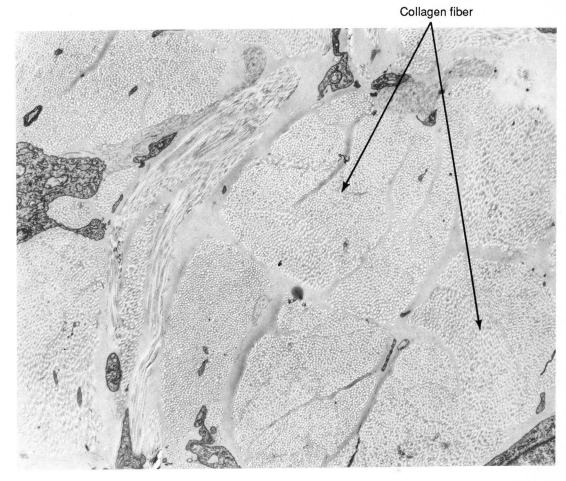

Figure 5–6. Electron micrograph of dense connective tissue showing a bundle of collagen fibers composed of individual smaller fibrils.

Collagen Biosynthesis & Degradation

The synthesis of collagen proceeds through the following steps, which are summarized in Fig 5–8:

(1) Polypeptide alpha chains are assembled on polyribosomes bound to rough endoplasmic reticulum membranes and injected into the cisternae as **preprocollagen** molecules. The signal peptide is clipped off, forming **procollagen.**

(2) Hydroxylation of proline and lysine occurs after these amino acids are incorporated into polypeptide chains. Hydroxylation begins after the peptide chain has reached a certain minimum length and is still bound to the ribosomes. The 2 enzymes involved are peptidyl proline hydroxylase and peptidyl lysine hydroxylase.

(3) Glycosylation of hydroxylysine occurs after its hydroxylation. Different collagen types have variable amounts of carbohydrate in the form of galactose or glycosylgalactose linked to hydroxylysine.

(4) Each alpha chain is synthesized with an extra length of peptides on both NH_2- and COOH-terminal ends called **registration peptides.** Registration peptides probably ensure that the appropriate alpha chains (α1, α2) assemble in the correct position as a triple helix (Fig 5–3). In addition, the extra peptides make the resulting **procollagen molecule** soluble and prevent its premature intracellular assembly and precipitation as collagen fibrils. Procollagen is transported as such out of the cell to the extracellular environment.

(5) Outside the cell, specific proteases called **procollagen peptidases** remove the registration peptides. This altered protein, known as **tropocollagen,** is capable of assembling into polymeric collagen fibrils. The hydroxyproline residues contribute to the stability of the tropocollagen triple helix, forming hydrogen bonds between its polypeptide chains.

(6) In collagen types I and III, fibrils aggregate spontaneously to form fibers. Proteoglycans and structural glycoproteins play an important role in the

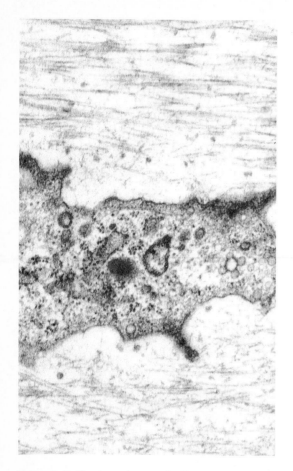

Figure 5–7. Electron micrograph of hyaline cartilage matrix showing the fine collagen fibrils of collagen type II interspersed with abundant amorphous ground substance. Transverse striations of the fibrils are barely visible because of the interaction of collagen with chondroitin sulfate. In the center is a portion of a chondrocyte. Compare the appearance of these fibrils with those of fibrocartilage (see Fig 7–10). × 14,000.

aggregation of tropocollagen to form fibrils and in the formation of fibers from fibrils.

(7) Fibrillar structure is reinforced by the formation of covalent cross-links between tropocollagen molecules. This process is catalyzed by the action of the enzyme **lysyl oxidase** that also acts in the extracellular space.

The synthesis of collagen involves a cascade of unique posttranslational biochemical modifications of the original procollagen polypeptide. All these modifications are crucial to the structure and function of normal mature collagen. These modifications are carried out by a series of different enzymes and cofactors, each of which is specifically designed for a particular role in the construction of the final product. Because there are so many steps in collagen biosyn-

thesis, there are many points at which the process may be interrupted or changed by faulty enzymes or by disease processes.

It should not be surprising, therefore, that a large number of pathologic conditions have been described that are directly attributable to insufficient or abnormal collagen synthesis. Table 5–3 lists examples of the many disorders due to collagen biosynthesis failure. In addition to disorders caused by faulty collagen synthesis, several diseases have been described that result from an overaccumulation of collagen. In **progressive systemic sclerosis,** almost all organs may present an excessive accumulation of collagen **(fibrosis).** This occurs mainly in the skin, digestive tract, muscles, and kidneys, causing inflexibility of the involved organs. **Keloid** is a local swelling caused by abnormal amounts of collagen that form in scars of the skin. Keloids, which occur most often in individuals of black African descent, can be a troublesome clinical problem to manage since they can be disfiguring and since excision is almost always followed by recurrence.

The degradation of collagen is simpler than its synthesis and is initiated by specific enzymes called **collagenases.** These enzymes are known to cut the collagen molecule into 2 parts that are susceptible to further degradation by nonspecific proteases.

Collagen Fibers

Collagen fibers are the most numerous fibers in connective tissue. Fresh collagen fibers are colorless strands, but when present in great numbers they cause the tissues in which they lie to be white (eg, in tendons and aponeuroses).

The orientation of the elongated tropocollagen molecules in these fibers makes them birefringent. When fibers containing collagen are stained with an acidic dye composed of elongated molecules (eg, Sirius red) that binds to collagen in a parallel array to its molecules, the collagen's normal birefringence increases considerably. Because this increase in birefringence occurs only in oriented collagen structures, it is used as a specific method for their detection (see Fig 5–10).

Collagen fibers are inelastic and, because of their molecular configuration, have a tensile strength greater than steel. Consequently, collagen imparts a unique combination of flexibility and strength to the tissues in which it lies.

Collagen fibers consist of closely packed thick fibrils with an average diameter of 75 nm (Fig 5–9) in mammals. The diameter of the fibers depends on the number of fibrils they contain. In many parts of the body, collagen fibers are organized in a parallel array, forming **collagen bundles** (Fig 5–5).

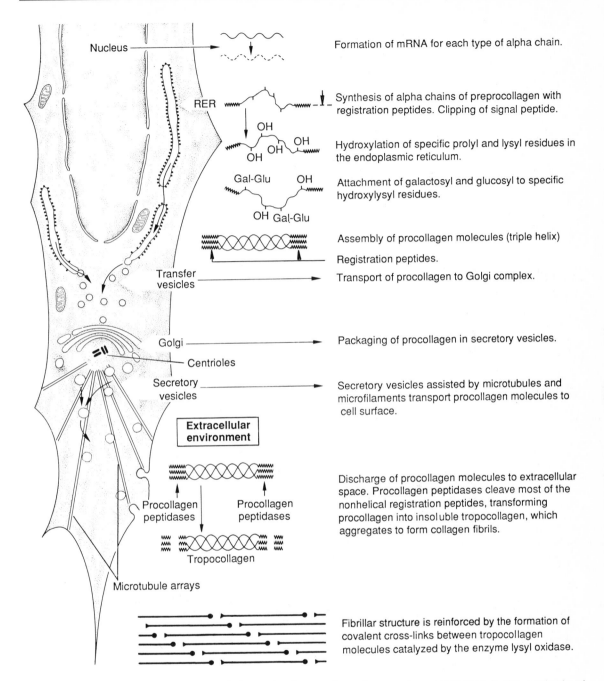

Nucleus — Formation of mRNA for each type of alpha chain.

RER — Synthesis of alpha chains of preprocollagen with registration peptides. Clipping of signal peptide.

OH — Hydroxylation of specific prolyl and lysyl residues in the endoplasmic reticulum.

Gal-Glu OH — Attachment of galactosyl and glucosyl to specific hydroxylysyl residues.

Assembly of procollagen molecules (triple helix)

Registration peptides.

Transfer vesicles — Transport of procollagen to Golgi complex.

Golgi — Packaging of procollagen in secretory vesicles.

Centrioles

Secretory vesicles — Secretory vesicles assisted by microtubules and microfilaments transport procollagen molecules to cell surface.

Extracellular environment

Procollagen peptidases   Procollagen peptidases

Tropocollagen — Discharge of procollagen molecules to extracellular space. Procollagen peptidases cleave most of the nonhelical registration peptides, transforming procollagen into insoluble tropocollagen, which aggregates to form collagen fibrils.

Microtubule arrays

Fibrillar structure is reinforced by the formation of covalent cross-links between tropocollagen molecules catalyzed by the enzyme lysyl oxidase.

Figure 5–8. Schematic representation of the molecular events and organellar participation in the synthesis of collagen.

Table 5–3. Examples of clinical disorders resulting from defects in collagen synthesis.

Disorder	Defect	Symptoms
Ehlers-Danlos type IV	Faulty transcription or translation of type III	Aortic and/or intestinal rupture
Ehlers-Danlos type VI	Faulty lysine hydroxylation	Augmented skin elasticity, rupture of eyeball
Ehlers-Danlos type VII	Decrease in pro-collagen peptidase activity	Increased articular mobility, frequent luxation
Scurvy	Lack of vitamin C (cofactor for proline hydroxylase)	Ulceration of gums, hemorrhages
Osteogenesis imperfecta	Change of one nucleotide in genes for collagen type I	Spontaneous fractures, cardiac insufficiency

Because of their long and tortuous course, the morphologic characteristics of collagen fibers are better studied in spread preparations than in histologic sections. Mesentery is frequently used for this purpose; when spread on a slide, it is sufficiently thin to be stained and examined under the microscope. Mesentery consists of a central portion of connective tissue lined on both surfaces by a simple squamous epithelium, the mesothelium. The collagen fibers in a spread preparation appear as elongated and tortuous cylindrical structures of indefinite length and a diameter that varies from 1 to 20 μm (Figs 5–10 and 5–11).

Seen in the light microscope, collagen fibers are acidophilic; they stain pink with eosin, blue with Mallory's trichrome stain, green with Masson's trichrome stain, and red with Sirius red.

Reticular Fibers

Reticular fibers are extremely thin, with a diameter between 0.5 and 2 μm. They form an extensive network in certain organs. They are not visible in hematoxylin and eosin preparations but can be easily

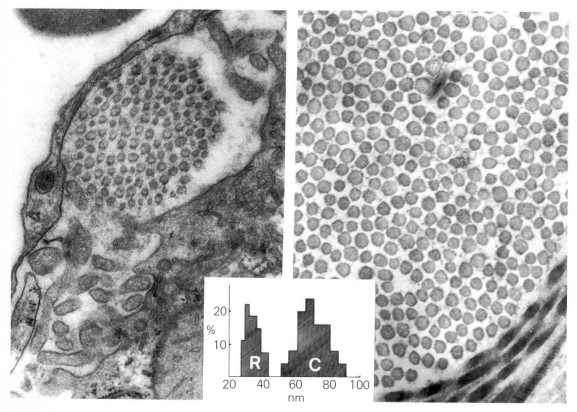

Figure 5–9. Electron micrograph of cross-sectional appearance of reticular **(left)** and collagen **(right)** fibers. Note that each fiber type is composed of numerous smaller collagen fibrils. Reticular fibers (R) comprise fibrils of significantly narrower diameter than collagen (C; see histogram inset); in addition, the constituent fibrils reveal an abundant surface-associated granularity not present on regular collagen fibrils **(right)**. × 70,000.

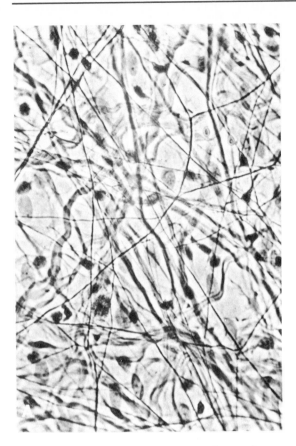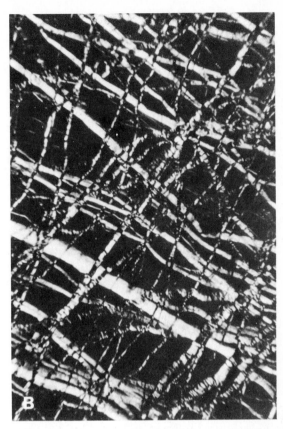

Figure 5–10. A: Whole mesentery spread on a microscope slide. The preparation was stained by the Weigert method for elastic fibers and photographed under the phase contrast microscope. The thin, taut filaments are elastic fibers that branch and form a woven network. Collagen fibers are the thick and wavy structures. × 200. **B:** A similar preparation stained with Sirius red and observed with polarization microscopy. Collagen fibers are the only structures revealed. The birefringence of collagen is due to the tight packing and paracrystalline assembly of its tropocollagen subunits. × 300.

stained black by impregnation with silver salts. Because of their affinity for silver salts, they are called **argyrophilic** (from Greek, *argyros*, silver + *philein*) fibers (Fig 5–12).

Reticular fibers are also PAS-positive. Both PAS-positivity and argyrophilia are considered to be due to the high content of glycoproteins associated with these fibers. Reticular fibers have 6–12% hexoses as opposed to 1% in collagen fibers. Immunocytochemical and histochemical evidence reveals that reticular fibers (in contrast to collagen fibers, which consist of collagen type I) are composed mainly of collagen type III in association with other types of collagen, glycoproteins, and proteoglycans. They are formed by loosely packed, thin (average, 45-nm) fibrils (Fig 5–9) bound together by abundant small interfibrillar bridges probably composed of proteoglycans and glycoproteins. Because of their small diameter, reticular fibers have a weak birefringence when stained with Sirius red and observed by means of polarizing microscopy.

Reticular fibers are particularly abundant in smooth muscle, endoneurium, and the framework of hematopoietic organs (eg, spleen, lymph nodes, red bone marrow) and constitute a network around the cells of parenchymal organs (eg, liver, kidney, endocrine glands). During embryogenesis, inflammatory processes, and wound healing, most connective tissues have an abundance of reticular fibers, but these are subsequently replaced by regular collagen fibers.

The small diameter and the loose disposition of reticular fibers create a flexible network in organs that are subjected to changes in form or volume such as the arteries, spleen, liver, uterus, and intestinal muscle layers.

Reticular fibers, considered at one time to be immature collagen fibers, are separate entities with characteristic biochemical, morphologic, functional, and pathologic features.

Ehlers-Danlos type IV disease, considered a deficiency of collagen type III, is characterized by

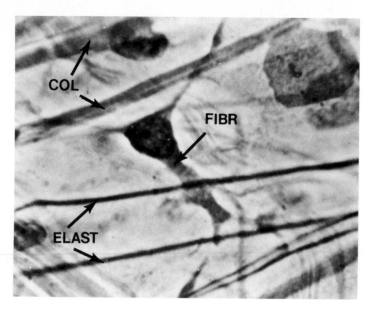

Figure 5–11. Phase contrast photomicrograph of a piece of mesentery spread on a glass slide. Shown are a fibroblast (FIBR), collagen fibers (COL), and elastic fibers (ELAST). H&E stain, × 800.

arterial and intestinal ruptures (Table 5–3). Both structures are rich in reticular fibers.

The Elastic Fiber System

This system is composed of three types of fibers—oxytalan, elaunin, and elastic. The structures of the elastic fiber system develop through three successive stages that can be observed in both embryonic and adult tissues. In the initial stages, the fiber is composed of a bundle of thin, glycoprotein-containing microfibrils. These **oxytalan fibers** can be found in the zonule fibers of the eye (Fig 24–14) and in the dermis (Fig 18–8). In the next stage of development, an irregular deposition of the protein **elastin** appears between the oxytalan fibers forming the **elaunin fibers.** These structures are found around sweat glands and in the dermis. During the third stage, elastin gradually accumulates until it occupies the center of the fiber

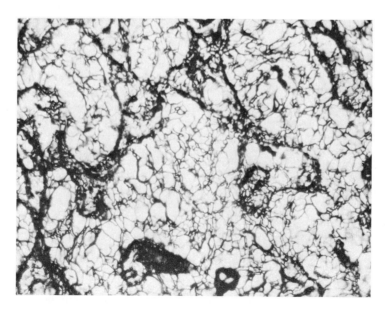

Figure 5–12. Section from a lymph node stained with silver. Note the thin black lines representing the argyrophilic reticular fibers. × 200.

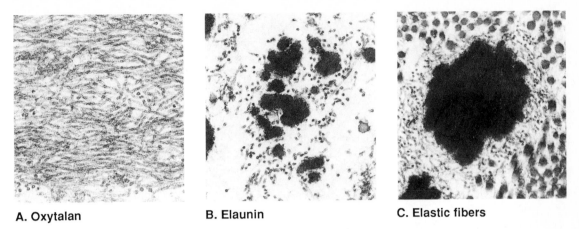

A. Oxytalan　　　　**B. Elaunin**　　　　**C. Elastic fibers**

Figure 5–13. Electron-microscope observations of developing elastic fibers. **A:** In early stages of formation, developing fibers consist of numerous small glycoprotein microfibrils. **B:** With further development amorphous elastin is found among the microfibrils. **C:** The amorphous elastin accumulates, ultimately occupying the center of an elastic fiber delineated by microfibrils. Note the collagen fibrils, seen in cross section, at upper left. (Courtesy of GS Montes.)

bundles, which are further surrounded by a thin sheath of microfibrils. These are the **elastic fibers,** the most numerous component of the elastic fiber system.

While oxytalan fibers are highly resistant to tension, elastic fibers yield elastically to tension. Elastin is responsible for the pronounced elasticity of elastic fibers, which are some five times more elastic than a typical rubber band. The elastic fiber system, by using different proportions of microfibrils and elastin, thus comprises a family of fibers whose variable func-

Stretch ⇅ Relax
Single elastin molecule
Cross-link

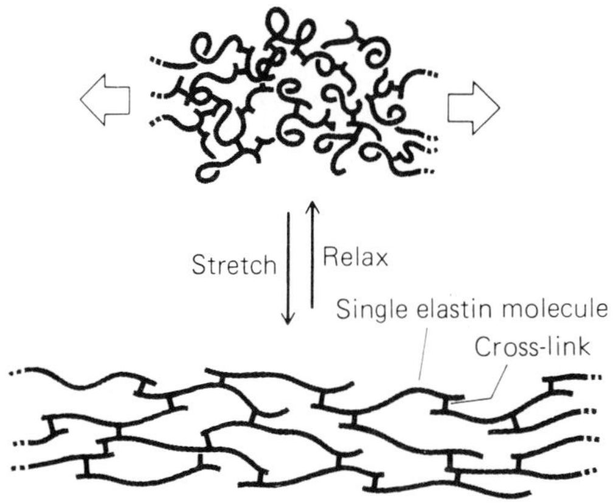

Figure 5–14. Elastin molecules are joined together by covalent bonds to generate an extensive cross-linked network. Because each elastin molecule in the network can expand and contract like a random coil, the entire network can stretch and recoil like a rubber band. (Reproduced, with permission, from Alberts B et al: *Molecular Biology of the Cell,* Garland, 1983.)

tional characteristics are adapted to local tissue requirements.

Elastin is secreted as proelastin, a globular molecule of MW 70,000 that polymerizes, producing the amorphous rubberlike glycoprotein called elastin that predominates in the mature fibers (Fig 5–13C). It is produced by fibroblasts in skin and tendon and by smooth muscle cells in the large blood vessels with elastic tissue. Elastin is resistant to boiling, acid and alkali extraction, and digestion by the usual proteases. It is easily hydrolyzed by pancreatic **elastase.** All this is apparently due to its tertiary and quaternary structure, stabilized by hydrophobic interactions between the nonpolar peptide chains.

The amino acid composition of elastin resembles that of collagen in that elastin is rich in glycine and proline. Elastin contains 2 unusual amino acids, **desmosine** and **isodesmosine,** formed by covalent reactions among 4 lysine residues. This effectively cross-links elastin and is thought to account for the rubberlike qualities of this protein. A model that illustrates the elasticity of elastin is presented in Fig 5–14.

Elastin also occurs in a nonfibrillar form as **fenestrated membranes** (elastic laminae) present in the walls of some blood vessels.

CELLS

Some cells of connective tissue, such as fibroblasts and adipose cells, are produced locally and remain there; others, such as leukocytes, come from other territories and can be transient inhabitants of connective tissue. These cells have various functions, which are summarized in Table 5–4.

Table 5–4. Functions of connective tissue cells.

Cell Type	Main Product or Activity	Main Function
Fibroblast, chondroblast, osteoblast, odontoblast	Production of fibers and ground substance	Structural
Plasma cell	Production of antibodies	Immunologic
Lymphocyte	Production of immuno-competent cells	Immunologic
Eosinophilic leukocyte	Phagocytosis of antigen-antibody complex	Immunologic
Macrophages, neutrophilic leukocyte	Phagocytosis of foreign substances, phagocytosis of bacteria	Defense
Mast cells, basophilic leukocyte	Liberation of pharmacologically active substances (eg, histamine)	Defense; pharmacologically active substances
Adipose cell	Storage of neutral fats, heat production	Energy reservoir; heat production

Cells of the connective tissue interact, creating complex mechanisms that help defend the organism from invasion. Thus, macrophages can influence antibody production by lymphocyte-derived plasma cells. Lymphocytes and mast cells can also produce substances that participate in the inflammatory process.

Fibroblasts

The fibroblast is the cell most commonly found in connective tissue. It is responsible for the synthesis of fibers and amorphous intercellular substance. Two stages of activity—active and quiescent—in this cell are observed. The cell with intense synthetic activity is morphologically distinct from the quiescent fibroblast that is found scattered within the matrix it has already synthesized. Some histologists reserve the term **fibroblast** to denote the active cell and call the quiescent cell a **fibrocyte.**

The active fibroblast has an abundant and irregularly branched cytoplasm. Its nucleus is ovoid, large, and pale-staining, with fine chromatin and a prominent nucleolus. The cytoplasm is rich in rough endoplasmic reticulum, and the Golgi complex is well developed (Figs 5–15 and 5–16).

The fibrocyte, a smaller cell than the fibroblast, tends to be spindle-shaped. It has fewer processes than the fibroblast; a smaller, darker, elongated nucleus; an acidophilic cytoplasm; and a small amount of RER. When it is adequately stimulated, the fibrocyte may revert to the fibroblast state, and its synthetic activities are reactivated. This occurs during wound healing, and in such instances the cell reassumes the form and appearance of a fibroblast. In addition, the **myofibroblast,** a cell with features of both fibroblasts and smooth muscle, is observed during wound healing. These cells have the morphologic characteristics of a fibroblast, but contain increased amounts of actin microfilaments and myosin. Their activity is responsible for wound closure following tissue injury, a process called **wound contraction.**

Fibroblasts synthesize collagen, reticular and elastic fibers, and the glycosaminoglycans and glycoproteins of the amorphous intercellular substance. In adults, fibroblasts in connective tissue rarely undergo division. Mitoses are observed only when the organism requires additional fibroblasts, eg, when connective tissue is damaged.

Macrophages: The Mononuclear Phagocyte System

These cells were discovered and initially characterized by their phagocytic capacity. When a vital dye such as trypan blue or India ink is injected into an animal, these cells engulf and accumulate it in their cytoplasm in the form of granules or vacuoles visible in the light microscope. Macrophages derive mainly from precursor cells from the bone marrow that divide, producing **monocytes** (from Greek, *monos,* single, + *kytos*) that circulate in the blood. In a second step, these cells migrate into the connective tissue where they mature and are called **macrophages.** Tissue macrophages can proliferate locally, producing more such cells.

Macrophages, which are distributed throughout the body, are present in most organs and constitute the **mononuclear phagocyte system.** In certain regions, macrophages have special names, eg, Kupffer cells in the liver, microglial cells in the central nervous system. Osteoclasts in bone tissue are also part of the mononuclear phagocyte system. To be classified as components of this system, phagocytes must be derived from bone marrow stem cells, have characteristic morphologic features, and exhibit relatively intense phagocytic activity mediated by immunoglobulins or serum complement. At one time, most of the body's macrophages were considered to be constituents of what was referred to as the **reticuloendothelial system.** Certain components of this system are excluded from the mononuclear phagocyte system, notably the reticular cells of lymphoid organs. Conversely, a few cell types not originally considered components of the reticuloendothelial system (eg, alveolar macrophages of the lung, microglia) are included in the mononuclear phagocyte system.

Although mononuclear phagocytes have a wide spectrum of morphologic features that correspond to their state of functional activity and to the tissue they inhabit, they are characterized by an irregular surface with pleats, protrusions, and indentations—a morphologic expression of their active pinocytotic and phagocytic activities. They generally have a well-

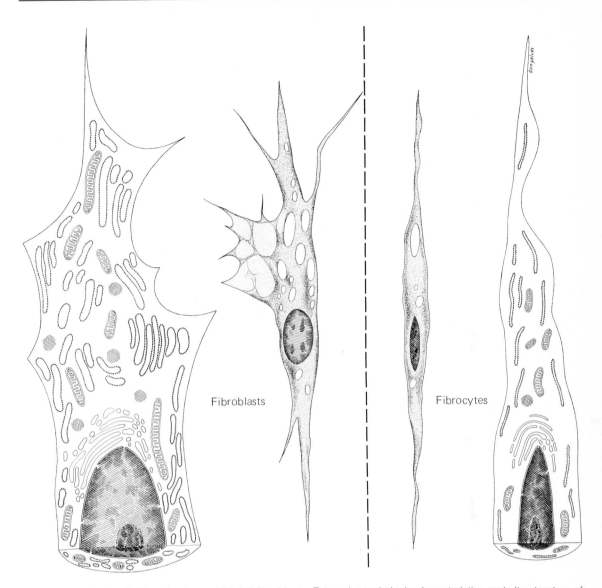

Figure 5–15. Active **(left)** and quiescent **(right)** fibroblasts. External morphologic characteristics and ultrastructure of each cell are shown. Fibroblasts that are actively engaged in synthesis are richer in mitochondria, lipid droplets, Golgi complex, and rough endoplasmic reticulum than are quiescent fibroblasts, often called fibrocytes.

developed Golgi complex, many lysosomes, and a prominent rough endoplasmic reticulum (Fig 5–17). In the process of monocyte-to-macrophage transformation, there is an increase in protein synthesis and cell size. An increase in the Golgi complex as well as in the number of lysosomes, microtubules, and microfilaments is also apparent. Macrophages measure between 10 and 30 μm and usually have an oval or kidney-shaped nucleus located eccentrically. Macrophages are long-living cells and may survive for months in the tissues. When adequately stimulated, these cells may increase in size, forming **epithelioid**

(*epi* + *thele* + Greek, *eidos,* resemblance) cells, or several may fuse to form **multinuclear giant cells**—cell types usually found only in pathologic conditions (Fig 5–18).

The major functions of macrophages are the ingestion of particles and their digestion by the lysosomes and the secretion of an impressive array of substances that participate in defensive and reparative functions. Ingestion is performed by surrounding the particle with thin extensions of the cell surface that ultimately fuse, isolating the particle within a phagocytic vacuole. Next, lysosomes fuse with the phagocytic vacuole

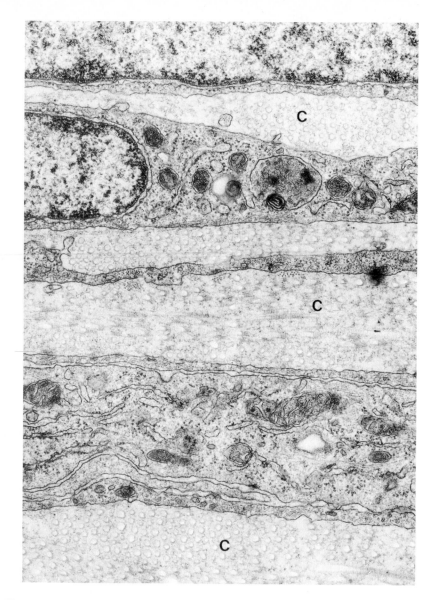

Figure 5–16. Electron micrograph revealing portions of several flattened fibroblasts in dense connective tissue. Abundant mitochondria, rough endoplasmic reticulum, and vesicles distinguish these cells from the less active fibrocytes. Multiple strata of collagen fibrils (C) lie among the fibroblasts. × 30,000.

and digest the contents. The currently accepted hypothesis regarding the mechanism of phagocytosis is summarized in Fig 5–19. In addition to this function, macrophages participate in the immune system of the body; there is evidence that these cells influence activation of the immune response. They also participate in cell-mediated resistance to infection by bacteria, viruses, protozoa, fungi, and metazoa (eg, parasitic worms); in cell-mediated resistance to tumors; and in the destruction of aged erythrocytes, extrahepatic bile production, and iron and fat metabolism.

The diversity of macrophage morphologic characteristics extends to its metabolism, which also varies according to this cell's functional activity and environment. Thus, lung macrophages exhibit a high level of aerobic glycolysis (probably related to the high oxygen tension available locally), whereas peritoneal macrophages have a high level of anaerobic glycolysis.

When macrophages are stimulated (by injection of foreign substances or by infection), they

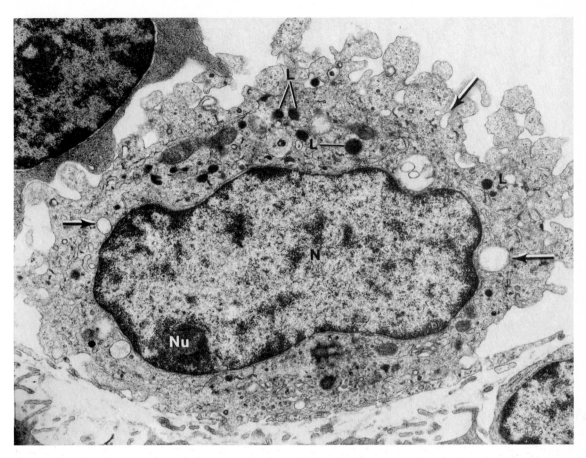

Figure 5–17. Electron micrograph of a macrophage. Note the secondary lysosomes (L), the nucleus (N), and the nucleolus (Nu). The arrows point to phagocytic vacuoles.

change their morphology and metabolism. Under these conditions, they are called **activated macrophages** and acquire characteristics not present in their nonactivated state. Thus activated, macrophages, in addition to showing an increase in their capacity for phagocytosis and intracellular digestion, exhibit enhanced metabolic and lysosomal enzyme activity. Activated macrophages can also secrete several substances that participate in inflammation and repair (eg, collagenase) and exhibit increased tumor cell-killing capacity (Fig 5–20).

Mast Cells

Mast cells are oval to round connective tissue cells, 20–30 μm in diameter, whose cytoplasm is filled with basophilic granules. The rather small and spherical nucleus is centrally situated; it is frequently obscured by the cytoplasmic granules (Fig 5–21).

The electron microscope reveals a few small spherical mitochondria, short cisternae of rough endoplasmic reticulum, and a well-developed Golgi complex.

The secretory granules are 0.3–0.5 μm in diameter and are limited by a membrane. Their interior is heterogeneous in appearance, with a prominent scroll-like substructure (Fig 5–22). The principal function of mast cells is the storage of chemical mediators of the inflammatory response.

Mast cell granules are metachromatic because of their content of glycosaminoglycans. **Metachromasia** is a property of certain basic aniline dyes (eg, toluidine blue) in which the stained material takes on a different color (purple-red) from that of the applied dye (blue). Other constituents of mast cell granules are histamine, neutral proteases, and eosinophil chemotactic factor of anaphylaxis (ECF-A). Mast cells also release leukotrienes (formerly known as slow-reacting substance of anaphylaxis: SRS-A), but these substances are not stored in the cell. Rather, they are synthesized from membrane phospholipids and immediately released upon appropriate stimulation.

There are at least 2 populations of mast cells in connective tissues. One type is called the **connective**

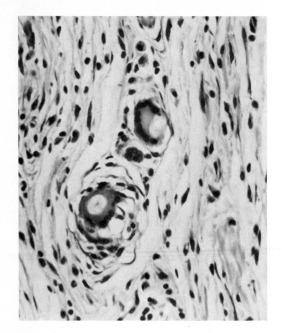

Figure 5-18. Photomicrograph of 2 foreign body giant cells. In their cytoplasm, both cells contain phagocytized material that appears lightly stained. Many nuclei can be seen at the periphery of these cells. H&E stain, × 320.

tissue mast cell, in which the proteoglycan in the granules is mainly heparin, a substance with anticoagulant activity. In the second type, termed **mucosal mast cells,** the granules contain chondroitin sulfate instead of heparin. The 2 types also react differently to pharmacologic agents.

Mast cells originate from stem cells in the bone marrow. Although they are, in many respects, similar to basophilic leukocytes, they have a separate stem cell and are not the basophils found in connective tissue. Likewise, basophils are not circulating mast cells.

The surface of mast cells contains specific receptors for IgE, a type of immunoglobulin produced by plasma cells. Most IgE molecules are fixed on the surface of mast cells and blood basophils; very few remain in the plasma.

Release of the chemical mediators stored in mast cells promotes the allergic reactions known as **immediate hypersensitivity reactions** because they occur within a few minutes after penetration by antigen of an individual previously sensitized to the same or a very similar antigen. There are many examples of immediate hypersensitivity reaction; a dramatic one is **anaphylactic shock,** a potentially fatal condition. It may occur, for example, when a person is injected with tetanus antitoxin months after having had one or more injections of it. The process of ana-

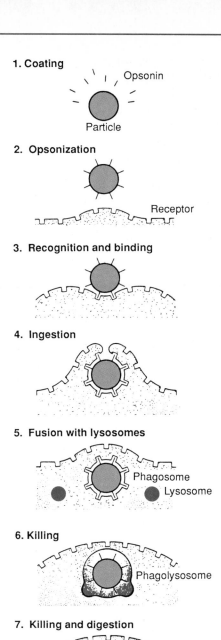

Figure 5-19. Phagocytosis of foreign particles. **1:** Coating of a foreign particle by substances such as immunoglobulins (opsonins) for which the phagocyte has receptors. **2:** Binding of opsonized particle to phagocyte. **3** and **4:** Uptake of the opsonized particle involves sequential interaction of phagocyte membrane receptors with the particle ("zippering"). Subsequent events include fusion of the phagocytic vacuole with lysosomes and killing and digestion of the foreign particle (**5, 6,** and **7**). (Redrawn and reproduced, with permission, from Stites DP, Stobo JD, Wells JV [editors]: *Basic & Clinical Immunology,* 6th ed. Appleton & Lange, 1987.)

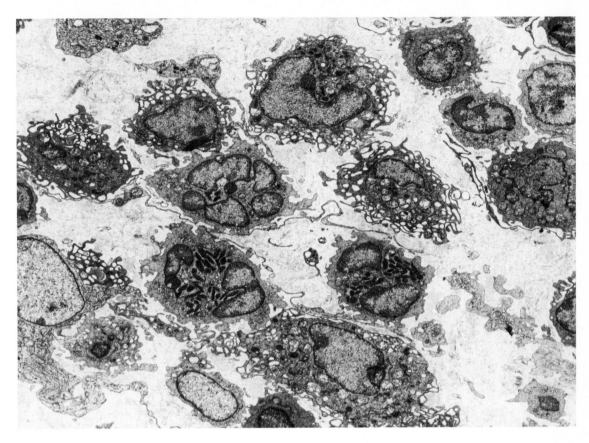

Figure 5–20. Electron micrograph of several macrophages and two eosinophils in a region immediately adjacent to a tumor. This figure illustrates the participation of macrophages in tissue reaction to tumor invasion.

phylaxis consists of the following sequential events: The first exposure to an antigen (allergen), such as tetanus antitoxin or bee venom, results in production of the IgE class of immunoglobulins (antibodies) by plasma cells. IgE is avidly bound to the surfaces of mast cells. A second exposure to the antigen results in binding of the antigen to IgE on the mast cells. This event triggers release of the mast cell granules, liberating histamine, heparin, leukotrienes, and ECF-A (Fig 5–23).

Histamine causes contraction of smooth muscle (mainly of the bronchioles), dilates blood capillaries, and increases their permeability. Leukotrienes produce slow contractions in smooth muscle, and ECF-A attracts blood eosinophils. Heparin is a blood anticoagulant, but blood clotting remains normal in humans during anaphylactic shock. Any liberated histamine is inactivated immediately after release.

Mast cells are widespread in the human body but are particularly abundant in the dermis and digestive and respiratory tracts. Mast cells are typical of cells that liberate pharmacologically active substances which act locally and therefore are classified as **paracrine cells** (defined in Chapter 4).

Plasma Cells

Plasma cells are few in number in connective tissue in most areas of the body. They are numerous in sites subject to penetration by bacteria and foreign proteins (eg, intestinal mucosa) and in areas where there is chronic inflammation.

Plasma cells are large, ovoid cells that have a basophilic cytoplasm owing to their richness in rough endoplasmic reticulum (Figs 5–24 and 5–25). The juxtanuclear Golgi complex and the centrioles occupy a region that appears pale in regular histologic preparations.

The nucleus of the plasma cell is spherical and eccentrically placed, containing compact, coarse heterochromatin alternating with lighter areas of approximately equal size. This configuration resembles the face of a clock with the heterochromatin clumps corresponding to the numerals. Thus, the nucleus of a plasma cell is commonly described as having a clock-face appearance (Fig 5–26).

Plasma cells are responsible for the synthesis of the antibodies found in the bloodstream. Antibodies are specific globulins produced by the organism in response to penetration by antigens. Each antibody is specific for the one antigen that gave rise to its production and reacts specifically with it, although it is possible for an antibody to cross-react with antigens possessing similar molecular configurations. The results of the antibody-antigen reaction are variable. Its capacity to neutralize harmful effects caused by antigens is important. When an antigen is a toxin (eg, tetanus, diphtheria), it may lose its capacity to do harm when it combines with its respective antibody.

Immunofluorescence and cytochemical techniques have demonstrated that after injection of an antigen, the corresponding antibody appears first in the cytoplasm of the plasma cell. Electron-microscope studies have shown that the first intracellular site in which antibodies appear is the cisternae of the rough endoplasmic reticulum.

Many of the antibodies synthesized by the plasma cells are specific for bacterial antigens and thus protect the body against these microorganisms. Since bacteria are never found inside plasma cells but are instead engulfed by the macrophages, it was thought that there was a mechanism by which the plasma cell

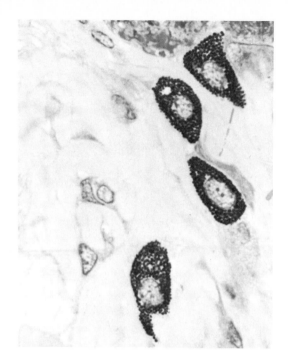

Figure 5–21. Thin section of connective tissue. Four mast cells appear with their conspicuous granules, stained by toluidine blue. × 800.

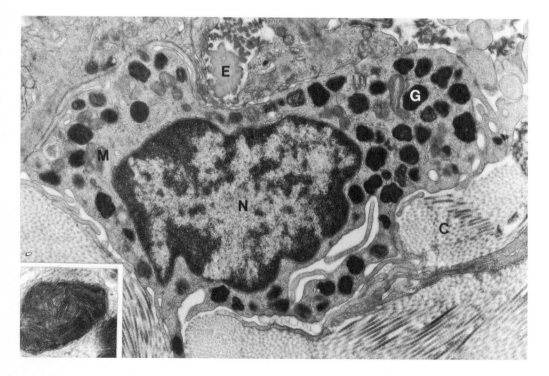

Figure 5–22. Electron micrograph of a human mast cell. The granules (G) contain heparin and histamine. Note the characteristic scroll-like structures within the granules. M, mitochondrion; N, nucleus; C, collagen fibrils; E, elastic fibril. **Inset:** Higher magnification view of a mast cell granule. (Courtesy of MC Williams.) × 14,700; Inset, × 44,600.

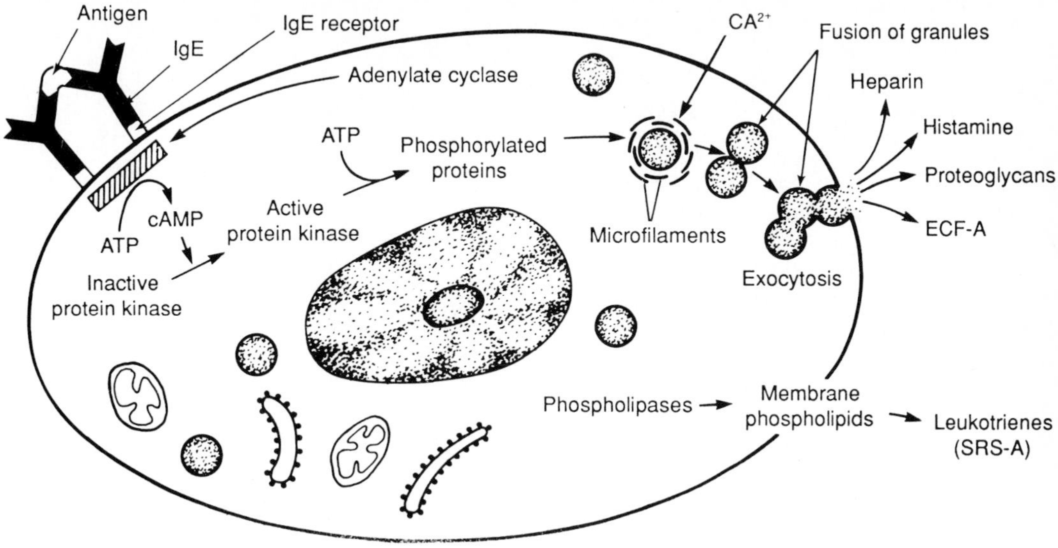

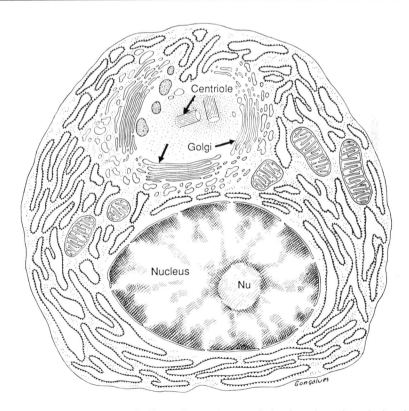

Figure 5–23. Mast-cell secretion. After a second exposure to an antigen (eg, bee venom), IgE molecules bound to surface receptors are cross-linked by the antigen. This activates adenylate cyclase and results in the phosphorylation of certain proteins. At the same time, Ca^2 enters the cell. These events lead to intracellular fusion of specific granules and exocytosis of their contents. In addition, phospholipases act on membrane phospholipids to produce leukotrienes. The process of extrusion does not damage the cell, which remains viable and synthesizes new granules.

Figure 5–24. Ultrastructure of a plasma cell. The cell contains a well-developed rough endoplasmic reticulum, with dilated cisternae containing gamma globulins (antibodies). In plasma cells, the secreted proteins do not aggregate into secretory granules. Nu, nucleolus. (Redrawn and reproduced, with permission, from Ham AW: *Histology*, 6th ed. Lippincott, 1969.)

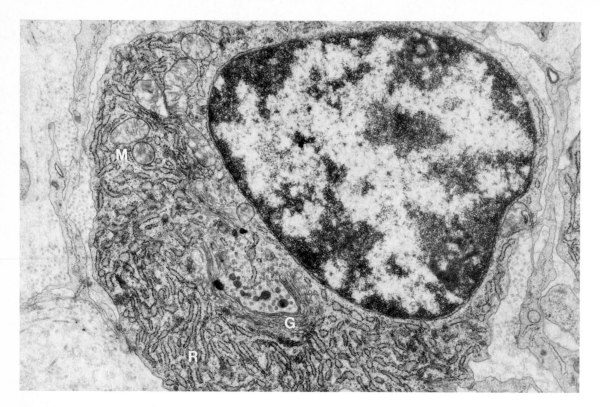

Figure 5–25. A plasma cell seen under the electron microscope. The micrograph shows the abundance of rough endoplasmic reticulum (R). Observe that many cisternae are dilated. M, mitochondria; G, Golgi complex. × 18,000.

learned about the nature of the bacterial antigens present in the macrophage. Although the process by which this information is transmitted has not been completely elucidated, electron-microscope studies have shown that cellular contact occurs between macrophages and the presumed precursor plasma cells (see Chapters 13 and 14). This suggests a transfer of information-bearing substances (Fig 5–27).

Some antigens must establish contact with macrophages in order to stimulate the production of antibody-forming plasma cells. Other antigens act directly on plasma cell precursors (B lymphocytes). In such instances, the resulting plasma cells synthesize antibodies without assistance from macrophages. Plasma cells seldom divide; their average life is 10–20 days.

Adipose Cells

Adipose cells (adipocytes; from Latin, *adeps*, fat, + Greek, *kytos*) are connective tissue cells that have become specialized for storage of neutral fats or for the production of heat. Often called **fat cells,** they are discussed in detail in Chapter 6.

Leukocytes

Leukocytes (from Greek, *leukos*, white, + *kytos*) or white blood corpuscles, are frequently found in connective tissue. In general, they migrate across capillary and venule walls from the blood. There is a continuous movement of leukocytes from blood to connective tissue, and this process (diapedesis) increases greatly during inflammation. These cells do not move back into the blood after having resided in connective tissue.

A. Neutrophils: These cells are characterized by the variable lobulation of their nuclei. They exhibit 2 types of granules containing both enzyme and nonenzyme proteins that function mainly in the killing and digestion of bacteria. Neutrophils are attracted to sites of acute inflammation and form cell aggregates that are characteristic of specific types of inflammation. Accumulations of dead neutrophils form pus.

B. Eosinophils: The main morphologic characteristics of eosinophils (from Greek, *eos*, dawn, + *philein*) are the eosinophilic granules in their cytoplasm (lysosomes). Electron-microscope examination shows that these granules are membrane-bound and, in their interior, possess a flat crystalloid embedded in a granular substance. The nucleus of these cells usually has 2 lobes (Fig 5–28).

The number of eosinophils increases during the course of allergic, parasitic, and other types of diseases.

The injection of antigenic protein causes an increase in the number of eosinophils in the injected area. This attraction is due to the complex formed by the reaction of the injected protein and its antibody. The antigen-antibody complex is promptly phagocytosed by eosinophils, although these cells are not very active in the phagocytosis of bacteria and foreign particles.

Substances secreted by eosinophils are involved in allergic reactions. Both mast cells and basophils release **eosinophil chemotactic factors** (ECF-A and ECF-C) that attract these cells to allergic inflammatory areas. Under these conditions, eosinophils release the enzymes **arylsulfatase** and **histaminase** (probably from their granules), which cleave 2 of the main mediators involved in the allergic reaction, leukotriene C (formerly known as SRS-A) and histamine. Eosinophils thus can exert a negative feedback control in allergic processes not only by removing the antigen-antibody complexes through phagocytosis but also by hydrolyzing mediators.

C. Basophils: Basophils are a form of leukocyte that contains granules similar in composition and function to those of mast cells. Basophils, the only source of histamine in blood, also play a role in allergic phenomena. Blood from allergic individuals releases histamine when placed in contact with allergens.

D. Lymphocytes: Connective tissue lymphocytes (from Latin, *lympha*, + Greek, *kytos*) have a diameter of 6–8 μm (small lymphocytes). They have a small amount of slightly basophilic cytoplasm and a

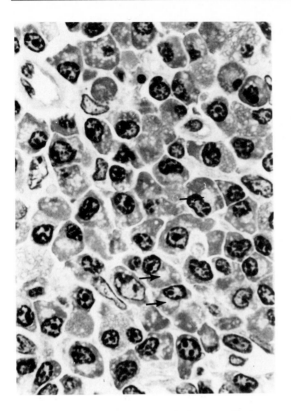

Figure 5–26. Photomicrograph of plasma cells (arrowheads). Observe the coarse chromatin and light juxtanuclear area corresponding to the region of the Golgi complex and centriole. Compare with Figs 5–24 and 5–25. × 600.

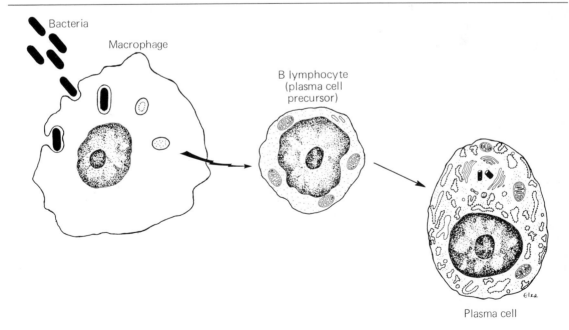

Bacteria

Macrophage

B lymphocyte (plasma cell precursor)

Plasma cell

Figure 5–27. Possible relationships between macrophages and plasma cells. It has been shown that some kind of information passes from macrophages to plasma cell precursors.

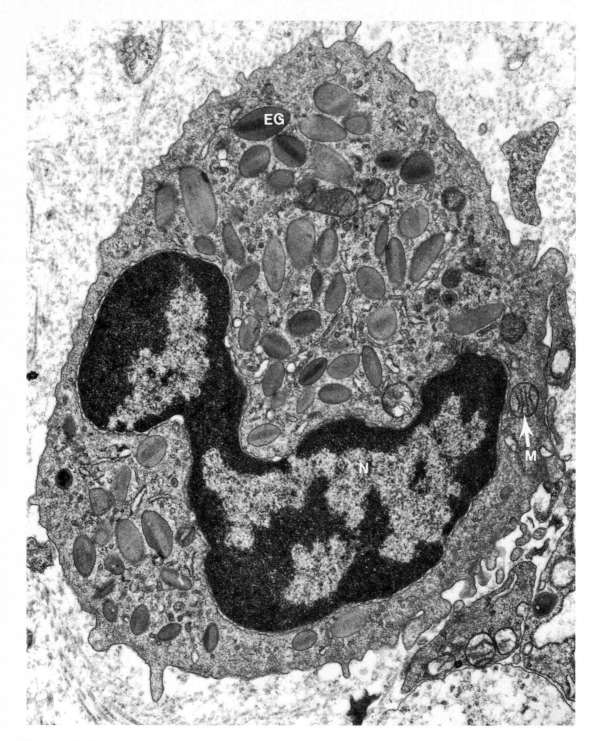

Figure 5–28. Electron micrograph of an eosinophil from human connective tissue. Typical eosinophilic granules are clearly seen. Each granule has a disk-shaped electron-dense crystal that appears surrounded by a matrix enveloped by a unit membrane. EG, eosinophil granule; N, nucleus; M, mitochondria. × 20,000.

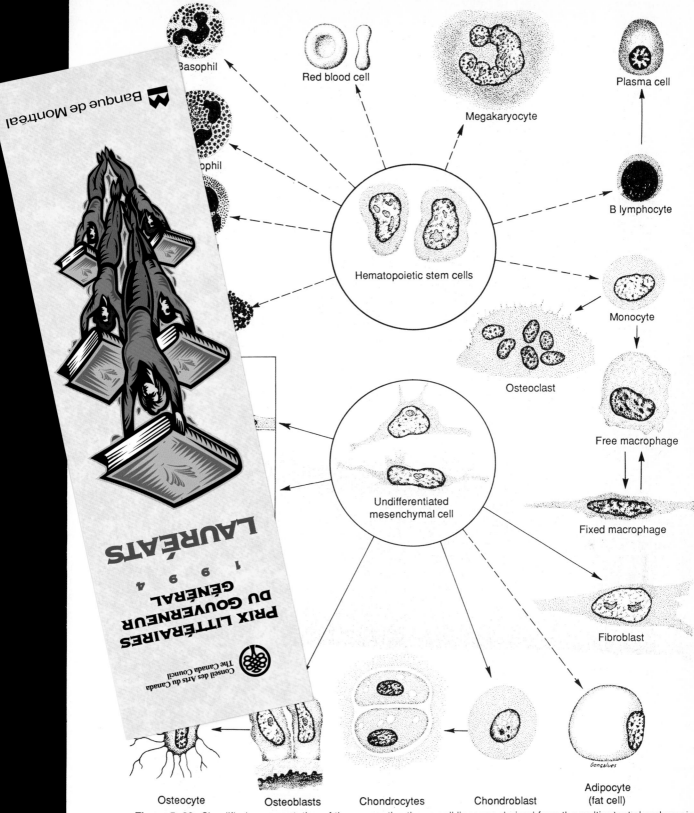

Basophil

Red blood cell

Megakaryocyte

Plasma cell

...ophil

Hematopoietic stem cells

B lymphocyte

Monocyte

Osteoclast

Free macrophage

Undifferentiated
mesenchymal cell

Fixed macrophage

Fibroblast

Gonçalves

Osteocyte

Osteoblasts

Chondrocytes

Chondroblast

Adipocyte
(fat cell)

Figure 5–29. Simplified representation of the connective tissue cell lineages derived from the multipotential embryonic mesenchyme cell. Dotted arrows indicate that intermediate cell types exist between the examples illustrated. The 2 cells in the rectangle are epithelial cells that still maintain some mesenchymal characteristics. Note that the cells are not drawn in proportion to actual sizes (eg, adipocyte, megakaryocyte, and osteoclast cells are significantly larger than other illustrated cells).

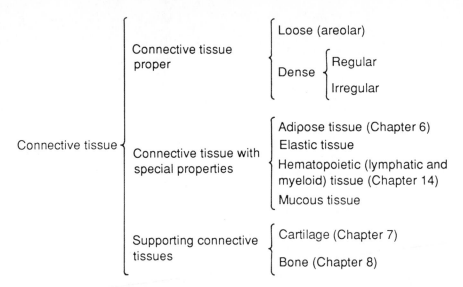

Figure 5–30. Simplified scheme classifying the principal types of connective tissue. These are discussed in the chapters indicated.

large, dark nucleus with condensed chromatin that sometimes shows an indentation. The nucleolus is not visible under the light microscope.

The lymphocytes of connective tissue represent a heterogeneous population. Some have a long life span (many months to several years), whereas others live for only a short time (a few days or weeks). Two main functional types have been recognized: the **T lymphocytes,** which are responsible for initiating cell-mediated immune responses and have a long life; and the **B lymphocytes,** which, when stimulated by an antigen, divide several times and generate plasma cells that in turn secrete antibodies specific to the antigen. Lymphocytes, which are found in large numbers, are characteristic of sites of chronic inflammation.

The relationships among cells found in different types of connective tissue are shown in Fig 5–29. For further discussions of lymphocytes, see Chapters 12, 13, and 14.

TYPES OF CONNECTIVE TISSUE

There are several types of connective tissue that consist of the basic components already described—fibers, cells, and ground substance. The names given to the different types denote either the component that predominates in the tissue or a structural characteristic of the tissue. Note that the classification shown in Fig 5–30 does not include all possible types of connective tissue.

Connective Tissue Proper

There are 2 classes of connective tissue proper: loose and dense.

A. Loose Connective Tissue: This tissue, also called **areolar** tissue, is the more abundant of the 2 types. It fills spaces between fibers and muscle sheaths, supports epithelial tissue, and forms a layer that ensheathes the lymphatic and blood vessels. Loose connective tissue is also found in the papillary layer of the dermis, in the hypodermis, in the serosal linings of peritoneal and pleural cavities, and in glands and the mucous membranes (wet membranes that line the hollow organs) supporting the epithelial cells.

Loose connective tissue comprises all the main components of connective tissue proper (Fig 5–31). The most numerous cells are fibroblasts and macrophages, but all the other types of connective tissue cells are present also. Collagen, elastic, and reticular fibers appear in this tissue, though the proportion of reticular fibers is small. A major constituent of loose connective tissue is the amorphous ground substance.

Loose connective tissue has a delicate consistency; it is flexible, very well vascularized, and not very resistant to stress.

B. Dense Connective Tissue: This type of tissue consists of the same components found in loose connective tissue, but there is a clear predominance of collagen fibers and fewer cells. Dense connective tissue is less flexible and far more resistant to stress than is loose connective tissue. It is known as **dense irregular** connective tissue when the collagen fibers are arranged in bundles without a definite orientation. The collagen fibers form a 3-dimensional network in this tissue and provide resistance to stress from all directions (Fig 5–32). This type of tissue is encountered in such areas as the dermis.

The collagen bundles of **dense regular** connective

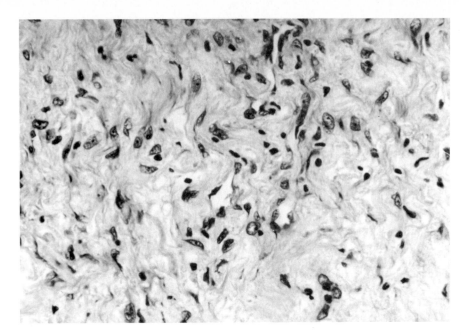

Figure 5–31. Section of loose connective tissue. Note the abundance of cells, most of which are fibroblasts. × 400.

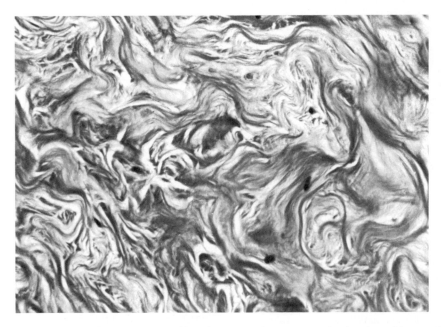

Figure 5–32. Dense irregular connective tissue. This tissue contains many randomly oriented large collagen fibers, sparse ground substance, and few cells. H&E stain, × 320.

tissue are arranged according to a definite pattern. The collagen fibers of this tissue are formed in response to prolonged stresses exerted in the same direction; they consequently offer great resistance to traction forces.

Tendons are the most common example of dense regular connective tissue. These elongated cylindrical structures attach striated muscle to bone; they are white and inextensible by virtue of their richness in collagen fibers. They have parallel, closely packed bundles of collagen separated by a small quantity of amorphous intercellular substance. Their fibrocytes contain elongated nuclei parallel to the fibers and sparse cytoplasmic folds that envelop portions of the collagen bundles. Their cytoplasm is rarely revealed in hematoxylin and eosin stains—not only because it is sparse but also because it stains the same color as the fibers (Figs 5–33 and 5–34).

The collagen bundles of the tendons (primary bundles) aggregate into larger bundles (secondary bundles) that are enveloped by loose connective tissue containing blood vessels and nerves. Externally, the tendon is surrounded by a sheath of dense connective tissue. In some tendons, this sheath is made up of 2

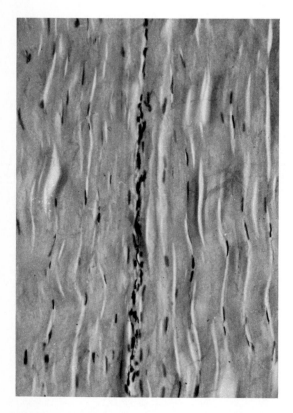

Figure 5–33. Dense regular connective tissue (longitudinal section through a tendon). There are numerous collagen bundles in parallel array, and fibrocyte nuclei are seen between the collagen bundles. H&E stain, × 320.

layers, both lined by squamous cells of mesenchymal origin. One layer is fixed to the tendon, and the other lines the neighboring structures. A cavity containing a viscous fluid (similar to synovial fluid) is formed between the 2 layers. This fluid, which contains water, proteins, glycosaminoglycans, glycoproteins, and ions, is a lubricant that permits an easy sliding movement of the tendon within its sheath.

Elastic Tissue

Elastic tissue is composed of bundles of thick, parallel elastic fibers. The space between these fibers is occupied by thin collagen fibers and flattened fibroblasts. The abundance of elastic fibers in this tissue confers on it a typical yellow color and great elasticity. Elastic tissue, which occurs infrequently, is present in the yellow ligaments of the vertebral column and in the suspensory ligament of the penis.

Reticular Tissue

Reticular tissue is a specialized loose connective tissue variation that provides the architectural framework of the myeloid (bone marrow) and lymphoid (lymph nodules and nodes, spleen) hematopoietic (often spelled hemopoietic) organs. In this form of connective tissue, **reticular cells** elaborate a fine matrix of branched reticular fibers. Reticular cells are simply fibroblasts specialized for secreting the constituents of reticular fibers. The reticular cells are dispersed along this matrix and ensheathe the reticular fibers and ground substance with cytoplasmic processes. The resulting cell-lined trabecular system creates a spongelike structure (Fig 5–35) within which cells and fluids of a given organ are readily mobile.

In addition to the reticular cells, cells of the mononuclear phagocyte system are strategically dispersed along the trabeculae. These cells monitor the flow of materials through the sinuslike spaces and phagocytotically remove antigens and other forms of cellular debris.

Mucous Tissue

Mucous tissue has an abundance of amorphous ground substance composed chiefly of hyaluronic acid. It is a jellylike tissue containing collagen fibers and a few elastic or reticular fibers. The cells in this tissue are mainly fibroblasts. Mucous tissue is the principal component of the umbilical cord, where it is referred to as **Wharton's jelly.** It is also found in the pulp of young teeth.

HISTOPHYSIOLOGY

Connective tissues have the functions of support, packing, storage, transport, defense, and repair. The functions of support and packing are obvious—epithelial, muscular, and nerve tissues are associated with connective tissue that supports and fills the

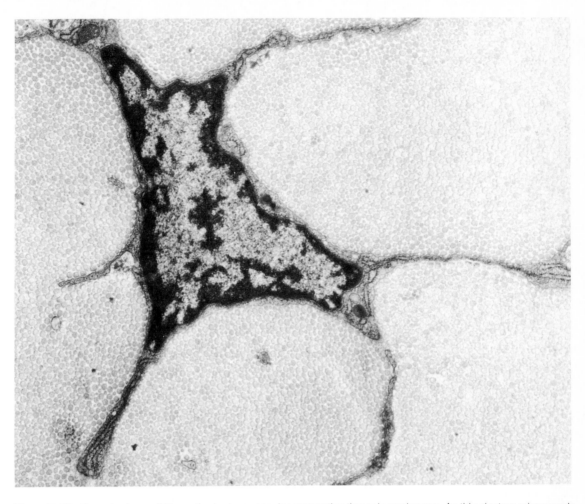

Figure 5–34. The cytoplasm of fibrocytes in dense regular connective tissue is rarely seen. As this electron micrograph reveals, the sparse cytoplasm of the fibrocyte is subdivided into numerous thin cytoplasmic processes that interdigitate among the coarse collagen fibers. Note that the thick collagen fibers are composed of smaller parallel collagen fibrils of various diameters. × 25,000.

tissue spaces between their cells. The support function is carried out mainly by connective tissue fibers.

Fibers, predominantly composed of collagen, constitute tendons, aponeuroses, capsules of organs, and membranes that envelop the central nervous system (meninges). They also make up the trabeculae and walls inside several organs, forming the most resistant component of the stroma (support tissue) of these organs.

Storage

Lipids, which are important nutritional reserves, are stored in adipose tissue (see Chapter 6). In addition, because of its richness in glycosaminoglycans, loose connective tissue stores water and electrolytes. The most abundant electrolyte is sodium. Although only a small percentage of connective tissue consists

of plasma proteins, it is estimated that because of its wide distribution as much as one-third of the plasma proteins of the body are stored in the intercellular connective tissue matrix.

Defense

Several defense mechanisms depend upon the cells and intercellular components of connective tissue. This tissue contains a number of cell types, each with several functions (summarized in Table 5–4), creating a complex network of activities that can initiate and regulate defense mechanisms in the body. One of these important mechanisms has been extensively studied; it is called **inflammation.**

This process is a vascular and cellular defen-

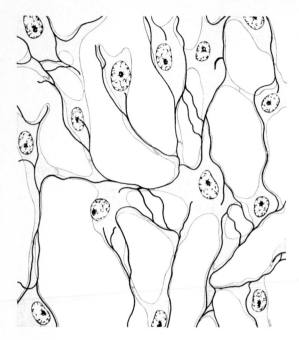

Figure 5–35. Schematic drawing of reticular connective tissue showing only the fixed cells and the fibers (free cells are not represented). Reticular fibers are enveloped by the cytoplasm of reticular cells; the fibers, however, are extracellular, being separated from the cytoplasm by the cell membrane. Within the sinuslike spaces, cells and tissue fluids of the organ are freely mobile.

sive reaction against foreign substances, in most cases, against pathogenic bacteria or irritating chemical substances. The classic signs of inflammation were first enunciated by Celsus (first century AD) as redness and swelling with heat and pain (rubor et tumor cum calore et dolore). Much later, disturbed function (functio laesa) was added as the fifth cardinal sign.

Inflammation begins with local release of **chemical mediators of inflammation,** substances of different origin (mainly from cells and blood plasma proteins) that induce the main events characteristic of this reaction, eg, **increase of blood flow** and **vascular permeability, chemotaxis,** and **phagocytosis.**

Increase of vascular permeability is caused by the action of vasoactive substances; an example is histamine, which is liberated from mast cells and basophilic leukocytes. Histamine promotes the permeability of endothelial cells, mainly in capillaries and venules (see Chapter 11). Increases of vascular flow and permeability are responsible for local swelling (edema), redness, and heat. Pain is due mainly to the action of chemical mediators. **Chemotaxis** (from Greek, *chemeia,* alchemy, + *taxis,* orderly arrange-

ment), the phenomenon by which specific cell types are attracted by chemical substances, is responsible for the migration of large quantities of specific cell types to regions of inflammation.

As a consequence of chemotaxis, leukocytes cross the walls of venules and capillaries, invading the inflamed area. This migration is called **diapedesis.**

During the initial or **acute phase** of inflammation, the neutrophils predominate; when the inflammation persists and enters the **chronic phase,** the cell population changes. The main types of cells in the chronic phase are lymphocytes and macrophages, which come from the blood, and plasma cells, which originate from B lymphocytes. Macrophages in the area of inflammation represent wandering connective tissue cells that have migrated to that site, or they may differentiate from monocytes that arrive via the circulation.

The cells in the inflamed area engulf the remains of the cells and fibers altered by this process and participate in the production of antibodies against invading microorganisms. Surrounding connective tissue frequently forms a retaining fibrous wall, or capsule, around the inflammation.

Repair

Connective tissue has great regenerative capacity, and the areas destroyed by inflammation or traumatic injury are easily repaired. The spaces left by injuries to tissues whose cells do not divide (eg, cardiac muscle) are filled by connective tissue, which forms a scar. The healing of surgical incisions depends on the reparative capacity of connective tissue. The main cell involved in repair is the fibroblast.

Transport

There is a close association between blood capillaries, lymphatic capillaries, and connective tissue. These vessels, except in nerve tissue, are always ensheathed by connective tissue. Consequently, the connective tissue carries nutrients from the blood to various tissues in the body and moves metabolic wastes from the cells to the blood.

Hormonal Effects

Different hormones influence the metabolism of connective tissue. An example is the hormone **cortisol (hydrocortisone),** which is produced by the cortical layer of the adrenal gland and inhibits the synthesis of fibers by connective tissue cells. **Adrenocorticotropic hormone (ACTH),** released by the pituitary, which stimulates the production of cortisol, has the same effect. Injection of either cortisol or ACTH has a detrimental effect on wound healing. These hormones suppress or attenuate the inflammatory process; their action is also directed against the cells of the connective tissue (lymphocytes, plasma cells, etc).

Hypothyroidism causes an accumulation of glycosaminoglycans in connective tissues. Adult hypothyroidism is called **myxedema (mucous edema)** and is associated with an excess of glycosaminoglycans in the connective tissue.

Nutritional Factors

Vitamin C (ascorbic acid) deficiency leads to **scurvy,** a disease characterized by generalized degeneration of connective tissue. In the absence of this vitamin, fibroblasts synthesize defective collagen and the defective fibers are not replaced. This leads to a generalized degeneration of connective tissue that becomes more pronounced in areas where collagen renewal takes place at a faster rate. The periodontal ligament that holds teeth in their sockets exhibits a relatively high collagen turnover; consequently, this ligament is markedly affected by scurvy, which leads to a loss of teeth. Some bacteria of the genus *Clostridium* that cause gas gangrene produce collagenase, which greatly increases the invasive power of these microorganisms. Ascorbic acid is a cofactor for proline hydroxylase, which is essential for the normal synthesis of collagen. In this step of hydroxylation, iron, molecular oxygen, and α-ketoglutarate are also necessary. Changes in the concentration of these substances within the cell also influence the rate of collagen biosynthesis. The roles of vitamins A, C, and D in connective tissue are also discussed in Chapter 8.

Renewal of Collagen

Collagen is a stable protein, and its renewal is very slow. Its **turnover rate** is different in different anatomic structures. The collagen of tendons is renewed very slowly or not at all, whereas the collagen of loose connective tissue is renewed more rapidly.

REFERENCES

Deyl Z, Adam M: *Connective Tissue Research: Chemistry, Biology and Physiology,* Riss, 1981.

Gay S, Miller EJ: *Collagen in the Physiology and Pathology of Connective Tissue.* Gustav Fischer, 1978.

Hay ED (editor): *Cell Biology of Extracellular Matrix.* Plenum, 1982.

Junqueira LCU, Montes GS: Biology of collagen proteoglycan interaction. *Arch Histol Jpn* 1983;**46:**589.

Kefalides NA, Alper R, Clark CC: Biochemistry and metabolism of basement membranes. *Int Rev Cytol* 1979;**61:**167.

Krstić RV: *Illustrated Encyclopedia of Human Histology.* Springer-Verlag, 1984.

Mathews MB: *Connective Tissue, Macromolecular Structure and Evolution.* Springer-Verlag, 1975.

Montes GS et al: Collagen distribution in tissues. In: *Ultrastructure of the Connective Tissue Matrix.* Ruggieri A, Motta PM (editors). Martinus Nijhoff, 1984.

Prockop DJ et al: The biosynthesis of collagen and its disorders. *N Engl J Med* 1979;**301:**13.

Sandberg LB et al: Elastin structure, biosynthesis, and relation to disease state. *N Engl J Med* 1981;**304:**556.

Van Furth R (editor): *Mononuclear Phagocytes: Functional Aspects.* 2 vols. Martinus Nijhoff, 1980.

6

Adipose Tissue

Adipose tissue is a special type of connective tissue in which adipose cells **(adipocytes)** predominate. These cells can be found isolated or in small groups within the connective tissue itself; most are found in large aggregates, making up the adipose tissue spread throughout the body. Adipose tissue is, in a sense, one of the largest organs in the body. In men of normal weight, adipose tissue represents 15–20% of the body weight; in women of normal weight, 20–25% of body weight.

Adipose tissue is the largest repository of energy (in the form of triglycerides) in the body. The other organs that store energy (in the form of glycogen) are the liver and skeletal muscle. Since eating is a periodic activity and the supply of glycogen is limited, there must be a large store of calories that can be mobilized between meals. Because triglycerides are of lower density than glycogen and have a higher caloric value (9.3 kcal/g for triglycerides versus 4.1 kcal/g for carbohydrates), adipose tissue is a very efficient storage tissue. It is in a state of continuous turnover and is sensitive to both nervous and hormonal stimuli. Subcutaneous layers of adipose tissue help to shape the surface of the body, while deposits in the form of pads act as shock absorbers, chiefly in the soles and palms. Since fat is a poor heat conductor, it contributes to the thermal insulation of the body. Adipose tissue also fills up spaces between other tissues and helps to keep some organs in position.

There are 2 known types of adipose tissue; they present different localizations, structures, colors, and pathologies. **Unilocular (common** or **yellow)** adipose tissue is composed of cells that when completely developed contain one large central droplet of yellow fat in their cytoplasm. **Multilocular** (or **brown) adipose tissue** is composed of cells that contain numerous lipid droplets and abundant, brown mitochondria. Both types of adipose tissue have a rich blood supply.

UNILOCULAR ADIPOSE TISSUE

Cells of this tissue have only one large fat vacuole; they are the main energy depot for the organism.

The color of unilocular adipose tissue varies from white to dark yellow, depending on the diet; it is due

mainly to the presence of carotenoids dissolved in fat droplets of the cells. Almost all adipose tissue in adults is of this type. It is found throughout the human body except for the eyelids, the penis, the scrotum, and all of the auricle of the external ear but the lobule. The distribution and density of adipose deposits are determined by age and sex.

In the newborn, unilocular adipose tissue has a uniform thickness throughout the body. As the baby matures, it tends to disappear from some parts of the body and increase in others, since its distribution is partly regulated by sex hormones and adrenocortical hormones, which control the accumulation of fat and are largely responsible for male or female body contour.

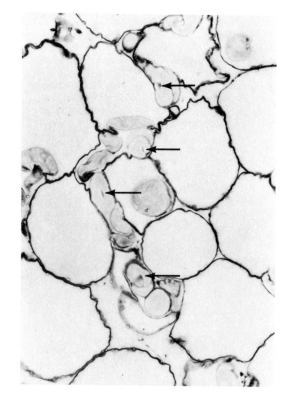

Figure 6–1. Photomicrograph of unilocular adipose tissue. The arrows show blood capillaries. H&E stain.

126

Histologic Structure

Unilocular adipose cells are spherical when isolated but are polyhedral in adipose tissue, where they are closely packed. Each cell is between 50 and 150 μm in diameter. Since lipid droplets are removed by the alcohol and xylol used in routine histologic techniques, each cell appears in standard microscope preparations as a thin ring of cytoplasm surrounding the vacuole left by the dissolved lipid droplet—the **signet ring cell.** Consequently, these cells have eccentric and flattened nuclei (Fig 6–1). The rim of cytoplasm that remains after removal of the stored triglycerides (neutral fats) may rupture and collapse, distorting the tissue structure.

The thickest portion of the cytoplasm surrounds the nucleus of these cells and contains a Golgi complex, filamentous and ovoid mitochondria, poorly developed cisternae of the rough endoplasmic reticulum, and free polyribosomes. The rim of cytoplasm surrounding the lipid droplet contains vesicles of smooth endoplasmic reticulum, occasional microtubules, and numerous pinocytotic vesicles. Electron-microscope studies reveal that each adipose cell usually possesses minute lipid droplets in addition to the single large one seen with the light microscope; the droplets are not surrounded by a membrane. Each adipose cell is surrounded by a basal lamina.

Unilocular adipose tissue is subdivided into incomplete lobules by a partition of connective tissue containing a rich vascular bed and network of nerves. Reticular fibers form a fine interwoven network that supports individual fat cells and binds them together.

Although blood vessels are not always apparent, adipose tissue is richly vascularized. Considering the amount of cytoplasm that exists in fat cells, the ratio of blood volume to cytoplasm volume is greater in adipose tissue than in striated muscle.

Histophysiology

The lipids stored in adipose cells are chiefly triglycerides, ie, esters of fatty acids and glycerol. Fatty acids stored by these cells have their origin in dietary fats that are brought to adipose tissue cells in the form of chylomicron triglycerides, in triglycerides synthesized in the liver and transported to adipose tissue in the form of **very low density lipoproteins** (VLDL), and by synthesis of free fatty acids and glycerol from glucose to form triglycerides in adipose cells.

Chylomicrons (from Greek, *chylos,* juice, + *micros,* small) are particles up to 3 μm in diameter formed in intestinal epithelial cells and transported in blood plasma and mesenteric lymph. They consist of a central core composed mainly of triglycerides and a small quantity of cholesterol esters surrounded by a

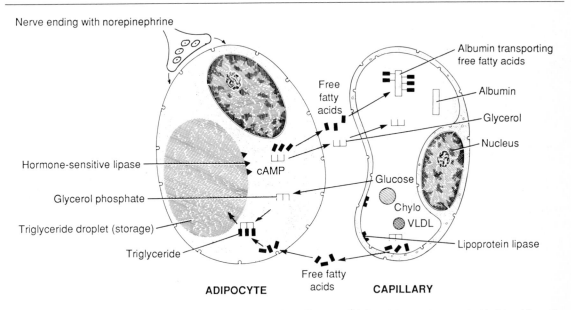

Figure 6–2. The process of lipid storage and release by the adipocyte. Triglycerides are transported in blood from the intestine and liver by lipoproteins known as chylomicrons (Chylo) and very low density lipoproteins (VLDL). In adipose tissue capillaries, these lipoproteins are partly broken down by lipoprotein lipase, releasing free fatty acids and glycerol. The free fatty acids diffuse from the capillary into the adipocyte, where they are reesterified to glycerol phosphate, forming triglycerides. These resulting triglycerides are stored in droplets until needed. Norepinephrine from nerve endings stimulates the cyclic AMP (cAMP) system (see Fig 4–16), which activates hormone-sensitive lipase. This hydrolyzes stored triglycerides to free fatty acids and glycerol. These latter substances diffuse into the capillary, where free fatty acids are bound to the hydrophobic moeity of albumin for transport to distant sites for use as an energy source.

stabilizing monolayer consisting of apolipoproteins, cholesterol, and phospholipids. Very low density lipoproteins have proportionately more lipid in their surface layer because they are smaller (greater surface-to-volume ratio), have different apolipoproteins at the surface, and contain a higher proportion of cholesterol esters to triglycerides when compared with chylomicrons. Chylomicrons and VLDL are hydrolyzed at the luminal surfaces of blood capillaries of adipose tissue by lipoprotein lipase, an enzyme synthesized by the adipocyte and transferred to the capillary cell membrane. Free fatty acids enter the adipocyte by mechanisms that are not completely understood. An active transport system as well as free diffusion seem to be involved. It is probable that the numerous pinocytotic vesicles seen at the surfaces of adipocytes are not involved. The fatty acids cross the following layers in passing from the endothelium into the adipose cell: (1) capillary endothelium, (2) capillary basal lamina, (3) connective tissue ground substance, (4) adipocyte basal lamina, and (5) adipocyte plasma membrane. The movement of fatty acids across the cytoplasm into the lipid droplet is incompletely understood but may utilize specific carrier proteins (Fig 6–2). Within the adipocyte, the fatty acids combine with an intermediate product of glucose metabolism, glycerol phosphate, to form triglyceride molecules. These are then deposited in the triglyceride droplets. Mitochondria and smooth endoplasmic reticulum are organelles that participate actively in the process of lipid uptake and storage.

Adipose cells can synthesize fatty acids from glucose, a process accelerated by insulin. Insulin also stimulates the uptake of glucose into the adipose cells and increases the synthesis of lipoprotein lipase.

Stored lipids are mobilized by humoral and neurogenic mechanisms, resulting in the liberation of fatty acids and glycerol into the blood. An enzyme known as **hormone-sensitive lipase** (triglyceride lipase) is activated by adenylate cyclase when the tissue is stimulated by norepinephrine. Norepinephrine is liberated at the endings of the postganglionic sympathetic nerves present in adipose tissue. The activated enzyme breaks down triglyceride molecules located mainly at the surface of the lipid droplets. The relatively insoluble fatty acids are transported in association with serum albumin to other tissues of the body, while the more soluble glycerol remains free and is taken up by the liver.

Growth hormone, glucocorticoids, prolactin, corticotropin, insulin, and thyroid hormone also have roles in different steps in the metabolism of adipose tissue.

Under circumstances of bodily need, mobilization of lipids does not occur in uniform proportion in all parts of the body. Subcutaneous, mesenteric, and retroperitoneal deposits are the first to be mobilized, while adipose tissue in the hands, feet, and retroorbital fat pads resists long periods of starvation. After such periods, unilocular adipose tissue loses nearly all its fat and becomes a tissue containing polyhedral or spindle-shaped cells with very few lipid droplets. These cells remain as quiescent adipocytes and do not modulate into fibroblasts or other types of connective tissue cells.

Both the unilocular and multilocular adipose tissues are richly innervated by the sympathetic division of the autonomic nervous system. In unilocular adipose tissue, nerve endings are found only in the walls of blood vessels; the adipocytes are not directly innervated. Multilocular fat cells do receive direct sympathetic innervation: Release of the neurotransmitter (norepinephrine) activates the hormone-sensitive lipase described above. This innervation plays an important role in the mobilization of fats when the body is subjected to long periods of fasting or severe cold.

Obesity in adults may result from an excessive accumulation of fat in unilocular tissue cells that become larger than usual (**hypertrophic obesity**). An increase in the number of adipocytes causes **hyperplastic obesity.**

Histogenesis

Adipose cells develop from mesenchymally derived lipoblasts. These cells have the appearance of

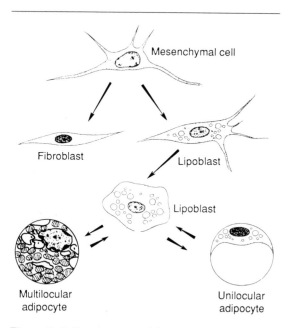

Figure 6–3. Development of fat cells. Undifferentiated mesenchymal cells are transformed into lipoblasts that accumulate fat and thus give rise to mature fat cells. When a large amount of lipid is mobilized by the body, mature unilocular fat cells return to the lipoblast stage. Undifferentiated mesenchymal cells also give rise to a variety of other cell types, including fibroblasts. The mature fat cell is actually larger than shown here in relation to the other cell types in this illustration.

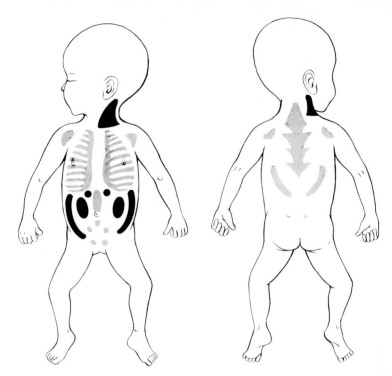

Figure 6–4. Distribution of adipose tissue. In a human newborn, multilocular adipose tissue constitutes 2–5% of the body weight and is distributed as shown. The black areas indicate multilocular adipose tissue; shaded areas, a mixture of multilocular and unilocular adipose tissue. (Modified, redrawn, and reproduced, with permission, from Merklin RJ: Growth and distribution of human fetal brown fat. *Anat Rec* 1974;**178**:637.)

fibroblasts but are able to accumulate fat in their cytoplasm. Lipid accumulations are at first isolated from one another but soon fuse to form the single larger droplet that is characteristic of unilocular tissue cells (Fig 6–3). Lipoblasts or immature adipose cells that contain more than one lipid droplet are said to be in the multilocular stage.

The human being is one of the few mammals born with fat stores; they begin to accumulate at the 30th week of gestation. After birth, the development of new adipose cells is common mainly around small blood vessels, where undifferentiated mesenchymal cells are usually found.

It is believed that during a finite postnatal period, nutritional and other influences can cause an increase in the number of adipocytes, but the cells do not increase in number after that period. They accumulate more lipid only under conditions of excess caloric intake (overfeeding). This early increase in the number of adipocytes may predispose an individual to hyperplastic obesity in later life.

MULTILOCULAR ADIPOSE TISSUE

Cells of this tissue have several fat vacuoles and transform stored chemical energy to heat when stimulated.

Multilocular adipose tissue is also called **brown fat** because of its color, which is due to both the large number of blood capillaries in this tissue and the numerous mitochondria (containing colored cytochromes) in the cells. Unlike unilocular tissue, which is present throughout the body, brown adipose tissue has a more limited distribution because it is more abundant in hibernating animals, it was improperly called the **hibernating gland.**

In rats and several other mammals, this tissue is found mainly about the shoulder girdle. In the human embryo and the newborn, multilocular adipose tissue is encountered in several areas and remains restricted to these locations after birth (Fig 6–4). It is greatly reduced in adulthood. The function of this tissue in humans appears to be of importance mainly in the first months of postnatal life, when it produces heat and thus protects the newborn against cold.

Histologic Structure

Multilocular tissue cells are polygonal and smaller than cells of unilocular adipose tissue. Their cytoplasm contains a great number of lipid droplets of different sizes (Figs 6–5 and 6–6), a spherical and central nucleus, and numerous mitochondria with abundant long cristae.

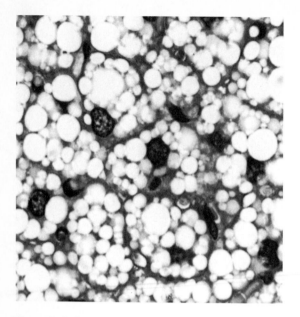

Figure 6–5. Photomicrograph of multilocular adipose tissue with its characteristic cells containing central spherical nuclei and multiple lipid droplets. × 1000.

Multilocular adipose tissue resembles an endocrine gland in that its cells assume an almost epithelial arrangement of closely packed masses associated with blood capillaries. This tissue is subdivided by partitions of connective tissue into lobules that are better delineated than in unilocular adipose tissue lobules. Cells of this tissue receive direct sympathetic innervation.

Histophysiology

The physiology of multilocular adipose tissue is understood best in the study of hibernating species.

In animals ending their hibernation period, or in newborn mammals (including humans) who are exposed to a cold environment, nerve impulses liberate norepinephrine into the tissue. This neurotransmitter activates the hormone-sensitive lipase present in adipose cells, promoting hydrolysis of triglycerides to fatty acids and glycerol. Liberated fatty acids are metabolized with a consequent increase in oxygen consumption and heat production, elevating the temperature of the tissue and warming the blood passing through it. Heat production is increased, because the mitochondria in cells of this tissue have a transmem-

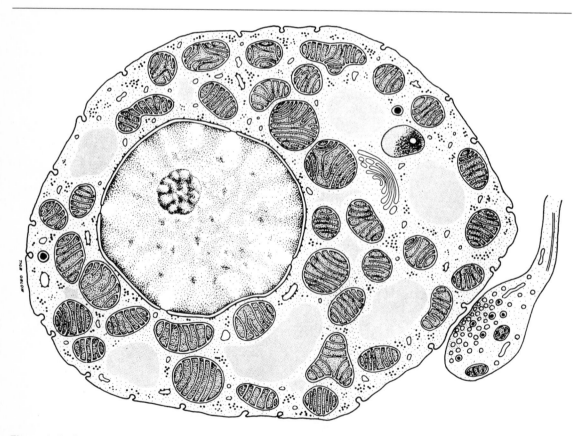

Figure 6–6. Drawing of multiocular adipose tissue. Observe the central nucleus, multiple fat droplets, and abundant mitochondria. Sympathetic nerve ending is present at the lower right.

brane protein called **thermogenin** in their inner membrane. This protein permits the backflow of protons previously transported to the intermembranous space without passing through the ATP synthetase system in the mitochondrial globular units. Consequently, the energy generated by proton flow is not used to synthesize ATP but is dissipated as heat. Warmed blood circulates throughout the body, heating it and carrying fatty acids not metabolized in the adipose tissue. These will be utilized by other organs.

> Thermogenin is reduced in quantity in obese animals and increased in animals submitted to low temperatures. Its increase may explain the presence of individuals who seem to be able to overeat without becoming obese and, conversely, its reduction may be related to obesity.

Histogenesis

Multilocular adipose tissue develops differently from unilocular tissue. The mesenchymal cells that constitute this tissue resemble epithelium (thus suggesting an endocrine gland) before they accumulate fat. Apparently there is no formation of multilocular adipose tissue after birth, nor is one type of adipose tissue transformed into another.

Tumors of Adipose Tissues

> Unilocular adipocytes can generate very common benign tumors called **lipomas.** Malignant adipocyte-derived tumors **(liposarcomas)** are among the more common tumors of connective tissue. Tumors of the multilocular adipose cells **(hibernomas)** have also been described.

REFERENCES

Angel A, Hollenberg CH, Roncari DAK (editors): *The Adipocyte and Obesity: Cellular and Molecular Mechanisms.* Raven Press, 1983.

Napolitano L: The differentiation of white adipose cells: An electron microscope study. *J Cell Biol* 1963;**18**:663.

Nedergaard J, Lindberg O: The brown fat cell. *Int Rev Cytol* 1982;**74**:310.

Renold AE, Cahill GF Jr (editors): *Handbook of Physiology.* Section 5: *Adipose Tissue.* American Physiological Society, 1965.

Slavin BG: The cytophysiology of mammalian adipose cells. *Int Rev Cytol* 1972;**33**:297.

Cartilage

Cartilage tissue is characterized by an extracellular matrix enriched with glycosaminoglycans and proteoglycans. These macromolecules interact with collagen and elastic fibers. Variations in the composition of these matrix components produce 3 types of cartilage.

Cartilage is a specialized form of connective tissue in which the extracellular matrix has a firm consistency. This matrix endows cartilage with the resilience that allows the tissue to bear mechanical stresses without permanent distortion. The main function of cartilage is to support soft tissues. Being smooth-surfaced and resilient, cartilage is a shock-absorbing and sliding area for joints, thus facilitating bone movements. Cartilage is also essential for the development and growth of long bones both before and after birth (see Chapter 8).

Cartilage consists of cells (**chondrocytes;** from Greek, *chondros,* cartilage, + *kytos*) and an extensive **extracellular matrix** composed of fibers and ground substance. Chondrocytes synthesize and secrete the extracellular matrix, and the cells themselves are located in matrix cavities called **lacunae.** Collagen, hyaluronic acid, proteoglycans, and small amounts of several glycoproteins are the principal macromolecules present in all types of cartilage matrix. Elastic cartilage, characterized by its great pliability, contains significant amounts of elastin in the matrix.

Since collagen and elastin are flexible, the firm gel-like consistency of cartilage depends upon electrostatic bonds that occur between collagen fibers and the glycosaminoglycan side chains of matrix proteoglycans. It also depends on the binding of water (solvation water) to the negatively charged glycosaminoglycan chains that extend from the proteoglycan core proteins. An example of the importance of matrix proteoglycans is observed after intravenous injection of papain in rabbits. Within hours after the injection of this protease, the cartilages supporting the ears of these animals lose their turgidity and the ears droop (Fig 7–1, inset). The loss of turgidity is due to digestion of proteoglycan core proteins and the consequent dissolution of glycosaminoglycan side chains (Fig 7–1).

As a consequence of different functional requirements, 3 forms of cartilage have evolved, each exhibiting variations in matrix composition. **Hyaline cartilage,** the most common form, possesses a matrix containing type II as the principal collagen type. The more pliable and distensible **elastic cartilage** possesses, in addition to collagen type II, an abundance of elastic fibers within its matrix. **Fibrocartilage,** present in regions of the body subject to great stress or the demands of weight bearing, is characterized by a matrix containing a dense network of coarse type I collagen fibers.

In all 3 types, cartilage is avascular and is nourished by diffusion of nutrients from capillaries in adjacent connective tissue (perichondrium) or by means of synovial fluid from joint cavities. In some instances, blood vessels traverse a cartilage to nourish other tissues, but these vessels do not supply nutrients to the cartilage. As might be expected of cells in an avascular tissue, chondrocytes exhibit low metabolic activity. Cartilage has no lymphatic vessels or nerves.

The **perichondrium** (Figs 7–2 and 7–5) is a capsulelike sheath of dense connective tissue that surrounds cartilage in most places, forming an interface between the cartilage and the tissue the cartilage supports. The perichondrium harbors the vascular supply for the avascular cartilage. Articular cartilage, which covers the surfaces of the bones of movable joints, is devoid of perichondrium and is sustained by the diffusion of oxygen and nutrients from the synovial fluid.

HYALINE CARTILAGE

Hyaline cartilage (Fig 7–2) is the most common and best studied of the 3 types.

Fresh hyaline cartilage is bluish-white and translucent. In the embryo, it serves as a temporary skeleton until it is gradually replaced by bone. Between the diaphysis and the epiphysis of growing long bones, the **epiphyseal plate,** composed of hyaline cartilage, is responsible for the longitudinal growth of bone (Fig 7–3).

In adult mammals, hyaline cartilage is located in the articular surfaces of the movable joints; the walls of larger respiratory passages (nose, larynx, trachea, bronchi); and the ventral ends of ribs, where they articulate with the sternum.

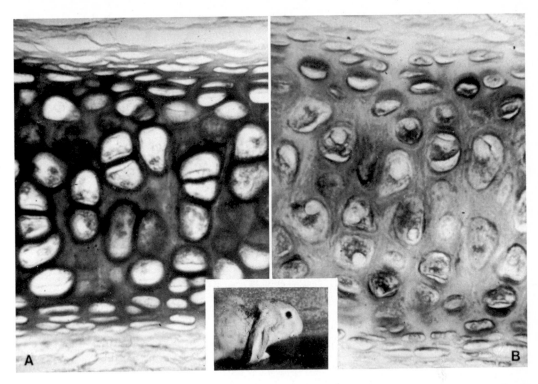

Figure 7–1. Sections of rabbit ear cartilage with its proteoglycan stained by alcian blue. **A** presents a section from a control animal; **B** is from an animal previously injected intravenously with papain, an enzyme that hydrolyzes the proteoglycan moiety of the cartilage matrix. Observe the decrease of proteoglycan content in the cartilage of the injected animal (less-intense staining by alcian blue). **Inset:** The collapsed ear of the papain-injected animal. This experiment dramatically illustrates the functional role of proteoglycans in cartilage matrix. × 600.

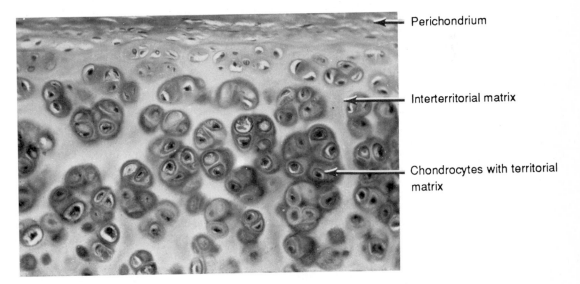

Figure 7–2. Photomicrograph of hyaline cartilage. Most chondrocytes are organized in isogenous groups. An enriched concentration of glycosaminoglycans in the matrix—the territorial, or capsular, matrix—is present around the chondrocytes. The upper part of the figure shows the perichondrium where fibroblasts may differentiate into chondrocytes during cartilage growth. H&E stain, × 300.

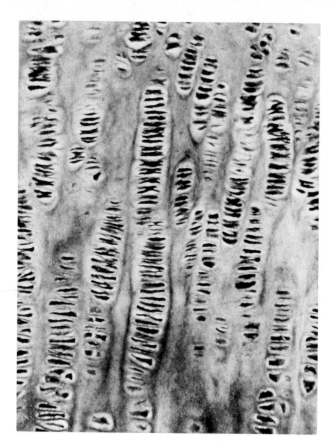

Figure 7–3. Photomicrograph of a portion of the epiphyseal plate cartilage. Large numbers of chondrocytes in the proliferative zone of this cartilage are arranged side by side in parallel columns. H&E stain, × 320.

Matrix

Forty percent of the dry weight of hyaline cartilage consists of collagen embedded in an amorphous intercellular substance. In routine histologic preparations, the collagen is indiscernible from the amorphous substance for 2 reasons: the collagen is in the form of fibrils, which have submicroscopic dimensions; and the refractive index of the fibrils is almost the same as that of the ground substance in which they are embedded.

Although hyaline cartilage fibrils have a 64 nm periodicity, this is not clearly seen in most fibrils from routine sections, for it is masked by its interaction with the proteoglycans (see Fig 5–7). Hyaline cartilage contains primarily type II collagen.

Cartilage proteoglycans contain chondroitin 4-sulfate, chondroitin 6-sulfate, and keratan sulfate, covalently linked to core proteins (Table 7–1). Up to 200 of these proteoglycans are noncovalently associated with long molecules of hyaluronic acid, forming **proteoglycan aggregates** that interact with collagen (Fig 7–4). The aggregates can be up to 4 μm in length. Structurally, proteoglycans resemble bottle brushes, the protein core being the stem and the radiating glycosaminoglycan chains the bristles.

The high content of solvation water bound to the negative charges of glycosaminoglycans acts as a shock absorber or biomechanical spring that is of great functional importance, especially in articular cartilages.

In addition to type II collagen and proteoglycan, an important component of cartilage matrix is the glycoprotein **chondronectin,** a macromolecule that pro-

Table 7–1. Approximate composition of cartilage proteoglycans (average molecular weight = 25 × 10⁶).*

Component	Number of Chains	Molecular Weight	Percent of Dry Weight
Core protein	1	200,000–350,000	7–12
Chondroitin sulfates	100	20,000	85
Keratan sulfate	50	5000	7

* Modified and reproduced, with permission, from Hardingham TE: Structure and associations of proteoglycans in cartilage. In: Amott S, Rees DA, Morris ER: *Molecular Biophysics of the Extracellular Matrix.* Humana Press, 1984.

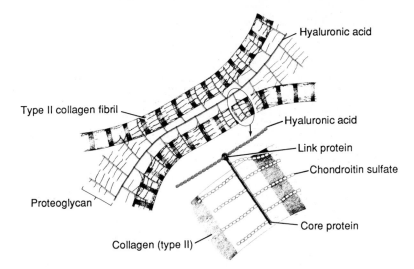

Figure 7–4. Schematic representation of molecular organization in cartilage matrix. Linking proteins noncovalently bind the protein core (lighter color) of proteoglycans to the linear hyaluronic acid molecules (darker color). The chondroitin sulfate side chains of the proteoglycan electrostatically bind to the collagen fibrils, forming a cross-linked matrix. The oval outlines the area enlarged in the lower part of the figure.

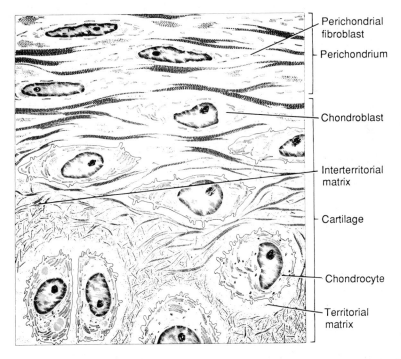

Figure 7–5. Diagram of the area of transition between the perichondrium and hyaline cartilage. As perichondrial cells differentiate into chondrocytes, they become round, with an irregular surface. Cartilage (interterritorial) matrix contains numerous fine collagen fibrils except around the periphery of the chondrocytes, where the matrix consists primarily of glycosaminoglycans; this region is called the capsular, or territorial, matrix.

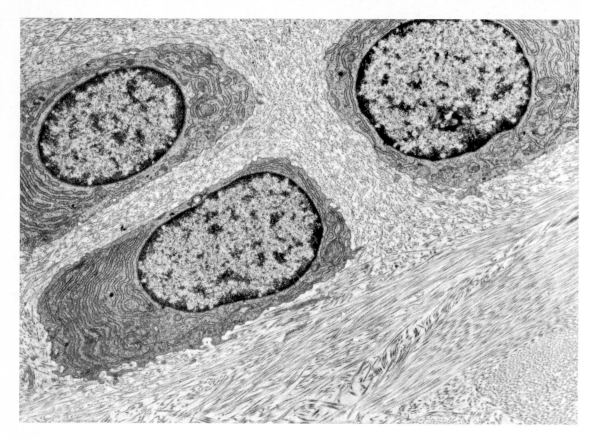

Figure 7–6. Electron micrograph of fibrocartilage, showing 3 chondrocytes in their lacunae. Observe the abundance of rough endoplasmic reticulum. These cells synthesize proteins for the cartilage matrix. Fine collagen fibers, sectioned in several planes, are prominent around the chondrocytes. × 3750.

motes the adherence of chondrocytes to matrix collagen. The cartilage matrix immediately surrounding each chondrocyte is rich in glycosaminoglycan and poor in collagen. This peripheral zone, called the **territorial,** or **capsular,** matrix, histochemically exhibits an intense basophilia, metachromasia, and greater PAS positivity than does the matrix located between the capsules, the **interterritorial matrix** (Figs 7–2 and 7–5).

Perichondrium

Except in the articular cartilage of joints, all hyaline cartilage is covered by a layer of dense connective tissue, the perichondrium, which is essential for the growth and maintenance of cartilage (Figs 7–2 and 7–5). It is rich in collagen type I fibers and contains numerous fibroblasts. Although cells in the inner layer of the perichondrium resemble fibroblasts, they are chondroblasts and easily differentiate into chondrocytes.

Chondrocytes

At the periphery of hyaline cartilage, young chondrocytes have an elliptic shape, with the long axis parallel to the surface. Farther in, they are round, 10–30 μm in diameter, and may appear in groups (Fig 7–2) of up to 8 cells originating from mitotic divisions of a single chondrocyte. These groups are designated **isogenous** (from Greek, *isos,* equal, + *genos,* family) **groups.** In epiphyseal plate cartilage, the proliferating chondrocytes are accumulated in rows (Fig 7–3).

Cartilage cells and the matrix shrink during histologic preparation, causing both the irregular shape of the chondrocytes and their retraction from the capsule. In living tissue, the chondrocytes fill the lacunae completely. The electron microscope reveals larger and more frequent indentations and protrusions in young chondrocytes (Fig 7–6). These structural characteristics increase their surface area, facilitating exchange with the extracellular medium; this has an important function in maintaining nutrition of these cells, since they are located at a distance from the bloodstream.

Mature chondrocytes have organelles typical of protein secretory cells—an elaborate rough endoplasmic reticulum and well-developed Golgi complex (Fig 7–10). They synthesize type II collagen, proteoglycans, and chondronectin.

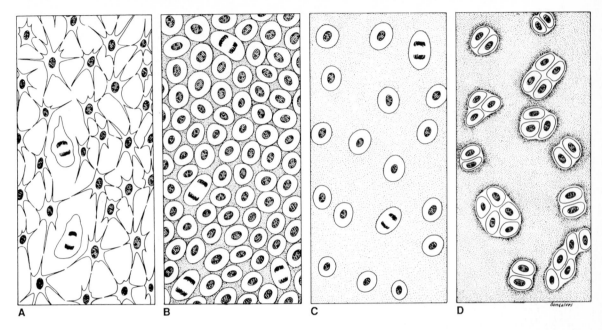

Figure 7–7. Histogenesis of hyaline cartilage. **A:** The mesenchyme, the precursor tissue of all types of cartilage. **B:** Mitotic proliferation of mesenchymal cells gives rise to a highly cellular tissue. **C:** Chondroblasts are separated from one another by the formation of a great amount of matrix. **D:** Multiplication of cartilage cells gives rise to isogenous groups, each surrounded by a condensation of territorial (capsule) matrix.

Histophysiology

Since cartilage is devoid of blood capillaries, chondrocytes respire under low oxygen tension. Hyaline cartilage cells metabolize glucose mainly by anaerobic glycolysis to produce lactic acid as the end product. Nutrients from the blood diffuse from the perichondrium to the more deeply placed chondrocytes. Because of this, the maximum width of the cartilage is limited. The nutrients diffuse through the solvation water of the matrix. There is almost no free water in cartilage matrix.

Chondrocyte function depends on a proper hormonal balance. The synthesis of sulfated glycosaminoglycans is accelerated by growth hormone, thyroxine, and testosterone. It is retarded by cortisone, hydrocortisone, and estradiol. Cartilage growth depends mainly upon the hypophyseal growth hormone, **somatotropin.** This hormone does not act directly on cartilage cells but promotes the synthesis of **somatomedin C** in the liver. Somatomedin C acts directly on cartilage cells, promoting their growth.

> Cartilage cells can give rise to benign (**chondroma**) or malignant (**chondrosarcoma**) tumors.

Histogenesis

Cartilage derives from the mesenchyme (Fig 7–7). The first modification observed is the rounding up of the mesenchymal cells, which retract their extensions, multiply rapidly, and form mesenchymal condensations. The cells formed by this direct differentiation of mesenchymal cells, now called **chondroblasts,** have a ribosome-rich basophilic cytoplasm. Synthesis and deposition of the matrix then begin to separate the chondroblasts from one another. The differentiation of cartilage takes place from the center outward; therefore, the more central cells have characteristics of chondrocytes while the peripheral cells are typical chondroblasts. The superficial mesenchyme develops into chondroblasts and fibroblasts of the perichondrium.

Growth

The growth of cartilage is attributable to 2 processes: **interstitial growth,** resulting from the mitotic division of preexisting chondrocytes; and **appositional growth,** resulting from the differentiation of perichondrial cells. In both cases, newly formed chondrocytes synthesize collagen fibrils and ground substance. Real growth is thus much greater than that from the simple increase in the number of cells. Interstitial growth is the less important of the 2 processes. It occurs only during the early phases of cartilage formation, when it increases tissue mass by expanding the cartilage matrix from within. Interstitial growth also occurs in the epiphyseal plates of long bones and within articular cartilage. In the epiphyseal plates, interstitial growth is important in increasing

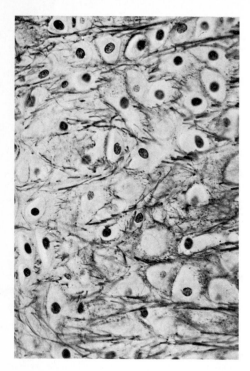

Figure 7–8. Photomicrograph of elastic cartilage, stained for elastic fibers. × 350.

the length of long bones and in providing a cartilage model for endochondral bone formation (see Chapter 8). In articular cartilage, as cells and matrix near the articulating surface are gradually worn away, the cartilage must be replaced from within, since there is no perichondrium here to add cells by apposition. It cartilage found elsewhere in the body, interstitial growth becomes less pronounced as the matrix becomes increasingly rigid from the cross-linking of matrix components. Cartilage then grows in girth only by apposition. Chondroblasts of the perichondrium proliferate and become chondrocytes once they have surrounded themselves with cartilaginous matrix and are incorporated into the existing cartilage (Figs 7–2 and 7–5).

Degenerative Changes

In contrast to other tissues, hyaline cartilage is subjected to the degenerative processes that increase with age. The most common is calcification of the matrix; this is preceded by an increase in the size and volume of the cells, followed by their death. Although calcification is a regressive alteration, it occurs normally in certain cartilages, providing a model for bone development. (See Endochondral Ossification, Chapter 8.) Asbestiform degeneration, frequent in aged cartilage, is due to the formation of localized aggregates of thick, abnormal collagen fibrils in this tissue.

Regeneration

Except in young children, damaged cartilage regenerates with difficulty and often incompletely. Regeneration occurs because of the activity of the

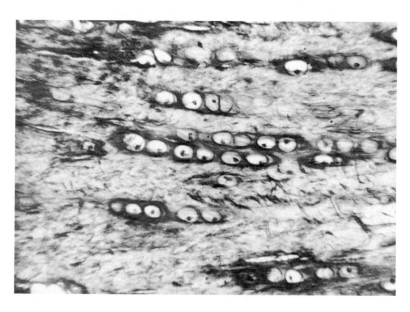

Figure 7–9. Photomicrograph of fibrocartilage. Observe rows of chondrocytes separated by collagen fibers. Picro-Sirius-hematoxylin, × 500.

perichondrium. When cartilage fractures, chondroblasts from the perichondrium invade the fractured area and generate new cartilage. In extensively damaged areas (and occasionally in small areas), the perichondrium, instead of forming new cartilage, generates a scar of dense connective tissue.

ELASTIC CARTILAGE

Elastic cartilage is found in the auricle of the ear, in the walls of the external auditory canals, in the auditory (eustachian) tubes, the epiglottis, and the cuneiform cartilage in the larynx.

Basically, elastic cartilage is identical to hyaline cartilage except that, in addition to collagen type II fibrils, it contains an abundant network of fine elastic fibers. Fresh elastic cartilage has a yellowish color caused by the presence of elastin in the elastic fibers, which may be demonstrated by standard elastin stains (eg, orcein; see Fig 7–8).

The chondrocytes of elastic and hyaline cartilage tissues are similar, and elastic cartilage is frequently found to be gradually continuous with hyaline cartilage. Like hyaline cartilage, elastic cartilage possesses a perichondrium. The presence of elastic fibers in the extracellular matrix makes elastic cartilage somewhat less susceptible to degenerative processes than hyaline cartilage.

FIBROCARTILAGE

Fibrocartilage has characteristics intermediate between those of dense connective tissue and hyaline cartilage. It is found in intervertebral disks, in attachments of certain ligaments to the cartilaginous surface of bones, and in the symphysis pubis. Fibrocartilage is always associated with dense connective tissue, and the border areas between these 2 tissues are not clear-cut but show a gradual transition.

Fibrocartilage contains chondrocytes similar to those of hyaline cartilage, either singly or in isogenous groups. The chondrocytes are very often arranged in long rows (Fig 7–9). Fibrocartilage matrix is acidophilic because it contains a great number of

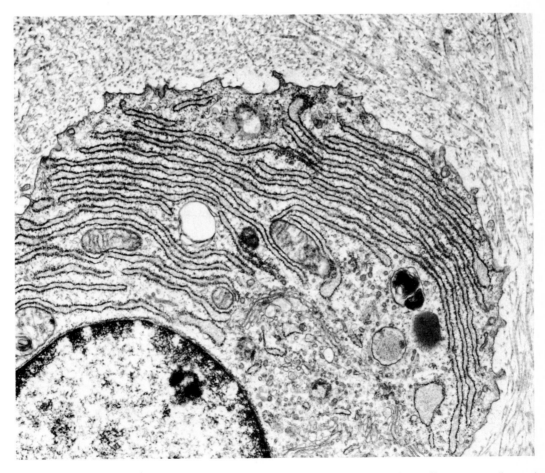

Figure 7–10. Electron micrograph of fibrocartilage. Observe the densely packed collagen fibers surrounding a chondrocyte. × 20,000.

coarse type I collagen fibers, which are easily seen under the microscope (Fig 7–10). The amorphous matrix is less abundant in this type of cartilage.

In fibrocartilage, the numerous collagen fibers either form irregular bundles between the groups of chondrocytes or are aligned in a parallel arrangement along the columns of chondrocytes (Fig 7–6). This orientation depends upon the stresses acting on fibrocartilage, since the collagen bundles take up a direction parallel to those stresses. There is no identifiable perichondrium in fibrocartilage.

INTERVERTEBRAL DISKS

Each intervertebral disk is situated between 2 vertebrae and held to them by means of ligaments. The disks have 2 components: the cartilaginous annulus fibrosus and the liquid nucleus pulposus. The intervertebral disk acts as a lubricated cushion that prevents adjacent vertebrae from being eroded by abrasive forces during movement of the spinal column. The liquid nucleus pulposus serves as a shock absorber to cushion the impact between adjacent vertebrae.

The **annulus fibrosus** has an external layer of dense connective tissue, but it is mainly composed of overlapping laminae of fibrocartilage in which collagen bundles are orthogonally arranged in adjacent layers. The multiple lamellae, with the 90-degree registration of type I collagen fibers in adjacent layers, provide the disk with an unusual resilience that enables it to withstand the pressures generated by impinging vertebrae. In tangential section, the disk presents a characteristic herringbone pattern as a result of the orthogonal alignment of collagen in alternating lamellae.

The **nucleus pulposus** is situated in the center of the annulus fibrosus. It is derived from the notochord and consists of a few rounded cells embedded in an amorphous viscous substance rich in hyaluronic acid and type II collagen fibrils. In children, the nucleus pulposus is large, but it gradually becomes smaller with age and is partially replaced by fibrocartilage.

Herniation of the Intervertebral Disk

Rupture of the annulus fibrosus, which most frequently occurs in the posterior region where there are fewer collagen bundles, results in expulsion of the liquid nucleus pulposus and a concomitant flattening of the disk. As a consequence, the disk frequently dislocates or slips from its position between the vertebrae. If it moves toward the spinal cord, it can compress the nerves and result in severe pain and neurologic disturbances. The pain accompanying a slipped disk may be perceived in areas innervated by the compressed nerve fibers—usually the lower lumbar region.

REFERENCES

Anderson DR: The ultrastructure of elastic and hyaline cartilage in the rat. *Am J Anat* 1964;**114**:403.
Chakrabarti B, Park JW: Glycosaminoglycans: Structure and interaction. *CRC Crit Rev Biochem* 1980;**8**:225.
Eyre DR, Muir H: The distribution of different molecular species of collagen in fibrous, elastic and hyaline cartilages of the pig. *Biochem J* 1975;**151**:595.
Hall BK (editor): *Cartilage*, Vol 1: *Structure, Function, and Biochemistry*. Academic Press, 1983.
Junqueira LCU et al: Quantitation of collagen-proteoglycan interaction in tissue sections. *Connect Tissue Res* 1980;**7**:91.
Reddy AH (editor): *Extracellular Matrix Structure and Functions*. Alan R Liss, 1985.
Stockwell RA: *Biology of Cartilage Cells*. Cambridge Univ Press, 1979.
Thomas L: Reversible collapse of rabbit ears after intravenous papain, and prevention of recovery by cortisone. *J Exp Med* 1956;**104**:245.
Zambrano NZ et al: Collagen arrangement in cartilages. *Acta Anat* 1982;**113**:26.

Bone

Bone is one of the hardest tissues of the human body, second only to cartilage in its ability to withstand stress. As the main constituent of the adult skeleton, it supports fleshy structures, protects such vital organs as those in the cranial and thoracic cavities, and harbors the bone marrow, where blood cells are formed. Bone also serves as a reservoir of calcium, phosphate, and other ions that can be released or stored in a controlled fashion to maintain constant concentrations of these important ions in body fluids.

In addition to these functions, bones form a system of levers that multiply the forces generated during skeletal muscle contraction, transforming them into bodily movements.

Bone is a specialized connective tissue composed of intercellular calcified material, the **bone matrix,** and 3 different cell types: **osteocytes** (from Greek, *osteon,* bone, + *kytos*), which are found in cavities **(lacunae)** within the matrix (Fig 8–1); **osteoblasts,** which synthesize the organic components of the matrix; and **osteoclasts,** which are multinucleated giant cells involved in the resorption and remodeling of bone tissue.

Since metabolites are unable to diffuse through the calcified matrix of bone, the exchanges between osteocytes and blood capillaries depend on cellular communication through the **canaliculi** (from Latin, *canalis,* canal), thin, cylindric spaces that perforate the matrix (Fig 8–2). These canaliculi permit the osteocytes to communicate via thin cytoplasmic (filopodial) processes with their neighbors, with the internal and external surfaces of the bone, and with the blood vessels traversing the matrix.

All bones are lined on both internal and external surfaces by layers of tissue containing osteogenic cells—**endosteum** on the inner surface and **periosteum** on the outer.

Because of its hardness, bone is difficult to section with the microtome; therefore, special techniques must be used for its study. One of these consists of grinding slices of bone with abrasives until they are thin enough to be translucent. The preparation thus obtained is referred to as a **ground section.** This technique does not preserve the cells but does permit detailed study of the matrix, its lacunae, and its canaliculi. Because of differences in refractive index between lacunae and canaliculi (which are both filled

with air in these preparations) and the medium used in mounting, light rays striking the lacunae and canaliculi are deflected and do not penetrate the objective lens of the microscope. Lacunae and canaliculi consequently appear black in ground sections (see Fig 8–2).

Another frequently used technique that permits the observation of the cells and organic matrix is based on the decalcification of bone preserved by standard fixatives. The mineral is removed by immersion in a dilute acid solution (eg, 5% nitric acid) or in a solution containing a calcium-chelating substance (eg, ethylenediamine-tetraacetic acid, EDTA). The decalcified tissue is then embedded, sectioned, and stained.

BONE CELLS

Osteoblasts

Osteoblasts are responsible for the synthesis of the organic components of bone matrix (type I collagen, proteoglycans, and glycoproteins). Deposition of the

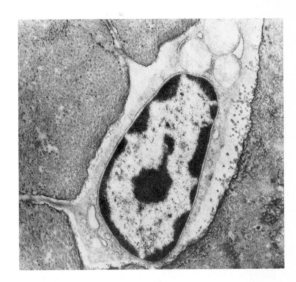

Figure 8–1. Section of bone tissue showing an osteocyte with its cytoplasmic processes surrounded by matrix. Ultrastructure compatible with a low level of synthetic activity is apparent in both nucleus and cytoplasm.

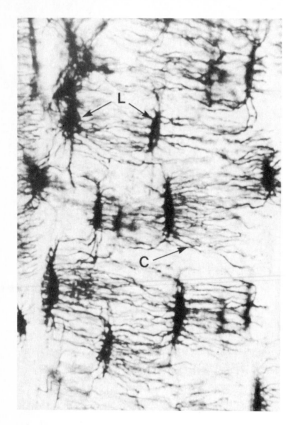

Figure 8–2. Photomicrograph of ground section of bone. Lacunae (L) and canaliculi (C) appear black. × 900.

the osteoblast layer and the previously formed bone. This process, **bone apposition,** is completed by subsequent deposition of calcium salts into the newly formed matrix.

The fluorescent antibiotic tetracycline interacts with great affinity with recently deposited mineralized bone matrix. Based on this interaction, a method was developed to measure the rate of bone apposition—an important parameter in the study of bone growth and the diagnosis of bone growth diseases. Tetracycline is administered twice to patients, with an interval of 5 days between injections. A bone biopsy is then performed and the sections studied with fluorescence microscopy. The distance between the 2 fluorescent layers is proportional to the rate of bone apposition. This procedure is of diagnostic importance in such diseases as **osteomalacia,** in which mineralization is impaired, and **osteitis fibrosa cystica,** in which increased osteoclast activity results in removal of bone matrix and fibrous degeneration.

The role of osteoblasts in secreting bone collagen has been studied by radioautography in animals injected with ^{3}H-glycine, an amino acid constituting one-third of the residues in collagen (Fig 8–4).

Osteocytes

Osteocytes, which derive from osteoblasts, lie in the lacunae situated between lamellae of matrix. Only one osteocyte is found in each lacuna. The thin, cylindrical canaliculi house cytoplasmic processes of osteocytes. Processes of adjacent cells make contact via gap junctions, and nutrients are passed in this way to the cells. Some molecular exchange between osteocytes and blood vessels also takes place through the small amount of extracellular substance located between osteocytes (and their processes) and the bone matrix. This exchange can provide support for a chain of about 15 cells.

When compared to osteoblasts, the flat, almond-shaped osteocytes exhibit a significantly reduced rough endoplasmic reticulum (Fig 8–1) and Golgi complex and more condensed nuclear chromatin. These cells are actively involved with the maintenance of the bony matrix. Death of the osteocytes is followed by resorption of this matrix.

Osteoclasts

Osteoclasts are very large, extensively branched motile cells. Dilated portions of the cell body (Fig 8–5) contain 5 to 50 or more nuclei. The branches of the cell are quite irregular and vary in both thickness and shape. In areas of bone undergoing resorption, osteoclasts are found to lie within enzymatically etched depressions in the matrix known as **Howship's lacunae.** Osteoclasts are derived from the fusion of

inorganic components of bone is also dependent on the presence of viable osteoblasts. They are exclusively located at the surfaces of bone tissue, side by side, in a way that resembles simple epithelium (Fig 8–3). When they are actively engaged in matrix synthesis, osteoblasts have a cuboidal to columnar shape, basophilic cytoplasm, and high alkaline phosphatase activity. When their synthesizing activity declines, they flatten, and cytoplasmic basophilia declines, as does alkaline phosphatase activity.

Osteoblasts have cytoplasmic processes that bring them into contact with neighboring osteoblasts. The processes are more evident when the cell begins to surround itself with matrix. Once surrounded by newly synthesized matrix, the osteoblast is referred to as an **osteocyte.** Lacunae and canaliculi appear, because the matrix is formed around a cell and its cytoplasmic extensions.

During matrix synthesis, osteoblasts have the ultrastructure of cells actively synthesizing proteins for export. Osteoblasts are polarized cells. Secretion of matrix components occurs at the cell surface, which is in contact with older bone matrix, producing a layer of new (but not yet calcified) matrix between

Osteoblast   Osteoclast   Osteocyte   Mesenchyme   Bone matrix   Newly formed matrix

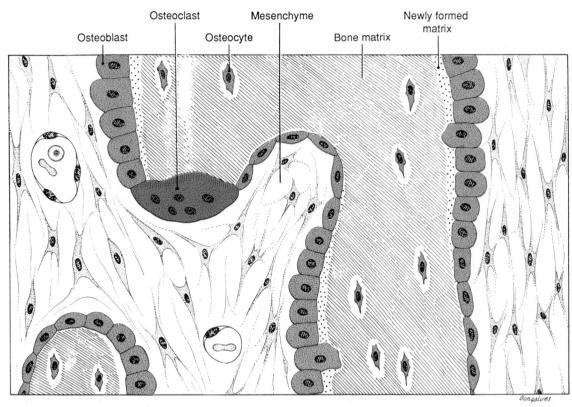

Figure 8–3. Drawing representing the events that occur during intramembranous ossification. Osteoblasts (lighter color) are synthesizing collagen, which forms a strand of matrix that traps cells. As this occurs, the osteoblasts gradually differentiate to become osteocytes. The lower part of the drawing shows an osteoblast being trapped in newly formed bone matrix.

blood-derived monocytes and thus belong to the mononuclear phagocyte system (Chapter 5).

Osteoclasts usually have acidophilic cytoplasm. In active osteoclasts, the surface-facing bone matrix is folded into irregular, often subdivided projections, forming a ruffled border. In addition to establishing a device whereby small particles may be easily trapped and subjected to enzymatic activity, this arrangement considerably increases the active resorptive area. Numerous free polysomes, some rough endoplasmic reticulum, abundant mitochondria, and a well-developed Golgi complex are found in addition to the great number of lysosomes present within the cell.

Crystals containing calcium have been observed in the spaces between the folds as well as in cytoplasmic vacuoles that probably derived from the surface membrane of the osteoclasts. Disintegrating collagen fibers have also been reported in the extracellular space close to the folds of the osteoclast, but they never occur within its cytoplasm. Osteoclasts secrete acid, collagenase, and other proteolytic enzymes that attack the bone matrix, liberate the calcified ground substance, and are actively engaged in elimination of debris formed during bone resorption.

BONE MATRIX

Inorganic matter represents about 50% of the dry weight of bone matrix. Calcium and phosphorus are especially abundant, but bicarbonate, citrate, magnesium, potassium, and sodium are also found. X-ray diffraction studies have shown that calcium and phosphorus form hydroxyapatite crystals with the composition $CA_{10}(PO_4)_6(OH)_2$. Significant quantities of amorphous (noncrystalline) calcium phosphate are also present. In electron micrographs, hydroxyapatite crystals of bone appear as plates measuring $40 \times 25 \times 3$ nm. They lie alongside the collagen fibrils but are surrounded by an amorphous ground substance. The surface ions of hydroxyapatite are hydrated, and a layer of water and ions forms around the crystal. This layer, the **hydration shell,** facilitates the exchange of ions between the crystal and the body fluids.

The organic matter is type I collagen and amorphous ground substance, which contains glycosaminoglycans associated with proteins. Several specific glycoproteins have been isolated from bone. Bone sialoprotein and osteocalcin contain several γ-carboxy-

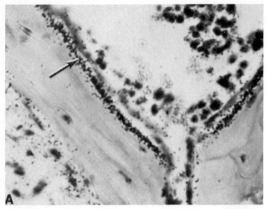

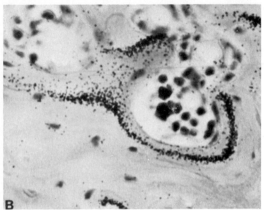

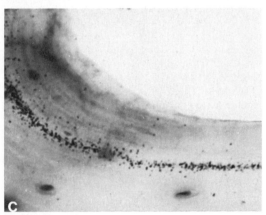

Figure 8–4. Radioautographs of bone tissue from mice injected with ³H-glycine and sacrificed at different intervals after the injection. **A:** From a mouse killed 4 hours after injection. At this time, the newly formed matrix, which contains ³H-glycine-labeled collagen synthesized by the osteoblasts, is strongly radioactive (arrow). Some radioactivity remains in the osteoblasts. Bone marrow cells (upper right) are also radioactive. **B:** From a mouse killed 7 days after injection. The radioactive band is deeper into the calcified matrix because of the subsequent accumulation of the nonradioactive collagen formed after utilization of all labeled glycine. **C:** From a mouse killed 45 days after injection. The radioactive band is more deeply situated in comparison with the sections from previous intervals. H&E stain, × 300.

glutamic acid residues; this causes them to bind calcium avidly and may be responsible for promoting calcification of bone matrix. Other tissues containing type I collagen are not normally calcified and do not contain these glycoproteins. Among the glycosaminoglycans of bone are chondroitin 4-sulfate, chondroitin 6-sulfate, and keratan sulfate. Because of its high collagen content, decalcified bone matrix intensely binds stains for collagen fibers.

The association of hydroxyapatite with collagen fibers is responsible for the hardness and resistance that are characteristic of bone. After a bone is decalcified, its shape is preserved, but it becomes as flexible as a tendon. Removal of the organic part of the matrix—which is mainly collagenous in nature—also leaves the bone with its original shape; however, it becomes fragile, breaking and crumbling easily when handled.

PERIOSTEUM & ENDOSTEUM

External and internal surfaces of bone are covered by layers of bone-forming cells and connective tissue called periosteum and endosteum.

The **periosteum** consists of an outer layer of collagen fibers and fibroblasts (Fig 8–6). Bundles of periosteal collagen fibers, called **Sharpey's fibers,** penetrate the bone matrix, binding the periosteum to bone. The inner, more cellular layer of the periosteum is composed of flattened cells with the potential to divide by mitosis and differentiate into osteoblasts. These **osteoprogenitor cells** are characterized by their location, their spindle shape, a small amount of rough endoplasmic reticulum, and their poorly developed Golgi complex. Autoradiographic studies demonstrate that these cells take up ³H-thymidine, which is subsequently encountered in osteoblasts. These cells play a prominent role in bone growth and repair.

The **endosteum** (Fig 8–6) lines all internal surfaces of cavities within the bone and is composed of a single layer of flattened osteoprogenitor cells and a very small amount of connective tissue. Therefore, the endosteum is considerably thinner than the periosteum.

The principal functions of periosteum and endosteum are nutrition of osseous tissue and provision of a continuous supply of new osteoblasts for repair or growth of bone. For these reasons, precautions are taken to preserve the periosteum and endosteum during bone surgery.

TYPES OF BONE

Microscopic examination of bone shows that 2 varieties exist: **primary, immature,** or **woven bone;** and **secondary, mature,** or **lamellar** (from Latin, diminutive of *lamina,* leaf) **bone.** Primary bone is the first bone tissue to appear in embryonic development

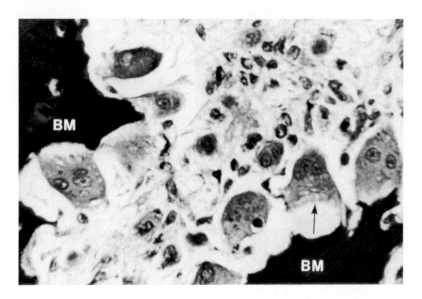

Figure 8–5. Photomicrograph of a bone section showing several osteoclasts. Observe the ruffled border (arrow). Bone matrix (BM) appears dark. The separation between some osteoclasts and the bone matrix is an artifact. Sirius red and hematoxyin stain, × 800.

and in fracture and other repair processes. It is characterized by random disposition of fine collagen fibers—in contrast to the organized lamellar disposition of collagen in secondary bone. Primary bone is temporary and is replaced in adults by secondary bone.

Gross observation of bone in cross section shows dense areas without cavities—corresponding to **compact bone**—and areas with numerous interconnecting cavities—corresponding to **cancellous (spongy) bone** (Fig 8–7). Under the microscope, however, both compact bone and the trabeculae separating the cavities of cancellous bone have the same basic histologic structure.

In long bones, the bulbous ends—called **epiphyses**—are composed of spongy bone covered by a thin layer of compact bone. The cylindrical part—**diaphysis** (from Greek, *dia,* through, + *phyein,* to bring forth)—is almost totally composed of compact bone, with a small component of spongy bone on its inner surface around the bone marrow cavity (Fig 8–14). Short bones usually have a core of spongy bone completely surrounded by compact bone. The flat bones that form the calvaria have 2 layers of compact bone called **plates** (tables), separated by a layer of spongy bone called the **diploë.**

The cavities of spongy bone and the marrow cavity in the diaphyses of long bones contain **bone marrow,** of which there are 2 kinds: **red bone marrow,** in which blood cells are forming; and **yellow bone marrow,** composed mainly of fat cells.

Primary Bone Tissue

The first bone tissue to appear is primary bone. It is temporary and is replaced in adults by secondary bone tissue except in a very few places in the body, eg, near the sutures of the flat bones of the skull, in tooth sockets, and in the insertions of some tendons.

In addition to the irregular array of collagen fibers, other characteristics of primary bone tissue are a smaller mineral content (it is more easily penetrated by x-rays) and a higher proportion of osteocytes than in secondary bone tissue.

Secondary Bone Tissue

Secondary bone is the variety usually found in adults. Characteristically, it shows collagen fibers arranged in lamellae (3–7 μm thick) that are parallel to each other or concentrically organized around a vascular canal. The whole complex of concentric lamellae of bone surrounding a canal containing blood vessels, nerves, and loose connective tissue is called a **haversian system** or **osteon** (Figs 8–6 and 8–8). Lacunae containing osteocytes are found between and occasionally within the lamellae. In each lamella, collagen fibers are parallel to each other. Surrounding each haversian system is a deposit of amorphous material called the **cementing substance** that consists of mineralized matrix with few collagen fibers.

In compact bone (eg, the diaphysis of long bones), the lamellae exhibit a typical organization consisting of **haversian systems, outer circumferential lamellae, inner circumferential lamellae,** and **interstitial**

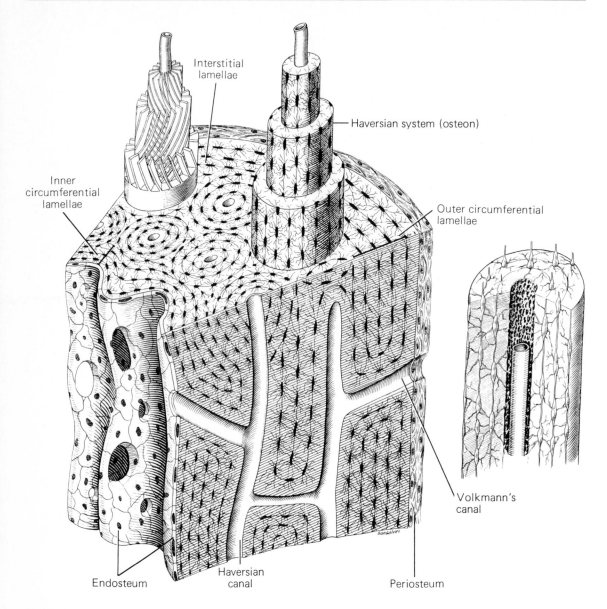

Figure 8–6. Schematic drawing of the wall of a long bone diaphysis. Observe the 4 types of lamellar bone: haversian system, outer and inner circumferential lamellae, and interstitial lamellae. The protruding haversian system on the left shows the orientation of collagen fibers in each lamella. At the right is a haversian system showing lamellae, a central blood capillary, and many osteocytes with their processes.

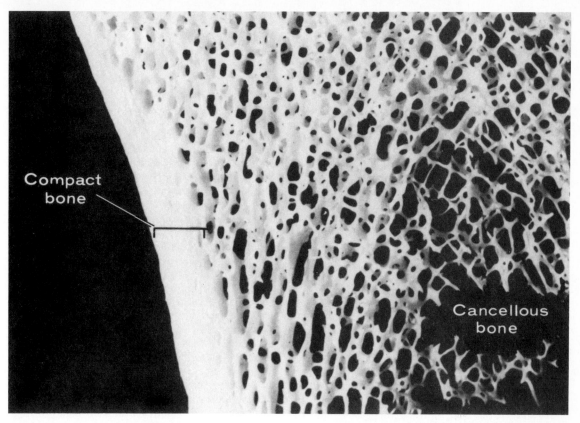

Figure 8–7. Thick ground section of tibia illustrating the cortical compact bone and the lattice of trabeculae of cancellous bone (Courtesy of DW Fawcett).

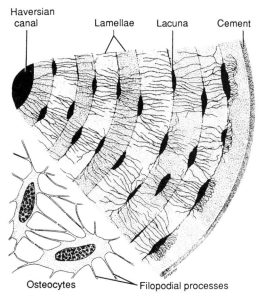

Figure 8–8. Schematic drawing of 2 osteocytes and part of a haversian system. Collagen fibers of contiguous lamellae are sectioned at different angles. Observe the numerous canaliculi that permit communication between lacunae and with the haversian canals. Although it is not apparent in this simplified diagram, each lamella actually consists of multiple lamellae in which the parallel arrays of collagen fibers in adjacent lamellae are oriented in different directions. The presence of large numbers of lamellae with differing fiber orientations provides the bone with great strength despite its light weight. (Redrawn and reproduced, with permission, from Leeson TS, Leeson CR: *Histology*, 2nd ed. Saunders, 1970.)

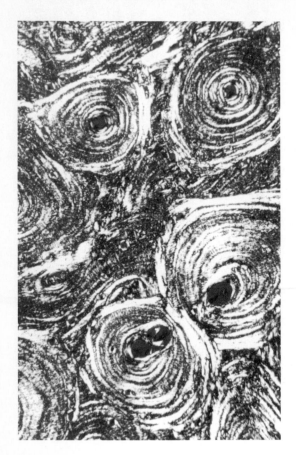

Figure 8–9. Transverse section of decalcified diaphysis; polarization microscopy showing the alternating light and dark bands of the haversian system. This alternating birefringence is due to the presence of collagen fibers disposed in different orientations in contiguous lamellae. × 150.

lamellae. The 4 types of lammelar bone are easily identified in cross section (Fig 8–6). Since the principal function of haversian systems is to bring nutrients to compact bone, it is not surprising to find that these systems are absent in the thin spicules of cancellous bone. Here, nutrients can diffuse into the bony tissue from surrounding blood capillaries.

Each haversian system is a long, often bifurcated cylinder parallel to the long axis of the diaphysis. It consists of a central canal surrounded by 4–20 concentric lamellae. Each endosteum-lined canal contains blood vessels, nerves, and loose connective tissue. The haversian canals communicate with the marrow cavity, the periosteum, and each other through transverse or oblique Volkmann's canals (Fig 8–6). Volkmann's canals do not have concentric lamellae; instead, they perforate the lamellae (Fig 8–6). All vascular canals found in bone tissue come into existence when matrix is laid down around preexisting blood vessels.

Examination of haversian systems with polarized light shows bright anisotropic layers alternating with dark isotropic layers (Fig 8–9). When observed under polarized light at right angles to their length, collagen fibers are birefringent (anisotropic). The alternating bright and dark layers are due to the orientation of collagen fibers in the lamellae. In each lamella, fibers are parallel to each other and follow a helical course. The pitch of the helix is, however, different for different lamellae, so that at any given point fibers from adjacent lamellae intersect at approximately right angles (Fig 8–6). Cross sections of a haversian system show transverse sections of collagen fibers in one lamella and oblique, almost longitudinal, sections of collagen fibers in the adjacent lamella. The structure of haversian systems as shown in the light microscope is compatible with these observations. In one lamella, the collagen fibers are sectioned transversely and appear granular; in the next, the fibers are sectioned obliquely and have an elongated appearance (Fig 8–8).

There is great variability in the diameter of haversian canals. Each system is formed by successive deposits of lamellae, starting from the periphery, so that younger systems have larger canals. Thus, in mature haversian systems, the most recently formed lamella is the one closest to the central canal.

During growth—and even in adult bone—there is continuous destruction and rebuilding of haversian systems, so that one often sees systems with only a few lamellae and a large central canal.

Inner and outer circumferential lamellae are, as their names indicate, located around the marrow cavity and immediately beneath the periosteum. Their lamellae have a circular distribution, with the marrow cavity as the center. There are more outer than inner circumferential lamellae (Fig 8–6).

Between the 2 circumferential systems are numerous haversian systems, and among the latter are triangular or irregularly shaped groups of parallel lamellae called **interstitial** (or intermediate) **lamellae.** These structures represent lamellae left by haversian systems destroyed during growth and remodeling of bone (Fig 8–10).

HISTOGENESIS

Bone can be formed in 2 ways: by direct mineralization of matrix secreted by osteoblasts (*intramembranous ossification*) or by deposition of bone matrix on a preexisting cartilage matrix (*endochondral ossification*).

In both processes, the bone tissue that appears first is primary or immature. Primary bone is a temporary tissue and is soon replaced by the definitive lamellar, or secondary, bone. During bone growth, areas of primary bone, areas of resorption, and areas of lamellar bone appear side by side. This combination of bone synthesis and removal (remodeling) occurs not

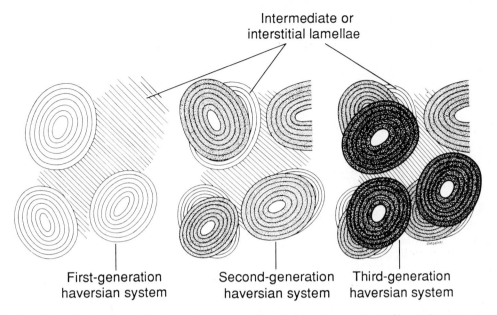

Intermediate or
interstitial lamellae

First-generation
haversian system

Second-generation
haversian system

Third-generation
haversian system

Figure 8–10. Schematic drawing of diaphyseal bone remodeling showing 3 generations of haversian systems and their successive contributions to the formation of intermediate, or interstitial, lamellae.

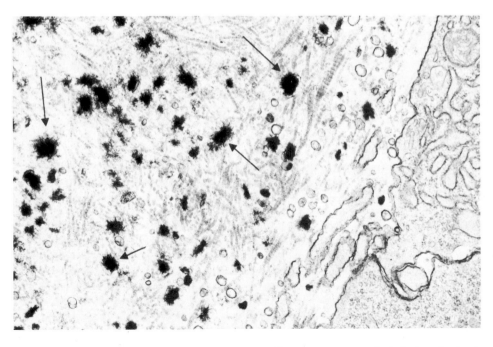

Figure 8–11. Calvarium in the early stage of mineral deposition. There are numerous foci of mineralization (arrows) in the collagen-rich matrix. × 18,000. (Courtesy of E Katchburian.)

only in growing bones but also throughout adult life, although its rate of change then is considerably slower.

Intramembranous Ossification

Intramembranous ossification, the source of most of the flat bones, is so called because it takes place within condensations of mesenchymal tissue. The frontal and parietal bones of the skull—as well as parts of the occipital and temporal bones and the mandible and maxilla—are formed by intramembranous ossification. This process also contributes to the growth of short bones and the thickening of long bones.

In the mesenchymal condensation layer, the starting point for ossification is called a **primary ossification center.** The process begins when groups of cells differentiate into osteoblasts. New bone matrix is formed and calcification follows (Fig 8–11), resulting in the encapsulation of some osteoblasts, which then become osteocytes (Fig 8–12). These islands of developing bone are known as **spicules.** The spicules are so called because of their appearance in histologic sections; they are sections of walls that delineate elongated cavities containing capillaries, bone marrow cells, and undifferentiated cells. Several such groups arise almost simultaneously at the ossification center, so that the fusion of the spicules gives the bone a spongy structure (Fig 8–13). The connective tissue that remains among the bone spicules is penetrated by growing blood vessels and additional undifferentiated mesenchymal cells, giving rise to the bone marrow cells.

Cells of the mesenchymal tissue condensation divide, giving rise to more osteoblasts, which are responsible for the continued growth of the ossification center. The several ossification centers of a bone grow radially and finally fuse together, replacing the original connective tissue. The fontanelles of newborn infants, for example, are soft areas in the skull that correspond to parts of the connective tissue not yet ossified.

In cranial flat bones, especially after birth, there is a marked predominance of bone formation over bone resorption at both the internal and the external surfaces. Thus, 2 layers of compact bone (internal and external plates) arise, whereas the central portion (diploë) maintains its spongy nature.

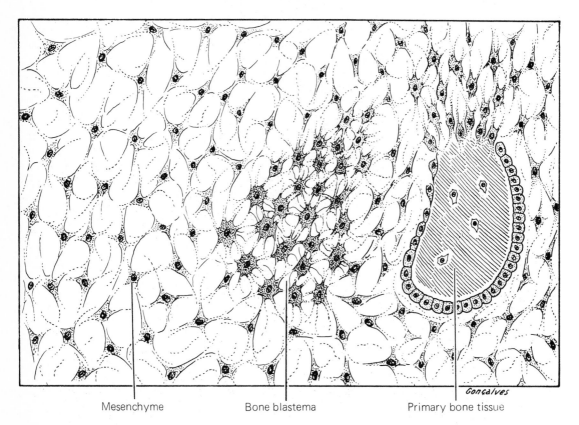

Mesenchyme   Bone blastema   Primary bone tissue

Gonçalves

Figure 8–12. The beginning of intramembranous ossification. Mesenchymal cells round up and form a blastema from which osteoblasts differentiate.

Bone   Osteo-   Osteo-
spicule   blast   clast

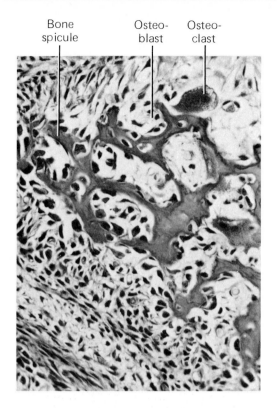

Figure 8–13. Photomicrograph of intramembranous ossification from the head of a young rat. Bone tissue shows osteocytes in lacunae. There are numerous osteoblasts and an osteoclast around the newly formed bone tissue. × 350.

That portion of the connective tissue layer which does not undergo ossification gives rise to the endosteum and the periosteum of intramembranous bone.

Endochondral Ossification

Endochondral (*endon* + *chondros*) ossification takes place within a piece of hyaline cartilage whose shape resembles a small version or model of the bone to be formed. This type of ossification is principally responsible for the formation of short and long bones (Fig 8–14).

Basically, endochondral ossification consists of 2 phases. The first phase is hypertrophy and destruction of the chondrocytes of the model of the bone, leaving expanded lacunae separated by septa of calcified cartilage matrix. In the second phase, an **osteogenic bud** consisting of osteoprogenitor cells and blood capillaries penetrates the spaces left by the degenerating chondrocytes. The osteoprogenitor cells give rise to osteoblasts, which cover the cartilaginous septa with bone matrix. The septa of calcified cartilage tissue thus serve as supports for the beginning of ossification (Fig 8–14).

Long bones are formed from cartilaginous models with dilatations (epiphyses) at each end of a cylindrical shaft (diaphysis). The first bone tissue to be formed appears by means of intramembranous ossification within the perichondrium surrounding the diaphysis (Fig 8–14). Thus, a hollow bone cylinder, the **bone collar,** is produced in the deep portions of the perichondrium surrounding the cartilage. From this point on, the perichondrium will be called the **periosteum** because it covers the newly developed bone. Within the forming bone collar, chondrocytes of the model begin to degenerate, since the new osseous collar prevents the diffusion of nutrients into the cartilage matrix. As the chondrocytes begin to degenerate, they lose their ability to maintain the matrix, calcium deposits form, and the cartilage becomes **calcified.**

Blood vessels of the osteogenic bud, coming from the periosteum through holes made by osteoclasts in the bone collar, penetrate the calcified cartilage matrix. Osteoprogenitor cells invade the area along with the blood vessels; they proliferate and give rise to osteoblasts. Osteoblasts form a continuous layer over the calcified cartilaginous matrix and start to synthesize bone matrix. Primary bone synthesis thus takes place over the remnants of calcified cartilage (Fig 8–15). Bone marrow stem cells are circulating in the blood and are brought into the forming bone by the osteogenic bud.

In histologic sections, calcified cartilage can be distinguished as basophilic, whereas the bone tissue deposited over it is acidophilic. As the bone matrix develops, calcified cartilage remnants are resorbed by the giant multinucleated cells similar to osteoclasts.

The ossification center described above, which appears in the diaphysis, is called the **primary ossification center** (Fig 8–14). Its rapid longitudinal growth ends by occupying the whole diaphysis, which then becomes composed completely of bone tissue. This expansion of the primary ossification center is accompanied by expansion of the periosteal bone collar, which also grows in the direction of the epiphyses. From the beginning of the formation of the ossification center, osteoclasts are active, and resorption of the bone occurs at the center, which results in formation of a hollow marrow cavity. This cavity grows toward the epiphyses as ossification continues toward the ends of the finally complete bone model.

At later stages in embryonic development, a **secondary ossification center** (Fig 8–14) arises at the center of each epiphysis; even within one bone, however, all centers do not develop simultaneously. The function of these centers is similar to that of the primary center, but their growth is radial instead of longitudinal. Furthermore, since the articular cartilage has no perichondrium, there is no equivalent of a bone collar formed here (Fig 8–14).

When the bone tissue that originated at the secondary centers occupies the epiphysis, cartilage remains

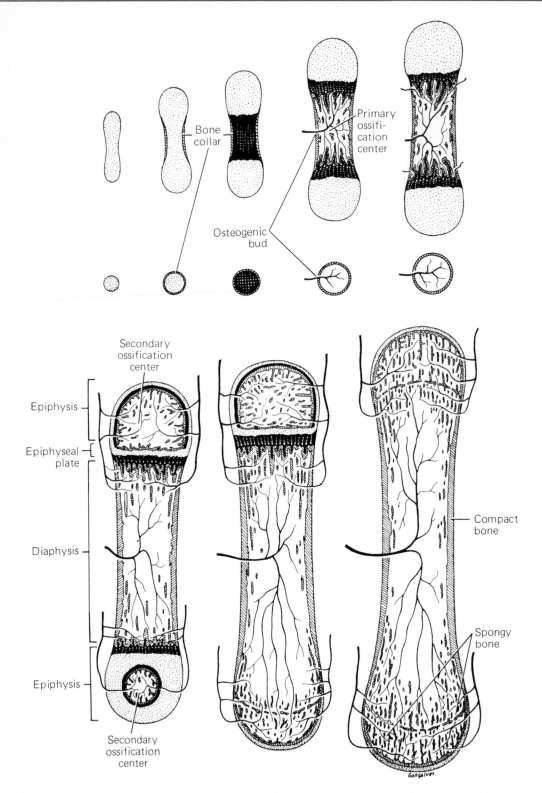

Figure 8–14. Formation of a long bone on a model made of cartilage. Hyaline cartilage is stippled; calcified cartilage is black, and bone tissue is indicated by oblique lines. The 5 small drawings in the middle row represent cross sections through the middle regions of the figures shown in the upper row. (For details, see text.) (Redrawn and reproduced, with permission, from Bloom W, Fawcett DW: *A Textbook of Histology*, 9th ed Saunders, 1968).

Remnants of cartilage matrix

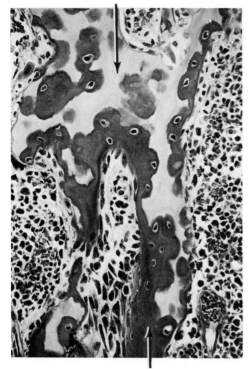

Bone tissue

Figure 8–15. Photomicrograph of endochondral ossification from the finger of a human fetus. Remnants of calcified cartilage matrix appear covered by dark primary bone tissue. Calcified cartilage matrix has no cells, while bone matrix contains many osteocytes. × 238.

restricted to 2 places: articular cartilage, which persists throughout adult life and does not contribute to bone formation; and **epiphyseal cartilage,** or the **epiphyseal plate,** which connects epiphysis to diaphysis (Figs 8–16 and 8–17). As the cartilage of the epiphyseal plate grows, it is replaced continuously by newly formed bone matrix mainly from the diaphyseal center. No further longitudinal growth of the bone takes place after the growth of the epiphyseal plate ceases.

Epiphyseal cartilage is divided into 5 zones (Fig 8–17), starting from the epiphyseal side of cartilage: (1) The **resting zone** consists of hyaline cartilage without morphologic changes in the cells. (2) In the **proliferative zone,** chondrocytes divide rapidly and form columns (isogenous groups) of stacked cells parallel to the long axis of the bone. (3) The **hypertrophic cartilage zone** contains large chondrocytes whose cytoplasm has accumulated glycogen. The resorbed matrix is reduced to thin septa between the chondrocytes. (4) Simultaneous

with the death of chondrocytes occurring in the **calcified cartilage zone,** the thin septa of cartilage matrix become calcified by the deposit of hydroxyapatite (Figs 8–16 and 8–17). (5) In the **ossification zone,** endochondral bone tissue appears. Blood capillaries and osteoprogenitor cells formed by mitosis of cells originating from the periosteum invade the cavities left by the chondrocytes. The osteoprogenitor cells form osteoblasts, which in turn form a discontinuous layer over the septa of calcified cartilage matrix. Over these septa, the osteoblasts deposit matrix (Fig 8–15).

The bone matrix calcifies, and some osteoblasts are transformed into osteocytes. In this way, **bone spicules** are formed with a central area of calcified cartilage and a superficial layer of primary bone tissue (Fig 8–16).

In summary, growth in length of a long bone occurs by proliferation of chondrocytes in the epiphyseal plate adjacent to the epiphysis. At the same

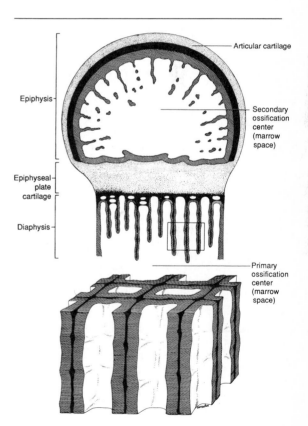

Figure 8–16. Schematic drawings showing the 3-dimensional shape of bone spicules in the epiphyseal plate area. Hyaline cartilage is stippled, calcifed cartilage is black, and bone tissue is shown in color. The upper drawing shows the region represented 3-dimensionally in the lower drawing. (Redrawn and reproduced, with permission, from Ham AW: *Histology,* 6th ed., Lippincott, 1969.)

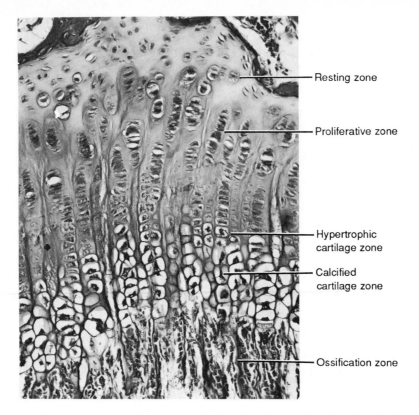

Resting zone

Proliferative zone

Hypertrophic
cartilage zone

Calcified
cartilage zone

Ossification zone

Figure 8–17. Photomicrograph of the epiphyseal plate, showing the changes that take place in the cartilage and the formation of bone spicules. H&E stain, × 110.

time, chondrocytes of the diaphyseal side of the plate hypertrophy; their matrix becomes calcified, and the cells die. Osteoblasts lay down a layer of primary bone on the calcified cartilage spicules. The rates of these 2 opposing events (proliferation and destruction) are approximately equal, and thus the epiphyseal plate does not change thickness. Instead, it is displaced away from the middle of the diaphysis, resulting in growth in length of the bone.

Mechanisms of Calcification

No generally accepted hypothesis now exists that explains the events occurring during calcium phosphate deposition on bone matrix.

It is known that calcification begins by the deposition of calcium salts on collagen fibrils, a process induced by proteoglycans and high affinity calcium binding glycoproteins **(osteonectin).** The deposition of calcium salts is probably accelerated by the ability of osteoblasts to concentrate them in intracytoplasmic vesicles and releasing, when necessary, their content to the extracellular medium.

Calcification is aided, in some unknown way, by alkaline phosphatase produced by osteoblasts and present at ossification sites.

BONE GROWTH & REMODELING

Bone growth is generally associated with partial resorption of preformed tissue and the simultaneous laying down of new bone (which exceeds the rate of bone loss). This permits the shape of the bone to be maintained while it grows. The rate of bone remodeling (bone turnover) is very active in young children, where it can be 200 times faster than in adults.

Cranial bones grow mainly because of the formation of bone tissue by the periosteum between the sutures and on the external bone surface. At the same time, resorption takes place on the internal surface. Since bone is an extremely plastic tissue, it responds to the growth of the brain and forms a skull of adequate size. The skull will be small if the brain does not develop completely and larger than normal in a person suffering from hydrocephalus, a disorder characterized by abnormal accumulation of spinal fluid and dilatation of the cerebral ventricles.

The growth of long bones is a complex process. The epiphyses increase in size owing to the radial growth of the cartilage, followed by endochondral ossification. In this way, the spongy part of the epiphysis increases.

The diaphysis (the bone formed between the 2

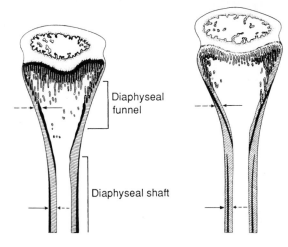

Diaphyseal funnel

Diaphyseal shaft

Figure 8–18. Drawings based on radioautographs of animals injected with radioactive phosphate at several intervals before being killed. Black areas indicate radioactive matrix, solid arrows indicate zones of bone deposition, and broken arrows indicate zones of bone resorption. In diaphyseal funnels, bone deposition occurs mainly at the internal surface; on the diaphysis, bone is laid down mainly on the outer surface. (Based on the work of CP Leblond et al. Redrawn and reproduced, with permission, from Greep RO, Weiss L: *Histology*, 3rd ed., McGraw-Hill, 1973.)

epiphyseal plates) consists initially of a bone cylinder. Because of the faster growth of the epiphyses, the extremities of the diaphysis soon become larger, forming 2 **diaphyseal funnels** separated by the **diaphyseal shaft.**

The diaphyseal shaft increases in length mainly as a result of the osteogenic activity of the epiphyseal plate; it increases in width as a result of the formation of bone by the periosteum on the external surface of the bone collar. At the same time, bone is removed from the internal surface, causing the bone marrow cavity to increase in diameter.

Because of the osteogenic activity of the endosteum, deposition of bone occurs on the internal surfaces (Fig 8–18) of both diaphyseal funnels. At the same time, bone is resorbed from opposite areas on the external surface. The narrow parts of the diaphyseal funnels therefore become gradually cylindrical; this is due mainly to the osteogenic activity of the epiphyseal plate (Fig 8–19). As a result of this process, the cylindrical diaphyseal shaft increases in length, and the 2 diaphyseal funnels grow farther apart as the bone lengthens. Gradually, osteogenic activity in the endosteum of the cylindrical portion of the diaphyseal funnel ceases, permitting the bone marrow cavity to maintain its diameter or to increase it slowly by resorption. As the central bone spicules become eroded to make room for the bone marrow cavity, the epiphyseal cartilage remains firmly at-

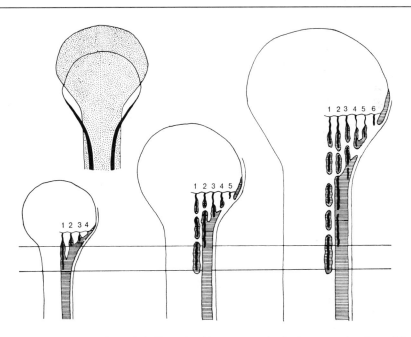

Figure 8–19. Growth of a long bone. **Upper left:** The role of bone resorption in the external surface of the funnel for bone growth. **Lower drawings:** Bone growth taking place by diaphyseal displacement. (Use the 2 parallel lines as reference.) Observe also how epiphyseal bone spicules contribute to the diaphyseal development; eg, spicule 2 is being incorporated into the diaphysis. (Based on the work of CP Leblond et al.)

tached to the diaphyseal funnel by means of the peripheral spicules (Figs 8–18 and 8–19).

In brief, it can be said that long bones become longer as a result of the activity of the epiphyseal plates and wider as a result of the apposition of bone formed by the periosteum. When the cartilage of the epiphyseal plate stops growing, it is replaced by bone tissue through the process of ossification. This closure of the epiphyses occurs around age 20. After that point, longitudinal growth of bones becomes impossible, although widening may still occur.

Fracture Repair

When a bone is fractured, the damaged blood vessels produce a localized hemorrhage with formation of a blood clot. Destruction of bone matrix and death of bone cells adjoining the fracture also occur.

During repair, the blood clot, cells, and damaged bone matrix are removed by macrophages. The periosteum and the endosteum around the fracture respond with intense proliferation of osteoprogenitor cells, which form a cellular tissue surrounding the fracture and penetrating between the extremities of the fractured bone (Fig 8–20A and B).

Primary bone is then formed by endochondral ossification of small cartilage fragments that appear in the connective tissue of the fracture.

Bone is also formed by means of intramembranous ossification. Therefore, areas of cartilage, intramembranous ossification, and endochondral ossification are encountered simultaneously in fractures. Repair progresses in such a way that irregularly formed trabeculae of primary bone temporarily unite the extremities of the fractured bone, forming a **bone callus** (Figs 8–20C and 8–21).

Normal stress imposed on the bone during repair and during the patient's gradual return to activity serves to remodel the bone callus. Since these stresses are identical to those that occurred during the growth of the bone, and thus influence its structure, remodeling of the callus reconstitutes the bone as it was prior to fracture. The primary bone tissue of the callus is gradually resorbed and replaced by secondary bone, resulting in restoration of the original bone structure (Fig 8–20D).

HISTOPHYSIOLOGY

Support & Protection

Bones form the skeleton, whose function is to bear the weight of the body. Voluntary (skeletal) muscles are inserted onto the bones via intercalation of the tendons with the connective tissue of the periosteum. Long bones constitute a system of levers that increase

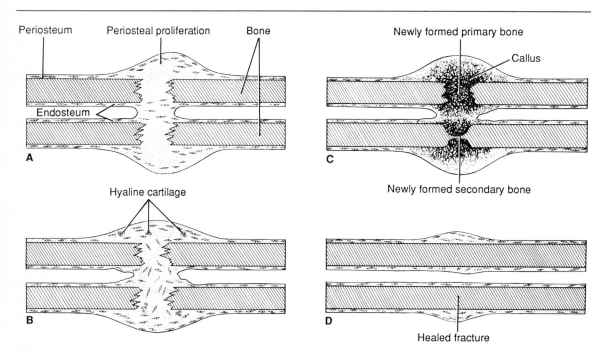

Figure 8–20. Repair of a fractured bone by formation of new bone tissue through periosteal and endosteal cell proliferation.

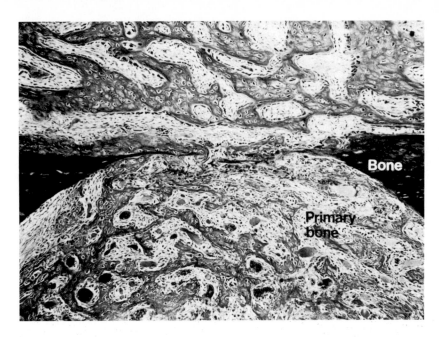

Figure 8–21. Photomicrograph of a mouse bone callus 7 days after fracture. The early callus contains mainly primary bone tissue made by cells originating in the periosteum. This micrograph corresponds with the callus area in Fig 8–20C. × 118.

the forces produced by muscular contractions. Bones protect the central nervous system (which is enclosed in the skull and the spinal canal), the bone marrow, and the thoracic contents.

Plasticity

In spite of its hardness, bone is capable of remodeling its internal structure according to the different stresses to which it is subjected. For example, the positions of the teeth in the jawbone can be modified by lateral pressures produced by orthodontic appliances. Bone formation takes place on the side where traction is applied and is resorbed where pressure is exerted (on the opposite side). In this way, teeth move within the jawbone while the alveolar bone is being remodeled. This capacity for reconstruction is characteristic of all bones.

Calcium Reserve

The skeletal contains 99% of the total calcium of the body and acts as a calcium reservoir. The concentration of calcium in the blood and in tissues is quite stable. There is a continuous interchange between blood calcium and bone calcium. The calcium absorbed from a meal, which would otherwise increase the blood calcium level, is rapidly deposited in bones or excreted in the feces or urine. Calcium in bones is mobilized when the concentration in blood decreases.

Bone calcium is mobilized by two mechanisms,

one rapid and the other slow. The first is the simple transference of ions from hydroxyapatite crystals to interstitial fluid—from which, in turn, calcium passes into the blood. This purely physical mechanism, which takes place mainly in spongy bone, is aided by the large surface area of the hydroxyapatite crystals. The younger, slightly calcified lamellae that exist even in adult bone (because of continuous remodeling) receive and lose calcium more readily. These lamellae are more important for the maintenance of calcium concentration in the blood than are the older, greatly calcified lamellae, whose role is mainly that of support and protection.

The second mechanism for mobilizing calcium depends on the action of hormones on bone. **Parathyroid hormone** activates and increases the number of cells (osteoclasts) promoting resorption of the bone matrix, with the consequent liberation of calcium.

Another hormone, **calcitonin,** which is synthesized by the parafollicular cells of the thyroid gland, inhibits matrix resorption. Its effect on bone, therefore, is the opposite of that of parathyroid hormone.

Since the concentration of calcium in tissues and blood must be kept constant, nutritional deficiency of calcium results in decalcification of bones; they then are more likely to fracture and are more transparent to x-rays. Decalcification of bone may also be caused by excessive production of parathyroid hormone (hyperparathyroidism), which results in intense resorption of bone, elevation of blood calcium levels, and abnormal deposits of calcium in several organs, mainly the kidneys and arterial walls.

Nutrition

Especially during growth, bone is sensitive to nutritional factors. Insufficient dietary protein causes a deficiency of amino acids and leads to reduced synthesis of collagen by osteoblasts. Deficiency of calcium leads to incomplete calcification of the organic bone matrix; it may be due either to the lack of calcium in the diet or to the lack of vitamin D, which is important for the absorption of calcium by the small intestine.

Calcium deficiency in children causes **rickets,** a disease in which the bone matrix does not calcify normally and the bone spicules formed by the epiphyseal plate become distorted by the normal strains of body weight and muscular activity. Consequently, ossification processes at this level are hindered and the bones not only grow more slowly but also become deformed.

Calcium deficiency in adults gives rise to **osteomalacia** (*osteon* + Greek, *malakia,* softness), characterized by deficient calcification of recently formed bone and partial decalcification of already calcified matrix. However, since adults have no epiphyseal cartilage, the deformation of long bones and retardation of growth that is characteristic of rickets in children does not occur, and of course growth is not affected. Osteomalacia may be aggravated during pregnancy, since the developing fetus requires a great deal of calcium.

Osteomalacia should not be confused with **osteoporosis,** a condition not related to nutrition. In the former, there is a decrease in the amount of calcium per unit of bone matrix. Osteoporosis, frequently found in immobilized patients and postmenopausal women, is a decrease in bone mass caused by decreased bone formation, increased bone resorption, or both. In osteoporosis, the ratio of mineral to matrix is normal.

In addition to the aforementioned effect on intestinal absorption, vitamin D has a direct effect on ossification, as has been demonstrated with in vitro experiments. Bone tissue cultivated in a medium rich in calcium but deficient in vitamin D does not calcify properly. Excessive amounts of vitamin D are toxic and give rise to calcification of many soft tissues.

Another vitamin that acts directly on bone is vitamin C, which is essential for collagen synthesis by both osteoblasts and osteocytes. Vitamin C deficiency interferes with bone growth and hinders repair of fractures by altering collagen deposition.

Hormonal Factors

In addition to parathyroid hormone and calcitonin, several other hormones act on bone.

The anterior lobe of the pituitary synthesizes growth hormone, which stimulates overall growth—but especially that of epiphyseal cartilage. Consequently, lack of growth hormone during the growing years causes **pituitary dwarfism;** an excess of growth hormone causes excessive growth of the long bones, resulting in **gigantism.** Adult bones cannot increase in length when stimulated by an excess of growth hormone because of the lack of epiphyseal cartilage, but they do increase in width by periosteal growth.

In adults, an increase in growth hormone causes **acromegaly,** a disease in which the bones—mainly the long ones—become very thick.

The sex hormones, both male (androgens) and female (estrogens), have a complex effect on bones and are, in a general way, stimulators of bone formation. They influence the time of appearance and the development of ossification centers.

Precocious sexual maturity caused by sex hormone-producing tumors or the administration of sex hormones retards bodily growth, since the epiphyseal cartilage is quickly replaced by bone. In hormone deficiencies caused by castration or by abnormal development of the gonads, epiphyseal cartilage remains functional for a longer period of time, resulting in tall stature.

Interrelationships Between Bone Cells

Radioautographic studies performed after the administration of ^{3}H-thymidine to young animals—whose bone cells proliferate rapidly—reveal that osteoblasts and osteocytes do not divide after having been formed from the **osteoprogenitor cell.** These studies also show that osteoblasts usually give rise to osteocytes that can remain as such for long periods (in secondary bone) or short periods (in primary bone). Both osteoblasts and osteocytes can revert to osteoprogenitor cells. The ability of the cells related to bone production to both turn over rapidly and modulate back to osteoprogenitor cells confers a high plasticity that permits the cells to adapt quickly to changing conditions.

Bone cells may escape the normal controls of proliferation and develop tumors. Benign bone cell tumors are called **osteomas;** malignant tumors are termed **osteosarcomas.** Primary bone is the only type of bone present in osteosarcomas; its presence is important for diagnosis. Most cases of osteosarcoma occur in children and adolescents, usually around the knee joint, and are more frequent in males than in females.

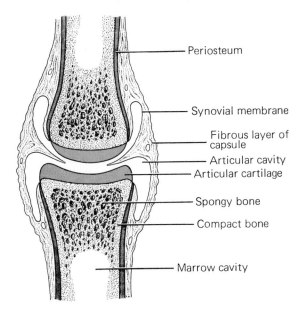

Figure 8–22. Schematic drawing of a diarthrosis. The capsule is formed by 2 parts: the external **fibrous layer** and the **synovial layer** (synovial membrane) that lines the articular cavity except for the cartilaginous areas.

JOINTS

Joints are regions where bones are capped and surrounded by connective tissues, holding the bones together and determining the type and degree of movement between them. Joints may be classified as **diarthroses,** which permit free bone movement, and **synarthroses** (from Greek, *syn,* together, + *arthrosis,* articulation), in which very limited or no movement occurs. There are 3 types of synarthroses, according to the type of tissue uniting the bone surfaces: **synostosis, synchondrosis,** and **syndesmosis.**

Synostosis

In these joints, bones are united by bone tissue and no movement takes place. In elderly people, this type of synarthrosis unites the skull bones. In children and young adults, these bones are united by dense connective tissue.

Synchondrosis

Synchondroses (*syn* + *chondros*) are articulations in which the bones are joined by hyaline cartilage. The epiphyseal plates of growing bones are one example. In the adult human, synchondrosis unites the first rib to the sternum.

Syndesmosis

As is the case with synchondrosis, a syndesmosis permits a certain amount of movement. The bones are joined by an interosseous ligament of dense connective tissue (eg, the pubic symphysis).

Diarthrosis

Diarthroses are joints that generally unite long bones and have great mobility, such as the elbow and knee joints. In a diarthrosis, ligaments and a capsule of connective tissue maintain the contact at the ends of the bone. The capsule encloses a sealed **articular cavity** that contains **synovial fluid,** a colorless, transparent, viscous fluid. Synovial fluid is a blood plasma dialysate with a high concentration of hyaluronic acid produced by B cells of the synovial layer. The sliding of articular surfaces covered by hyaline cartilage and having no perichondrium is facilitated by the lubricating synovial fluid, which also supplies nutrients and oxygen to the avascular articular cartilage (Figs 8–22 and 8–23).

The resilient articular cartilage is also a very efficient absorber of the intermittent mechanical pressures to which many joints are subjected. Proteoglycan molecules, found isolated or aggregated in

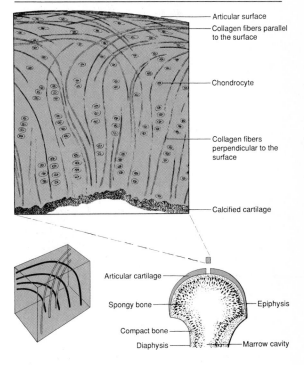

Figure 8–23. Articular surfaces of diarthroses are covered by hyaline cartilage that is devoid of perichondrium. The upper figure shows that in this cartilage, collagen fibers are first perpendicular and then parallel to the cartilage surface. Deeply located chondrocytes are globular and are arranged in vertical rows. Superficially placed chondrocytes are flattened; they are not organized in groups. The lower left drawing shows the organization of collagen fibers in articular cartilage in 3 dimensions.

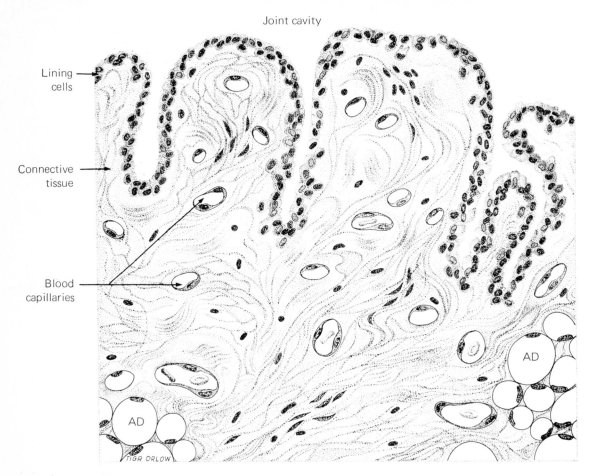

Figure 8–24. Histologic structure of the synovial membrane, with its lining cells in epitheloid arrangement. There is no basal lamina between the lining cells and the underlying connective tissue. This tissue is rich in blood capillaries and contains a variable amount of adipose cells (AD). (Reproduced, with permission, from Cossermelli W: *Reumatologia Basica*, Sarvier, 1971.)

a network, contain a large amount of water. These matrix components, rich in highly branched hydrophilic glycosaminoglycans, function as a biomechanical spring. When pressure is applied, water is forced out of the cartilage matrix into the synovial fluid. When water is expelled, another mechanism that contributes to cartilage resilience enters into play. This is the reciprocal electrostatic repulsion of the negatively charged carboxyl and sulfate groups in the glycosaminoglycan molecules. These charges are also responsible for separating the glycosaminoglycan branches, thus creating spaces to be occupied by water. When the pressure is released, water is attracted back into the interstices of the glycosaminoglycan branches. These water movements are brought about by the use of the joint. They are essential for nutrition of the cartilage, facilitating the interchange of O_2, CO_2, and other molecules between the synovial fluid and the articular cartilage.

The capsules of diarthroses (Fig 8–22) vary in structure according to the joint. Generally, however, this capsule is composed of 2 layers, one external (**fibrous layer**) and one internal (**synovial layer**).

The synovial layer is arranged in folds that occasionally penetrate deep into the interior of the articular cavity. The internal surface of the synovial membrane is usually lined by a layer of squamous or cuboidal cells. Underneath these cells is a layer of loose or dense connective tissue with areas of adipose tissue. The lining cells of the synovial membrane originate in the mesenchyme (Fig 8–24). They are separated from each other by a small amount of connective tissue ground substance (Fig 8–25).

Observations with the electron microscope have shown 2 cell types lining the synovial membrane (Fig 8–25). Some of these cells are intensely phagocytic; they have a structure similar to cells in the mononu-

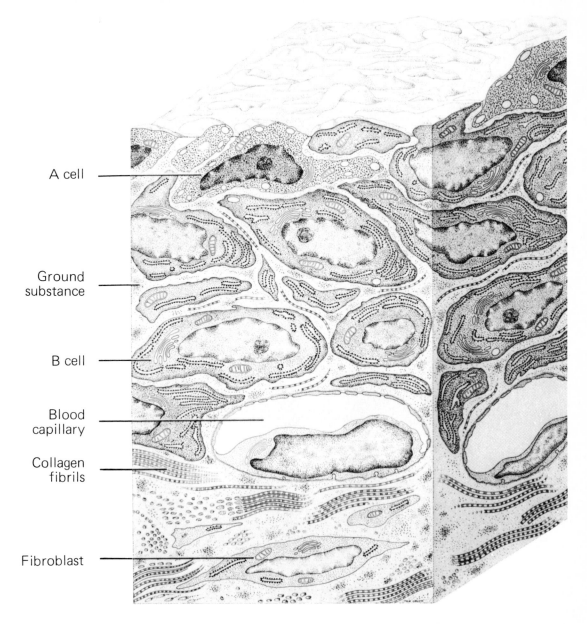

A cell

Ground
substance

B cell

Blood
capillary

Collagen
fibrils

Fibroblast

Figure 8–25. Schematic representation of the ultrastructure of synovial membrane. A and B cell types are separated by a small amount of connective tissue ground substance. No basal lamina is seen separating the lining cells from the connective tissue. Blood capillaries are of the fenestrated type, which facilitates exchange of substances between blood and synovial fluid.

clear phagocyte system and are called **A cells.** They have a large Golgi complex and many lysosomes but only a small amount of rough endoplasmic reticulum. The other cell type is called the **B cell** and resembles a fibroblast.

The fibrous layer is made of dense connective tissue that is better developed in parts subject to great strain. This layer envelops the ligaments of the joint and some of the tendons inserted into the bone near the joint.

REFERENCES

Bourne GH (editor): *The Biochemistry and Physiology of Bone,* 2nd ed. 4 vols. Academic Press, 1971–1976.

Ghadially FN: *Fine Structure of Synovial Joints.* Butterworth, 1983.

Gothlin G, Ericsson JLE: The osteoclast: Review of ultrastructure, origin and structure-function relationship. *Clin Orthop* 1976;**120**:201.

Hancox NM: *Biology of Bone.* Cambridge Univ Press, 1972.

Holtrop ME: The ultrastructure of bone. *Ann Clin Lab Sci* 1975;**5**:264.

Jotereau FV, LeDouarin NM: The developmental relationship between osteocytes and osteoclasts: A study using the quail-chick nuclear marker in endochondral ossification. *Dev Biol* 1978;**63**:253.

Termine JD et al: Osteonectin, a bone-specific protein linking mineral to collagen. *Cell* 1981;**26**:99.

Urist MR: *Fundamental and Clinical Bone Physiology.* Lippincott, 1980.

Nerve Tissue

9

The human nervous system contains at least 10 billion neurons. These basic building blocks of the nervous system have evolved from primitive neuroeffector cells that respond to various stimuli by contracting. In higher animals, contraction became the specialized function of muscle cells, and transmission of nerve impulses became the specialized function of neurons.

Nerve tissue is distributed throughout the body as an integrated communications network. Anatomically, the nervous system is divided into the **central nervous system,** consisting of the brain and the spinal cord; and the **peripheral nervous system,** composed of nerve fibers and small aggregates of nerve cells called **nerve ganglia.**

Structurally, nerve tissue consists of 2 cell-type classifications: **nerve cells,** or **neurons,** which usually show numerous long processes; and several types of **glial cells,** or **neuroglia** (from Greek, *neuron,* nerve, + *glia,* glue), which support and protect neurons and participate in neural activity, neural nutrition, and the defense processes of the central nervous system.

In the central nervous system, nerve cell bodies are concentrated in groups **(nuclei)** located at some distance from the tips of their processes. The brain and spinal cord are composed of **gray matter** and **white matter.** The former contains mainly nerve cell bodies and neuroglia as well as a complicated network of nerve cell processes. White matter does not contain nerve cell bodies; it consists of neuronal processes and neuroglia. It takes its name from the presence of **myelin,** a whitish material that envelops most of the neuronal processes. The brain stem exhibits zones containing both nerve cells and myelinated fibers, ie, both gray matter and white matter.

Neurons respond to environmental changes **(stimuli)** by altering electrical-potential differences that exist between the inner and outer surfaces of their membranes. Cells with this property (eg, neurons, muscle cells, some gland cells) are called **excitable,** or **irritable.** Neurons react promptly to stimuli with a modification of electrical potential that may be restricted to the place that received the stimulus or may be spread (propagated) throughout the neuron by the membrane. This propagation, called the **action potential,** or **nerve impulse,** transmits information to other neurons, muscles, and glands.

The 2 fundamental functions of the nervous system are to detect, analyze, integrate, and transmit all information generated by sensory stimuli (such as heat and light) and by mechanical and chemical changes that take place in the internal and external milieu; and to organize and coordinate, directly or indirectly, most functions of the body, especially the motor, visceral, endocrine, and mental activities.

DEVELOPMENT OF NERVE TISSUE

Nerve tissues develop from embryonic ectoderm that is induced to differentiate in this direction by the underlying notochord. First, a neural plate forms; then the edges of the plate thicken, forming the neural groove. The edges of the groove grow toward each other and ultimately fuse, forming the neural tube. This structure gives rise to the entire central nervous system, including neurons, glial cells, ependymal cells, and the epithelial cells of the choroid plexus.

Some cells lateral to the neural groove, making up the **neural crest,** undergo extensive migrations and give rise to most of the peripheral nervous system, as well as a number of other structures. Neural crest derivatives include the following: (1) chromaffin cells of the adrenal medulla (see Chapter 21); (2) melanocytes of skin and subcutaneous tissues (see Chapter 18); (3) odontoblasts (see Chapter 15); (4) cells of the pia mater and the arachnoid; (5) sensory neurons of cranial and spinal sensory ganglia; (6) postganglionic neurons of sympathetic and parasympathetic ganglia; (7) Schwann cells of peripheral axons; and (8) satellite cells of peripheral ganglia.

NEURONS

Nerve cells, or neurons, are independent anatomic and functional units with complex morphologic characteristics. They are responsible for the reception, transmission, and processing of stimuli; the triggering of certain cell activities; and the release of neurotransmitters and other informational molecules.

Most neurons consist of 3 parts: the **dendrites,** which are multiple elongated processes specialized in

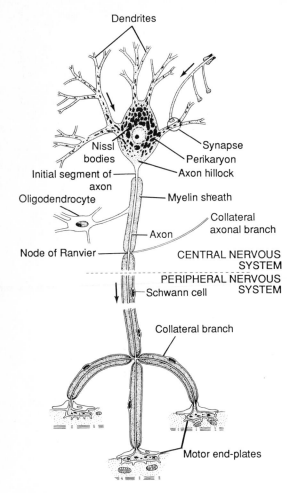

Figure 9–1. Schematic drawing of a Nissl-stained motor neuron. The myelin sheath is produced by oligodendrocytes in the central nervous system and by Schwann cells in the peripheral nervous system. The neuronal cell body has an unusually large, euchromatic nucleus with a well-developed nucleolus. The perikaryon contains Nissl bodies, which are also found in large dendrites. An axon from another neuron is shown at upper right. It has 3 end bulbs, one of which forms a synapse with the neuron. Note also the 3 motor end-plates, which transmit the nerve impulse to striated skeletal muscle fibers. Arrows show the direction of the nerve impulse.

receiving stimuli from the environment, from sensory epithelial cells, or from other neurons; the **cell body,** or **perikaryon** (from Greek, *peri,* around, + *karyon*) which represents the trophic center for the whole nerve cell and is also receptive to stimuli; and the **axon,** which is a single process specialized in generating or conducting nerve impulses to other cells (nerve, muscle, and gland cells). The distal portion of the axon is usually branched and constitutes the **terminal arborization.** Each branch of this arborization terminates on the next cell in dilatations called

end bulbs (boutons), which form a part of the **synapse.** Synapses transmit information to the next cell in the chain (Fig 9–1).

Neurons and their processes are extremely variable in size and shape (Fig 9–2). Perikaryons can be spherical, ovoid, or angular; some are very large, measuring up to 150 μm in diameter—large enough to be visible to the naked eye. Other nerve cells are among the smallest cells in the body; for example, the perikaryons of granule cells of the cerebellum are only 4–5 μm in diameter.

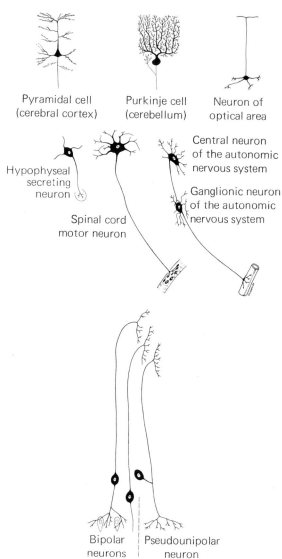

Figure 9–2. Diagrams of several types of neurons. The morphologic characteristics of neurons are very complex. All neurons shown here, except for the bipolar and pseudounipolar neurons, which are not very numerous in nerve tissue, are of the common multipolar variety.

According to the size and shape of their processes, most neurons can be placed in one of the following categories: **multipolar neurons,** which have more than 2 cell processes, one process being the axon and the others dendrites; **bipolar neurons,** with one dendrite and one axon; and **pseudounipolar neurons,** which have a single process that is close to the perikaryon and divides into 2 branches. The process then forms a T shape, with one branch extending to a peripheral ending and the other toward the central nervous system (Fig 9–2). In pseudounipolar neu-rons, stimuli that are picked up by the dendrites travel directly to the axon terminal without passing through the perikaryon.

Most neurons of the body are multipolar. Bipolar neurons are found in the cochlear and vestibular gan-glia as well as in the retina and the olfactory mucosa. Pseudounipolar neurons are found in the spinal gan-glia (the sensory ganglia located in the dorsal roots of the spinal nerves); they are also found in most cranial ganglia.

Neurons can also be classified according to their

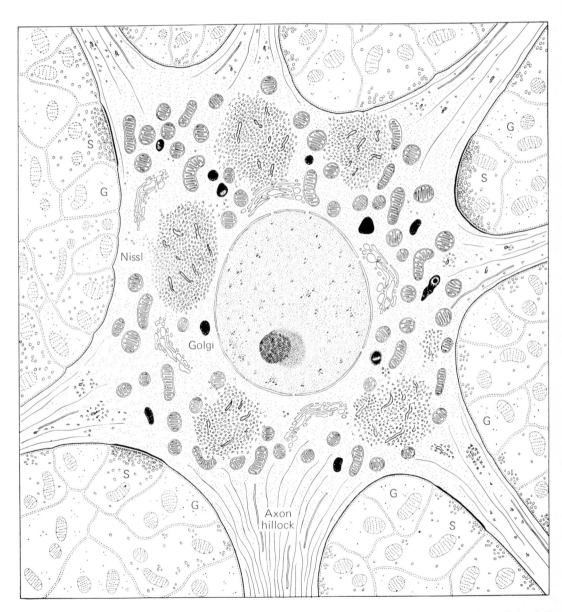

Figure 9–3. Ultrastructure of a neuron. The neuronal surface is completely covered either by synaptic endings of other neurons (S) or by processes of glial cells (G). At synapses, the neuronal membrane is thicker and is called the postsynaptic membrane. The neuronal process devoid of ribosomes (lower part of figure) is the axon hillock. The other processes of this cell are dendrites.

functional roles. **Motor (efferent) neurons** control effector organs such as muscle fibers and exocrine and endocrine glands. **Sensory (afferent) neurons** are involved in the reception of sensory stimuli from the environment and from within the body. **Interneurons** establish interrelationships among other neurons, forming complex functional chains or circuits (as in the retina).

During mammalian evolution there has been a great increase in the number and complexity of interneurons. Highly developed functions of the nervous system cannot be ascribed to simple neuron circuits; rather, they depend on complex interactions established by the integrated functions of many neurons.

In the central nervous system, nerve cell bodies are present only in the gray matter. White matter contains neuronal processes but no perikaryons. In the peripheral nervous system, perikaryons are found in ganglia and in some sensory regions (eg, olfactory mucosa).

PERIKARYON, OR SOMA

The perikaryon is the part of the neuron that contains the nucleus and surrounding cytoplasm, exclusive of the cell processes. It is primarily a trophic center, although it also has receptive capabilities. The perikaryon of most neurons receives a great number of nerve endings that convey excitatory or inhibitory stimuli generated in other nerve cells (Figs 9–3 and 9–6).

Nucleus

Most nerve cells have a spherical, unusually large, euchromatic (pale-staining) nucleus with a prominent nucleolus. Binuclear nerve cells are seen in sympathetic and sensory ganglia. The chromatin is finely dispersed, reflecting the intense synthetic activity of these cells.

Rough Endoplasmic Reticulum

Perikaryons contain a highly developed rough endoplasmic reticulum organized into aggregates of parallel cisternae. In the cytoplasm between the cisternae are numerous polyribosomes; these cells synthesize both structural proteins and proteins for transport. When appropriate stains are used, rough endoplasmic reticulum and free ribosomes appear under the light microscope as basophilic granular areas called **Nissl bodies** (Figs 9–1 and 9–4).

The number of Nissl bodies varies according to neuronal type and functional state. They are particularly abundant in large nerve cells such as motor neurons (Fig 9–4).

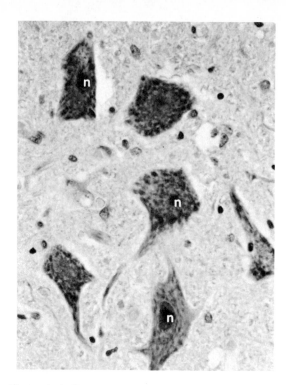

Figure 9–4. Photomicrograph of motor neurons from the human spinal cord. The cytoplasm contains a great number of Nissl bodies, making it difficult to see the cell nucleus (n). Although their cellular boundaries are not evident, nuclei of numerous glial and endothelial cells are present around the neurons. H&E stain, × 360.

Golgi Complex

The Golgi complex is located only in the perikaryon and consists of multiple parallel arrays of smooth cisternae arranged around the periphery of the nucleus. There are also a number of smaller, spherical vesicles that probably represent both transfer and secretory vesicles (Fig 9–3). With the use of osmic acid or silver impregnation techniques, the Golgi complex takes on the appearance of a network of irregular filaments.

Mitochondria

Mitochondria are found in neurons and are especially abundant in the axon terminals. They are scattered throughout the cytoplasm of the perikaryon.

Neurofilaments & Microtubules

Intermediate filaments with a diameter of 10 nm called **neurofilaments** are abundant in perikaryons and cell processes. Neurofilaments bundle together as a result of the action of certain fixatives. When impregnated with silver, they form **neurofibrils** that are visible with the light microscope. In tissue cultures under certain conditions, it is possible to see

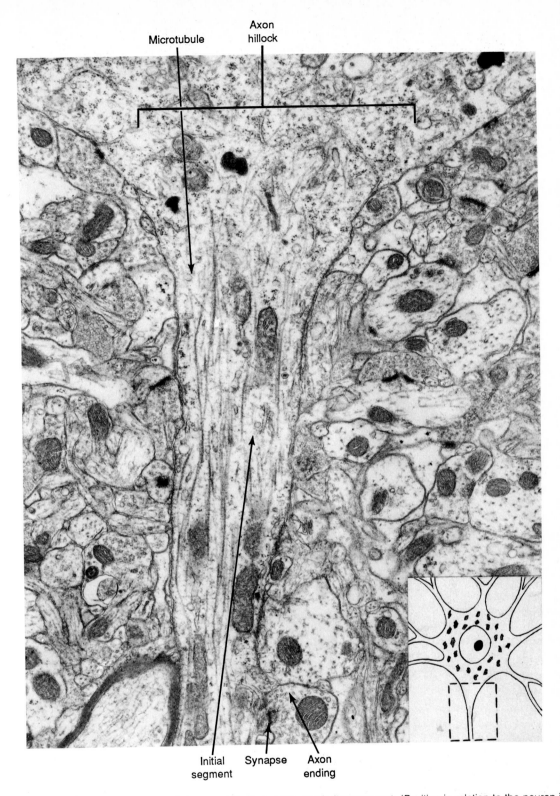

Microtubule   Axon
               hillock

Initial   Synapse   Axon
segment   ending

Figure 9–5. Electron micrograph of the axon hillock and the axon's first segment. (Position in relation to the neuron is indicated in the inset.) The axon hillock lacks ribosomes and endoplasmic reticulum. The parallel arrangement of microtubules in bundles is initiated in the axon hillock and becomes more pronounced in the initial segment of the axon. An axon ending synapses with the initial segment in the lower portion of the micrograph. Note that there is virtually no intercellular material in nerve tissue (see also Fig 9–3). × 26,000. (Courtesy of A Peters.)

neurofibril-like structures in living neurons. The neurofilaments can probably be seen because they are often aligned as closely packed, parallel bundles of filaments, although they are actually below the limit of resolution of the light microscope. The perikaryon also contains microtubules with a diameter of 24 nm that are identical to those found in many other cells (Fig 9–4). Nerve cells occasionally contain inclusions of pigments, such as **lipofuscin,** which is known to be a residue of undigested material by lysosomes, and **melanin,** which is of unknown significance.

DENDRITES

Most nerve cells have numerous dendrites, which considerably increase the receptive area of the cell. The aborization of dendrites makes it possible for one neuron to receive and integrate a great number of axon terminals from other nerve cells. It has been estimated that up to 200,000 axonal terminations establish functional contact with the dendrites of the Purkinje cell found in the cerebellum (Fig 9–2). That number may be even higher in other nerve cells. Bipolar neurons, with only one dendrite, are uncommon and are found only in special sites. Unlike axons, which maintain a constant diameter from one end to the other, dendrites become thinner as they subdivide into branches.

The composition of dendritic cytoplasm is similar to that of the perikaryon; however, dendrites are devoid of Golgi complexes. Nissl bodies and mitochondria are present except in very thin dendrites. Neurofilaments (10 nm) and microtubules (about 24 nm), also found in axons, are more numerous in dendrites. Dendrites are usually short and divide like the branches of a tree (arborization). In some instances, however, they assume other forms—for example, the characteristic dendrites of the cerebellar Purkinje cells branch in one plane only, assuming the shape of a fan (Fig 9–2) and increasing the surface area of each Purkinje cell from 250 μm^2 in early development to 27,000 μm^2 in the mature cell. Dendrites are usually covered by a large number of spines, small dendritic projections that represent sites of synaptic contact.

AXONS

Most neurons have only one axon; a very few have no axon at all. An axon is a cylindrical process that varies in length and diameter according to the type of neuron. Although some neurons have short axons, axons are usually very long processes. For example, axons of the motor cells of the spinal cord that innervate the foot muscles may have a length of up to 100 cm (about 40 inches).

All axons originate from a short pyramid-shaped region, the **axon hillock,** that usually arises from the perikaryon (Fig 9–3) but in a few cases originates

from the stem of a major dendrite. The axon hillock can be differentiated from dendrites by distinctive cytologic features. The rough endoplasmic reticulum and ribosomes found in perikaryons and dendrites do not extend into the axon hillock; in the axon hillock, the microtubules are arranged in fascicles or bundles (Figs 9–3 and 9–5). The plasma membrane of the axon is called the **axolemma** (*axon* + Greek, *eilema,* sheath); its contents are known as **axoplasm.**

In neurons that give rise to a myelinated axon, the portion of the axon between the axon hillock and the point at which myelination begins is called the **initial segment.** This is the site where various excitatory and inhibitory stimuli impinging on the neuron are algebraically summed, resulting in the "decision" to

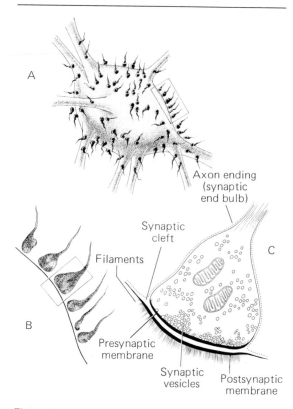

Figure 9–6. External morphologic features of a neuron and some of its processes. **A:** Axon endings from other neurons are shown in black. **B:** Enlargement of area outlined in **A. C:** Ultrastructure of the synapse outlined in **B.** At synaptic junctions the 2 cell membranes are separated by a slender space—the synaptic cleft. Presynaptic and postsynaptic membranes appear to be thicker than the neuronal membrane elsewhere. This is due to the accumulation of cytoplasmic proteins adjacent to these membranes. The axon ending shows 2 mitochondria as well as numerous synaptic vesicles that contain neurotransmitters. Liberation of the mediator substance transmits the nerve impulse from the presynaptic to the postsynaptic membrane. (Redrawn and reproduced, with permission, from De Robertis, Novinsky, Saez: *Biologia Celular,* 8th ed. El Ateneo [Buenos Aires], 1970.)

propagate—or not to propagate—an action potential, or nerve impulse. It is known that several types of ion channels are localized in the initial segment and that these channels are important in generating the propagating electrical-potential change that constitutes the action potential. The initial segment of the axon is characterized by the **dense undercoating,** a thin layer of electron-dense material beneath the plasma membrane. Microtubules and neurofilaments continue in fascicles from the axon hillock into the initial segment.

In contrast to dendrites, axons have a constant diameter and do not branch profusely. Occasionally, the axon, shortly after its departure from the cell body, gives rise to a branch that returns to the area of the nerve cell body. These branches are known as **collateral branches** (Fig 9–4).

Axonal cytoplasm (axoplasm) possesses a few mitochondria, microtubules, and neurofilaments and some cisternae of smooth endoplasmic reticulum. The absence of polyribosomes and RER emphasizes the dependence of the axon on the perikaryon for its maintenance. If an axon is severed, its peripheral parts degenerate and die.

SYNAPSES

When axons are artificially stimulated, they conduct the nerve impulse in both directions from the stimulation point. The impulse directed to the cell body, however, does not excite other neurons, and only the impulse reaching the final arborization of the axon, the axon terminal, can excite the next cell in the chain, be it neuron, muscle, or gland cell.

This dynamic polarization of the transmission of the nerve impulse depends on highly specialized structures called **synapses,** which are classically defined as the contact of one axon with the dendrites or perikaryon or, very rarely, the axon of another neuron. Synaptic contact also is established between neurons and muscle and gland cells. Most central nervous system synapses are between an axon and a dendrite **(axodendritic)** or between an axon and a cell body **(axosomatic).** But there are also synapses between dendrites **(dendrodendritic)** and between axons **(axoaxonic).** Synapses function by altering the membrane potential of neurons and other effector cells. The influence of a particular synapse on a neuron is related to its distance from the initial segment of the axon. Consequently, the influence of incoming information on neuronal activity is intimately related to the distribution and location, as well as number, of synapses on the dendritic tree and cell body.

Morphologically, several types of synapses can be identified. The axon terminal may form bulbous expansions, basketlike structures, or club-shaped terminations (Fig 9–6). These synaptic end bulbs are often called **boutons terminaux.** More often, the axon establishes several synapses along its course. In this case, there are enlargements along the axon, called

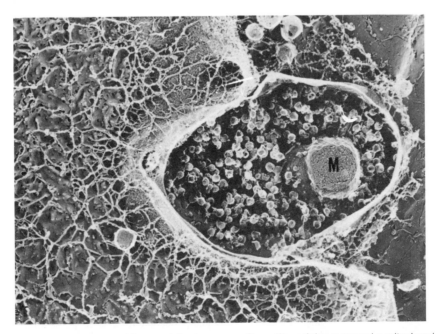

Figure 9–7. View of a rotary-replicated freeze-etched synapse. Synaptic vesicles surround a mitochondrion (M) in the axon terminal. × 25,000. (Reproduced, with permission, from Heuser JE, Salpeter SR: Organization of acetylcholine receptors in quick-frozen, deep-etched and rotary-replicated Torpedo postsynaptic membrane. *J Cell Biol* 1979;**82:**150.)

boutons en passage. The analysis of a synapse under the electron microscope shows that it is actually a specialized, localized region of contact between 2 cells (Figs 9–6 and 9–22). It is composed of a terminal membrane (presynaptic membrane), a region of extracellular space (**synaptic cleft**), and a postsynaptic membrane belonging to a dendrite, perikaryon, axon of another neuron, or membrane of a muscle or gland cell. At a synapse, the plasma membranes of the 2 neurons are usually separated by a distance of 20–30 nm (the synaptic cleft). These membranes are firmly bound together at the synaptic region, and in some instances, dense filaments form bridges between them. The plasma membranes of the 2 neurons appear to be thicker at the presynaptic and postsynaptic areas of the synapse than elsewhere. This apparent increase in membrane thickness is due to the accumulation of dense-staining cytoplasmic proteins beneath the membranes forming the synapse. Cytoplasmic filaments resembling those found in desmosomes are anchored to the inside of each of these membranes.

The cytoplasm in the endings of the terminal typically contains numerous **synaptic vesicles** (Figs 9–7 and 9–22) with a diameter of 20–65 nm, although some vesicles as large as 160 nm have been observed.

Synaptic vesicle shape and content have been correlated with the function of the synapse. Thus, round, clear vesicles are associated with acetylcholine-mediated excitatory transmission at the neuromuscular junction and at other sites in the central nervous system. Norepinephrine-secreting axons display vesicles with an overall diameter of 40–60 nm and a dense-staining core with a diameter of 15–25 nm.

Neurosecretory axons (eg, axons of the paraventricular and supraoptic nuclei of the hypothalamus that contain oxytocin, vasopressin, and their associated neurophysins) have larger secretory granules, 120–150 in diameter. Electron-dense material fills these granules with no intervening clear space.

Neurofilaments are infrequent, but mitochondria are numerous. The synaptic vesicles contain substances called **neurotransmitters** that are responsible for the transmission of the nerve impulse across the synapse. These mediators are liberated at the presynaptic membrane by exocytosis and act on the postsynaptic membrane to initiate an excitatory or inhibitory response. The membranes of synaptic vesicles that are incorporated into the presynaptic membranes undergo endocytosis and are reused to form new synaptic vesicles (see new vesicle formation in Fig 9–24).

> Events occurring at the neuromuscular synapse (junction) are of clinical importance in that by blocking transmission at this site with commonly used drugs, one can promote muscle relaxation during anesthesia, and reduction of muscle spasticity in certain neurologic conditions.

In addition to the chemical synapses described above, in which a chemical substance mediates the

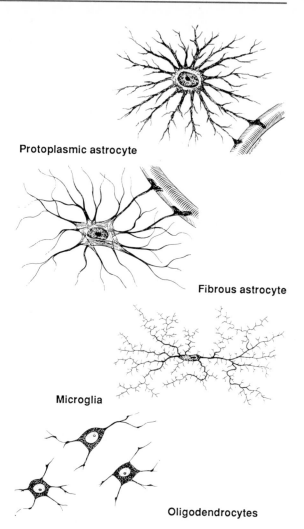

Protoplasmic astrocyte

Fibrous astrocyte

Microglia

Oligodendrocytes

Figure 9–8. Drawings of neuroglial cells as seen in slides stained by metallic impregnation. Observe that only astrocytes exhibit vascular end-feet, which cover the walls of blood capillaries.

transmission of the nerve impulse, there are also the electrical synapses. Here the nerve cells are linked through a gap junction (see Chapter 4) that permits the passage of ions from one cell to another, thus providing for their electrical coupling. Electrical synapses are less numerous than chemical synapses.

NEUROGLIA

Several cell types found in the central nervous system in association with the neurons are classified as **neuroglia (neuroglial, or glial, cells). Neuroglia separate neurons, form myelin, and have trophic and phagocytic functions.** The several types of neuroglia show morphologic and functional differences (Figs 9–8 and 9–9).

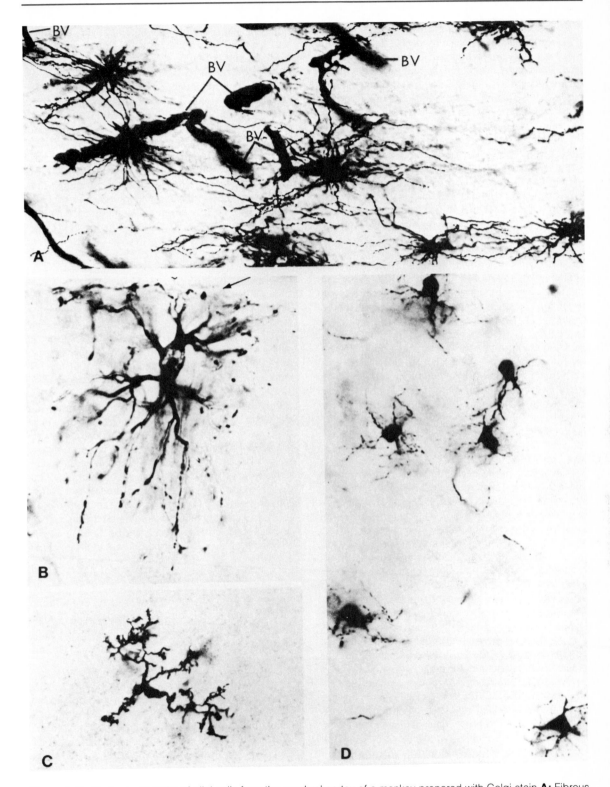

Figure 9–9. Photomicrographs of glial cells from the cerebral cortex of a monkey prepared with Golgi stain **A:** Fibrous astrocytes, showing blood vessels (BV). × 1000. **B:** Protoplasmic astrocyte showing brain surface **(arrow)**. × 1900. **C:** Microglial cell. × 1700. **D:** Oligodendrocytes. X 1900. (Reproduced, with permission, from Jones E, Cowan WM: The Nervous Tissue. In: *Histology: Cell and Tissue Biology*, 5th ed, Weiss L [editor]. Elsevier, 1983.)

Routine hematoxylin and eosin (H&E) preparations are not adequate to study neuroglia, since with this staining technique only their small nuclei (3–10 μm in diameter) can be seen among the larger nuclei of nerve cells (Fig 9–4). The cytoplasm and processes of the neuroglia are not identifiable, for it is impossible to distinguish them from the processes of the neurons. The neuroglia play an important role in the normal function of the nervous system. For the study of the morphologic characteristics of neuroglia, special procedures involving silver or gold impregnation techniques are used.

It has been estimated that in the central nervous system there are 10 glial cells for each neuron. Since neuroglia are much smaller, however, they occupy only about half the total volume of nervous tissue.

Neuroglia include several varieties: astrocytes, oligodendrocytes, microglia, and ependymal cells.

Neuroglial (glial) cells, which are not thought to generate action potentials or to form synapses with other cells, maintain the composition of fluids in the brain. Glial cells have receptors for neurotransmitters and exhibit peptides in common with some neurons; they thus help to control the chemical and electrical environment of the neurons. Unlike neurons, glial cells retain their ability to undergo mitosis throughout the life of the organism. Oligodendroglial cells form the myelin sheaths of axons in the central nervous system and are probably necessary for the maintenance and viability of neurons.

Astrocytes

Astrocytes (from Greek, *astron,* star, + *kytos*) are the largest of the neuroglia, possessing numerous long processes. They have spherical, centrally located nuclei that stain lightly (Fig 9–8). Many of their processes have expanded pedicles at their ends that attach to the walls of blood capillaries. These pedicles, called the **vascular feet,** or **vascular end-feet,** of the neuroglia, completely surround and ensheathe all vessels of the nourishing vascular network. Processes of astrocytes are also present at the periphery of the brain and spinal cord, forming a layer under the pia mater. This layer, which also contains processes of other neuroglia, separates the connective tissue of the pia mater from the nerve cells. Astrocytes provide some structural support for nervous tissue, and their extensions form a sealed barrier that protects the central nervous system. The nerve cells thus occupy the kind of sheltered and regulated environment necessary for the complex procedures involved in electrical signaling (see Fig 9–32). After injury to the central nervous system, astrocytes proliferate at the site of injury and form a type of scar tissue.

There are 2 types of astrocytes: protoplasmic, which are found in the gray matter of the brain and spinal cord; and fibrous, which are found chiefly in the white matter. In electron micrographs, astrocytes are identified by their light-staining, relatively organelle-free cytoplasm. Intermediate filaments, which are 10 nm in diameter and composed of glial fibrillar acidic protein, are abundant.

A. Protoplasmic Astrocytes: Protoplasmic astrocytes have abundant granular cytoplasm. Their processes have many branches, are shorter than those of fibrous astrocytes, and are relatively thick (Figs 9–8 and 9–9). Their processes envelop the surfaces of nerve cells, synaptic areas, and blood vessels.

B. Fibrous Astrocytes: Fibrous astrocytes have long, slender, smooth processes that branch infrequently. In special silver-stained preparations, their cytoplasm shows fibrillar material that is probably formed by the aggregation of 10-nm intermediate filaments (see Chapter 3) abundant in the cell bodies and processes of fibrous astrocytes (Figs 9–9 and 9–10).

Oligodendrocytes

Oligodendrocytes are much smaller than astrocytes, and their processes are less numerous and shorter than those present in other neuroglia (Fig 9–8). Their nuclei are smaller and stain more intensely than do the nuclei of astrocytes. The number of oligodendrocytes increases with the increasing complexity of the nervous system in different species. Human nerve tissue has the highest number per nerve cell.

Oligodendrocytes are found in both gray and white matter. In gray matter, they are localized mainly close to perikaryons. In white matter, oligodendrocytes appear in rows among the myelinated nerve fibers. Study of fetal nerve tissue with the electron microscope shows that the myelin sheath of central nervous system tissue is produced by the processes of oligodendrocytes. In this aspect of their function, the oligodendrocytes are analogous to the Schwann cells of peripheral nerves (Fig 9–11). Unlike Schwann cells, oligodendroglial cells can participate in the myelination of more than one axon (Fig 9–11).

The cytoplasm of oligodendrocytes is electron-dense and contains many mitochondria, a large Golgi complex, cisternae of rough endoplasmic reticulum, and numerous microtubules. These characteristics permit their identification in electron micrographs.

Microglia

Microglia are phagocytic cells that represent the mononuclear phagocyte system in nervous tissue. Their cell bodies are small, dense, and elongated. Their nuclei show highly condensed chromatin and an elongated shape along the axis of the cell body. The shape of the nuclei of microglia permits their identification in hematoxylin and eosin preparations; other neuroglia have spherical nuclei. Microglia have short processes covered by numerous small expansions, giving them a thorny appearance (Fig 9–8). While microglia are not numerous, they are found in both white and gray matter.

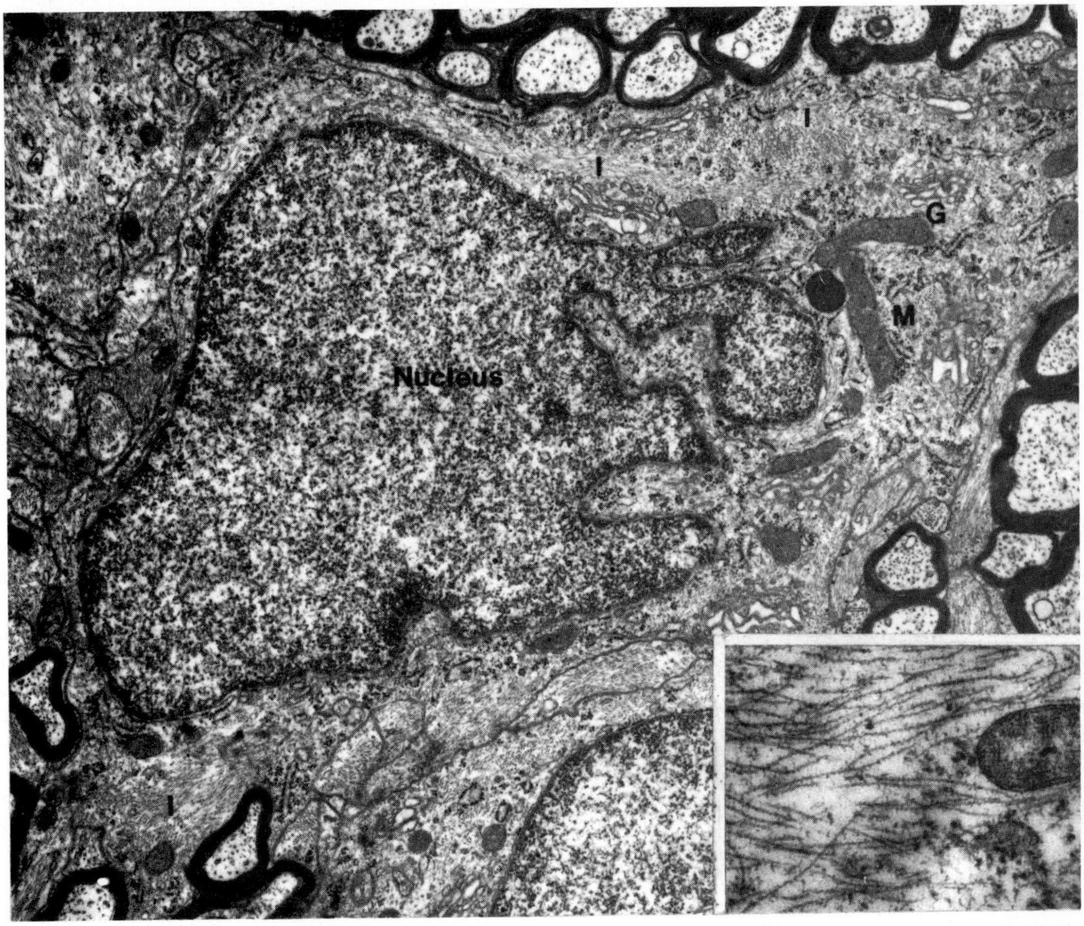

Figure 9–10. Electron micrograph of a fibrous astrocyte. G, Golgi complex; M, mitochondrion; I, intermediate (10-nm) filaments. × 12,000. The inset shows the abundant filaments in the cytoplasm. × 42,000. (Courtesy of A Peters.)

Ependymal Cells

Ependymal cells derive from the internal lining of the neural tube and retain their epithelial arrangement, while the other cells from the neural tube develop processes and give rise to neurons or neuroglia. Ependymal cells line the cavities of the brain and spinal cord and are bathed by the cerebrospinal fluid that fills these cavities. Most ependymal cells possess motile cilia that serve to produce movement of the cerebrospinal fluid.

Ependymal cells possess an abundance of mitochondria, an apical Golgi complex, and a sparse rough endoplasmic reticulum. The lateral surfaces of some ependymal cells exhibit gap junctions and zonulae adherentes, but in most areas of the brain, tight junctions (zonulae occludentes) are absent. Therefore, substances in the cerebrospinal fluid can come in contact with cells deep within the thick neuroepithelium.

The contour of the basal surface of the ependymal cell varies with its position in the brain or spinal cord. Most ependymal cells have a flattened base, but some have a long process that extends deep into the subjacent neural tissue. This latter type of cell is called a **tanycyte** and is conspicuous in the floor of the third ventricle. Here, the tanycyte may play a role in transferring chemical signals from cerebrospinal fluid to the primary capillary plexus of the hypophyseal-pituitary portal system (see Chapter 20).

Histophysiology

In the central nervous system, connective tissue layers form the enveloping protective and vascular coats (meninges) of the system. The very small amount of connective tissue that extends into the nerve tissue is restricted to sheaths that are present around the larger blood vessels. The supporting function of connective tissue is assumed by neuroglia. Because of their number and their long processes, astrocytes seem to be the most important supporting elements.

Glial cells, especially astrocytes, participate in the

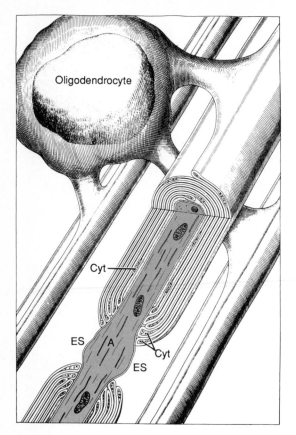

Figure 9–11. Myelin sheath of the central nervous system. The same oligodendrocyte forms myelin sheaths for several (3–50) nerve fibers. In the central nervous system, the nodes of Ranvier are somtimes covered by processes of other cells, or there is considerable extracellular space (ES) at that point. The axolemma shows a thickening where the cell membrane of the oligodendrocyte comes into contact with it. This limits the diffusion of materials into the periaxonal space between the axon and the myelin sheath. At upper left is a surface view of the cell body of an oligodendrocyte. Cyt, cytoplasm of glial cell; A, axon. (Redrawn and reproduced, with permission, from Bunge et al: *J Biophys Biochem Cytol* 1961;**10:**67.)

repair process following injury to the central nervous system. Repair consists of the proliferation of glial cells that fill the defect left by the degeneration of neurons and their processes. Astrocytes may also participate in the formation of the blood-brain barrier, although it is now generally believed that tight junctions between endothelial cells have the major role in preventing the indiscriminate access of circulating molecules to neural tissue.

Oligodendroglial cells are frequently found adjacent to neurons, and this association has given rise to the concept that oligodendroglial cells have a symbiotic relation with neurons. Cytochemical studies performed on neurons and satellite cells isolated by

microsurgery have shown a metabolic dependency between them. Any stimulus that alters the chemical composition of the nerve cell is also reflected in the satellite cell.

NERVE FIBERS

Nerve fibers consist of axons enveloped by special sheaths of ectodermal origin. Groups of nerve fibers constitute the tracts of the brain, spinal cord, and peripheral nerves. Nerve fibers exhibit differences in their enveloping sheaths, related to whether the fibers are part of the central or the peripheral nervous system.

Most axons in adult nerve tissue are covered by single or multiple folds of a sheath cell. In peripheral nerve fibers, the sheath cell is the **Schwann cell,** and in central nerve fibers it is the **oligodendrocyte.** Axons of small diameter are usually **unmyelinated nerve fibers** (Figs 9–12 and 9–16). Progressively thicker axons are generally ensheathed by increasingly numerous concentric wrappings of the enveloping cell. When enveloped by **myelin sheaths,** the fibers are known as **myelinated nerve fibers** (Fig 9–14).

> Myelin consists of many layers of modified cell membranes. These membranes have a higher proportion of lipids than do other cell membranes. Central nervous system myelin contains 2 major proteins: myelin basic protein and proteolipid protein. Several human demyelinating diseases are due to an insufficiency or lack of one or both of these proteins.

Axonal conduction of the nerve impulse is faster in axons with larger diameters and thicker myelin sheaths. Fresh myelinated fibers appear as white, homogeneous, glistening cylinders.

Myelinated Fibers

Embryologic studies have shown that the first step in myelin formation is axon penetration of an existing groove of the Schwann cell cytoplasm. The edges of the groove come together to form a **mesaxon,** so that the plasma membranes of the 2 edges fuse together on their outer surface. Next, through a process not yet fully understood, the mesaxon wraps itself around the axon several times, the number of turns determining the thickness of the myelin layer. Close examination of Fig 9–14 (bottom) reveals continuous dark lines alternating with more diffuse lines. The regular dark lines are called **major dense lines** and represent the line of fusion of *cytoplasmic* surfaces of Schwann cell membranes. The less regular lines are called **intraperiod lines** and are sites of close contact, but not fusion, of the *extracellular* surfaces of adjacent layers of Schwann cell membrane (Figs 9–11 and 9–13). After this process, both an internal and an external mesaxon can be seen (Figs 9–13 and

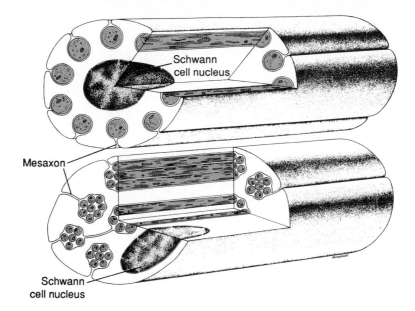

Figure 9–12. Above: The most frequent type of unmyelinated nerve fiber, in which isolated axons (shown in color) are surrounded by a Schwann cell and each axon has its own mesaxon. **Below:** Many very thin axons are sometimes found together, surrounded by the Schwann cell. In such cases, there is one mesaxon for several axons.

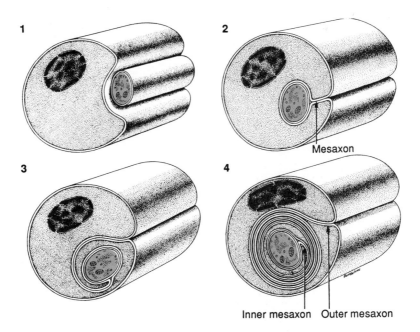

Figure 9–13. Four consecutive phases of myelin formation in peripheral nerve fibers.

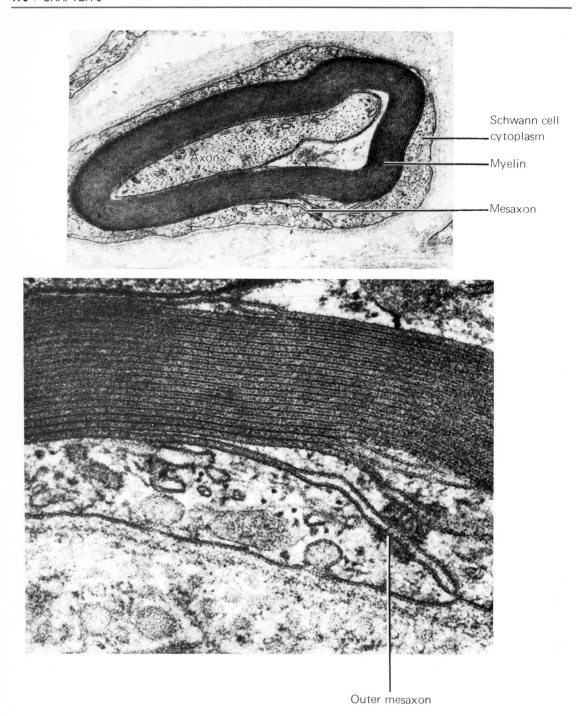

Figure 9–14. Electron micrographs of a myelinated nerve fiber. **Top:** × 20,000. **Bottom:** × 80,000.

9–14). The clefts of Schmidt-Lanterman are areas in which the cytoplasm of the Schwann cells is present within the myelin layer (Figs 9–15 and 9–16). These cytoplasmic areas were left behind during the winding process of the cytoplasm around the axon.

In myelinated fibers, the plasmalemma of the covering Schwann cell winds and wraps around the axon. The layers of membranes of the sheath cell unite and form myelin, a lipoprotein complex (Fig 9–13) whose lipid component can be partly removed by standard histologic procedures. Its presence can be demonstrated by osmium tetroxide, which preserves myelin and stains it black (Fig 9–14).

Each axon is surrounded by myelin formed by a series of Schwann cells. The myelin sheath shows gaps along its path called the **nodes of Ranvier** (Fig 9–15); these represent the spaces between adjacent Schwann cells along the length of the axon. Interdigitating processes of Schwann cells partially cover the node (Fig 9–16). The distance between 2 nodes is called an **internode** and consists of one Schwann cell. The length of the internode varies between 1 and 2 mm, depending on the diameter of the axon. The thickness of the myelin sheath varies according to the axonal diameters but it is constant along the length of a particular axon. Under the light microscope, the myelin sheath shows cone-shaped clefts called **clefts, or incisures, of Schmidt-Lanterman** that are actually helical cytoplasmic tunnels from the outside of the sheath to the inside. They represent distentions within the myelin layers caused by the localized presence of Schwann cell cytoplasm. This cytoplasm and, consequently, the clefts move up and down the sheath. Their apexes do not always point in the same direction (Fig 9–15).

There are no Schwann cells in the central nervous system; here, the myelin sheath is formed by the processes of the oligodendrocytes. Oligodendrocytes differ from Schwann cells in that different branches of one cell can envelop segments of several axons (Fig 9–11). The nodes of Ranvier may be uncovered in the central nervous system; Schmidt-Lanterman clefts are absent.

Unmyelinated Fibers

In both the central and peripheral nervous systems, not all axons are sheathed in myelin. In the peripheral system, all unmyelinated axons are enveloped within simple clefts of the Schwann cells (Fig 9–12). Unlike their association with individual myelinated axons, each Schwann cell can ensheathe many unmyelinated axons. Unmyelinated nerve fibers do not have nodes of Ranvier, since abutting Schwann cells are longitudinally united to form a continuous sheath.

The central nervous system is rich in unmyelinated axons; unlike those in the peripheral system, these axons are not sheathed. In the brain and spinal cord, unmyelinated axonal processes run free among the other neuronal and glial processes.

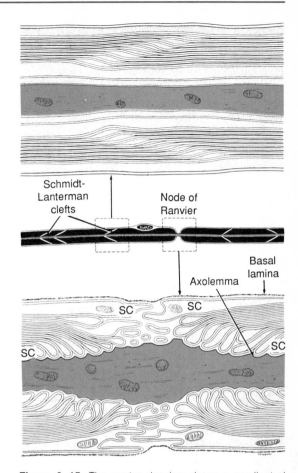

Figure 9–15. The center drawing shows a myelinated peripheral nerve fiber as seen under the light microscope. The process (shown in color) is the axon enveloped by the myelin sheath (shown in black) and by the cytoplasm of Schwann cells. A Schwann cell nucleus, the Schmidt-Lanterman clefts, and a node of Ranvier are shown. The upper drawing shows the ultrastructure of the Schmidt-Lanterman cleft. The cleft is formed by Schwann cell cytoplasm that is not displaced to the periphery during myelin formation. The lower drawing shows the ultrastructure of a node of Ranvier. Note the appearance of loose interdigitating processes of the outer leaf of the Schwann cells' cytoplasm (SC) and the close contact of the inner leaf of the cytoplasm with the axolemma. This acts as a sort of barrier to the movement of materials in and out of the periaxonal space between the axolemma and the membrane of the Schwann cell. The basal lamina around the Schwann cell is continuous. Covering the nerve fiber is a connective tissue layer—mainly reticular fibers—that forms the endoneurial sheath of the peripheral nerve fibers.

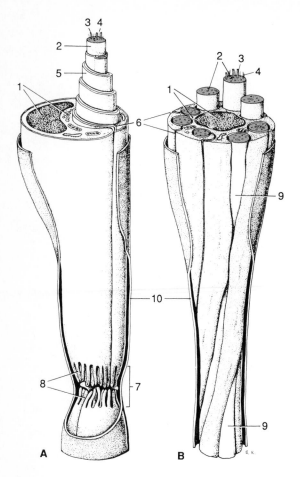

Figure 9–16. Schematic 3-dimensional drawings showing several ultrastructural features of a myelinated **(A)** and an unmyelinated **(B)** nerve fiber. 1, nucleus and cytoplasm of Schwann cell; 2, axon; 3, microtubule; 4, neurofilament; 5, myelin sheath; 6, mesaxon; 7, node of Ranvier; 8, interdigitating processes of Schwann cells at the node of Ranvier; 9, side view of an unmyelinated axon; 10, basal lamina. (Slightly modified and reproduced, with permission, from Krstić RV: *Ultrastructure of the Mammalian Cell.* Springer-Verlag, 1979.)

NERVES

In the peripheral nervous system, the nerve fibers are grouped in bundles to form the nerves. Except for a few very thin nerves made up of unmyelinated fibers, nerves have a whitish appearance because of their myelin content.

Nerves have an external fibrous coat of dense connective tissue called **epineurium,** which also fills the space between the bundles of nerve fibers. Each bundle is surrounded by the **perineurium,** a sleeve formed by layers of flattened epithelium-like cells. These cells of each layer of the perineural sleeve are joined at their edges by tight junctions, an arrangement that makes the perineurium a barrier to the passage of most macromolecules. Within the perineurial sheath run the Schwann cell-ensheathed axons and their enveloping connective tissue, the **endoneurium** (Fig 9–17). The endoneurium consists of a thin layer of reticular fibers (Figs 9–18 and 9–19). Endoneurial reticular fibers are probably produced by Schwann cells.

The nerves establish communication between brain and spinal cord centers and the sense organs and effectors (muscles, glands, etc). They possess afferent and efferent fibers in relation to the central nervous system. **Afferent** fibers carry the information obtained from the interior of the body and the environment to the central nervous system. **Efferent** fibers carry impulses from the central nervous system to the effector organs commanded by these centers. Nerves possessing only sensory fibers are called **sensory nerves;** those composed only of fibers carrying impulses to the effectors are called **motor nerves.** Most nerves have both sensory and motor fibers and are called **mixed nerves** (Fig 9–17); these nerves have both myelinated and unmyelinated axons (Fig 9–19).

AUTONOMIC NERVOUS SYSTEM

The autonomic nervous system is related to the control of smooth muscle, the secretion of some glands, and the modulation of cardiac rhythm. Its function is to make adjustments in certain activities of the body in order to maintain a constant internal environment (**homeostasis**; from Greek, *homiois*, like, + *stasis*, a standing). Although the autonomic nervous system is by definition a motor system, fibers that receive sensation originating in the interior of the organism accompany the motor fibers of the autonomic system.

Although the term **autonomic** implies that this part of the nervous system functions independently, this is not the case; its functions are constantly subject to the influences of conscious activity.

The concept of the autonomic nervous system is mainly functional. Anatomically, it is composed of collections of nerve cells located in the central nervous system, fibers that leave the central nervous system through cranial or spinal nerves, and nerve ganglia situated in the paths of these fibers. The term **autonomic** covers all the neural elements concerned with visceral function.

The first neuron of the autonomic chain is located in the central nervous system. Its axon forms a synapse with the second multipolar neuron in the chain, located in a ganglion of the peripheral autonomic system. The nerve fibers (axons) of the first neuron are called **preganglionic fibers;** the axons of the second neuron to the effectors—muscle or gland—are called **postganglionic fibers.**

The adrenal medulla is the only organ that receives

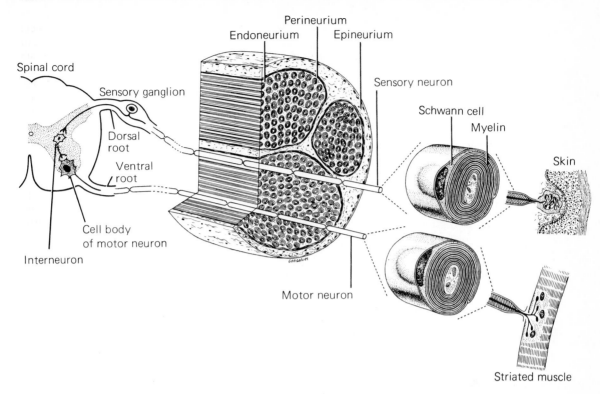

Figure 9–17. Schematic representation of a nerve and a reflex arc. In this example, the sensory stimulus starts in the skin and passes to the spinal cord via the dorsal root ganglion. The sensory stimulus then activates a motor fiber innervating skeletal muscle. Examples of the operation of this reflex are withdrawal of the finger from a hot surface and the knee-jerk reflex. (Slightly modified, redrawn, and reproduced, with permission, from Ham AW: *Histology*, 6th ed, Lippincott, 1969.)

preganglionic fibers, because the majority of the cells, after migration into the gland, differentiate into secretory cells rather than ganglion cells. Consequently, the innervation of the adrenal medulla is still preganglionic.

The autonomic nervous system is composed of 2 parts that differ both anatomically and functionally: the sympathetic system and the parasympathetic system (Fig 9–20).

Sympathetic System

The nuclei (nerve cell bodies) of the **sympathetic system** are located in the thoracic and lumbar segments of the spinal cord. The sympathetic system is also called the **thoracolumbar division** of the autonomic nervous system. The axons of these neurons—preganglionic fibers—leave the central nervous system by way of the ventral roots and white communicating rami of the thoracic and lumbar nerves. The ganglia of the sympathetic system form the paravertebral chain and plexuses situated near the viscera. The chemical mediator of the postganglionic fibers of the sympathetic system is **norepinephrine,** which is also produced by the adrenal medulla.

Parasympathetic System

The parasympathetic system has its nuclei in the medulla and midbrain and in the sacral portion of the spinal cord. The preganglionic fibers of these neurons leave through 4 of the cranial nerves (III, VII, IX, and X) and also through the second, third, and fourth sacral spinal nerves. The parasympathetic system is therefore also called the craniosacral division of the autonomic system.

The second neuron of the parasympathetic series is found in ganglia smaller than those of the sympathetic system; it is always located near or within the effector organs. These neurons are usually located in the walls of organs (eg, stomach, intestines), in which case the preganglionic fibers enter the organs and form a synapse there with the second neuron in the series.

The chemical mediator released by the pre- and postganglionic nerve endings of the parasympathetic system is **acetylcholine.** Acetylcholine is readily inactivated by the acetylcholinesterase—one of the reasons parasympathetic stimulation has both a more discrete and a more localized action than sympathetic stimulation.

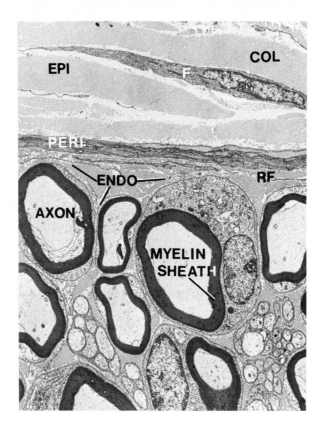

Figure 9–18. Electron micrograph of a cross section through a nerve, showing the epineurium (EPI), the perineurium (PERI) and the endoneurium (ENDO). The epineurium is a dense connective tissue rich in collagen fibers (COL) and fibroblasts (F). The perineurium is made up of several layers of flat cells tightly joined together to form a barrier to the penetration of the nerve by macromolecules. The endoneurium is composed mainly of reticular fibers (RF) synthesized by Schwann cells (SC). × 1200.

Distribution

Most of the organs innervated by the autonomic nervous system receive both sympathetic and parasympathetic fibers (Fig 9–20). Generally, in organs where one system is the stimulator, the other has an inhibitory action.

HISTOPHYSIOLOGY OF NERVE TISSUE

The integrative function of nerve tissue depends on the generation and conduction of nerve impulses and on the production of neurohormones by special nerve cells. (Neurohormones are discussed in Chapter 20.)

Axonal conduction of nerve impulses (action potentials) is one of the basic and better understood functions of nerve tissue. It has been long established that the key role in impulse conduction is played by the cell membrane.

Resting Potential

Intracellular ionic concentrations differ greatly from those found in extracellular fluids. The K^+ concentration inside a neuron is about 20 times greater than the concentration of this ion in the extracellular fluid. Conversely, Na^+ ions are about 10 times more concentrated outside the cell than inside. The cell membrane is much more permeable to K^+ than it is to any of the other ions. Potassium therefore tends to diffuse outward, down its concentration gradient. As a consequence, positive charges accumulate to the outer surface of the membrane and are balanced by the negative charge provided by impermeable macromolecules within the cell. This process continues until the diffusion force, provided by the concentration gradient, is just balanced by the increasing difficulty of moving a positive charge into an already positively charged region. At this point, there is no net movement of potassium ions. This separation of charge across the cell membrane is the **resting membrane potential.** Convention-

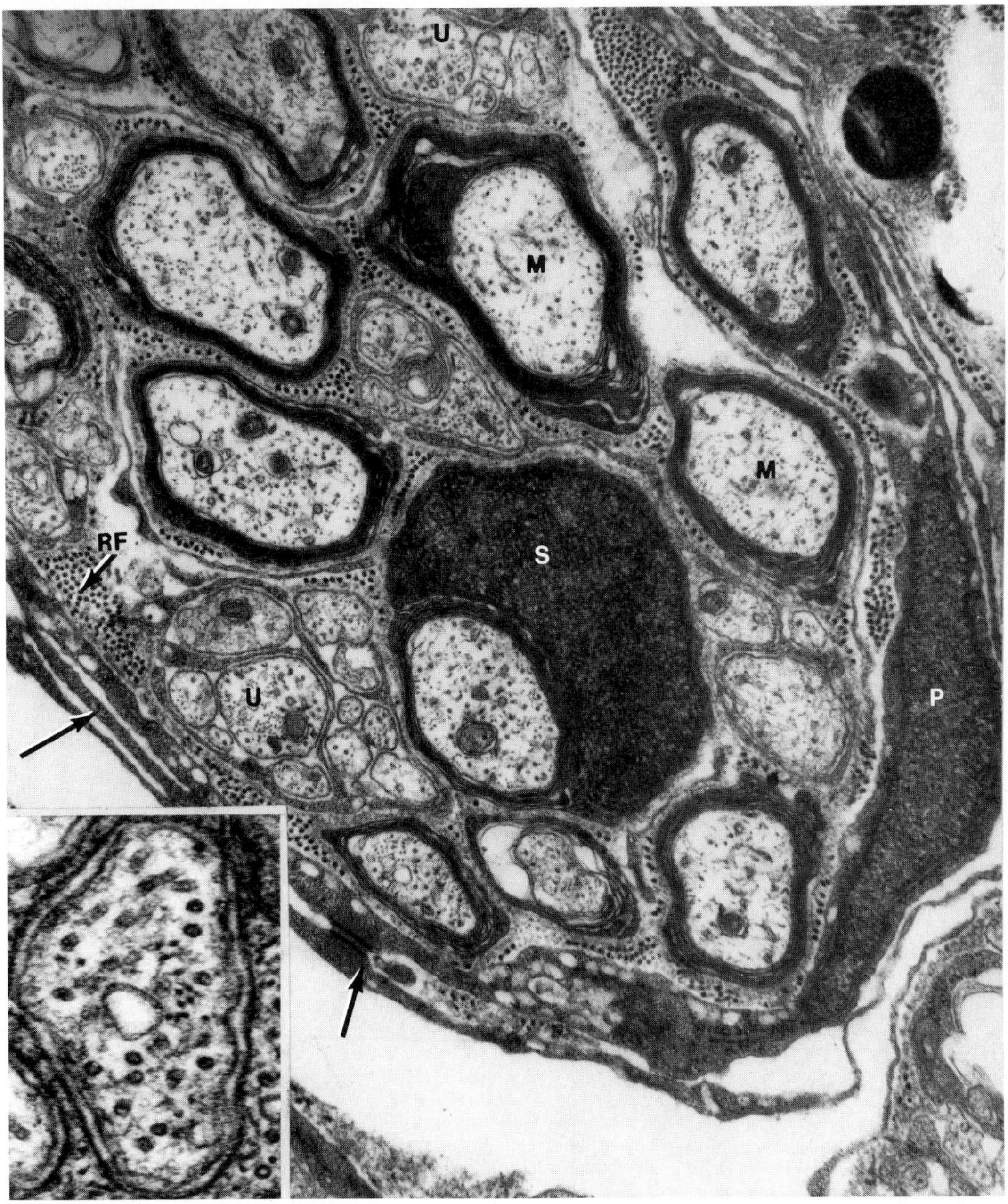

Figure 9–19. Electron micrograph of a peripheral nerve containing both myelinated (M) and unmyelinated (U) nerve fibers. The reticular fibers (RF) seen in cross section belong to the endoneurium. Near the center of the figure is a Schwann cell nucleus (S). the perineurial cells (P, arrows) form a barrier that controls access of materials to nerve tissue. × 30,000. The inset shows part of an axon, where numerous neurofilaments and microtubules are seen in cross section. × 60,000.

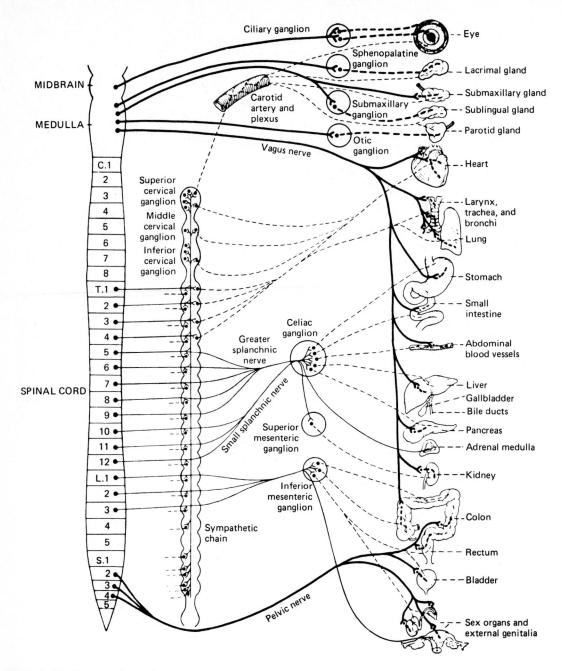

Figure 9–20. Diagram of the efferent autonomic pathways. Preganglionic neurons are shown as solid llines, postganglionic neurons as dotted lines. The heavy lines are parasympathetic fibers; the light lines are sympathetic fibers. (Slightly modified and reproduced, with permission, from Youmans W: *Fundamentals of Human Physiology*, 2nd ed. Year Book, 1962.)

ally, the external medium (extracellular fluid) is considered to be at ground potential (0 volts); the interior of the cell is from 40 to 100 mV negative with respect to the exterior.

The concentration differences are maintained by a group of "pumps" that use the energy in ATP to actively transport ions. The best known is the Na^+/K^+-ATPase, which exchanges internal Na^+ ions for external K^+ ions.

Action Potential

Plasma membranes of neurons and muscle cells (and some other cells) contain integral membrane proteins that function as ion-selective channels. At any one time, these channels can be in one of 3 states—open, closed, or inactivated. Because the transition from the closed to the open state is governed by the membrane potential, the channels are termed **voltage-gated channels.**

In the resting neuron, the membrane potential is about -90 mV, as indicated in Fig 9–21 (left electrode pair), and most of the sodium and potassium channels are in the closed state. One result of excitatory synaptic input on the postsynaptic cell is partial depolarization of the cell; ie, the membrane potential is displaced toward 0 volts. When this depolarization reaches a critical level, called the **threshold** (-70 mV in our example), sodium channels open, allowing sodium ions to enter. This has the effect of further depolarizing the cell and causing more sodium channels to open, resulting in reversal of the membrane potential at this site (right electrode pair in Fig 9–21). This explains the upward swing of the curve in the lower half of Fig 9–21. Sodium channels now un-

dergo spontaneous inactivation and remain in this state for 1–2 milliseconds.

Also as a result of membrane potential changes, potassium channels open but more slowly and for more prolonged periods of time. This has the effect of bringing the membrane potential back to its original level and even below it (**hyperpolarization**) (Fig 9–21). This sequence of events, the **action potential,** is an all-or-nothing event, since only stimuli above threshold will evoke it and the action potential is of constant amplitude and duration. After 1–2 milliseconds (the **refractory period**), the channels return to their original states and the membrane can again respond to a stimulus. Axons can generate action potentials up to 1000 times per second.

Propagation of action potential–The sodium ions that enter the cell at a particular site not only serve to depolarize that site, but can also diffuse longitudinally and depolarize adjacent sites. Diffusion toward the cell body (**antidromic** [from Greek, *antidromein,* to run in a contrary direction] **spread**) has no effect, because the sodium channels are inactivated. Diffusion of sodium ions toward the synaptic end of the axon (**orthodromic spread**), however, does depolarize the adjacent region of the membrane, leading to the generation of an action potential at this new site. This leads to a rapid, constant amplitude signal being propagated down the axon (away from the cell body), with frequency being the only information encoded.

Myelinated axons are structurally adapted for rapid conduction of the action potential. Since most of their surface is encased in an insulating layer of myelin, only the nodes of Ranvier are exposed to the extracellular environment and thus available to complete the ionic circuits necessary for the generation of action potentials. In addition, sodium and potassium channels are concentrated at the nodes, with very few channels being found in the internodal axonal membranes. Therefore, the depolarization required for an action potential is conducted quickly from one node to the next (**saltatory conduction**). As a result of myelination, an action potential is conducted much more rapidly over a myelinated axon (1–100 m/s) than it is over unmyelinated axons (0.6–2 m/s). In addition, less energy is required by the pumps to reestablish the ionic gradients, although the changes in ionic concentration resulting from the propagation of an action potential are very small.

The energy used in the conduction of the impulse is restored by an increase in axonal metabolism, with enhanced oxygen consumption and heat production.

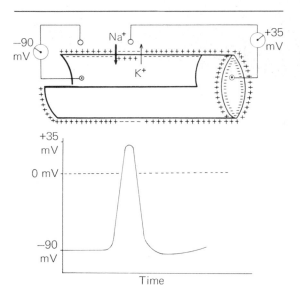

Figure 9–21. Diagrammatic representation of resting and action potentials in an axon.

Nerve impulse conduction can be blocked by cold, heat, or pressure on the nerve fiber. More complete blocking is obtained by application of local anesthetics.

According to their conduction velocities, nerve fibers can be divided into 3 classes: A, B, and C. Type A fibers are myelinated, have large diameters and long internodes, and conduct impulses with higher velocity (15–100 m/s). Type B fibers have smaller diameters, shorter internodes, and medium conduction velocity (3–14 m/s). Type C fibers are thin and unmyelinated, with slow conduction velocity (0.5–2 m/s).

Nerve impulses are transmitted from one neuron to another or to an effector cell by the neurotransmitters liberated at synapses (Figs 9–22 and 9–23). When an action potential invades an axonal terminus, or ending, calcium ions are allowed to enter the ending. Ca^{2+} ions facilitate the fusion of synaptic vesicles containing a neurotransmitter (eg, acetylcholine) with the presynaptic membrane. The transmitter (about 10,000 molecules of acetylcholine per vesicle) is released by exocytosis into the synaptic cleft. It diffuses across the cleft and binds to receptors on the postsynaptic membrane, leading to increased ionic permeability of this membrane, its depolarization, and generation of an action potential in the postsynaptic cell.

After performing its function, the excess acetylcholine is removed by the degradative action of the enzyme acetylcholinesterase. This enzyme is secreted from cells and is bound to the basal lamina in the synaptic cleft. The entire process is very rapid and can occur in a few milliseconds.

Other neurotransmitters exist (with their appropriate mechanisms of disposal). This function has been demonstrated for gamma-aminobutyric acid (GABA), glutamic acid, dopamine, serotonin (5-hydroxytryptamine, 5-HT), and glycine.

In mammals, gamma-aminobutyric acid is localized exclusively in the central nervous system, and it may function as an inhibitory chemical transmitter. There is a class of peptide neurotransmitters that are potent inhibitors of pain receptors. **Endorphins** and

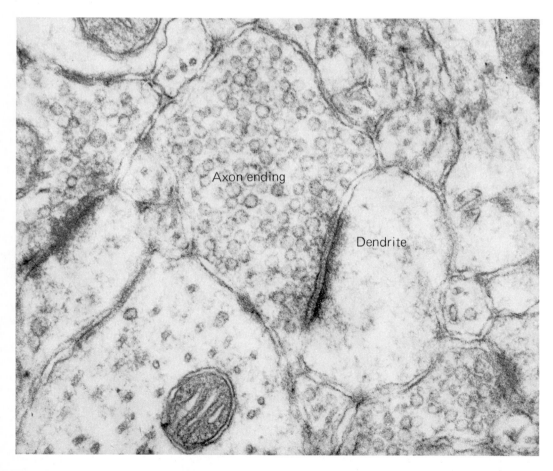

Figure 9–22. Electron micrograph of cerebral cortex. Near the center of the figure is a synapse between one axon ending and a dendrite. The postsynaptic (dendritic) membrane shows a greater accumulation of electron-dense material than does the presynaptic (axonal) membrane. This is an asymmetric, or type 1, synapse. The axon ending contains numerous synaptic vesicles. × 90,000. (Courtesy of A Peters.)

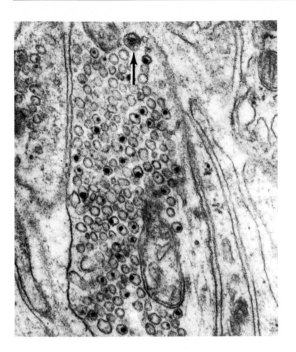

Figure 9–23. Adrenergic nerve ending. There are many 50-nm-diameter vesicles with dark, electron-dense cores containing norepinephrine. × 40,000. (Courtesy of A Machado.)

enkephalins are natural brain peptides exhibiting morphinelike analgesic powers that may also regulate behavior. Several peptide hormones such as cholecystokinin, vasoactive intestinal polypeptide, and bombesin, originally described in the digestive tract where they are produced by DNES cells (see Chapter 4), have been localized in different areas of the central nervous system. They may participate in the regulation of neurotransmitters. Current concepts of the production, liberation, and inactivation of the 2 best known chemical mediators are summarized in Figs 9–24 and 9–25.

The abundance of RNA in the perikaryon suggests intense protein synthesis, which has been confirmed by radioautographic studies using ^{3}H-leucine and other labeled amino acids. Because axons do not contain ribosomes, all the proteins in these processes are synthesized in the perikaryon and moved down the axon by an energy-requiring mechanism known as **axonal transport.** Newly synthesized and labeled protein molecules migrate down the axons (anterograde transport) at several speeds, but there are 2 main rates: a fast rate in the range of hundreds of millimeters per day and a slow rate in the range of several millimeters per day. The fast transport mechanism moves membranes, mitochondria, and synaptic vesicles, among other things, down the axon from their site of formation in the neuron cell body. Substances such as actin, tubulins, metabolic enzymes, and neurofilament proteins are transported at the slow rate. Agents that disrupt microfilaments and microtubules greatly slow both the fast and slow anterograde transport systems. Experimental evidence has been presented to show that transport of protein also occurs in a centripetal direction (retrograde transport) from the axon to the perikaryon. Thus, receptors and synaptic membrane proteins are removed from the periphery and shipped back to the cell body, where they can be reused. Enzymatic markers, such as peroxidase, that are captured by axon terminals and transported to the perikaryon have been used extensively to study the physiology and morphology of the nervous system.

A trophic function has been ascribed to the nervous system of mammals for the structures it innervates. It is known that denervation of organs such as glands and muscles can lead to their atrophy, with functional and morphologic recuperation after reinnervation. Whether the atrophy is solely a consequence of disuse is an open question. In lower vertebrates, peripheral nerves have a trophic function that is not dependent on the nerve impulse.

DEGENERATION & REGENERATION OF NERVE TISSUE

Neurons do not divide, and their degeneration represents a permanent loss. Neuronal processes in the central nervous system are, within very narrow limits, replaceable by growth through the synthetic activity of their perikaryons. Peripheral nerve fibers can also regenerate if their perikaryons are not destroyed.

Death of a nerve cell is limited to its perikaryon and processes. The neurons functionally connected to the dead neuron do not die, except for those with only one link. In this latter instance, the isolated neuron undergoes **transneuronal degeneration.**

In contrast to nerve cells, neuroglia of the central nervous system and Schwann cells and ganglionic satellite cells of the peripheral nervous system are able to divide by mitosis. Spaces in the central nervous system left by nerve cells lost by disease or injury are invaded by neuroglia.

Since nerves are widely distributed throughout the body, they are often subjected to injury. When a nerve axon is transected, degenerative changes take place, followed by a reparative phase.

In a wounded nerve fiber, it is important to distinguish the changes occurring in the proximal segment from those in the distal segment. The proximal segment maintains its continuity with the trophic center (perikaryon) and frequently regenerates. The distal segment, separated from the nerve cell body, degen-

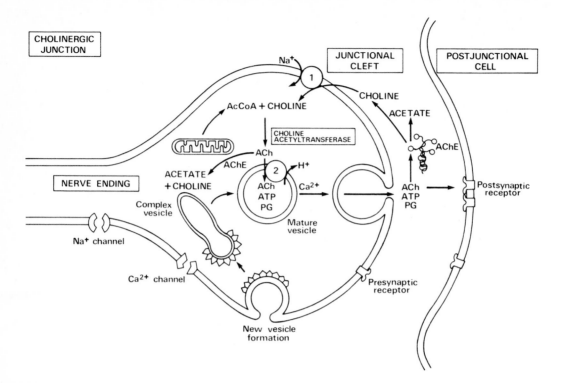

Figure 9–24. Schematic illustration of a generalized cholinergic junction (not to scale). Two cellular structures, the cholinergic nerve terminal (on the left) and the postjunctional cell (at right), are separated by the junctional (synaptic) cleft. Choline is transported into the nerve terminal by a carrier (1) that also transports sodium ion, using the sodium gradient for energy. This transport can be inhibited by hemicholinium. Inside the nerve terminal, choline combines with activated acetate (AcCoA) in a reaction catalyzed by choline acetyltransferase to form acetylcholine (ACh). Storage vesicle formation is initiated by the deposition of clathrin molecules on the inner surface of the terminal membrane (the fencelike structure on the new vesicle). A complex vesicle is formed from molecules pinched off from the surface. Eventually, this gives rise to a mature storage vesicle. ACh is transported into the storage vesicle by the action of a carrier (2) that uses the outward flux of protons as its source of energy. ATP and proteoglycan (PG) are also stored in the vesicle. Release of the transmitter occurs when an action potential carried down the axon by the action of voltage-sensitive sodium channels invades the nerve's terminals. Voltage-sensitive calcium channels in the terminal membrane open, allowing an influx of calcium. The increase in intracellular calcium causes fusion of the vesicles with the surface membrane, resulting in an exocytotic expulsion of ACh, ATP, and proteoglycan into the junctional cleft. This step is blocked by botulin. ACh reaching prejunctional and postjunctional receptors modifies the function of the corresponding cell. (Note that some cholinergic junctions appear to lack prejunctional receptors.) ACh also diffuses into contact with acetylcholinesterase (AChE), a polymeric enzyme that splits ACh into choline and acetate. At some cholinergic junctions, a polypeptide cotransmitter, vasoactive intestinal polypeptide (VIP), is released along with ACh into the junctional cleft. (Reproduced, with permission, from Katzung BG [editor]: *Basic & Clinical Pharmacology*, 4th ed. Appleton & Lange, 1989.)

erates totally and is removed by tissue macrophages (Fig 9–26).

Axonal injury causes the following changes in the perikaryon: **chromatolysis,** ie, dissolution of Nissl substances with a consequent decrease in cytoplasmic basophilia; an increase in the volume of the perikaryon; and migration of the nucleus to a peripheral position in the perikaryon. The proximal segment of the axon degenerates close to the wound for a short distance, but growth starts as soon as debris is removed by macrophages.

In the nerve stub distal to the injury, both the axon

(now separated from its trophic center) and the myelin sheath degenerate completely, and their remnants, excluding their connective tissue and perineurial sheaths, are removed by macrophages (Fig 9–26B). While these regressive changes take place, Schwann cells proliferate within the remaining connective tissue sleeve, giving rise to solid cellular columns. These rows of Schwann cells serve as guides to the sprouting axons formed during the reparative phase.

After these regressive changes, the proximal segment of the axon grows and branches, forming sev-

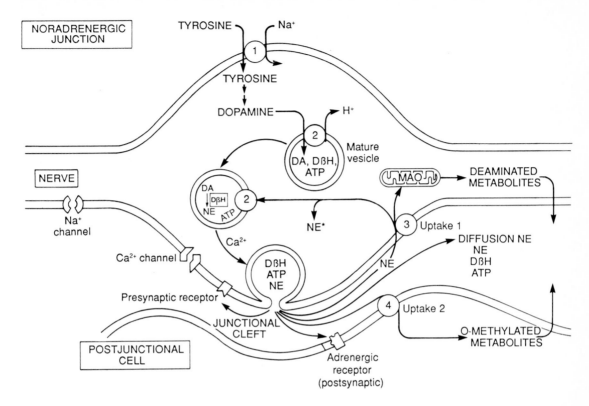

Figure 9–25. Schematic diagram of a neuroeffector junction of the peripheral sympathetic nervous system. The nerves terminate in complex networks with varicosities, or enlargements, that form synaptic junctions with effector cells. Some of the processes occurring in the noradrenergic varicosity—eg, new vesicle formation—are analogous to those in cholinergic terminals. Tyrosine is transported into the noradrenergic varicosity by a carrier (1) that is linked to sodium uptake. Tyrosine is decarboxylated to dopa and then hydroxylated to form dopamine (DA) in the cytoplasm. Dopamine is transported into the vesicle by a carrier mechanism (2) that can be blocked by reserpine. The same carrier transports norepinephrine (NE) and several other amines into these granules. Dopamine is converted to norepinephrine through the catalytic action of dopamine β-hydroxylase (DβH). ATP is also present in high concentration in the vesicle. Release of the transmitter occurs when an action potential is conducted to the varicosity by the action of voltage-sensitive sodium channels. Depolarization of the varicosity membrane opens voltage-sensitive calcium channels and results in an increase in intracellular calcium. The elevated calcium facilitates exocytotic fusion of vesicles with the surface membrane and expulsion of norepinephrine, ATP and some of the dopamine β-hydroxylase. Release is blocked by drugs such as guanethidine and bretylium. Norepinephrine reaching either pre- or postsynaptic receptors modifies the function of the corresponding cells. Norepinephrine also diffuses out of the cleft, or it can be transported into the cytoplasm of the varicosity (uptake 1 [3], blocked by cocaine, tricyclic antidepressants) or into the postjunctional cell (uptake 2 [4]). The nonvesicular norepinephrine (NE* can be released by tyrosine and a variety of other indirectly acting adrenergic agonists. (Reproduced, with permission, from Katzung BG [editor]: *Basic & Clinical Pharmacology*, 4th ed. Appleton & Lange, 1989.)

eral filaments that progress in the direction of the columns of Schwann cells (Fig 9–26C). Only fibers that penetrate these Schwann cell columns will continue to grow and reach an effector organ (Fig 9–26D).

When there is an extensive gap between the distal and proximal segments, or when the distal segment disappears altogether (as in the case of amputation of a limb), the newly grown nerve fibers may form a swelling or neuroma that can be the source of spontaneous pain (Fig 9–26E).

Regeneration is functionally efficient only when the fibers and the columns of Schwann cells are directed to the correct place. The possibility is good, however, since each regenerating fiber gives origin to several processes, and each column of Schwann cells receives processes from several regenerating fibers.

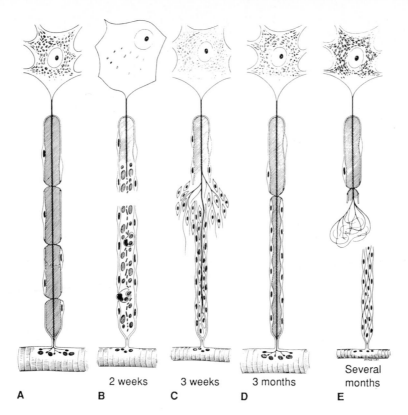

2 weeks   3 weeks   3 months   Several months

A   B   C   D   E

Figure 9–26. Main changes that take place in an injured nerve fiber. **A:** Normal nerve fiber, with its perikaryon and effector cell (striated skeletal muscle). Note the position of the neuron nucleus and the amount and distribution of Nissl bodies. **B:** When the fiber is injured, the neuronal nucleus moves to the cell periphery, and Nissl bodies become greatly reduced in number. The nerve fiber distal to the injury degenerates along with its myelin sheath. Debris is phagocytosed by macrophages. **C:** The muscle fiber shows a pronounced denervation atrophy. Schwann cells proliferate, forming a compact cord penetrated by the growing axon. The axon grows at the rate of 0.5–3 mm/per day. **D:** Here, the nerve fiber regeneration was successful. Note that the muscle fiber was also regenerated after receiving nerve stimuli. **E:** When the axon does not penetrate the cord of Schwann cells, its growth is not organized. (Redrawn and reproduced, with permission, from Willis RA, Willis AF: *The Principles of Pathology and Bacteriology,* 3rd ed. Butterworth, 1972.)

In an injured mixed nerve, however, if regenerating sensory fibers grow into columns connected to motor end-plates that were occupied by motor fibers, the function of the muscle will not be reestablished.

GANGLIA

Ganglia are usually ovoid structures encapsulated by dense connective tissue and associated with nerves. An aggregation of nerve cell bodies outside the central nervous system is called a **nerve ganglion.**

Two types of nerve ganglia can be distinguished on the basis of differing morphology and function: **dorsal root ganglia** (sensory), which occur at the dorsal (posterior) root of the spinal nerves and also in the path of some cranial nerves; and **autonomic ganglia,** which are associated with nerves of the autonomic system.

Intramural ganglia are very small, consisting of only a few nerve cells; they are located within viscera, especially the walls of the digestive tract (Fig 15–32). All intramural ganglia belong to the parasympathetic system.

A capsule of connective tissue surrounding each ganglion is continuous with the connective tissue within it and with the perineurium and epineurium of the pre- and postganglionic nerves.

In ganglia, the body of each ganglion cell is enveloped by a layer of small cuboidal glial cells called **satellite cells** (Fig 9–27). A thin fibrous layer of connective tissue envelops each satellite-cell-encapsulated perikaryon.

Dorsal Root Ganglia

These ganglia are located in the dorsal roots of the spinal nerves and in the paths of some cranial nerves. Their function is to carry to the central ner-

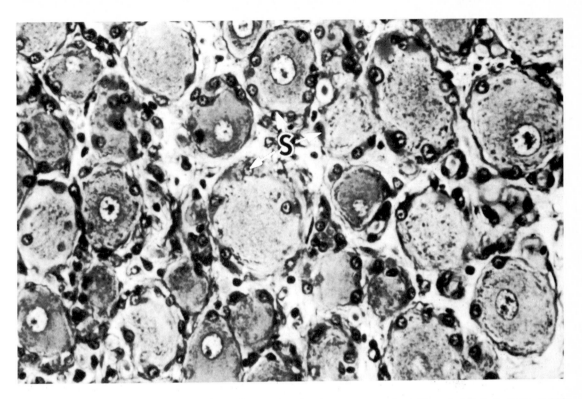

Figure 9–27. Photomicrograph of a spinal ganglion section showing neurons and satellite cells (S). Azan stain, × 300. (Reproduced, with permission, from Junqueira LC, Carneiro J: *Histologie.* Schiebler TH, Peiper U [translators]. Springer-Verlag, 1984.)

vous system impulses generated by various sensory receptors.

Dorsal root ganglia have pseudounipolar neurons whose T-shaped process sends one branch to the periphery and the other to the central nervous system. The 2 branches of the single T-shaped process constitute one axon, and the peripheral branch has a dendritic arborization. In this instance, the dendrites are not expansions of the cell body but of an axon. The nerve impulse goes directly from the periphery to the central nervous system, bypassing the perikaryon. The perikaryons of pseudounipolar neurons therefore do not receive nerve impulses, and their function is exclusively trophic. The single axonal process of this cell makes several irregular turns around the cell body before its bifurcation, which occurs outside the capsule of satellite cells.

The ganglia from the acoustic nerve are the only cranial ganglia whose cells are bipolar.

Autonomic Ganglia

Autonomic ganglia appear as bulbous dilatations in autonomic nerves. Some are located within certain organs, especially in the walls of the digestive tract, where they constitute the intramural ganglia. Autonomic ganglia usually have multipolar neurons, which may appear star-shaped in histologic sections (Fig 9–28). As with craniospinal ganglia, autonomic ganglia have neuronal perikaryons with fine Nissl bodies. The neurons of autonomic ganglia are frequently enveloped by a usually incomplete layer of satellite cells.

GRAY MATTER & WHITE MATTER

The central nervous system is composed of both white and gray matter. White matter contains myelinated and unmyelinated fibers, oligodendrocytes, fibrous astrocytes, and microglial cells. Its characteristic white color is a clue to the predominance of myelinated nerve fibers. Gray matter contains unmyelinated and myelinated fibers (mostly the former), perikaryons, protoplasmic astrocytes, oligodendrocytes, and microglial cells.

In cross sections of the spinal cord, white matter is peripheral and gray matter is central, assuming the shape of an H (Fig 9–29). In the horizontal bar of this H is an opening, the central canal, which is a remnant of the lumen of the embryonic neural tube lined by ependymal cells. The gray matter of the vertical bars of the H forms the anterior horns;

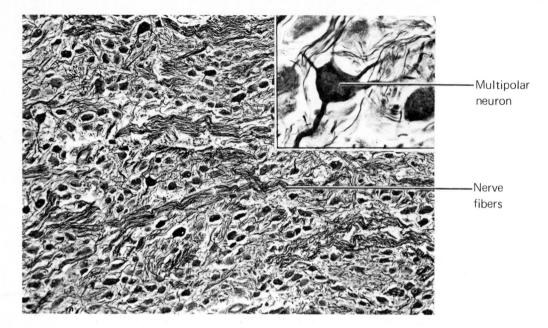

Figure 9–28. Photomicrographs of a silver-stained section from an autonomic nerve ganglion. Neurons and nerve fibers appear black. × 80. The inset shows a multipolar neuron. × 250.

these contain motor neurons whose axons make up the ventral roots of the spinal nerves. Gray matter also forms the posterior horns, which receive sensory fibers from neurons in the spinal ganglia (dorsal roots).

Spinal cord neurons are large and multipolar, especially in the anterior horns, where large motor neurons are found (Fig 9–29).

The cerebellum has 2 hemispheres separated by the **vermis.** The surface of the cerebellum has many furrows (**sulci**) perpendicular to the vermis. These furrows divide the organ into lobules, each of which has a superficial layer of gray matter (cortex) and a core of white matter (Fig 9–30).

The cerebellar cortex has 3 layers: an outer molecular layer, a central layer of Purkinje cells, and an inner granule layer (Fig 9–31). The neurons of the granule layer are the smallest in the human body (5 μm in diameter) and have a typical structure. Each granule cell (**cerebellar granule**) has 3–6 dendrites

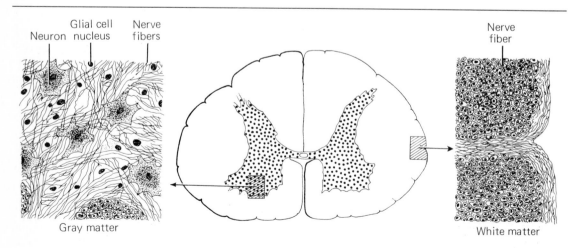

Figure 9–29. Center: Cross section through the spinal cord.

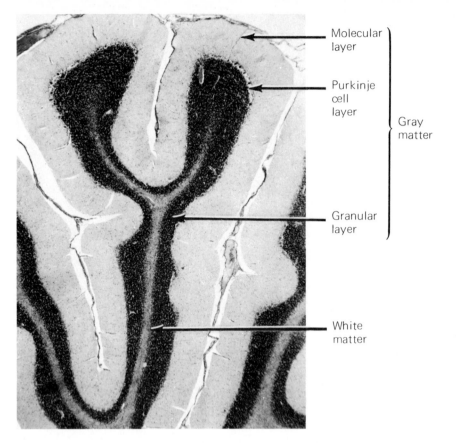

Figure 9–30. Photomicrograph of a portion of cerebellum. Each lobule contains a core of white matter and 3 layers of gray matter: granular, Purkinje, and molecular. H&E stain, × 28.

and, as usual, one axon. The Purkinje cells are quite large, and their dendrites divide repeatedly in one plane, forming a sort of fan (Fig 9–2). The most superficial layer of the cerebellum (the molecular layer) has few perikaryons and many unmyelinated nerve fibers.

Like the cerebellum, the cerebrum also has a cortex of gray matter and a central area of white matter in which are found nuclei of gray matter. The surface of the cerebrum is increased by many **gyri,** which are elevations separated by depressions (sulci). The cytology of the cerebral cortex varies according to the area. The majority of the cells of the cortex have perikaryons that are pyramidal, stellate, or spindle-shaped.

MENINGES

The central nervous system is protected by the skull and the vertebral column. It is also encased in membranes of connective tissue called the **meninges.**

Starting with the outermost layer, the meninges are named **dura mater, arachnoid,** and **pia mater.** The

arachnoid and the pia mater are linked together and are often considered as a single membrane called the **pia-arachnoid** (Fig 9–32).

Dura Mater

The dura mater is the external meninx, composed of dense connective tissue continuous with the periosteum of the skull. The dura mater that envelops the spinal cord is separated from the periosteum of the vertebrae by the **epidural space,** which contains thin-walled veins, loose connective tissue, and adipose tissue.

The dura mater is always separated from the arachnoid by the thin **subdural space.** The internal surface of all dura mater, as well as its external surface in the spinal cord, is covered by simple squamous epithelium of mesenchymal origin (Fig 9–32).

Arachnoid

The arachnoid has 2 components: a layer in contact with the dura mater and a system of trabeculae connecting that layer with the pia mater. The cavities between the trabeculae form the **subarachnoid**

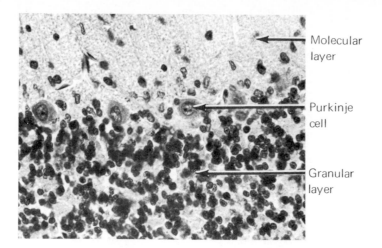

Molecular layer

Purkinje cell

Granular layer

Figure 9–31. Photomicrograph of cerebellar cortex. The staining procedure used does not reveal the unusually large dendritic arborization of the Purkinje cell, which is illustrated in Fig 9–2. H&E stain, × 250.

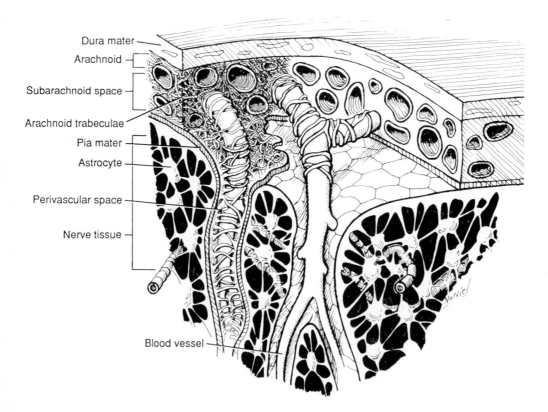

Dura mater

Arachnoid

Subarachnoid space

Arachnoid trabeculae

Pia mater

Astrocyte

Perivascular space

Nerve tissue

Blood vessel

Figure 9–32. Drawing of the meninges. The blood vessel arising from the subarachnoid space penetrates the nerve tissue and is partly enveloped by the pia mater.

space, which is filled with cerebrospinal fluid and is completely separated from the subdural space. The subarachnoid space communicates with the ventricles of the brain via the unpaired median aperture and the paired lateral apertures.

The arachnoid is composed of connective tissue devoid of blood vessels. Its surfaces are covered by the same type of simple squamous epithelium that covers the dura mater. Since, in the spinal cord, the arachnoid has fewer trabeculae, it can be more clearly distinguished there from pia mater.

In some areas, the arachnoid perforates the dura mater, forming protrusions that terminate in venous sinuses in the dura mater. These protrusions, which are covered by endothelial cells of the veins, are called **arachnoid villi.** Their function is to reabsorb cerebrospinal fluid into the blood of the venous sinuses.

Pia Mater

The pia mater is a loose connective tissue containing many blood vessels. Although it is located quite close to the nerve tissue, it is not in contact with nerve cells or fibers. Between the pia mater and the neural elements is a thin layer of neuroglial processes, adhering firmly to the pia mater.

The pia mater follows all the irregularities of the surface of the central nervous system and penetrates it to some extent along with the blood vessels. Pia mater is covered by squamous cells of mesenchymal origin.

Blood vessels penetrate the central nervous system through tunnels covered by pia mater and called the

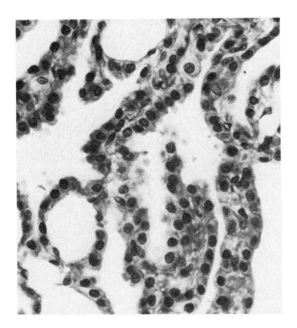

Figure 9–33. Photomicrograph of the choroid plexus. The numerous folds are covered by simple cuboidal epithelium. H&E stain, × 400.

perivascular spaces (Fig 9–32). The pia mater disappears before the blood vessels are transformed into capillaries. In the central nervous system, the blood capillaries are completely covered by expansions of the neuroglial cell processes.

Blood-Brain Barrier

The **blood-brain barrier** is a functional barrier that prevents the passage of certain substances from the blood to nerve tissue. Intravenously injected trypan blue, for example, appears in the intercellular spaces of all tissues except the central nervous system.

The blood-brain barrier results from the reduced permeability that is a property of blood capillaries of nerve tissue. Occluding junctions, which provide continuity between the endothelial cells of these capillaries, represent the main structural component of the barrier. The cytoplasm of these endothelial cells does not have the fenestrations found in many other locations, and very few pinocytotic vesicles are observed. It is also possible that expansions of neuroglial cell processes that envelop the capillaries are partly responsible for their low permeability.

CHOROID PLEXUS & CEREBROSPINAL FLUID

Choroid Plexus

The choroid plexus consists of invaginated folds of pia mater that penetrate the interior of the ventricles. It is found in the roofs of the third and fourth ventricles and in part in the walls of the lateral ventricles.

The choroid plexus is composed of loose connective tissue of the pia mater, covered by a simple cuboidal or low columnar epithelium that is continuous with the ependyma in other regions of the brain (Fig 9–33). The epithelial cells possess numerous irregular microvilli with dilated free ends. Their cytoplasm is rich in mitochondria, and there are junctional complexes near the free ends.

The connective tissue of the choroid plexus is quite cellular, containing many macrophages. The endothelium of its fenestrated capillaries has pores closed by thin diaphragms. The endothelial cells are held together by tight junctions. The epithelial and endothelial cells form the blood-cerebrospinal fluid barrier that is responsible for the difference in composition between blood plasma and cerebrospinal fluid.

The main function of the choroid plexus is to elaborate cerebrospinal fluid, a thin watery fluid actively secreted by the epithelial cells covering the plexuses.

Cerebrospinal Fluid

Cerebrospinal fluid contains only a small amount of solids and completely fills the ventricles, central canal of the spinal cord, subarachnoid space, and perivascular space. It is important for the metabolism of the central nervous system and acts as a protective device, forming a liquid layer in the subarachnoid space. This layer cushions the nerve tissue against trauma.

Adult humans have about 140 mL of cerebrospinal fluid in the cerebral ventricles and the subarachnoid space. The fluid is clear, has a low density (1.004–1.008 g/mL), and is very low in protein content. A few desquamated cells and 2–5 lymphocytes per milliliter are also present. The ionic composition of cerebrospinal fluid is very close to that of plasma, ie, high sodium and chloride but low potassium concentrations. It is produced by ultrafiltration and diffusion from the blood as well as by active transport across epithelial cells of the choroid plexus. Between 600 and 700 mL of cerebrospinal fluid are produced each day.

Cerebrospinal fluid circulates through the ventricles, from which it passes into the subarachnoid space. Here, arachnoid villi provide the main pathway for absorption of cerebrospinal fluid into the venous circulation. Lymphatic vessels are not present in nervous tissue.

A decrease in the absorption of cerebrospinal fluid or blockage of outflow from the ventricles results in the condition known as **hydrocephalus.**

REFERENCES

Alberts B, et al: *Molecular Biology of the Cell*, 2nd ed. Garland, 1989.

Axelrod J: Neurotransmitters. *Sci Am* (June) 1974;**230**:58.

Brightmann MW et al: The blood-brain barrier to proteins under normal and pathological conditions. *J Neurol Sci* 1970;**10**:215.

Heuser JE, Reese TS: Evidence for recycling of synaptic vesicle membrane during transmitter release at the frog neuromuscular junction. *J Cell Biol* 1973;**57**:315.

Heuser JE, Reese TS: Structural changes after transmitter release at the frog neuromuscular junction. *J Cell Biol* 1981;**88**:564.

Hubbard JI (editor): *The Peripheral Nervous System.* Plenum Press, 1974.

Jacobson M, Hunt RK: The origins of nerve-cell specificity. *Sci Am* (Feb) 1973;**228**:26.

Keynes RD: Ion channels in the nerve-cell membrane. *Sci Am* (March) 1979;**240**:126.

Landon DN (editor): *The Peripheral Nerve.* Chapman & Hall, 1976.

Morell P, Norton WT: Myelin. *Sci Am* (May) 1980;**242**:88.

Palay SL, Chan-Palay V: *Cerebellar Cortex, Cytology and Organization.* Springer-Verlag, 1974.

Peters A, Palay SL, Webster HF: *The Fine Structure of the Nervous System: The Neurons and Supporting Cells.* Saunders, 1976.

Reichardt LF, Kelly RB: A molecular description of nerve terminal function. *Annu Rev Biochem* 1983;**52**:871.

Schwartz JH: Axonal transport: Components, mechanisms, and specificity. *Annu Rev Neurosci* 1979;**2**:467.

Sears TA (editor): *Neuronal-Glial Cell Interrelationships.* Springer-Verlag, 1982.

Shepherd GM: Microcircuits in the nervous system. *Sci Am* (Feb) 1978;**238**:93.

Stevens CF: The neuron. *Sci Am* (March) 1979;**241**:55.

Muscle Tissue

10

Muscle tissue is composed of differentiated cells containing contractile proteins. **The structural biology of these proteins generates the forces necessary for cellular contraction, which drives movement within certain organs and the body as a whole.** Most muscle cells are of mesodermal origin, and their differentiation occurs mainly by a gradual process of lengthening, with simultaneous synthesis of myofibrillar proteins.

Three types of muscle tissue can be distinguished in mammals on the basis of morphologic and functional characteristics (Fig 10–1), and each type of muscle tissue has a structure adapted to its physiologic role. **Skeletal muscle** is composed of bundles of very long, cylindrical, multinucleated cells that show cross-striations. Their contraction is quick, forceful, and usually under voluntary control. It is caused by the interaction of thin actin filaments and thick myosin filaments whose molecular configuration allows them to slide upon one another. The forces necessary for sliding are generated by weak interactions in the bridges that bind actin to myosin.

Cardiac muscle also has cross-striations and is composed of elongated, branched individual cells that lie parallel to each other. At sites of end-to-end contact are the **intercalated disks,** structures found only in cardiac muscle. Cardiac muscle contraction is involuntary, vigorous, and rhythmic. **Smooth muscle** consists of collections of fusiform cells that, in the light microscope, do not show striations. Their contraction process is slow and not subject to voluntary control.

Some muscle cell organelles have names that differ from their counterparts in other cells. Thus, the cytoplasm of muscle cells (excluding the myofibrils) is called **sarcoplasm,** and the smooth endoplasmic reticulum is called **sarcoplasmic reticulum.** The **sarcolemma** is the cell membrane or plasmalemma.

SKELETAL MUSCLE

Skeletal muscle consists of **muscle fibers,** bundles of very long (up to 30 cm) cylindrical multinucleated

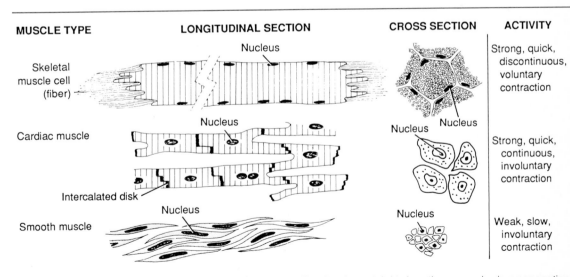

Figure 10–1. Diagram of the structure of the 3 muscle types. The drawings at right show these muscles in cross section. Skeletal muscle is composed of large, elongated, multinucleated fibers. Cardiac muscle is composed of irregular branched cells bound together longitudinally by intercalated disks. Smooth muscle is an agglomerate of fusiform cells. The density of the packing between the cells depends on the amount of extracellular connective tissue present.

cells with a diameter of 10–100 μm. Multinucleation results from the fusion of embryonic mononucleated myoblasts (muscle cell precursors). The oval nuclei are usually found at the periphery of the cell under the cell membrane. This characteristic nuclear location is helpful in distinguishing skeletal muscle from cardiac and smooth muscle, both of which have centrally located nuclei.

The variation in diameter of skeletal muscle fibers depends on such factors as the specific muscle and the age and sex, state of nutrition, and physical training of the individual. It is a common observation that exercise enlarges the musculature and decreases fat depots. The increase in muscle thus obtained is caused by formation of new myofibrils and a pronounced growth in the diameter of individual muscle fibers. This process, characterized by augmentation of cell volume, is called **hypertrophy** (from Greek, *hyper*, above, + *trophe*, nourishment); tissue growth by increase in the number of cells is termed **hyperplasia** (*hyper* + Greek, *plasis*, molding). Hyperplasia, which does not occur in either skeletal or cardiac muscle, does take place in smooth muscle, whose cells have not lost the capacity to divide by mitosis. It is rather frequent in many organs such as the uterus, where both hyperplasia and hypertrophy occur during pregnancy.

Organization of Skeletal Muscle

The masses of fibers that make up the different types of muscle are not grouped in random fashion but are arranged in regular bundles surrounded by the **epimysium** (*epi* + Greek, *mys*, muscle) an external sheath of dense connective tissue surrounding the entire muscle (Fig 10–2). From the epimysium, thin septa of connective tissue extend inward, surrounding the bundles of fibers within a muscle. The connective tissue around each bundle of muscle fibers is called the **perimysium** (*peri* + *mys*). Each muscle fiber is itself surrounded by a delicate layer of connective tissue, the **endomysium**, composed

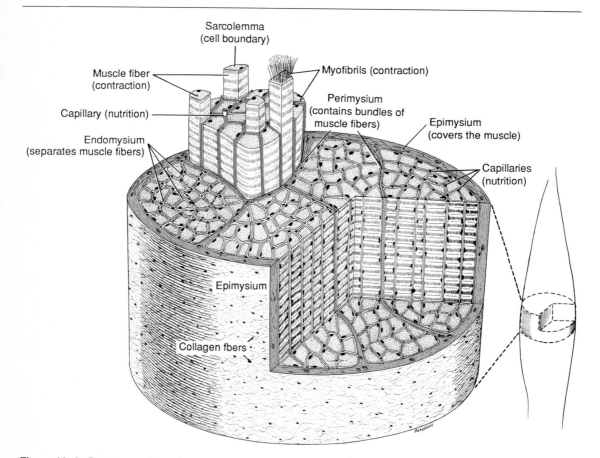

Figure 10–2. Structure and function of skeletal muscle. The drawing at right shows the area of muscle detailed in the enlarged segment. Color highlights endomysium, perimysium, and epimysium.

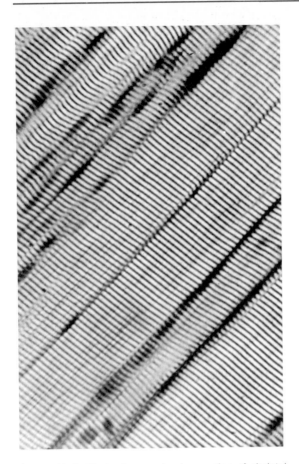

Figure 10–3. Photomicrograph of a section of skeletal muscle observed with the polarizing microscope. The appearance of the A bands as bright birefringement stripes is due to the highly ordered myosin molecules of the thick filaments. The I bands are dark. × 700.

mainly of a basal lamina and reticular fibers (Fig 10–2).

One of the most important roles of connective tissue is that of mechanical transmission of the forces generated by contracting muscle cells, since in most instances, individual muscle cells do not extend from one end of a muscle to the other.

Blood vessels penetrate the muscle within the connective tissue septa and form a rich capillary network that runs between and parallel to the muscle fibers. The capillaries are of the continuous type, and lymphatics are found in the connective tissue.

Some muscles taper off at their extremities, where a myotendinous junction is formed. The electron microscope shows that in this transitional region, collagen fibers of the tendon insert themselves into complex infoldings of the plasmalemma of the muscle fibers.

Organization of Skeletal Muscle Fibers

As observed with the light microscope, longitudinally sectioned muscle cells or fibers, when stained with hematoxylin and eosin, show cross-striations of alternating light and dark bands (Figs 10–3 and 10–4). The darker bands are called **A bands** (**anisotropic,** ie, birefringent in polarized light); the lighter bands are called **I bands** (**isotropic,** ie, does not alter polarized light). In the electron microscope, one can observe that each I band is bisected by a dark transverse line, the **Z line.** The smallest repetitive subunit of the contractile apparatus, the **sarcomere,** extends from Z line to Z line (Figs 10–5 and 10–6) and is about 2.5 μm long in resting muscle.

The sarcoplasm is filled with long cylindrical filamentous bundles called **myofibrils.** The myofibrils, which have a diameter of 1–2 μm and run parallel to the long axis of the muscle fiber, consist of an end-to-end chainlike arrangement of sarcomeres (Figs 10–5 and 10–6). The lateral registration of sarco-

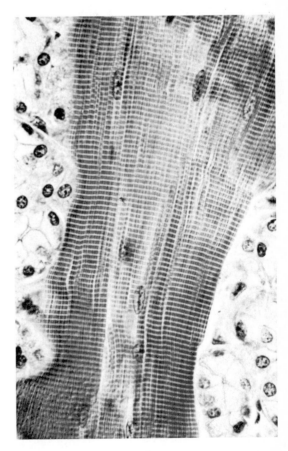

Figure 10–4. Photomicrograph of a section of the tongue of a rat, showing the transverse (cross) striations of the longitudinally cut skeletal muscle fibers. × 700.

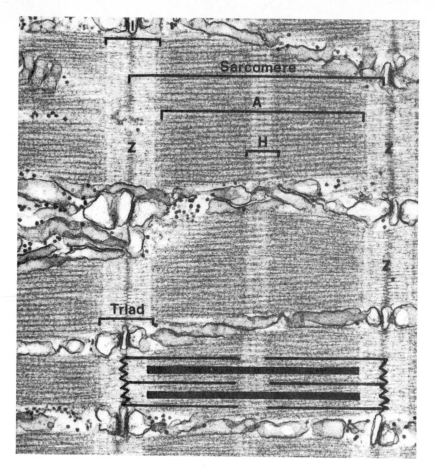

Figure 10–5. Electron micrograph of skeletal muscle of a tadpole. Observe the sarcomere with its A, I, and H bands and Z line. The position of the thick and thin filaments in the sarcomere is shown schematically in the lower part of the figure. As illustrated here, triads in amphibian muscle are aligned with the Z line in each sarcomere. In mammalian muscle, however, each sarcomere exhibits 2 triads, one at each A–I band interface (see Fig 10–11). × 35,700. (Courtesy of KR Porter.)

meres in adjacent myofibrils causes the entire muscle fiber to exhibit a characteristic pattern of transverse striations.

Studies within the electron microscope reveal that this sarcomere pattern is due mainly to the presence of 2 types of filaments—thick and thin—that lie parallel to the long axis of the myofibrils in a symmetric pattern.

The thick filaments are 1.6 μm long and 15 nm wide; they occupy the A band, the central portion of the sarcomere. The thin filaments run between and parallel to the thick filaments and have one end attached to the Z line (Figs 10–5 and 10–6). Thin filaments are 1.0 μm long and 8 nm wide. As a result of this arrangement, the I bands consist of the portions of the thin filaments that do not overlap the thick filaments. The A bands are mainly composed of thick filaments in addition to portions of overlapping thin filaments. Close observation of the A band

shows the presence of a lighter zone in its center, the **H band,** that corresponds to a region consisting only of the rodlike portions of the myosin molecule (Figs 10–5 and 10–6). Bisecting the H band is the **M line,** a region where lateral connections are made between adjacent thick filaments (Fig 10–6). The major protein of the M line is creatine kinase. Creatine kinase catalyzes the transfer of a phosphate group from phosphocreatine, a storage form of high-energy phosphate groups, to ADP, thus providing the supply of ATP necessary for muscle contraction.

Thin and thick filaments overlap for some distance within the A band. As a consequence, a cross section in the region of filament overlap shows each thick filament surrounded by 6 thin filaments in the form of a hexagon (Figs 10–6 and 10–7).

Striated muscle filaments contain at least 4 main proteins: actin, tropomyosin, troponin, and myosin. Thin filaments are composed of the first 3 proteins,

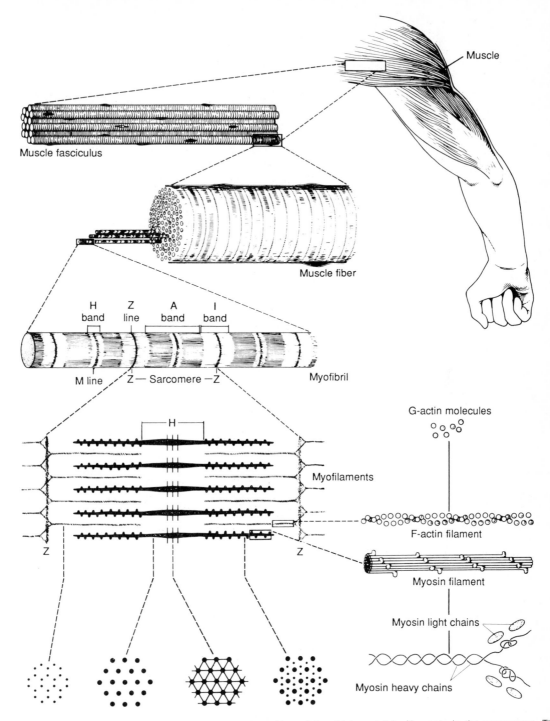

Figure 10–6. Diagram illustrating the structure and position of the thick and thin filaments in the sarcomere. The molecular structure of these components is shown at right. (Drawing by Sylvia Colard Keene. Reproduced, with permission, from Bloom W, Fawcett DW: *A Textbook of Histology,* 9th ed, Saunders, 1968.)

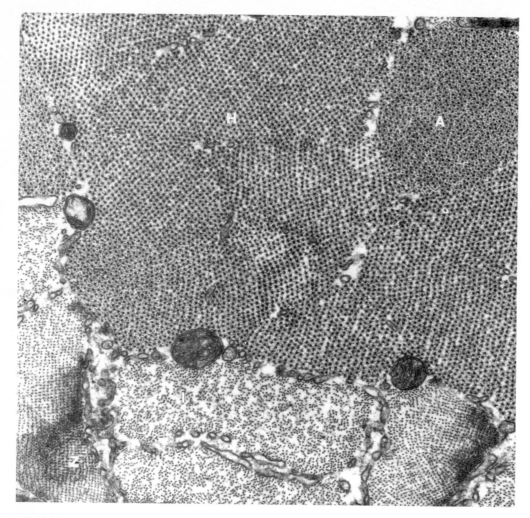

Figure 10–7. Transverse section of skeletal muscle myofibrils illustrating some of the features diagrammed in Fig 10–6. Z, Z line; I, I band; A, A band; H, H band. × 36,000.

while thick filaments consist primarily of myosin. Myosin and actin together represent 55% of the total protein of striated muscle.

Actin is present as long filamentous (F-actin) polymers consisting of 2 strands of globular (G-actin) monomers, 5.6 nm in diameter, twisted around each other in a double helical formation (Fig 10–6). A notable characteristic of all G-actin molecules is their structural asymmetry. When G-actin molecules polymerize to form F-actin, they bind back to front, producing a filament with distinguishable polarity (Fig 10–8). Each G-actin monomer contains a binding site for myosin (Fig 10–9). Actin filaments, which anchor perpendicularly on the Z line, exhibit opposite polarity on each side of the line (Fig 10–6). The protein α-actinin, a major component of the Z line, is thought to anchor the actin

filaments to this region. α-actinin and desmin (an intermediate-filament protein) are believed to tie adjacent sarcomeres together, thus keeping the myofibrils in register.

Tropomyosin is a long, thin molecule about 40 nm in length and containing 2 polypeptide chains. These molecules are bound head to tail, forming filaments that run over the actin subunits alongside the outer edges of the groove between the 2 twisted actin strands (Fig 10–8).

Troponin is a complex of 3 subunits: **TnT,** which strongly attaches to tropomyosin; **TnC,** which binds calcium ions; and **TnI,** which inhibits the actin-myosin interaction. A troponin complex is attached at one specific site on each tropomyosin molecule (Fig 10–8).

In thin filaments, each tropomyosin molecule spans

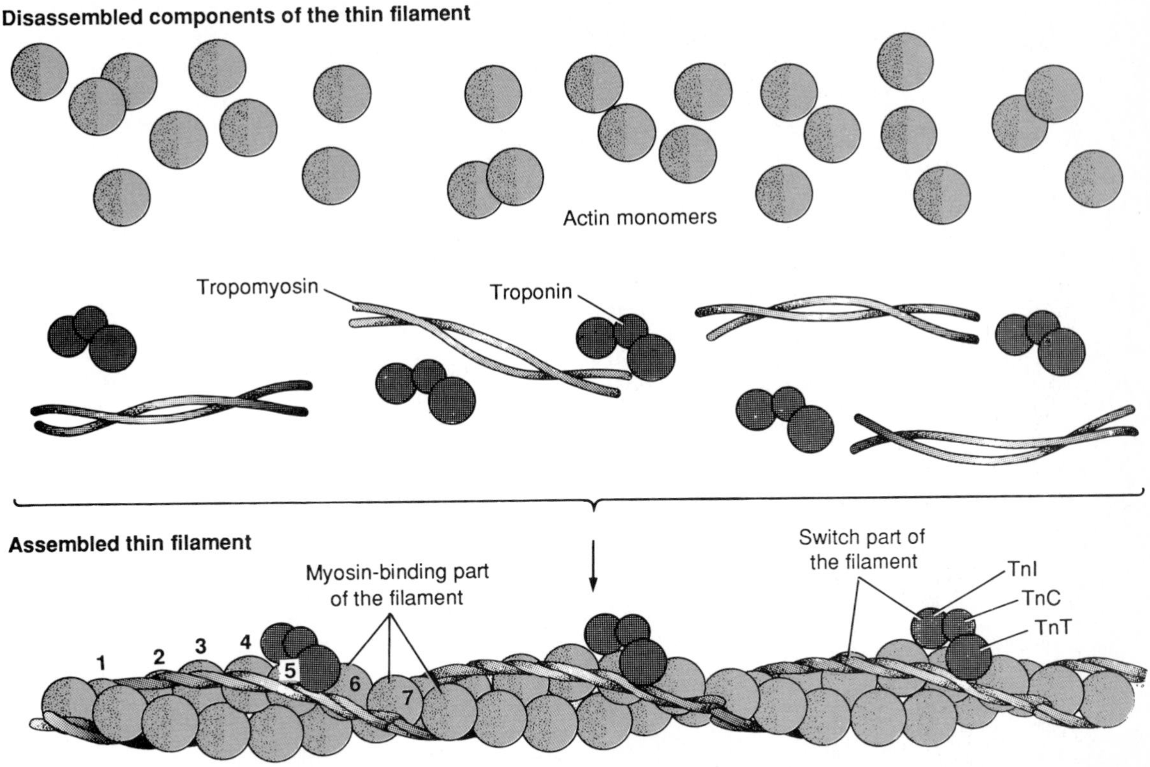

Disassembled components of the thin filament

Figure 10–8. Schematic representation of the thin filament, showing the spatial configuration of the 3 major protein components—actin (shown in color), tropomyosin, and troponin (black). The individual components in the top part of the drawing are shown in polymerized form in the bottom portion. The globular actin molecules are polarized (dark and light areas) and polymerize in one direction. Observe that each tropomyosin molecule extends over 7 actin molecules. TnI, TnC, TnT, see text (under *Troponin*).

7 G-actin molecules and has one troponin complex bound to its surface (Fig 10–8).

Myosin is a much larger complex (MW ~ 500,000). Myosin can be dissociated into 2 identical heavy chains and 2 pairs of light chains. Myosin heavy chains are thin, rodlike molecules (150 nm long and 2–3 nm thick) made up of 2 heavy chains twisted together. Small globular projections at one end of each heavy chain form the heads, which have ATP binding sites as well as the enzymatic capacity to hydrolyze ATP (ATPase activity) and the ability to bind to actin. The 4 light chains are associated with the head (Fig 10–6). When subjected to brief proteolysis, myosin heavy chains can be cleaved into 2 fragments, **light** and **heavy meromyosin.** The light fragment represents the greater part of the rodlike portion of the molecule; heavy meromyosin represents its globular projection plus a small part of the rod. Several hundred myosin molecules are arranged within each thick filament with their rodlike portions overlapping and their globular heads directed toward either end.

Analysis of thin sections of striated muscle shows the presence of cross-bridges between thin and thick filaments. These bridges are known to be formed by the head of the myosin molecule plus a short part of its rodlike portion. These bridges are considered to be directly involved in the conversion of chemical into mechanical energy (Fig 10–9).

Transverse Tubule System

The depolarization of the sarcoplasmic reticulum membrane, which results in the release of Ca^{2+} ions, is initiated at a specialized myoneural junction on the surface of the muscle cell. Surface-initiated depolarization signals would have to diffuse throughout the cell to effect Ca^{2+} release from internal sarcoplasmic reticulum cisternae. In larger muscle cells, the diffusion of the depolarization signal would lead to a wave of contraction, with peripheral myofibrils, contracting prior to more centrally positioned myofibrils. To provide for a uniform contraction, skeletal muscle possesses a system of **transverse (T) tubules** (Fig 10–10). These fingerlike invaginations of the sarcolemma form a complex anastomosing network of tubules that encircle the boundaries of the A–I bands of

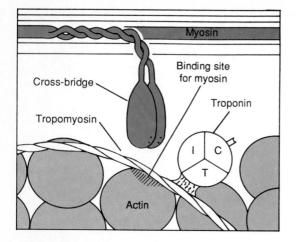

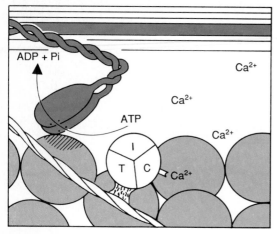

Figure 10–9. Initiation of muscle contraction occurs by the binding of Ca^{2+} to the TnC unit of troponin, which exposes the myosin binding site on actin (cross-hatched area). In a second step, the myosin head binds to actin and the ATP breaks down into ADP, yielding energy, which produces a movement of the myosin head. As a consequence of this change in myosin, the bound thin filaments slide over the thick filaments. This process, which repeats itself many times during a single contraction, leads to a complete overlapping of the actin and myosin and a resultant shortening of the whole myofiber. (Reproduced, with permission, from Ganong WF: *Review of Medical Physiology,* 14th ed. Appleton & Lange, 1989.)

each sarcomere in every myofibril (Figs 10–11 and 10–12).

Adjacent to opposite sides of each T tubule are expanded **terminal cisternae** of the sarcoplasmic reticulum. This specialized complex, consisting of SR-T tubule-SR components, is known as the **triad** (Figs 10–5, 10–11, and 10–12). At the triad, depolarization of the sarcolemma-derived T tubules is transmitted to the sarcoplasmic reticulum.

Sarcoplasmic Reticulum

As described above, muscle contraction depends on the availability of Ca^{2+} ions, and muscle relaxation is related to an absence of Ca^{2+}. The sarcoplasmic reticulum (SR) specifically regulates calcium flow, which is necessary for rapid contraction and relaxation cycles. Cytologically, the sarcoplasmic reticulum system consists of a branching network of smooth endoplasmic reticulum cisternae surrounding each myofibril (Fig 10–12). Following a neurally mediated depolarization of the sarcoplasmic reticulum membrane, Ca^{2+} ions concentrated within the sarcoplasmic reticulum cisternae are passively released into the vicinity of the overlapping thick and thin filaments, whereupon they bind to troponin and allow bridging between actin and myosin. When the membrane depolarization ends, the sarcoplasmic reticulum acts as a calcium sink and actively transports the Ca^{2+} back into the cisternae; this results in the cessation of contractile activity.

Mechanism of Contraction

Resting sarcomeres consist of partially overlapping thick and thin filaments. During contraction, both the thick and thin filaments retain their original length. Since contraction is not caused by a shortening of individual filaments, it must be the result of an increase in the amount of overlap between the filaments. The **sliding filament** hypothesis of muscle contraction proposed by Huxley (mentioned earlier), has received the most widespread acceptance.

The following is a brief description of how actin and myosin interact during a contraction cycle. At rest, ATP binds to the ATPase site on the myosin heads, but the rate of hydrolysis is very slow. Myosin requires acitn as a cofactor in order to break down ATP rapidly and release energy. In a resting muscle, myosin cannot associate with actin, because the binding sites for myosin heads on actin molecules are covered by the troponin-tropomyosin complex on the F-actin filament (Fig 10–9, top). When sufficiently high concentrations of calcium ions are available, however, they bind to the TnC subunit of troponin. The spatial configuration of the 3 troponin subunits changes and drives the tropomyosin molecule deeper into the groove of the actin helix (Fig 10–9). This exposes the myosin-binding site on the globular actin components, so that actin is free to interact with the head of the myosin molecule.

The binding of calcium ions to the TnC unit corresponds to the stage at which myosin-ATP is converted into the active complex. As a result of bridging between the myosin head and the G-actin subunit of the thin filament, the ATP is split into ADP and Pi, and energy is released. This activity leads to a deformation, or bending, of the head and a part of the rodlike portion (hinge region) of the myosin (Fig 10–9). Since the actin is bound to the myosin, movement of the myosin head pulls the actin past the my-

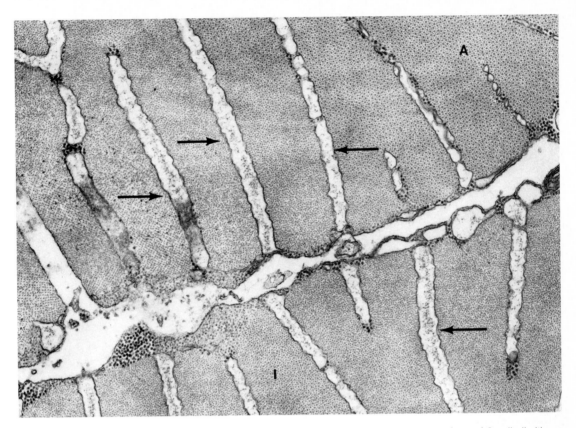

Figure 10–10. Electron micrograph of a transverse section of fish muscle, showing the surface of 2 cells limiting an intercellular space. Observe the invaginations of the sarcolemma, forming the tubules of the T system (arrows). The dark, coarse granules in the cytoplasm **(lower left)** are glycogen particles. **Upper right:** (A), the section passes through the A band, showing thick and thin filaments. **Lower left:** (I), the I band is sectioned, showing only thin filaments. × 60,000. (Courtesy of KR Porter.)

osin filament. The result is that the thin filament is drawn farther into the A band.

Although a large number of myosin heads extend from the thick filament, at any one time during the contraction only a small number of heads align with available actin binding sites. As the bound myosin heads move the actin, however, they provide for alignment of new actin-myosin bridges. The old actin-myosin bridges detach only after the myosin binds a new ATP molecule; this action also resets the myosin head and prepares it for another contraction cycle. If no ATP is available, the actin-myosin complex becomes stable; this accounts for the extreme muscular rigidity **(rigor mortis)** that occurs after death. A single muscle contraction is the result of hundreds of bridge-forming and bridge-breaking cycles. The contraction activity that leads to a complete overlap between thin and thick filaments continues until Ca^{2+} ions are removed and the troponin-tropomyosin complex again covers the myosin binding site.

During contraction, the I band decreases in size as

thin filaments penetrate the A band. The H band—the part of the A band with only thick filaments—diminishes in width as the thin filaments completely overlap the thick filaments. A net result is that each sarcomere, and consequently the whole cell (fiber), is greatly shortened (Fig 10–13).

Innervation

Myelinated motor nerves branch out within the perimysial connective tissue, where each nerve gives rise to several terminal twigs. At the site of innervation, the nerve loses its myelin sheath and forms a dilated termination (terminal bouton) that sits within a trough on the muscle cell surface. This structure is called the **motor end-plate** or **myoneural junction.** (Fig 10–13). At this site the axon is covered by a thin cytoplasmic layer of Schwann cells. Within the axon terminal are numerous mitochondria and synaptic vesicles, the latter containing the neurotransmitter **acetylcholine** (described in Chapter 9). Between the axon and the muscle is a space, the **synaptic cleft,** in which lies an amorphous basal lamina matrix. At the junc-

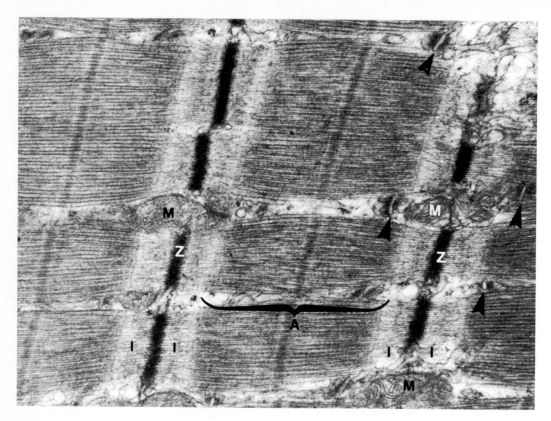

Figure 10–11. Electron micrograph of a longitudinal section of the skeletal muscle of a monkey. Note the mitochondria (M) between adjacent myofibrils. The arrowheads indicate triads—2 for each sarcomere in this muscle—located at the A–I band junction. A, A band; I, I band; Z, Z line. × 40,000. (Reproduced, with permission, from Junqueira LCU, Salles LMM: *Ultra-Estrutura e Função Celular.* Edgard Blücher, 1975.)

tion, the sarcolemma is thrown into numerous deep **junctional folds.** In the sarcoplasm below the folds lie several nuclei and numerous mitochondria, ribosomes, and glycogen granules.

When an action potential invades the motor end-plate, acetylcholine is liberated from the axon terminal, diffuses through the cleft, and binds to acetylcholine receptors in the sarcolemma of the junctional folds. Binding of the transmitter makes the sarcolemma more permeable to sodium, which results in **membrane depolarization.** Excess acetylcholine is hydrolyzed by the enzyme cholinesterase bound to the synaptic cleft basal lamina. Acetylcholine breakdown is necessary to avoid prolonged contact of the transmitter with receptors present in the sarcolemma.

The depolarization initiated at the motor end-plate is propagated along the surface of the muscle cell and deep into the fibers via the transverse tubule system. At each triad, the depolarization signal is passed to the sarcoplasmic reticulum and results in the release of Ca^{2+}, which initiates the contraction cycle. When depolarization ceases, the Ca^{2+} is actively transported back into the sarcoplasmic reticulum cisternae and the muscle relaxes.

Myasthenia gravis is an autoimmune disorder characterized by progressive muscular weakness caused by a reduction in the number of functionally active acetylcholine receptors in the sarcolemma of the myoneural junction. Circulating antibodies bind to the acetylcholine receptors in the junctional folds and inhibit normal nerve-muscle communication. As the body attempts to correct the condition, membrane segments with affected receptors are internalized, digested by lyosomes, and replaced by newly formed receptors. These receptors, however, are again made unresponsive to acetylcholine by the same antibodies, and the disease follows in its progressive course.

A single nerve fiber (**axon**) can innervate one muscle fiber, or it may branch and be responsible for innervating up to 160 or more muscle fibers. In the case of multiple innervation, a single nerve fiber and

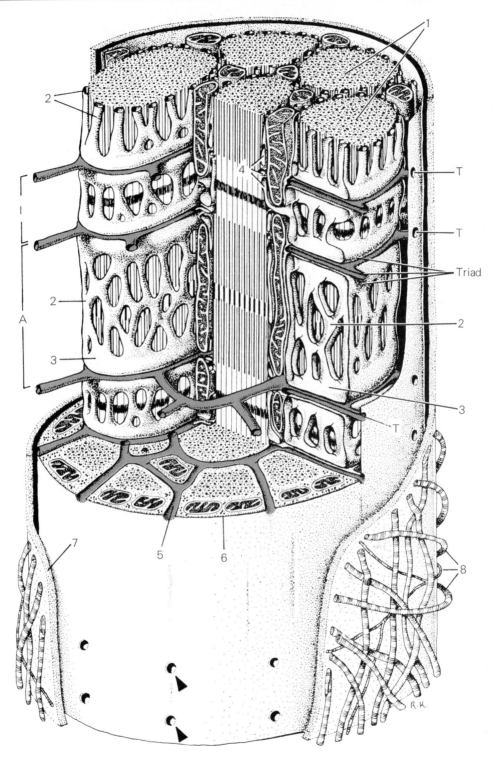

Figure 10–12. Diagram of a segment of mammalian skeletal muscle. The sarcolemma and muscle fibrils are partially cut, showing the following components: The invaginations of the T system (shown in color; T and 5) occur at the level of transition between the A and I bands twice in every sarcomere. They associate with terminal cisternae of the sarcoplasmic reticulum (3), forming triads. Abundant mitochondria (4) lie between the myofibrils. The cut surface of the myofibrils (1) shows the thin and thick filaments. Surrounding the sarcolemma are a basal lamina (7) and reticular fibers (8). (Reproduced, with permission, from Krstić RV: *Ultrastructure of the Mammalian Cell*. Springer–Verlag, 1979.)

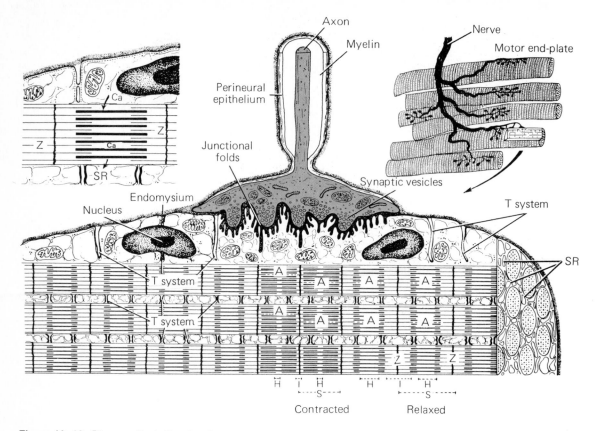

Figure 10–13. Diagram illustrating the ultrastructure of the motor end-plate and the mechanism of muscle contraction. The upper right drawing shows branching of a small nerve with a motor end-plate for each muscle fiber. The structure of one of the bulbs of an end-plate is highly enlarged in the center drawing. Observe that the axon terminal bud contains synaptic vesicles. The region of the muscle cell membrane covered by the terminal bud exhibits clefts and ridges called **junctional folds.** The axon (shown in color) loses its myelin sheath and dilates, establishing close, irregular contact with the muscle fiber. Muscle contraction begins with the release of acetylcholine from the synaptic vesicles of the end-plate. This neurotransmitter causes a local increase in the permeability of the sarcolemma. The process if propagated to the rest of the sarcolemma, including its invaginations (all of which constitute the T system), and is transferred to the sarcoplasmic reticulum (SR). The increase of permeability in this organelle liberates calcium ions that trigger the sliding filament mechanism of muscle contraction. Thin filaments slide between the thick filaments and reduce the distance between the Z lines. This produces a reduction in the size of all bands except the A band.

all the muscles it innervates are called a **motor unit.** Individual striated muscle fibers do not show graded contraction—they contract either all the way or not at all. In order to vary the force of contraction, the fibers within a muscle bundle should not all contract at the same time. Since muscles are broken up into motor units, the firing of a single nerve motor axon will generate tension proportional to the number of muscle fibers innervated by that axon. Thus, the number of motor units and the variable size of each unit can control the intensity of a muscle contraction. The ability of a muscle to perform delicate movements is dependent on the size of its motor units. For example, because of the fine control required by eye muscles, each of their fibers is innervated by a different nerve fiber. In larger mus-

cles exhibiting coarser movements, such as those of the limb, a single profusely branched axon innervates a motor unit that consists of more than 100 individual muscle fibers.

System of Energy Production

Skeletal muscle cells are highly adapted for discontinuous production of mechanical work through the release of chemical energy and must have depots of energy to cope with bursts of activity. The most readily available energy is stored in the form of ATP and phosphocreatine, both of which are energy-rich phosphate compounds. Chemical energy is also available in glycogen depots, which constitute about 0.5–1% of muscle weight. Muscle tissue obtains energy to be stored in phosphocreatine and

ATP from the breakdown of fatty acids and glucose. In the resting muscle or during its recovery after contraction, the major substrate is fatty acids. Fatty acids are broken down to acetate by the enzymes of β-oxidation, located in the mitochondrial matrix. Acetate is then further oxidized by the citric acid cycle, with the resulting energy being conserved in the form of ATP. Fatty acids are the main energy source in the skeletal muscle of endurance athletes, such as long-distance runners. When skeletal muscles are subjected to a short-term (sprint) exercise, they rapidly metabolize glucose (coming mainly from muscle glycogen stores) to lactate, causing an oxygen debt that is repaid during the recovery period. It is the lactate formed during this form of exercise that causes cramping and pain in skeletal muscles.

From the morphologic, histochemical, and functional point of view, we can classify skeletal muscle fibers into 3 types: red, white, and intermediate. **Red fibers** have a high content of red pigments (myoglobin and mitochondrial cytochromes), which are responsible for the dark red color. They contract at a slower rate than do white fibers but are capable of continuous and vigorous activity. Their energy derives mainly from oxidative phosphorylation, and these fibers contain great numbers of mitochondria. These are the fibers in both mammalian limbs and the breast muscles of migrating birds. The long muscles of the human back, adapted for long, slow, posture-maintaining contractions, are also an example of red muscle.

White fibers have a low content of myoglobin; they have fewer mitochondria and, consequently, less cytochrome. They are larger in diameter than red fibers. The breast muscles of chickens and turkeys as well as the extraocular muscles of the human eye consist of these fibers. They contract rapidly but cannot support continuous heavy work. The energy for their activity is derived mainly from anaerobic glycolysis. **Intermediate fibers** have characteristics that lie between the 2 described above. In humans, skeletal muscles are frequently composed of mixtures of these 3 types of fibers, as shown in Fig 10–14.

The differentiation of muscle into red, white, and intermediate fiber types is controlled by its innervation. In experiments where the nerves to red and white fibers are cut, crossed, and allowed to regenerate, the myofibers change their morphology and physiology in order to conform to the innervating nerve. Simple denervation of muscle will lead to fiber atrophy and paralysis.

Other Components of the Sarcoplasm

Glycogen is found in abundance in the sarcoplasm in the form of coarse granules (see Fig 10–10). It

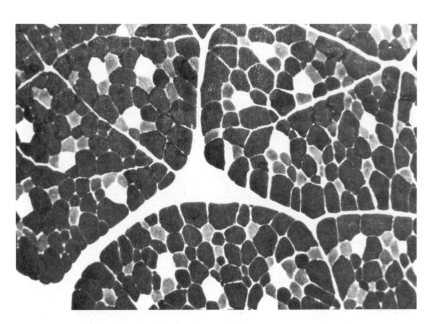

Figure 10–14. Transverse section of a striated muscle of the eye (rectus lateralis), stained by the histochemical technique for demonstrating myosin ATPase, showing 3 types of fibers in the muscle. This method shows that white fibers are large and dark-staining (high ATPase activity), red fibers are small and appear gray, and intermediate fibers are seen as pale areas in the section. (Reproduced, with permission, from Khan MA et al: A calcium-citrophosphate technique for the histochemical localization of myosin ATPase. *Stain Technol* 1972;**47**:277.)

serves as a depot of energy that is mobilized during muscle contraction.

Another component of the sarcoplasm is **myoglobin,** an oxygen-binding protein similar to hemoglobin that is principally responsible for the dark red color of some muscles. Myoglobin acts as an oxygen-storing pigment necessary for the high oxidative phosphorylation level in this type of fiber. For obvious reasons, it is present in great amounts in the muscle of deep-diving ocean mammals (eg, seals, whales). Muscles that must maintain activity for prolonged periods usually are red and have a high myoglobin content.

Mature muscle cells have negligible amounts of rough endoplasmic reticulum and ribosomes, an observation that is consistent with the low level of protein synthesis occurring in this tissue.

Muscle spindles are described in Chapter 24.

CARDIAC MUSCLE

During development, the splanchnic mesoderm cells of the primitive heart tube align into chainlike arrays. Rather than fusing into syncytial (*syn* + *kytos*) cells, as in the development of skeletal muscle, cardiac cells form complex junctions between their extended processes. Cells within a chain often bifurcate, or branch, and bind to cells in adjacent chains. Consequently, the heart consists of tightly knit bundles of cells, interwoven in a fashion that provides for a characteristic wave of contraction that leads to a wringing out of the heart ventricles.

Mature cardiac muscle cells are approximately 15 μm in diameter and from 85 to 100 μm in length. They exhibit a cross-striated banding pattern identical to that of skeletal muscle. Unlike multinucleated skeletal muscle, however, each cardiac muscle cell possesses only 1 or 2 centrally located pale-staining nuclei. Surrounding the muscle cells is a delicate sheath of endomysial connective tissue containing a rich capillary network.

A unique and distinguishing characteristic of cardiac muscle is the presence of darkly staining transverse lines that cross the chains of cardiac cells at irregular intervals (Fig 10–15). These **intercalated disks** represent junctional complexes found at the in-

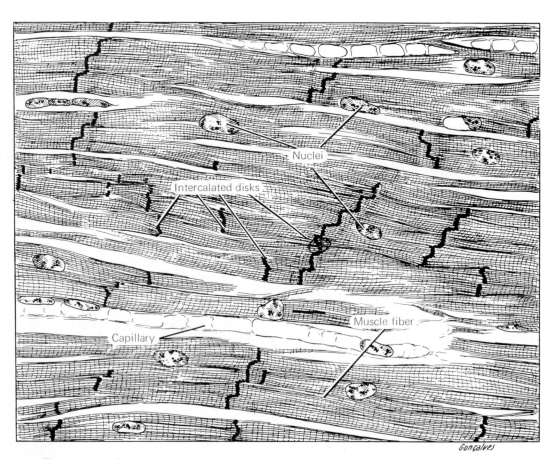

Figure 10–15. Diagram of a section of heart muscle, showing central nuclei and intercalated disks.

terface between adjacent cardiac muscle cells (Figs 10–16, 10–17, and 10–18). The junctions may appear as straight lines or may exhibit a steplike pattern. Two regions can be distinguished in the steplike junctions—a **transverse portion,** which runs across the fibers at right angles, and a **lateral portion** running parallel to the myofilaments. There are 3 main junctional specializations within the disk. **Fasciae**

adherentes, the most prominent membrane specialization in transverse portions of the disk, serve as anchoring sites for actin filaments of the terminal sarcomeres. Essentially, they represent **hemi-Z bands. Maculae adherentes** (desmosomes) bind the cardiac cells together to prevent their pulling apart under constant contractile activity. On the lateral portions of the disk, **gap junctions** provide ionic continuity be-

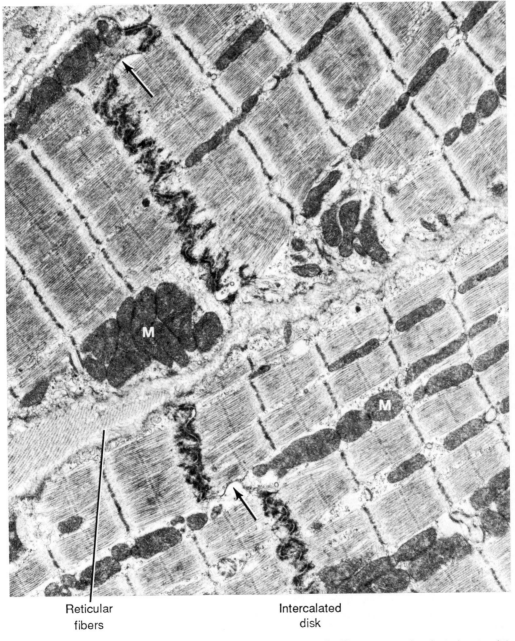

Reticular
fibers

Intercalated
disk

Figure 10–16. Longitudinal section of portions of 2 cardiac muscle cells. The transversely oriented parts of the intercalated disk consist of a fascia adherens and numerous desmosomes (T). The longitudinal parts (arrows) contain gap junctions. Mitochondria (M) are numerous. Reticular fibers (R) are seen between the 2 cells. × 18,000. (Reproduced, with permission, from Junqueira LCU, Salles LMM: *Ultra-Estrutura e Função Celular.* Edgard Blücher, 1975.)

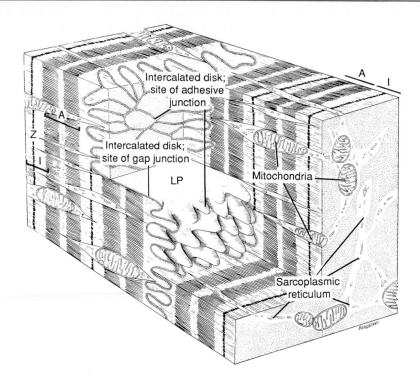

Figure 10–17. Ultrastructure of heart muscle in the region of an intercalated disk. Contact between cells is accomplished by interdigitation in the transverse region; it is smooth in the longitudinal plane (LP). (Redrawn and reproduced, with permission, from Marshall JM. The heart. In: *Medical Physiology*, 13th ed, Vol 2, Mountcastle VB [editor]. Mosby, 1974. Based on the results of Fawcett DW, McNutt NS: *J Cell Biol* 1969;**42:**1, modified from Poche R, Lindner E: *Zellforsch Mikrosk Anat* 1955;**43:**104.)

tween adjacent cells (Fig 10–18). The significance of ionic coupling is that chains of individual cells behave as a syncytium, allowing the signal to contract to pass in a wave from cell to cell.

The structure and function of the contractile proteins in cardiac cells is virtually the same as in skeletal muscle (Fig 10–19). The T tubule system and sarcoplasmic reticulum, however, are not as regularly arranged in the cardiac myocytes. The T tubules are more numerous and larger in ventricular muscle than in skeletal muscle. Cardiac T tubules are found at the level of the Z band rather than at the A-I junction (as in mammalian skeletal muscle). The sarcoplasmic reticulum is not as well developed and wanders irregularly through the myofilaments. As a consequence, discrete myofibrillar bundles are not present.

Triads are not common in cardiac cells, since the T tubules are generally associated with only one lateral expansion of sarcoplasmic reticulum cisternae. Thus, heart muscle characteristically possesses **diads** composed of one T tubule and one sarcoplasmic reticulum cisterna.

Cardiac muscle cells contain numerous mitochondria, which occupy 40% or more of the cytoplasmic volume (Fig 10–19), reflecting the need for contin-

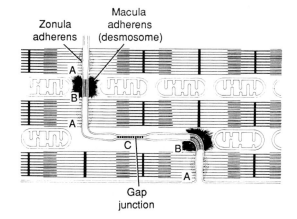

Figure 10–18. Diagrammatic representation of junctional specializations making up the intercalated disk. **Fascia** (or **zonula**) **adherens** (A) in the transverse portions of the disk serves to anchor actin filaments of the terminal sarcomeres to the plasmalemma. **Maculae adherentes,** or **desmosomes** (B), found primarily in the transverse portions of the disk, bind cells together, preventing their separation during contraction cycles. **Gap junctions** (C), restricted to longitudinal portions of the disk—the area subjected to the least stress—ionically couple cells and provide for the spread of contractile depolarization.

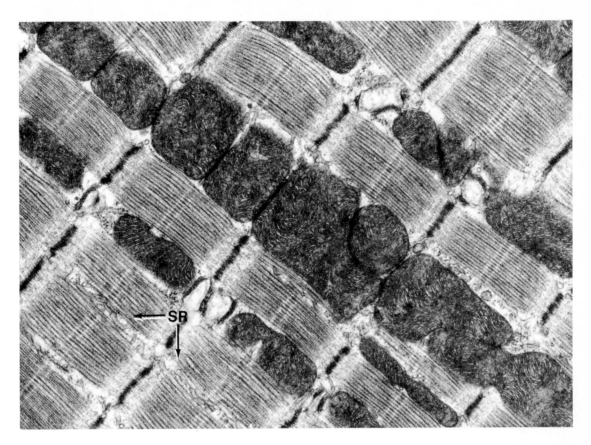

Figure 10–19. Electron micrograph from a longitudinal section of heart muscle. Observe the striation pattern and the alternation of myofibrils and mitochondria rich in cristae. Note the sarcoplasmic reticulum (SR), the specialized calcium-storing smooth endoplasmic reticulum. × 30,000.

uous aerobic metabolism in heart muscle. By comparison, only about 2% of a skeletal muscle fiber is occupied by mitochondria. Fatty acids, transported to cardiac muscle cells by lipoproteins, are the major fuel of the heart. Fatty acids are stored as triglycerides in the numerous lipid droplets seen in cardiac muscle cells. A small amount of glycogen is present; this can be broken down to glucose and utilized for energy production during periods of stress. Lipofuscin pigment granules (aging pigment), often seen in long-lived cells, are found near the nuclear poles of cardiac muscle cells.

A few differences in structure exist between atrial and ventricular muscle. The arrangement of myofilaments is the same in the 2 types of cardiac muscle, but atrial muscle has markedly fewer T tubules, and the cells are somewhat smaller. Membrane-limited granules, each about 0.2–0.3 μm in diameter, are found at both poles of cardiac muscle nuclei, and in association with Golgi complexes in this region. These granules are most abundant in muscle cells of the right atrium (approximately 600/cell), but they are also found in the left atrium, the ventricles, and several other places in the body. These atrial granules contain the high-molecular-weight precursor of a hormone known as **atrial natriuretic factor, auriculin,** or **atriopeptin.** Atrial natriuretic factor acts on the kidneys to cause sodium and water loss (natriuresis and diuresis). This hormone thus opposes the actions of aldosterone and antidiuretic hormone, whose effects on kidneys result in sodium and water conservation.

The rich autonomic nerve supply to the heart and the rhythmic impulse-generating and conducting structures are dealt with in Chapter 11.

SMOOTH MUSCLE

Smooth muscle is composed of elongated, nonstriated cells (Fig 10–20), each of which is enclosed by a basal lamina and a network of reticular fibers (Figs 10–21 and 10–22). The last 2 components serve to combine the force generated by each smooth muscle fiber into a concerted action, eg, peristalsis in the intestine.

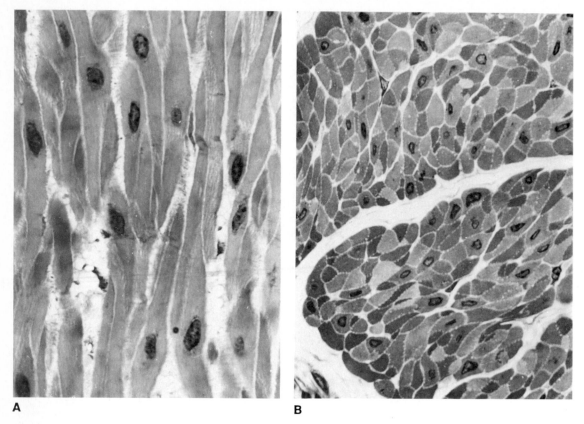

A   **B**

Figure 10–20. Photomicrographs of urinary bladder. Smooth muscle cells are sectioned longitudinally **(A)** and transversely **(B)**. Note the reticular fibers around the bundles of smooth muscle cells.

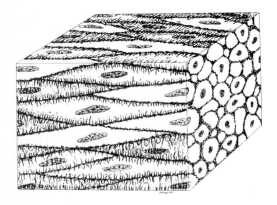

Figure 10–21. Diagram of a segment of smooth muscle. All cells are surrounded by a net of reticular fibers. In cross section, these cells exhibit variable diameters.

Smooth muscle cells are fusiform; ie, they are largest at their midpoints and taper toward their ends. They may be from 20 μm in small blood vessels to 500 μm in the pregnant uterus. During pregnancy, uterine smooth muscle cells undergo marked increase in size and number. Each cell has a single nucleus located in the center of the broadest part of the cell. To achieve closest packing, the narrow part of one cell lies adjacent to the broad part of neighboring cells (Fig 10–21). When such an arrangement is viewed in cross section, one sees a range of diameters with only the largest profiles containing a nucleus (Figs 10–20 and 10–21). The borders of the cell become scalloped when smooth muscle contracts, and the nucleus becomes folded or has the appearance of a corkscrew.

Concentrated at the poles of the nucleus are mitochondria, free ribosomes, cisternae of rough endoplasmic reticulum, and the Golgi complex.

A rudimentary sarcoplasmic reticulum is present; it consists of a closed system of membranes, similar to the sarcoplasmic reticulum of striated muscle. T tubules are not present in smooth muscle cells.

The characteristic contractile activity of smooth

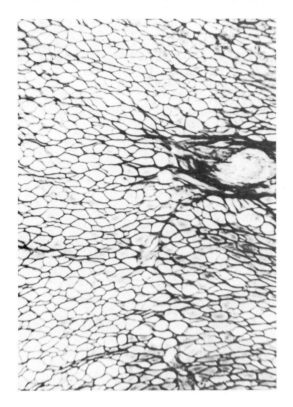

Figure 10–22. Transverse section of smooth muscle impregnated with silver to stain the reticular fibers. These structures form a network that surrounds the muscle cells not stained by this method. **Right:** an arteriole surrounded by thicker collagen fibers. × 300.

muscle is related to the structure and organization of its actin and myosin filaments, which do not exhibit the paracrystalline organization present in striated muscles (Fig 10–23). In smooth muscle cells, bundles of myofilaments crisscross obliquely through the cell, forming a latticelike network. These bundles consist of 5–7-nm thin filaments containing actin and tropomyosin, and 12–16-nm thick filaments consisting of myosin. Unlike the myosin filaments in skeletal muscle, which have a bare central region with myosin heads on each end, smooth muscle myosin has heads all along its length and bare regions at the ends of the filaments. This morphologic feature reflects polarity differences in the organization of myosin molecules. The molecular organization of the myosin filaments allows much greater actin overlap and a greater degree of contraction in smooth muscle. Both structural and biochemical studies reveal that smooth muscle actin and myosin contract by sliding filament mechanism similar to that which occurs in striated muscles.

An influx of Ca^{2+} is involved in the initiation of contraction in smooth muscle cells. The myosin of smooth muscle, however, interacts with actin only when its light chain is phosphorylated. For this reason, and because troponin is absent, the contraction mechanism in smooth muscle differs somewhat from skeletal and cardiac muscle. Ca^{2+} in a smooth muscle complexes with **calmodulin,** a calcium-binding protein that is also involved in contraction of nonmuscle cells. The Ca^{2+}-calmodulin complex activates myosin light-chain kinase, the enzyme responsible for the phosphorylation of myosin.

Factors other than calcium affect the activity of myosin light-chain kinase and thus influence the degree of contraction of smooth muscle cells. Contraction or relaxation may be regulated by hormones that act via cyclic AMP (cAMP). When levels of cAMP increase, myosin light-chain kinase is activated, myosin is phosphorylated, and the cell contracts. A decrease in cAMP has the opposite effect, decreasing contractility. The action of sex hormones upon uterine smooth muscle is another example of nonneural control. Estrogens increase cAMP and promote the phosphorylation of myosin and the contractile activity of uterine smooth muscle. Progesterone has an opposite effect. It decreases cAMP, promotes dephosphorylation of myosin, and relaxes uterine musculature.

Smooth muscle cells have an elaborate array of 10-nm intermediate filaments coursing through their cytoplasm. **Desmin (skeletin)** has been identified as the major protein of intermediate filaments in all smooth muscles, and **vimentin** occurs as an additional component in vascular smooth muscle. Two types of **dense bodies**—membrane-associated and cytoplasmic—are seen in smooth muscle. Both contain α-actinin and are thus similar to the Z lines of striated muscles. Both thin and intermediate filaments insert into dense bodies that transmit contractile force to adjacent smooth muscle cells and their surrounding network of reticular fibers.

The degree of innervation in a particular bundle of smooth muscle is dependent upon the function and the size of that muscle. Smooth muscle is innervated by both sympathetic and parasympathetic nerves of the autonomic system. Elaborate neuromuscular junctions like those in skeletal muscle are not present in smooth muscle. Frequently, autonomic nerve axons terminate in a series of dilatations in the endomysial connective tissue.

In general, smooth muscle occurs in large sheets such as are found in the walls of hollow viscera, eg, the intestines, uterus, and ureters. Their cells possess abundant gap junctions and a relatively poor nerve supply. These muscles function in syncytial fashion and are called **visceral smooth muscles.** In contrast, the **multiunit smooth muscles** have a rich innervation and can produce such very precise and graded contractions as those occurring in the iris of the eye.

Smooth muscle usually has spontaneous activity in the absence of nervous stimuli. Its nerve supply there-

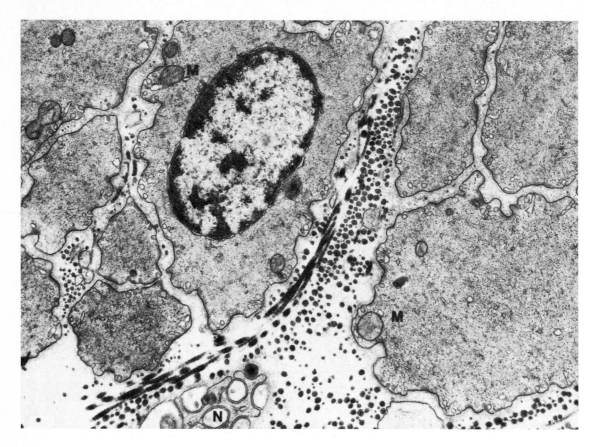

Figure 10–23. Electron micrograph of a transverse section of smooth muscle. The cells have variable diameters and many pinocytotic vesicles on their surface. Thick and thin filaments are not organized into myofibrils, and there are few mitochondria (M). Between the cells are collagen fibrils and a small unmyelinated nerve (N). × 6650.

fore has the function of modifying activity rather than initiating it, eg, as in skeletal muscle. Smooth muscle receives both adrenergic and cholinergic nerve endings that act antagonistically, stimulating or depressing its activity. In some organs, the cholinergic endings activate and the adrenergic nerves depress; in others the reverse occurs.

In addition to contractile activity, smooth muscle cells have also been shown to synthesize collagen, elastin, and proteoglycans, extracellular products normally associated with the function of fibroblasts. The elaborate rough endoplasmic reticulum and well-developed Golgi complex are organellar correlates reflecting this synthetic behavior.

REGENERATION OF MUSCLE TISSUE

The 3 types of adult muscle exhibit varying potentials for regeneration after injury.

Cardiac muscle has virtually no regenerative capacity beyond early childhood. Defects or damage (eg, infarcts) in heart muscle are generally replaced by proliferation of connective tissue, forming myocardial scars.

In skeletal muscle, although the nuclei in the syncytium are incapable of undergoing mitosis, the tissue undergoes regeneration. The source of regenerating cells is believed to be the **satellite cells.** Satellite cells are a sparse population of mononucleated spindle-shaped cells that lie within the basal lamina surrounding each mature muscle fiber. Because of their intimate apposition with the surface of the muscle fiber, they can be identified only with the electron microscope. They are considered to be inactive myoblasts that persist after muscle differentiation. Following injury or certain other stimuli, the normally quiescent satellite cells become activated, proliferating and fusing to form new skeletal muscle fibers. A similar activity of satellite cells has been implicated in muscle hypertrophy, where they fuse with their parent fibers to increase muscle mass following extensive exercise.

Smooth muscle is also capable of a modest regen-

erative response. Following injury, viable mononucleated smooth muscle cells undergo mitosis and provide for the replacement of the damaged tissue.

REFERENCES

Alberts B et al: *Molecular Biology of the Cell,* 2nd ed. Garland, 1989.

Bourne GH (editor): *The Structure and Function of Muscle.* Academic Press, 1972.

Bülbring E, Bolton TB (editors): Smooth muscle. *Br Med Bull* 1979;**35**:127.

Campion DR: The muscle satellite cell: A review. *Int Rev Cytol* 1984;**87**:225.

Cantin M, Genest J: The heart as an endocrine gland. *Sci Am* (Feb) 1986;**254**:76.

Cohen C: The protein swtich of muscle contraction. *Sci Am* (Nov) 1975;**233**:36.

Gabella G, Blundell D: Nexuses between smooth muscle cells of the guinea-pig ileum. *J Cell Biol* 1979;**82**:239.

Heuser JE. Reese TS: Evidence for recycling of synaptic vesicle membrane during transmitter release at the frog neuromuscular junction. *J Cell Biol* 1973;**57**:315.

Huxley HE: Molecular basis of contraction in cross-striated muscles and relevance to motile mechanisms in other cells. In: *Muscle and Nonmuscle Motility.* Vol 1. Stracher A (editor). Academic Press, 1983.

Sommer JR, Johnson EA: A comparative study of Purkinje fibers and ventricular fibers. *J Cell Biol* 1968;**36**:497.

The circulatory system consists of the blood and lymphatic vascular systems. The blood vascular system is composed of the following structures:

The heart, whose function is to pump the blood.

The arteries, a series of efferent vessels that become smaller as they branch and whose function is to carry the blood, with nutrients and oxygen, to the tissues.

The capillaries, a diffuse network of thin tubules that anastomose profusely and through whose walls the interchange between blood and tissues takes place.

The veins, which represent the convergence of the capillaries into a system of larger channels that convey products of metabolism, CO_2, etc, toward the heart.

The lymphatic vascular system begins in blind-ended tubules, the lymphatic capillaries, that anastomose to form vessels of steadily increasing size; these terminate in the blood vascular system, emptying into the large veins near the heart. The function of the lymphatic system is to return to the blood the fluid of the tissue spaces. Upon entering the lymphatic capillaries, this fluid contributes to the formation of the liquid part of the lymph; by passing through the lymphoid organs, it contributes to the circulation of lymphocytes and other immunologic factors.

By distributing hormones and nutrients to the cells and tissues of the body and transporting waste products to excretory organs, the circulatory system, along with the nervous system, contributes to the integrated functioning of the entire organism.

GENERAL STRUCTURE OF BLOOD VESSELS

All blood vessels have a number of structural features in common, although in the smallest vessels (capillaries and venules) the 3 tunics (described below) are greatly simplified. Blood vessels are structurally adapted according to physiologic requirements. Therefore, pulmonary arteries (low-pressure system) have thinner walls than do systemic arteries (high-pressure system) such as the carotid or renal arteries.

It should also be noted that there are no absolute criteria for distinguishing between large arteries, medium-sized arteries, and arterioles. Blood vessels constitute a continuous system, and some overlapping of classifications is to be expected.

Tunics

Blood vessels are usually composed of the following layers, or tunics (from Latin, *tunica,* coat) (Fig 11–1):

A. Tunica Intima: The intima consists of a layer of **endothelial cells** lining the vessel's interior surface. These cells rest on a basal lamina and have a turnover rate of 1% per day. (See under *Capillaries,* below, for a description of endothelial cells.) Beneath the endothelium is the **subendothelial layer,** consisting of loose connective tissue that may contain occasional smooth muscle cells. Both the connective tissue fibers and smooth muscle cells, when present, tend to be arranged longitudinally.

B. Tunica Media: The media consists chiefly of concentric layers of helically arranged smooth muscle cells (Fig 11–2). Interposed among the smooth muscle cells are variable amounts of elastic and reticular fibers and proteoglycans. Smooth muscle cells are the cellular source of this extracellular matrix. In arteries, the media is separated from the intima by an **internal elastic lamina.** This lamina, composed of elastin, has gaps **(fenestrae)** that allow substances to diffuse to and nourish cells deep in the vessel wall. In larger arteries, a thinner **external elastic lamina** is often found separating the media from the outer tunica adventitia. In capillaries and postcapillary venules, the media is represented by cells called **pericytes** (see under *Capillaries,* below).

C. Tunica Adventitia: The adventitia consists principally of longitudinally oriented collagen and elastic fibers (Fig 11–2). Collagen in the adventitia is type I; in the media, rich in reticular fibers, collagen is mainly type III. The adventitial layer gradually becomes continuous with the enveloping connective tissue of the organ through which the vessel is running.

Vasa Vasorum

In large vessels, vasa vasorum (vessels of the vessel) branch profusely in the adventitia and the outer

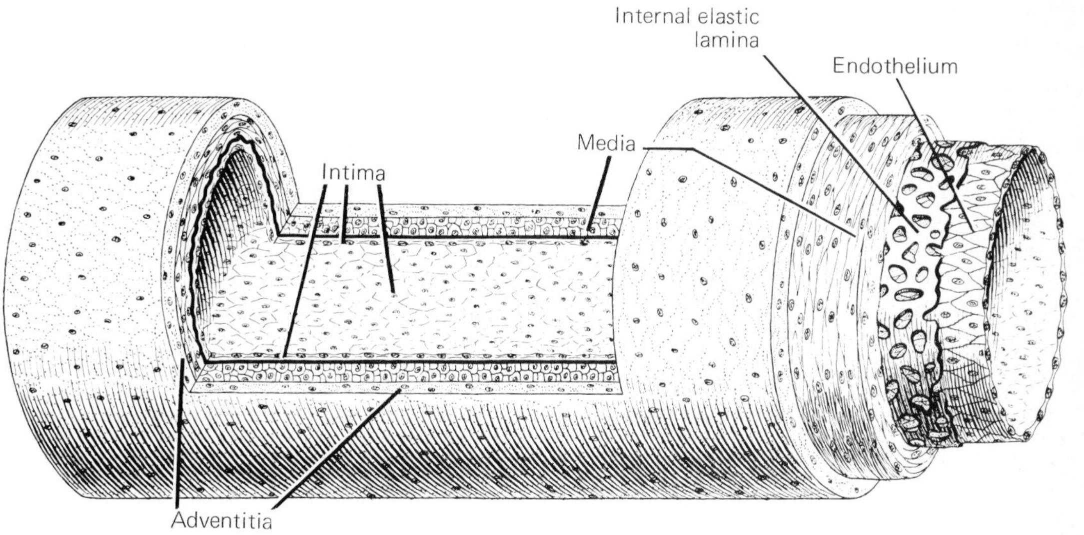

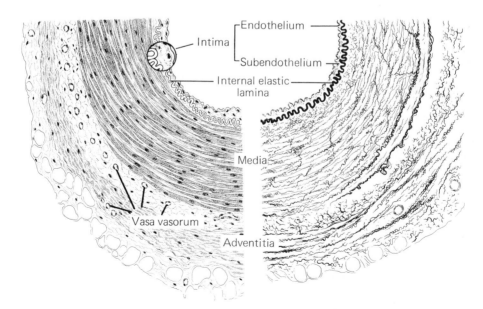

Figure 11–1. Drawing of a medium-sized muscular artery, showing its layers. Although the usual histologic preparations cause the layers to appear thicker than shown here, experimental work indicates that the drawing is more closely similar to the in vivo architecture of the vessel. After death, the vessel contracts, the layers become thicker, and the lumen becomes smaller and corrugated (as seen in Fig 11–8).

Figure 11–2. Comparative diagrams of a muscular artery prepared by H&E staining **(left)** and Weigert's staining method for elastic structures **(right).** The tunica media comprises a mixture of smooth muscle cells and reticular and elastic fibers. The adventitia and the outer part of the media have small blood vessels (vasa vasorum) and elastic and collagenous fibers.

part of the media (Fig 11–2). The vasa vasorum provide metabolites to the adventitia and the media in larger vessels, since the layers are too thick to be nourished solely by diffusion from the lumen. These vessels are more frequent in veins than in arteries. This greater abundance of vasa vasorum can be attributed to the paucity of oxygen and nutritional substances in venous blood. Vasa vasorum can arise from branches of the artery they supply or from neighboring arteries.

Although **lymphatic capillaries** can penetrate the media of veins, they are present in arteries only in the adventitia. This difference in distribution is probably related to differences in transmural pressures. The higher pressure across an arterial wall would tend to collapse a lymphatic capillary located near the arterial lumen, rendering it useless.

Innervation

Most blood vessels that contain smooth muscle in their walls are supplied with a profuse network of unmyelinated sympathetic nerve fibers (**vasomotor nerves**) whose neurotransmitter is norepinephrine. Discharge of norepinephrine from these nerves results in vasoconstriction. Because these efferent nerves generally do not enter the media of arteries, the neurotransmitter must diffuse for several micrometers to affect smooth muscle cells of the media. Gap junctions between smooth muscle cells of the media propagate the response to the neurotransmitter to the inner layers of muscle cells. In veins, nerve endings are found in both the adventitia and the media, but the overall density of innervation is less than that encountered in arteries. Arteries in skeletal muscle also receive a cholinergic vasodilator nerve supply.

Afferent (sensory) nerve endings in arteries include the **baroreceptors** (pressure receptors [from Greek, *baros,* weight, + Latin, *recipio,* to receive]) in the carotid sinus and the arch of the aorta as well as **chemoreceptors** of the carotid and aortic bodies.

SPECIFIC STRUCTURE OF BLOOD VESSELS

It is customary to divide the circulatory system into the **macrovasculature** (vessels > 0.1 mm in diameter) and the **microvasculature** (vessels visible only with the light microscope). The microvasculature is particularly important because of its participation in the interchange between the circulatory system and surrounding tissues in both normal and inflammatory processes.

Capillaries

Capillaries that have structural variations permit different levels of metabolic exchange between blood and surrounding tissues.

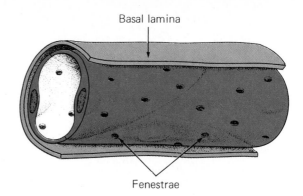

Figure 11–3. Diagram of the structure of a capillary with fenestrae in its wall; note that not all capillaries have perforated walls. The sectioned portion at left consists of 2 endothelial cells, and a basal lamina (lighter color) surrounds the capillary.

Capillaries are composed of a single layer of **endothelial cells** of mesenchymal origin rolled up in the form of a tube and enclosing a cylindrical space. The average diameter of capillaries is small, varying from 7 to 9 μm. Their length usually varies from 0.25 mm to 1 mm, the latter being characteristic of muscle tissue. In a few instances (eg, adrenal cortex, renal medulla), capillaries can be up to 50 mm long. The total length of capillaries in the human body has been estimated at 96,000 km (60,000 miles). When cut transversely, their walls are observed to consist of portions of one or more cells (Fig 11–3). The external surfaces of these cells usually rest on a basal lamina, a product of endothelial origin.

In general, endothelial cells are polygonal and about 10 × 30 μm when viewed face on; they are elongated in the direction of blood flow. The nucleus causes the cell to bulge into the capillary lumen. A small Golgi complex is present at the nuclear poles, a few mitochondria are evident, and free ribosomes as well as a few cisternae of rough endoplasmic reticulum are seen. Intermediate filaments (9–11 nm in diameter) are found in the perinuclear region. The presence of abundant microfilaments in endothelial cell cytoplasm is believed to be related to the proposed contractility of endothelial cells (Fig 11–4). The cell tapers toward the margins, where it may be 0.2 μm or less in thickness. Endothelial cells are held together by zonulae occludentes and an occasional desmosome. Gap junctions are also present. Junctions of the zonula occludens type are present between most endothelial cells and are of physiologic importance. Such junctions offer variable permeability to the macromolecules that play a significant role in both normal physiologic and pathologic conditions.

Junctions between endothelial cells of venules are the loosest. It is at this location that the char-

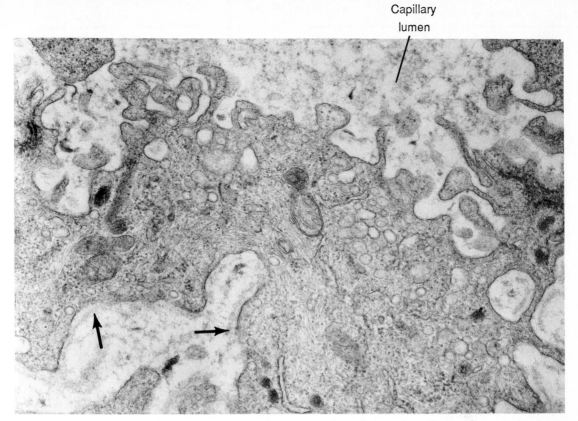

Figure 11–4. Electron micrograph of a section of a continuous capillary. Observe the ruffled appearance of its interior surface, the large and small pinocytotic vesicles, and numerous microfilaments in the cytoplasm. The arrows show the basal lamina. Reduced slightly from × 30,000.

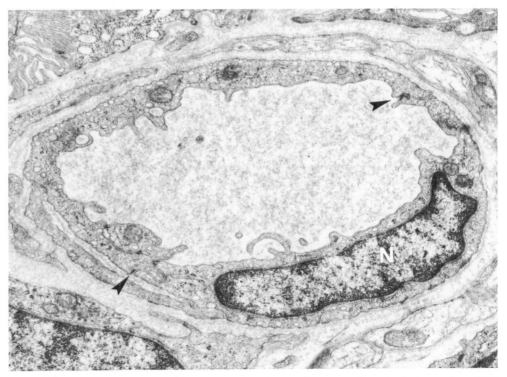

Figure 11–5. Electron micrograph of a transverse section of a continuous capillary. Note the nucleus (N) and the junctions between neighboring cells (arrowheads). Numerous pinocytotic vesicles are evident. × 10,000.

acteristic loss of fluid from the circulatory system occurs during the inflammatory response, leading to edema.

There are **pericytes** (from Greek, *peri,* around, + *kytos*), mesenchymal cells with long cytoplasmic processes that partly surround the endothelial cells, at various locations along capillaries and small venules. Enclosed in their own basal lamina, which may fuse with that of the endothelial cells, these perivascular cells have great potential for transformation into other cells. The presence of myosin, actin, and tropomyosin in pericytes strongly suggests that these cells also have a contractile function. Pericytes constitute the tunica media of these small vessels.

A thin layer of reticular fibers that encompasses capillaries and postcapillary venules is the equivalent of the adventitia of larger blood vessels.

Capillaries can be grouped into 4 types, depending on the structure of the endothelial cells and the presence or absence of a basal lamina.

(1) The **continuous,** or **somatic, capillary** (Fig 11–5) is characterized by the absence of fenestrae in its wall. This type of capillary is found in all kinds of muscle tissue, connective tissue, exocrine glands, and nervous tissue. Numerous pinocytotic vesicles, approximately 70 nm in greatest diameter, are present on both surfaces of muscle capillaries; they also appear as isolated vesicles in the cytoplasm of these cells. These vesicles are responsible for the transport of macromolecules in both directions across the endothelial cell. Few or no pinocytotic vesicles are encountered in the continuous capillaries supplying most parts of the nervous system. This feature, in part, accounts for the existence of the **blood-brain barrier** (see Chapter 9).

(2) Fenestrated, or **visceral, capillaries** are characterized by the presence of large fenestrae in the walls of endothelial cells. These fenestrae are 60–80 nm in diameter and are closed by a diaphragm that is thinner than a cell membrane (Figs 11–3 and 11–6) and does not have the trilaminar structure of a unit membrane (Fig 3–3). A continuous basal lamina is present. Fenestrated capillaries are encountered in tissues where rapid interchange of substances occurs between the tissues and the blood, as in the kidney, the intestine, and the endocrine glands. Macromolecules injected into the bloodstream can cross the capillary wall through these fenestrae to enter the tissue spaces. This seems to be as important a mechanism of transcapillary transport as is pinocytotic transport (see Chapter 4).

(3) The third type of capillary is again a fenestrated capillary, but in this case no diaphragms are present to close the openings (Fig 19–9). A very thick basal lamina separates this endothelium from the overlying epithelial cells (podocytes). This type of capillary is

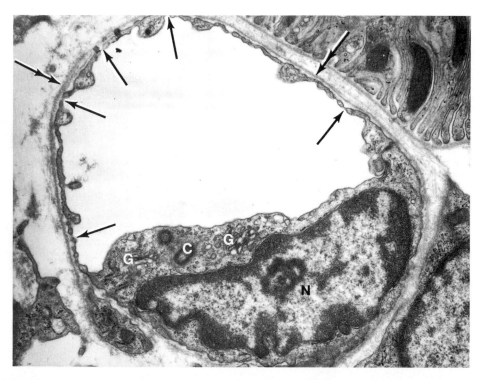

Figure 11–6. A fenestrated capillary in the kidney. Arrows indicate fenestrae closed by diaphragms. In this cell the Golgi complex (G), nucleus (N), and 2 centrioles (C) can be seen. Note the continuous basal lamina on the outer surface of the endothelial cell (double arrows). × 20,000. (Courtesy of J Rhodin.)

characteristic of the renal glomerulus (see Chapter 19).

(4) The fourth type of capillary, the **sinusoidal capillary** (Fig 14–14), has a torturous path and greatly enlarged diameter (30–40 μm), which slows the circulation of blood. There are multiple fenestrations (no diaphragms) in the endothelial cell wall (Figs 14–14 and 16–14). Macrophages are located either among or outside the cells of the endothelium. The basal lamina is often discontinuous. Sinusoidal capillaries are found mainly in the liver and in hematopoietic organs such as the bone marrow and spleen. The interchange between blood and tissues is thus greatly facilitated by the structure of the capillary wall.

As illustrated in Fig 11–7, capillaries anastomose freely, forming a rich network that interconnects the small arteries and veins. The arterioles branch into small vessels surrounded by a discontinuous layer of smooth muscle, the **metarterioles.** These branch into capillaries that form a network with a high surface area to facilitate the exchange of materials between the tissues and blood. Constriction of metarterioles helps to regulate but does not completely stop the circulation in capillaries, and it maintains pressure differences in the arterial and venous systems. There is a simple ring of smooth muscle cells, or sphincter, at the point where capillaries originate from the metarteriole. This **precapillary sphincter** can completely stop the blood flow within the capillary. The entire network does not always function simultaneously, and the number of functional and open capillaries depends not only on the state of contraction of the metarterioles but also on arteriovenous anastomoses that enable the arterioles to empty directly into venules, as illustrated in Fig 11–7. These interconnections are abundant in skeletal muscle and the skin of the hands and feet. When vessels of the arteriovenous anastomosis contract, all the blood must pass through the capillary network. When they relax, some blood flows directly to a vein instead of circulating in the capillaries. Capillary circulation is controlled by neural and hormonal stimulation.

The richness of the capillary network is related to the metabolic activity of the tissues and represents a transition zone between the high-pressure system (arterial) and low-pressure system (venous). Tissues with high metabolic rates, such as the kidney, liver, and cardiac and skeletal muscle, have an abundant capillary network; the opposite is true of tissues with low metabolic rates, such as smooth muscle and dense connective tissue.

An idea of the importance of the capillaries can be gained by noting that in the human body the surface area of the capillary network approaches 6000 m^2. Its total diameter is approximately 800 times larger than the aorta. A unit volume of fluid within a capillary is exposed to a larger surface area than is the same volume in the other parts of the system. The flow of

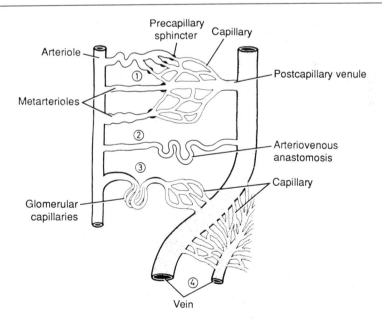

Figure 11–7. Types of microcirculation formed by small blood vessels. The usual sequence of arteriole→metarteriole→ capillary→venule and vein is shown at (1). An arteriovenous anastomosis is shown at (2), and an arterial portal system as is present in the kidney glomerulus is shown at (3). A venous portal system such as occurs in the liver is shown at (4). (Reproduced, with permission, from Krstić RV: *Illustrated Encyclopedia of Human Histology.* Springer-Verlag, 1984.)

blood in the aorta averages 320 mm/s; in the capillaries, about 0.3 mm/s. The capillary system can thus be compared with a lake where a full-flowing river enters and leaves; because of their thin walls and slow blood flow, the capillaries are a favorable place for the exchange of water, solutes, and macromolecules between blood and tissues.

Functions of capillaries. Capillaries perform at least 3 important functions. They serve as a selective permeability barrier, a synthetic and metabolic system, and a nonthrombogenic container for blood.

1. Permeability—Capillaries (and postcapillary venules) are often referred to as **exchange vessels,** since it is at these sites that oxygen, carbon dioxide, substrates, and metabolites are transferred from blood to the tissues and from the tissues to blood. Permeability of capillary walls varies with the size and charge of the permeating molecules and with the structure of the endothelial cell. The mechanism by which the interchange of materials between blood and tissue occurs is not clear. Researchers have postulated the existence of 2 sizes of pores in capillary walls. The smaller pores are thought to have a diameter of 9–11 nm and the larger pores a diameter of 50–70 nm. Three possible morphologic equivalents of these physiologic pores are intercellular junctions and clefts between neighboring endothelial cells, fenestral diaphragms in fenestrated capillaries, and large numbers of pinocytotic vesicles that are thought to cross the endothelial cells of most capillaries.

It is generally agreed that small hydrophobic and hydrophilic molecules (eg, oxygen, carbon dioxide, glucose) can diffuse or be actively transported across the plasmalemma of capillary endothelial cells. These substances are then transported by diffusion to the opposite cell surface where they are discharged into the extracellular space. Water and some other hydrophilic molecules, less than 1.5 nm in diameter and below 10,000 in molecular weight, can cross the capillary wall by diffusing through the intercellular junctions (paracellular pathway). The **intercellular junction** is now believed to be the morphologic counterpart of the **small pore** postulated by physiologic studies. The **large pore** of the physiologist is almost certainly represented morphologically by the **fenestrae** or **pinocytotic vesicles** of endothelial cells.

Abnormal states, such as inflammation induced by bacteria, chemical substances, and poisons (eg, snake or bee venom), apparently alter the permeability of the junctions between endothelial cells. Capillary and postcapillary venular permeability is greatly increased, and electron-dense colloidal substances can be observed to pass from capillary and small venule lumens into surrounding tissues by traversing the endothelial cell junctions. Leukocytes leave the bloodstream by passing between endothelial cells and entering the tissue spaces by a process called **diapedesis.** Opening of these junctions seems to be mediated by locally liberated pharmacologically active substances, such as **histamine** and **bradykinin,** that increase vascular permeability and can also play a conspicuous role in inflammation.

The observation that some drugs, given intravenously, do not reach the brain, although such penetration occurs in almost all other tissues of the body, gave rise to the concept of the **blood-brain barrier.** This phenomenon was initially studied by intravenous administration of dyes that readily escape from capillaries to surrounding tissues. Careful study of brain capillaries showed that not only do they have few pinocytotic vesicles and lack fenestrae, but that occluding junctions between their endothelial cells do not permit the passage of macromolecules used as tracers. These properties would appear to explain the barrier. Other blood-tissue barriers of physiologic and pathologic importance are the blood-ocular barrier, blood-thymus barrier, blood-nerve barrier, and blood-testicular-semiferous-tubule barrier.

2. Metabolic functions—Capillary endothelial cells can metabolize a wide variety of substrates. Although lung capillaries have been the most intensively studied, the results presented here are not restricted to pulmonary capillaries.

a. Activation—Conversion of angiotensin (from Greek, *angeion,* vessel, + *tendere,* to stretch) I to angiotensin II (see Chapter 19).

b. Inactivation—Conversion of bradykinin, serotonin, prostaglandins, norepinephrine, thrombin, etc, to biologically inert compounds.

c. Lipolysis—Breakdown of lipoproteins to yield triglycerides (energy) and cholesterol (substrates for steroid-hormone synthesis and membrane structure).

3. Antithrombogenic function—When endothelial cells desquamate, the uncovered subendothelial connective tissue induces the aggregation of blood platelets. Subsequent fibrin coagulation forms solid masses called **thrombi** that can grow and obstruct vascular flow, a potentially life-threatening condition. Endothelial cells, when present, prevent contact of platelets with the subendothelial connective tissue, exerting an antithrombogenic effect (see Chapter 12).

Arteries

These structures transport blood to tissues. They resist changes in blood pressure in their initial portions and regulate blood flow in their terminal portions.

Arteries are classified according to their size into arterioles, muscular arteries of medium or large diameter, and large, elastic arteries. In general, the walls of arteries are thicker than the walls of veins of the same overall diameter (Fig 11–8).

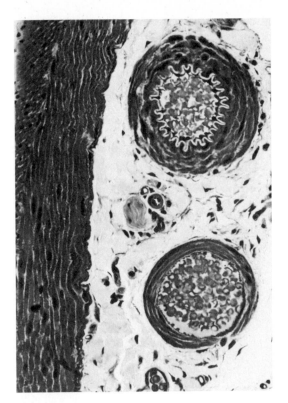

Figure 11–8. Photomicrographs of sections of a small muscular artery **(top)** and a venule **(bottom).**

A. Arterioles: These are generally less than 0.5 mm in diameter and have relatively narrow lumens. The lumen is lined by endothelial cells similar to those of continuous capillaries.

An important difference is the presence of rod-shaped granules, about 3 μm long but only 0.1 μm wide. These are the **Weibel-Palade granules** found only in endothelial cells of vessels larger than capillaries. These granules contain a protein of the blood coagulation mechanism known as van Willebrand's factor (factor VIII). Deficiency of this group of proteins results in impaired platelet adhesion to injured endothelium and in prolonged bleeding. It is among the causes of **hemophilia.**

The subendothelial layer is very thin, and an internal elastic lamina is lacking except in the largest arterioles. The media is muscular and generally composed of 1–5 circularly arranged layers of smooth muscle cells. The adventitia is thin and shows no external elastic lamina (Fig 11–8).

B. Muscular Arteries: Most of the named arteries in the human body are **muscular arteries** (Figs 11–2, 11–8, 11–9, and 11–10). The intima is similar to that described for arterioles except that the subendothelial layer is somewhat thicker and a few smooth muscle cells may be present. An internal elastic lamina is prominent (Figs 11–9 and 11–10). The media may contain up to 40 layers of smooth muscle cells, although the number of layers diminishes as the artery becomes smaller. These cells are intermingled with variable numbers of elastic lamellae (depending on the size of the vessel) as well as reticular fibers and proteoglycans. An external elastic lamina is present

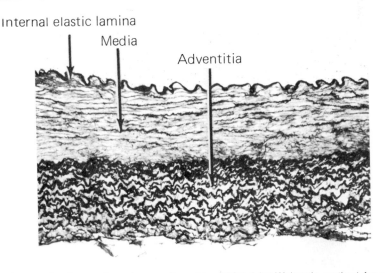

Internal elastic lamina

Media

Adventitia

Figure 11–9. Photomicrograph of a section of muscular artery stained by Weigert's method for elastic structures. × 110.

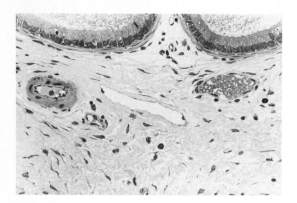

Figure 11–10. Photomicrograph of a small venule **(right)** and a small arteriole **(left)**. Walls of the arteries are thicker than those of the veins.. A lymphatic vessel is present between the arteriole and venule. Note the capillary next to the small arteriole and the field of loose connective tissue that surrounds the vessels.

in larger muscular arteries. The adventitia consists of collagen and elastic fibers, a few fibroblasts, and adipose cells. Lymphatics, vasa vasorum, and nerves are also found in the adventitia, and these structures may penetrate to the outer part of the media.

C. Large Elastic Arteries: These include the aorta and its large branches. They have a yellowish color from the accumulation of elastin in the media. This type of artery has the following characteristics:

The intima is thicker than the corresponding tunic of a muscular artery. The subendothelial layer is thick. The connective tissue fibers of the subendothelial layer display a longitudinal orientation and play an important role in the distortion of the endothelial layer of cells during rhythmic contractions and dilations of the vessel. An internal elastic lamina, although present, may not be easily evident, since it is similar to the elastic laminae of the next layer.

The media consists of a series of concentrically arranged perforated elastic laminae whose number increases with age (there are 40 in the newborn, 70 in the adult). Once formed, elastic structures usually become metabolically inert (shown by radioautographic studies), especially in older animals. These laminae become progressively thicker because of the deposit of elastin. Between the elastic laminae are smooth muscle cells, reticular fibers, and ground substance consisting mainly of chondroitin sulfate.

The tunica adventitia, which does not show an external limiting lamina, is relatively underdeveloped and contains elastic and collagen fibers.

D. Histophysiology of Arteries: The large arteries are called **conducting arteries,** since their major function is to transport blood away from the heart.

These arteries also serve to smooth out the large fluctuations in pressure created by the heartbeat. During ventricular contraction **(systole),** the elastic laminae of conducting arteries are stretched and reduce the pressure change. During ventricular relaxation **(diastole),** ventricular pressure drops to a low level, but the elastic rebound of conducting arteries helps maintain arterial pressure. As a consequence, arterial pressure and blood flow decrease and become less variable as the distance from the heart increases (Fig 11–11).

The function of medium-sized arteries, also known as **distributing arteries,** is to furnish blood to the various organs. The muscular layer in distributing arteries can control the flow of blood to various organs by contracting or not contracting (as a result of local chemical or more generalized neural input).

Blood vessels undergo progressive and gradual changes from birth to death, and it is difficult to say where the normal growth processes end and the processes or involution begin. Each artery exhibits its own aging pattern. The coronary artery is the one that changes most precociously, beginning at about 20 years of age. Other arteries begin to be modified only after age 40. When the media of an artery is weakened by an embryonic defect, disease, or lesion, the wall of the artery gives way, dilating extensively. As this process progresses, it becomes an **aneurysm** and can result in rupture of the wall. The importance of type III collagen in arterial structure is illustrated by the observation that in Ehlers-Danlos syndrome (a genetic deficiency of the synthesis of type III collagen), the main cause of death is spontaneous aortic rupture.

Atherosclerotic lesions are characterized by focal thickening of the intima, proliferation of smooth muscle cells and extracellular connective tissue elements, and the deposit of cholesterol in smooth muscle cells and macrophages. When heavily loaded with lipid, these cells are referred to as **foam cells** and form the macroscopically visible fatty streaks and plaques that characterize **atherosclerosis** (from Greek, *athere,* gruel, + *skleros,* hard). These changes may extend to the inner part of the tunica media, and the thickening may become so great as to occlude the vessel. Coronary arteries are among those most prone to atherosclerosis. It should be noted that uniform thickening of the intima is believed to be a normal phenomenon of aging.

Certain arteries irrigate only definite areas of specific organs, and obstruction results in **necrosis** (death of the tissues from a lack of metabolites). These are **infarcts** that occur commonly in the heart, kidneys, cerebrum, and certain other organs. In other regions, such as the skin, arteries anastomose frequently, and the obstruc-

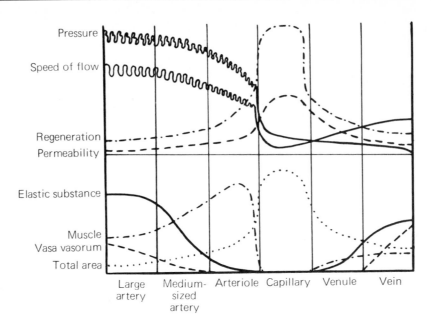

Figure 11–11. Graph showing the relationship between the characteristics of blood circulation and the structure of the blood vessels. The arterial blood pressure and rapidity of flow decrease and become more constant as distance from the heart increases. This coincides with a reduction in the number of elastic fibers and an increase in the number of smooth muscle cells in the arteries. The graphs illustrate the gradual changes in vessel structure and their biophysical properties. Regenerative capacity and permeability are higly developed in the capillaries. (Reproduced, with permission, from Cowdry EV: *Textbook of Histology.* Lea & Febiger, 1944.)

tion of one artery does not lead to tissue necrosis, because blood flow is maintained.

The polypeptide **angiotensin** contributes to the regulation of blood pressure by binding initially to vascular endothelial cells. This endothelial stimulus is later transmitted to arterial smooth muscle cells, stimulating their contraction and thus causing an increase in blood pressure. Morphologic studies have revealed that endothelial cells exhibit processes that extend across the internal elastic lamina and contact the smooth muscle cells.

Carotid-Bodies

Small structures encountered near the bifurcation of the common carotid artery act as chemoreceptors sensitive to low oxygen tension, high carbon dioxide concentration, and low arterial blood pH. Carotid bodies consist of glomus cells (type I cells) and sheath cells (type II cells) surrounded by a rich vascular supply whose capillaries are of the fenestrated type. Most of the nerves of the carotid body (95% in the rat) are afferent fibers. The glomus cells contain numerous dense-core vesicles that store dopamine, norepinephrine, and serotonin. It remains controversial whether the glomus cell or the afferent nerve endings are the principal chemoreceptor elements. Aortic bodies and jugular glomera are similar in structure to the

carotid body and are thought to have a similar function.

Arteriovenous Anastomoses

Direct communication between arterial and venous circulation is often observed. These arteriovenous anastomoses are distributed through the body and generally occur in small vessels. The luminal diameters of anastomotic vessels vary with the physiologic condition of the organ. Changes in diameter serve to regulate blood pressure, flow, and temperature and the conservation of heat in particular areas (Fig 11–7). By injecting microspheres of a size that will obliterate the capillaries, it is possible to calculate that about one-third of the blood flow in the ear of a rabbit can pass through arteriovenous anastomoses. In addition to these direct communications, there are more complex structures, **glomera**—mainly in fingerpads, fingernail beds, and ears. In these structures, the arterioles that are continuous with venules lose their internal elastic membranes and acquire a thick layer of concentrically arranged smooth muscle cells. This muscle layer forms a sheath that partly or completely surrounds the lumen of a vessel. Contraction of this layer can promote the complete or partial transitory closure of blood vessels. The glomera have an important role in controlling the circulation in various organs. They also participate in such physiologic phenomena as menstruation, erection, thermoregulation, and the regulation of blood pressure. The arteriovenous anastomoses are richly innervated by the sympathetic and parasympathetic nervous systems. Control of this activity appears to be mainly neural.

Veins

These structures return blood to the heart, aided by the action of smooth muscle and specialized valves.

When considered as a functional unit, all the veins can be classified as capacitance vessels because more than 70% of the total blood volume is in this portion of the cardiovascular system at any one time. As with arteries, it is customary to arbitrarily classify the veins into venules and veins of small, medium, and large size.

Venules are small, with a diameter of 0.2–1 mm. They are characterized by an intima composed of endothelium, a thin media that may consist of from none to a few cell layers of smooth muscle, and an adventitial layer. This last is the thickest layer and is composed of connective tissue rich in collagenous fibers. Venules have thin walls (Fig 11–10) when compared with an artery of comparable overall diameter. Venules with luminal diameters up to 50 μm have the structure and other biologic features of capillaries, eg, participation in inflammatory processes

and interchange of metabolites between blood and tissues.

With the exception of the main trunks, most veins are **small** or **medium-sized veins,** with a diameter of 1–9 mm. The intima usually has a thin subendothelial layer, but this may at times be absent. The media consists of small bundles of smooth muscle cells intermixed with reticular fibers and a delicate network of elastic fibers. The collagenous adventitial layer is well developed (Fig 11–12).

Large veins have a well-developed tunica intima. The media is much thinner, with few layers of smooth muscle cells and abundant connective tissue. The adventitial layer is the thickest and best developed tunic in veins. Cardiac muscle is present in the adventitia of the venae cavae and pulmonary veins for a short distance before they empty into the heart. In large, unsupported abdominal veins (eg, mesenteric vein) or in other large veins that lie below the level of the heart, the adventitia frequently contains longitudinal bundles of smooth muscle (Fig 11–13). This adventitial muscle serves to strengthen the wall and prevent distention of the vessel. The circular and longitudinal arrangement of smooth muscle in these vessels may oppose the action of gravity by providing a peristaltic pumping of the blood up to the heart. Unlike arteries, small or medium-sized veins have valves in their interior. These structures consist of 2 semilunar folds of

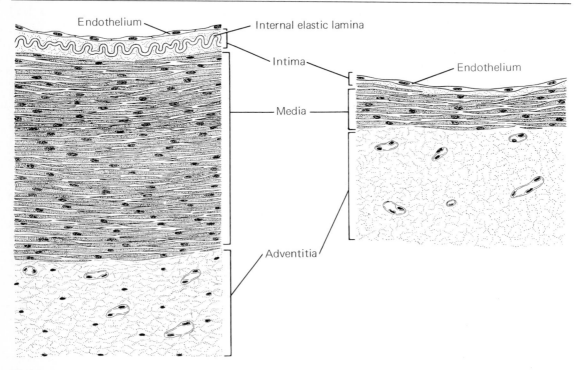

Figure 11–12. Diagram comparing the structure of a muscular artery **(left)** and accompanying vein **(right).** Note that the tunica intima and tunica media are highly developed in the artery but not in the vein.

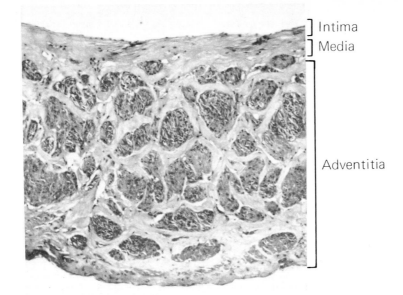

] Intima
] Media

Adventitia

Figure 11–13. Photomicrograph of a section of a larger vein. Observe the well-developed adventitia with characteristic longitudinal smooth muscle bundles. H&E stain, × 100.

the tunica intima that project into the lumen. They are composed of elastic connective tissue and are lined on both sides by endothelium. The valves, which are especially numerous in veins of the limbs, direct the venous blood toward the heart. The propulsive force of the heart is reinforced by contraction of skeletal muscles that surround these veins.

Heart

The heart is a muscular organ that contracts rhythmically, pumping the blood through the circulatory system. It is also responsible for producing a hormone called **atrial natriuretic factor.** Its walls consist of 3 tunics: the internal, or **endocardium;** the middle, or **myocardium;** and the external, or **pericardium** (from Greek, *peri* + *kardia,* heart). The heart's fibrous central region, the **fibrous skeleton,** serves as the base of the valves as well as the site of origin and insertion of the cardiac muscle cells.

A. Tunics: The **endocardium** is homologous with the intima of blood vessels. It consists of a single layer of squamous endothelial cells resting on a thin subendothelial layer of loose connective tissue containing elastic and collagen fibers as well as some smooth muscle cells. Between the endocardium and the myocardium is a layer of connective tissue (often termed the **subendocardial layer**), which consists of veins, nerves, and branches of the impulse-conducting system of the heart (Purkinje cells).

The **myocardium** is the thickest of the tunics of the heart and consists of cardiac muscle cells (see Chapter 10) arranged in layers that surround the heart

chambers in a complex spiral manner. A large number of these layers insert themselves into the fibrous cardiac skeleton. The arrangement of these muscle cells is extremely varied, so that in histologic preparations of a small area, cells are seen oriented in many directions. The muscle cells of the heart are grouped into 2 populations: contractile cells and the impulse-generating and conducting cells that generate and conduct the electrical signal initiating the heartbeat.

The **epicardium** is the serous covering of the heart, forming the visceral layer of the pericardium. Externally, it is covered by simple squamous epithelium (mesothelium) supported by a thin layer of connective tissue. A subepicardial layer of loose connective tissue contains veins, nerves, and nerve ganglia. The adipose tissue that generally surrounds the heart accumulates in this layer.

B. Fibrous Skeleton: The fibrous skeleton of the heart is composed of dense connective tissue. Its principal components are the **septum membranaceum, the trigona fibrosa,** and the **annuli fibrosi.** These structures consist of a dense connective tissue, with thick collagen fibers oriented in various directions. Certain regions contain nodules of fibrous cartilage.

C. Valves: The cardiac valves consist of a central core of dense fibrous connective tissue (containing both collagen and elastic fibers), lined on both sides by endothelial layers. The bases of the valves are attached to the annuli fibrosi of the fibrous skeleton.

D. Structures that Control Heartbeat: The impulse-generating and conducting system of the heart consists of several structures that make it possible for the atria and ventricles to beat in succession and thus permit the heart to function as an efficient pump. The **sinoatrial node** is the pacemaker of the heart, in that it has the most rapid rhythmic activity (Fig 11–14). It is located close to the entrance of the superior vena cava into the right atrium. The nodal cells are modified cardiac muscle cells, smaller than atrial muscle cells and with fewer myofibrils. Nodal cells are concentrically arranged around a large nodal artery. Internodal tracts of specialized cells conduct the electrical depolarization of the sinoatrial node to the **atrioventricular node.** This mass of specialized cardiac muscle cells lies beneath the endocardium of the septal wall of the right atrium. The nodal cells are similar to those of the sinoatrial node. In addition, there are large arterioles present as well as considerable amounts of adipose tissue.

The **atrioventricular bundle of His** is formed by **Purkinje cells** (Fig 11–15) that penetrate the fibrous skeleton and then divide to form the **right** and **left bundle branches.** The left bundle again divides to form 2 fascicles. These bundles of Purkinje cells travel in the subendocardial layer to the apex of the heart, where they reverse their direction and begin giving off side branches that make contact with ordinary (working) cardiac muscle cells via gap junctions. This arrangement allows the stimulus for ventricular contraction to be rapidly conducted to the apex of the heart, which must contract first to eject blood from the ventricles. The wave of contraction then sweeps toward the base of the heart (pulmonary valve and aortic valve). Purkinje cells have a diameter considerably greater than that of ordinary cardiac muscle cells.

Both the parasympathetic and sympathetic divisions of the autonomic system contribute to innervation of the heart and form widespread plexuses at the base of the heart. Ganglionic nerve cells and nerve fibers are present in the regions close to the sinoatrial and atrioventricular nodes. Although these nerves do not affect generation of the heartbeat, a process attributed to the sinoatrial (pacemaker) node, they do

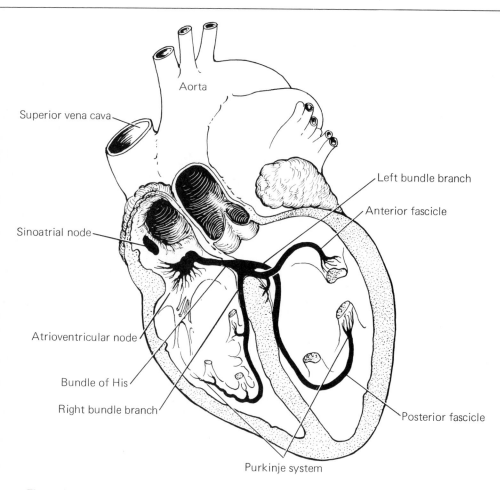

Figure 11–14. Diagram of the heart, showing the impulse-generating and conducting system.

Connective tissue

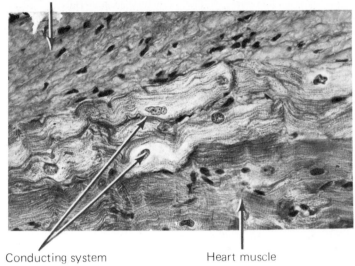

Conducting system   Heart muscle

Figure 11–15. The Purkinje cells of the conducting system of the heart are characterized by a reduced number of myofibrils present mainly in the periphery of the muscle cell. Purkinje cells are held together by intercalated disks. The light area around the nuclei of the conducting cells is caused by local accumulation of glycogen. H&E stain, × 400.

affect heart rhythm. Stimulation of the parasympathetic division (vagus nerve) promotes a slowing of the heartbeat, while stimulation of the sympathetic nerve accelerates the rhythm of the pacemaker.

Lymphatic Vascular System

The human body has, in addition to blood vessels, a system of endothelium-lined thin-walled channels that collect fluid from the tissue spaces and return to the blood. This fluid is called lymph; unlike the blood, it circulates in only one direction—toward the heart.

The **lymphatic capillaries** originate in the various tissues as thin, blind-ended vessels that consist of a single layer of endothelium. Lymphatic capillaries have no fenestrations in their endothelial cells or a

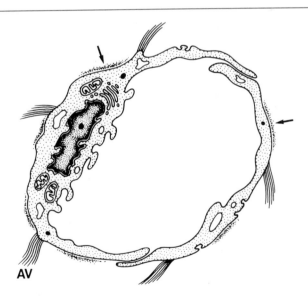

Figure 11–16. Structure of a lymphatic capillary at the electron microscope level. Note the overlapping free borders of endothelial cells, the discontinuous basal lamina (arrows), and the attachment of anchoring fibrils. (Courtesy of J James.)

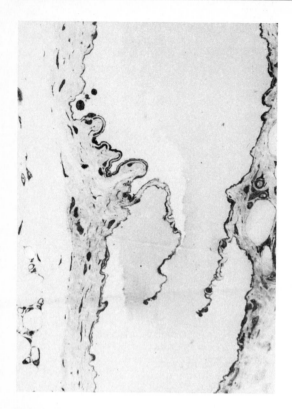

Figure 11–17. Longitudinal section of a lymphatic vessel. Note the prominent internal valve assuring unidirectional flow of lymph.

zonula occludens between neighboring cells, and they have almost no basal lamina.

These capillaries are held open by numerous microfibrils of the elastic fiber system (see Fig 5–13), which also bind them firmly to the surrounding connective tissue (Fig 11–16). Lymphatic capillaries absorb some of the electrolytes and proteins that continuously leave the blood capillaries. Contraction of their endothelial cells permits large amounts of tissue fluid to enter the lymphatic system.

The thin lymphatic vessels ultimately converge and end up as 2 large trunks, the **thoracic duct** and the **right lymphatic duct,** which empty into the junction of the left internal jugular vein with the left subclavian vein and into the confluence of the right subclavian vein and the right internal jugular vein. Interposed in the path of the lymphatic vessels are lymph nodes, whose morphology and functions are discussed in Chapter 14. With rare exceptions such as the nervous system and the bone marrow, a lymphatic system is found in almost all organs.

The larger lymphatic vessels have a structure similar to that of veins except they have thinner walls and lack a clear-cut separation between the 3 layers (intima, media, and adventitia). Like veins, they have

numerous internal valves (which are more numerous in lymphatic vessels). The lymphatic vessels are dilated and assume a nodular, or beaded, appearance between the valves.

As in veins, lymphatic circulation is aided by the action of external forces (eg, contraction of surrounding skeletal muscle) on their walls. These forces act discontinuously, and unidirectional lymph flow occurs mainly as a result of the presence of many valves in these vessels (Fig 11–17). Contraction of smooth muscle in the walls of larger lymphatic vessels also helps propel lymph toward the heart.

The large-sized **lymphatic ducts** (thoracic duct and right lymphatic duct) have a structure similar to that of a vein, with a reinforcement of smooth muscle in the middle layer. In this layer, the muscle bundles are longitudinally and circularly arranged, with longitudinal fibers predominating (Fig 11–18). The adventitia is relatively underdeveloped. As with arteries and veins, large lymphatic ducts contain vasa vasorum and a rich neural network.

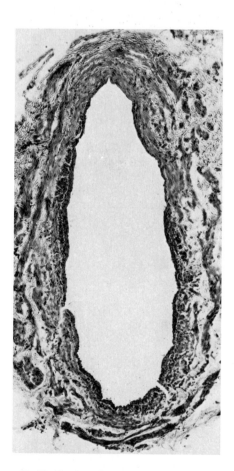

Figure 11–18. Section of the thoracic duct. H&E stain, × 200. (Reproduced, with permission, from Junqueira LC, Carneiro J: *Histologie,* Schiebler TH, Peiper U [translators]. Springer-Verlag, 1984.)

Tumors of Blood Vessels

Most malignant tumors of blood vessels derive from endothelial cells (**angiosarcomas** [*angeion + sarkos + oma*]) or from pericytes (**hemangiopericytomas** [from Greek, *haima*, blood, + *angeion + peri + kytos + oma*]). The presence of factor VII, localized by immunohistochemistry, is characteristic of endothelial-cell-derived tumors; tumors arising from pericytes do not contain this protein.

REFERENCES

Challice CE, Viragh S (editors): *Ultrastructure of the Mammalian Heart*. Academic Press, 1973.

Cliff WJ: *Blood Vessels*. Cambridge Univ Press, 1976.

Johnson PC: *Peripheral Circulation*. Wiley, 1978.

Joyce NE et al: Contractile proteins in pericytes. *J Cell Biol* 1985;**100**:1387.

Leak LV: Normal anatomy of the lymphatic vascular system. In: *Handbuch der Allgemeine Pathologie*. Meessen H (editor). Springer-Verlag, 1972.

Rhodin JAG: Architecture of the vessel wall. In: *Handbook of Physiology*. Section 2: Cardiovascular System. Vol 2. American Physiological Society, 1980.

Richardson JB, Beaulines A: The cellular site of action of angiotensin. *J. Cell Biol* 1971;**51**:419.

Simionescu N: Cellular aspects of transcapillary exchange. *Physiol Rev* 1983;**63**:1536.

Thorgeirsson G, Robertson AL Jr: The vascular endothelium: Pathobiologic significance. *Am J Pathol* 1978; **93**:802.

Wagner D, Marder J: Biosynthesis of von Willebrand protein by human endothelial cells: Processing steps and their intracellular localization. *J Cell Biol* 1984;**99**:2123.

Blood consists of the cells and fluid (about 5.5 L in an adult human male) within the closed circulatory system that flow in a regular unidirectional movement, propelled mainly by the rhythmic contractions of the heart. It is made up of 2 parts: **formed elements,** or blood cells, and **plasma** (Greek, *plasma*), the liquid in which the former are suspended. The formed elements are **erythrocytes,** or red blood cells; **platelets;** and **leukocytes,** or white blood cells.

If blood is removed from the circulatory system, it will clot. This clot contains formed elements and a clear yellow liquid called **serum,** which separates from the coagulum.

Blood collected and kept from coagulating by the addition of anticoagulants (heparin, citrate, etc) separates, when centrifuged, into layers that reflect its heterogeneity (Fig 12–1). The **hematocrit** is an estimation of the volume of packed erythrocytes per unit volume of blood. The normal value is 40–50% in the adult male. In the adult female, it is 35–45% and diminishes by physiologic hemodilution during pregnancy. The value is approximately 35% in a child up to age 10 years and 45–60% in the newborn. The hematocrit is normally higher in venous blood than in arterial blood because of the hydration of red cells and their increase in size.

The translucent, yellowish, and somewhat viscous supernatant obtained when whole blood is centrifuged is the plasma of the blood. The formed elements of the blood separate into 2 easily distinguishable layers. The lower layer represents 42–47% of the entire volume of blood present in the hematocrit tube. It is red and is made up of erythrocytes. The layer immediately above (1% of the blood volume), which is white or grayish in color, is called the **buffy coat** and consists of leukocytes. This separation occurs because the leukocytes are less dense than the erythrocytes. Covering the leukocytes is a fine layer of platelets not distinguishable by the naked eye.

Leukocytes, which have diversified functions (Table 12–1), constitute one of the body's chief defenses against infection. They circulate through the body via the blood vascular system. Crossing the capillary wall, these cells become concentrated rapidly in the tissues, where they display their defensive capabilities. The blood vascular system is a distributing vehicle. It transports oxygen (O_2; see Fig 12–2) and

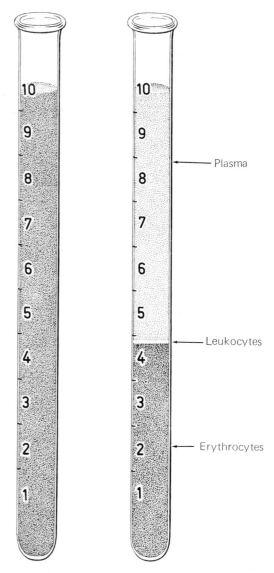

Figure 12–1. Hematocrit tubes with blood. **Left:** Before centifugation. **Right:** After centrifugation. The red blood cells represent 43% of the blood volume in the centrifuged tube. Between the sedimented red blood cells and the supernatant light-colored plasma is a thin layer of leukocytes; this layer is called the buffy coat.

Table 12-1. Products and Functions of the Blood Cells.

Cell Type	Main Products	Main Functions
Erythrocytes	Hemoglobin.	CO_2 and O_2 transport.
Neutrophils (terminal cells)	Specific granules and modified lysosomes (azurophilic granules).	Phagocytosis of bacteria.
Eosinophils (terminal cells)	Specific granules, pharmacologically active substances.	Defense against parasitic helminths. Modulation of inflammatory processes.
Basophils (terminal cells)	Specific granules containing histamine and heparin.	Release of histamine and other inflammation mediators.
Monocytes (not terminal cells)	Granules with lysosomal enzymes.	Generation of mononuclear-phagocyte system cells in tissues. Phagocytosis and digestion of protozoa and virus and senescent cells.
B Lymphocytes	Immunoglobulins.	Generation of antibody-producing terminal cells (plasmocytes).
T Lymphocytes	Substances that kill cells. Substances that control the activity of other leucocytes (interleukins).	Killing of virus-infected cells.
Natural killer cells (cytotoxic T cell)	Substances that promote perforations in the cell membrane of target cells (thereby killing them).	Killing of some tumor and virus-infected cells.
Platelets	Blood-clotting factors.	Clotting of blood.

carbon dioxide (CO_2) among other substances. O_2 is bound mainly to the hemoglobin of the erythrocytes, while CO_2, in addition to being bound to the proteins of the erythrocytes (mainly hemoglobin), is also carried in solution in the plasma as CO_2 or in the form of HCO_3^-.

The plasma transports nutrients from their site of absorption or synthesis, distributing them to different areas of the organism. It also transports *metabolic residues*, which are removed from the blood by the excretory organs. Blood, as the distributing vehicle for the hormones, permits the exchange of chemical messages between distant organs for normal cellular func-

tion. It further participates in the regulation of body temperature and in acid-base and osmotic balance.

Composition of Plasma

Plasma is an aqueous solution containing substances of small or large molecular weight that make up 10% of its volume. The plasma proteins account for 7% of the volume and the inorganic salts for 0.9%; the remainder of the 10% consists of several organic compounds—amino acids, vitamins, hormones, lipoproteins, etc—of differing origins.

Through the capillary walls, the low-molecular-weight components of plasma are in equilibrium with the interstitial fluid of the tissues. The composition of plasma is usually an indicator of the mean composition of the extracellular fluids in general.

The main plasma proteins are **albumin; alpha, beta,** and **gamma globulins;** and **fibrinogen.** Albumin is the main component and has a fundamental role in maintaining the osmotic pressure of the blood. The gamma globulins are antibodies and are called **immunoglobulins.** Fibrinogen is necessary for the formation of fibrin in the final step of coagulation.

Several substances that are insoluble or only slightly soluble in water can be transported by the plasma because they combine with albumin or with the alpha and beta globulins. For example, lipids are insoluble in the plasma but combine with the hydrophobic portions of protein molecules. Since the protein molecules also have hydrophilic parts, the lipid-protein complex is soluble in water.

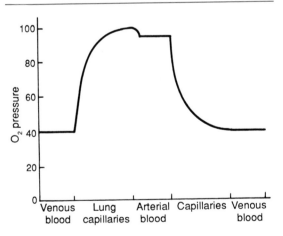

Figure 12-2. Blood oxygen content in each type of blood vessel. The amount of oxygen (O_2 pressure) is highest in arteries and lung capillaries; it decreases in tissue capillaries, where exchange takes place between blood and tissues.

Staining of Blood Cells

Blood cells are generally studied in smears or films prepared by spreading a drop of blood in a thin layer on a microscope slide (Fig 12-3). The blood should

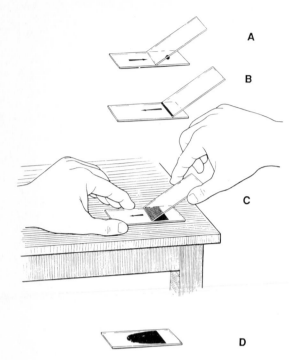

Figure 12–3. Preparation of a blood smear. **A:** A drop of blood is placed on a microscope slide. A second slide is moved over the first at an angle of 45 degrees. **B:** When the slide's edge touches the blood drop, the blood spreads along the edge. **C:** With a uniform movement of the oblique slide, a thin film of blood is spread on the horizontal slide. **D:** After air drying, slides are fixed and stained.

be evenly distributed over the slide and allowed to dry rapidly in air. In such films the cells are clearly visible and distinct from one another. Their cytoplasm is spread out, facilitating observation of their nuclei and cytoplasmic organization.

Blood smears are routinely stained with special dye mixtures first discovered by Dimitri Romanovsky and modified by other investigators. In 1891, Romanovsky observed that a mixture of solutions of methylene blue and eosin in certain proportions stained the nuclei of leukocytes and malarial parasites purple. Other components of the cell may stain pink from eosin binding or shades of red-blue resulting from the binding of **azures.** Azures are oxidation products of methylene blue and, like it, are positively charged. Positively charged dyes are known as *basic dyes.* Eosin is a negatively charged dye and is therefore called an *acidic dye.* Some information about the net charge of cellular constituents can thus be obtained by observing their affinity for acidic or basic dyes.

Stains currently used to study blood cells differ slightly in the proportions of their components and in the way methylene blue is oxidized. Each is named for the investigator who first introduced the particular modification. Leishman's, Wrights, and Giemsa's stains are examples of modified stains collectively known as Romanovsky-type mixtures.

FORMED ELEMENTS OF BLOOD

Erythrocytes

Red blood cells, which are anucleate, are packed with the oxygen-carrying protein, hemoglobin. Under normal conditions, these cells never leave the circulatory system.

Most mammalian erythrocytes (red blood cells) are described as biconcave disks without nuclei (Fig 12–4). When suspended in an isotonic medium, human erythrocytes are 7.5 μm in diameter, 2.6 μm thick at the rim, and 0.8 μm thick in the center. However, when dried and stained to make a routine blood film, they shrink to 7.2–7.4 μm in diameter and 1.9 μm in thickness at the rim (Fig 12–5). The biconcave shape provides erythrocytes with a large surface-to-volume ratio, thus facilitating gas exchange.

The normal concentration of erythrocytes in blood is approximately 3.9–5.5 million/μL in women and 4.1–6 million/μL in men (Table 12–2).

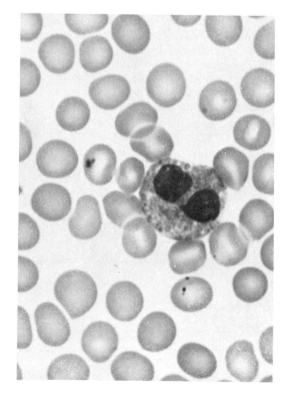

Figure 12–4. Photomicrograph of a Leishman-stained human blood smear, showing numerous erythrocytes and one granulocyte (eosinophil). × 1300.

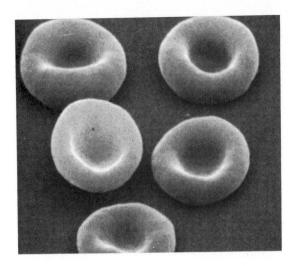

Figure 12–5. Scanning electron micrograph of normal human erythrocytes. Note their biconcave shape. Reproduced from × 6500.

A decreased concentration of red cells in the blood is usually associated with **anemia.** An increased number of red cells (**erythrocytosis** or **polycythemia**) may be a physiologic adaptation—it is found, for example, in people who live at high altitudes, where oxygen tension is low. Polycythemia, often associated with diseases of varying degrees of severity, increases blood viscosity; when severe, it can impair circulation of blood through the capillaries. Polycythemia might be better characterized as an increased hematocrit, ie, an increased volume occupied by erythrocytes (Fig 12–1).

Erythrocytes with diameters greater than 9 μm are called **macrocytes,** and those with diameters less than 6 μm are called **microcytes.** The presence of a high

Table 12–2. Size and number of human blood cells.

Cell	Size	Number*
Erythrocytes	6.5–8 μm (mean = 7.5 μm)	4.1–6 × 10⁶/μL (males) 3.9–5.5 × 10⁶μL (females)
Leukocytes		6000–10,000/μL
Neutrophil	12–15 μm	60–70%
Eosinophil	12–15 μm	2–4%
Basophil	12–15 μm	0–1%
Lymphocyte	6–18 μm	20–30%
Monocyte	12–20 μm	3–8%
Platelets	2–4 μm	200,000–400,000/μL

* Some references give these values per cubic millimeter (mm³). Microliters and cubic millimeters are identical units.

percentage of erythrocytes with greatly varying sizes is called **anisocytosis** (from Greek, *aniso*, uneven, + *kytos*).

The erythrocyte is quite flexible, a property that permits it to adapt to the irregular shapes and small diameters of capillaries. Observations in vivo show that when traversing the angles of capillary bifurcations, erythrocytes containing normal adult hemoglobin (HbA) are easily deformed and frequently assume a cuplike shape.

Erythrocytes are surrounded by a plasmalemma; which, because of its ready availability, is the best-known membrane of any cell. It consists of about 40% lipid (phospholipids, cholesterol, glycolipids, etc), 50% protein, and 10% carbohydrate. About half the proteins span the lipid bilayer and are known as **integral membrane proteins** (see Chapter 3). Several **peripheral proteins** (Fig 3–4A) are associated with the inner surface of the erythrocyte membrane. These seem to serve as a membrane skeleton that determines the unusual shape of the red blood cell. They also permit the flexibility of the membrane necessary for the large changes in shape that occur when the erythrocyte passes through capillaries. Because red blood cells are not rigid, the viscosity of blood remains low.

In their interiors, erythrocytes contain a 33% solution of hemoglobin, the oxygen-carrying protein that accounts for their acidophilia. In addition, there are enzymes of the glycolytic and hexose-monophosphate shunt pathways of glucose metabolism.

Inherited alterations in hemoglobin molecules are responsible for several pathologic conditions, of which **sickle cell disease** is an example. This inherited disorder is caused by a mutation of one nucleotide (**point mutation**) in the DNA of the gene for the β chain of hemoglobin. The triplet GAA (for glutamic acid) is changed to GUA, which specifies valine. As a result, the translated hemoglobin differs from the normal one by the presence of valine in the place of glutamic acid. The consequences of this single amino acid substitution are profound, however. When the altered hemoglobin (called HbS) is deoxygenated, it polymerizes and forms aggregates that give the erythrocyte a characteristic sickle shape (Fig 12–6). The sickled erythrocyte is inflexible, has a shortened life span that leads to profound anemia, and is much more viscous than normal cells. The resultant viscosity of the blood retards or even stops the flow through capillaries, leading to severe oxygen shortage (**anoxia**) in tissues.

Combined with oxygen or carbon dioxide, hemoglobin forms **oxyhemoglobin** or **carbaminohemoglobin,** respectively. The reversibility of these combinations is the basis for the gas-transporting ca-

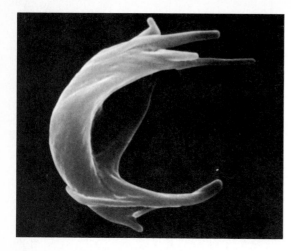

Figure 12–6. Scanning electron micrograph of a distorted red blood cell from a person who is homozygous for the HbS gene (sickle cell disease). Reproduced from × 6500.

pability of hemoglobin. The combination of hemoglobin with carbon monoxide (**carboxyhemoglobin**) is irreversible, however, resulting in a reduced capacity to transport oxygen.

> **Anemia** is a pathologic condition characterized by blood concentrations of hemoglobin below normal values. Although anemias are usually associated with a decreased number of red blood cells, it is also possible for the number of cells to be normal—but for each cell to contain a reduced amount of hemoglobin (**hypochromic anemia**). Anemia may be caused by loss of blood (hemorrhage); insufficient production of red blood cells by the bone marrow; production of red blood cells with insufficient hemoglobin, usually related to iron deficiency in the diet; or accelerated blood cell destruction.

Erythrocytes recently released by the bone marrow into the bloodstream often contain ribosomal RNA (rRNA), which, in the presence of supravital dyes (eg, brilliant cresyl blue), can be precipitated and stained. Under these conditions, the younger erythrocytes, called **reticulocytes** (see Fig 13–6), may have a few granules or a netlike structure in their cytoplasm.

> Reticulocytes normally constitute about 1% of the total number of circulating red blood cells; this is the rate at which erythrocytes are replaced daily by the bone marrow. Increased numbers of reticulocytes indicate an increased demand for oxygen-carrying capacity, which may be caused by such factors as hemorrhage or a recent ascent to high altitude.

The process by which reticulocytes are released from the bone marrow into the circulation is not completely understood.

Red blood cells lose their mitochondria, ribosomes, and many cytoplasmic enzymes during maturation from reticulocytes to adult erythrocytes, a process that takes 24–48 hours. This breakdown of organelles and enzymes is not mediated by lysosomal enzymes. Instead, a group of ATP-dependent enzymes, present in the cytoplasm, are responsible for the disappearance of proteins and organelles during erythrocyte development. The source of energy for erythrocytes is glucose, 90% of which is anaerobically degraded to lactate. The remaining 10% is aerobically utilized through the hexose-monophosphate shunt pathway. Because erythrocytes do not have a nucleus or other organelles necessary for protein synthesis, they do not synthesize hemoglobin.

Human erythrocytes survive in the circulation for about 120 days. This period is measured by labeling young erythrocytes with ^{14}C-glycine or ^{15}N-glycine and determining their survival. Worn-out erythrocytes are removed from the circulation by macrophages of the spleen and bone marrow. The signal for removal seems to be the appearance of defective complex oligosaccharides attached to integral membrane proteins of the plasmalemma.

Sometimes—mainly in disease states—nuclear fragments (containing DNA) remain in the erythrocyte after extrusion of its nucleus, which occurs late

Table 12–3. Granule composition in human granulocytes.

Cells	Specific Granules	Azurophilic Granules
Neutrophils	Alkaline phosphatase Collagenase Lactoferrin Lysozyme (2/3)	Acid phosphatase α-Mannosidase Arylsulfatase β-Galactosidase β-Glucuronidase Cathepsin 5′Nucleotidase Elastase Collagenase Myeloperoxidase Lysozyme Acidic mucosubstances Cationic antibacterial proteins
Eosinophils	Acid phosphatase Arylsulfatase β-Glucuronidase Cathepsin Phospholipase RNAase Eosinophilic peroxidase Major basic protein	
Basophils	Eosinophilic chemotactic factor Heparin Histamine Peroxidase	

in its development (see Chapter 13). These nuclear remnants are Feulgen-positive and stain with basic dyes.

Leukocytes

White blood cells are not permanent components of blood; they migrate to the tissues, where they perform multiple functions. On the basis of the type of granule in their cytoplasm and the shape of the nucleus, white blood cells are classified into 2 groups: **granulocytes** (polymorphonuclear leukocytes) and **agranulocytes** (mononuclear leukocytes). Granulocytes (from Latin, *granulum*, granule, + Greek, *kytos*) possess 2 types of granules: the **specific granules** that bind either neutral or acidic components of the Romanovsky-type dye mixture and have specific functions; and the **azurophilic granules.** Azurophilic (azure + Greek, *philein*) granules stain purple and are considered to be lysosomes. Specific and azurophilic granules contain the enzymes listed in Table 12–3. In addition, the nucleus has 2 or more lobes. Granulocytes include the **neutrophils, eosinophils,** and **basophils. Agranulocytes** do not have specific granules, but they do contain varying numbers of azurophilic granules that bind the azure dyes of the stain. The nucleus is round or indented. This group includes the **lymphocytes** and **monocytes.**

The size and frequency (differential count) of blood leukocytes are presented in Table 12–2.

Leukocytes are involved in the cellular and humoral defense of the organism against foreign material. They are spherical, nonmotile cells when in suspension in the circulating blood, but are capable of becoming flattened and motile on encountering a solid substrate. Leukocytes leave the capillaries by passing between endothelial cells and penetrating the connective tissue **(diapedesis).** The population of leukocytes in connective tissue is so great that they are considered normal cellular components of that tissue.

The number of leukocytes per microliter of blood in the normal adult is 6000–10,000; at birth, it varies between 15,000 and 25,000, and by the fourth day it falls to 12,000. At 4 years, the average is around 8000, with a maximum normal limit of 12,000. The white count reaches normal adult values at about 12 years of age. There is a qualitative variation within the white cell population depending on age; at birth there is a preponderance of neutrophils, but by the second week lymphocytes constitute about 60% of the leukocytes and predominate until age 4, when the granulocytes and lymphocytes are equal in number. There follows a progressive increase in the percentage of granulocytes, and the percentages typical of the adult (60–70%) are reached at 14–15 years. Not only the percentage but also the absolute number of each cell type per unit of blood volume must be taken into consideration when studying physiologic and pathologic variations in the number of blood cells.

Neutrophils (Polymorphonuclear Leukocytes)

These cells constitute 60–70% of circulating leukocytes. They are 12–15 μm in diameter, with a nucleus consisting of 2–5 lobes (usually 3 lobes) linked by fine threads of chromatin (Fig 12–7). The immature neutrophil (band form) has a nonsegmented nucleus in the shape of a horseshoe.

The nuclei of all granulocytes have a similar chromatin pattern, in which dense masses of heterochromatin are distributed on the inner surface of the nuclear envelope (Fig 12–8). Zones of loosely arranged euchromatin are located mainly in the center of the nucleus.

> Neutrophils with more than 5 lobes are called **hypersegmented** and typically represent old cells. Although the maturation of the neutrophil parallels the increase in the number of nuclear lobes under normal conditions, this relationship is not absolute. In some pathologic conditions, young cells appear with 5 or more lobes.

In females, the inactive X chromosome appears as a drumsticklike appendage on one of the lobes of the nucleus (Fig 12–7). This is not obvious in all neutrophils, however. The cytoplasm of the neutrophil contains 2 types of granules. The more abundant are the **specific granules,** which are small (near the limit of resolution of the light microscope) granules that show multiple forms (rounded to elongated) (Fig 12–8). Most neutrophilic specific granules are spherical (0.1 μm in diameter), but a few rod-shaped forms (0.1 × 1 μm) can be seen in the electron microscope.

The second granule population in neutrophils consists of azurophilic granules about 0.5 μm in diameter. These are primary lysosomes and contain the enzymes listed in Table 12–3.

In fully differentiated neutrophils, approximately one-third of the granules are azurophilic; the remainder are specific granules. Neutrophils also contain glycogen in their cytoplasm.

Glycogen is broken down to yield energy via the glycolytic and hexose-monophosphate shunt pathways of glucose oxidation. The citric acid cycle is less important, as might be expected in view of the paucity of mitochondria in these cells. The ability of neutrophils to survive in an anaerobic environment is highly advantageous, since they can kill bacteria and help clean up debris in poorly oxygenated regions, eg, inflamed or necrotic tissue.

Neutrophils are short-lived cells with a half-life of 6–7 hours in blood and a life span of 1–4 days in connective tissues. They then die, whether or not they have engaged in phagocytosis; they are therefore considered terminal cells. Eosinophils and basophils are also terminal cells, while monocytes and lymphocytes can go through several cycles of activity before dying. Because of this short life span, terminal cells do not produce additional granules, and the protein synthetic apparatus is poorly developed.

Neutrophils constitute a defense against invasion by microorganisms, especially bacteria. They are active phagocytes of small particles and have sometimes been called **microphages** to distinguish them from **macrophages,** which take up larger particles. These cells are inactive and spherical while circulating but change shape upon adhering to a solid substrate, over which they migrate via pseudopodia. The cells move at a speed of 19–36 μm/min.

The particle to be phagocytized by the neutrophil is surrounded by pseudopodia that fuse around it; thus, the particle eventually occupies a vacuole (phagosome) delimited by a membrane derived from the cell surface. Immediately thereafter, specific granules fuse with and discharge their contents into the phagosome. By means of proton pumps in the phagosome membrane, the pH of the vacuole is lowered to about 4.0. Then the azurophilic granules (primary lysosomes) discharge their enzymes into the acid environment, where killing and digestion of the bacterium are accomplished.

During phagocytosis, a burst of oxygen consumption occurs and leads to the formation of superoxide anions and hydrogen peroxide (H_2O_2). Superoxide (O_2^-) is a free radical formed by the loss of one electron from O_2. Together with myeloperoxidase and halide ions, these form a powerful cytotoxic system. This system may act by adding bulky halide groups (Cl^-, I^-) to essential proteins and thus interfering with their function. Strong oxidizing agents are also

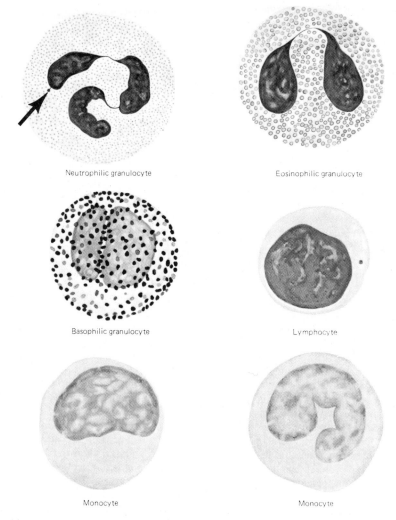

Neutrophilic granulocyte Eosinophilic granulocyte

Basophilic granulocyte Lymphocyte

Monocyte Monocyte

Figure 12–7. The 5 types of human leukocytes. The drawings were made from blood smears stained by the Romanovsky technique. Monocyte nuclei can present these 2 extreme forms. The neutrophil shows the drumsticklike appendage (sex chromatin; arrow) present in females. The same figure is shown in color on the color plate following page 246.

formed (eg, hypochlorite) that can inactivate proteins. These agents are effective against bacteria, fungi, viruses, and mammalian cells. Lysozyme has the function of specifically cleaving a bond in the peptidoglycan that forms the cell wall of some gram-positive bacteria, thus causing their death. Lactoferrin avidly binds iron; since this is a crucial element in bacterial nutrition, lack of available iron leads to bacterial death. The acid environment of phagocytic vacuoles can itself cause the death of certain microorganisms. A combination of these mechanisms will kill most microorganisms. Dead neutro-

phils, bacteria, and semi-digested material form a viscous, usually yellow collection of fluids called **pus.**

Lysosomal enzymes of the azurophilic granules hydrolyze the dead bacterium to its constituent small molecules. These diffuse out of the cell and provide small amounts of nutrients to surrounding tissues.

Eosinophils

Eosinophils are far less numerous than neutrophils, constituting only 2–4% of leukocytes in normal blood. The cell has a diameter of 12–15 μm and

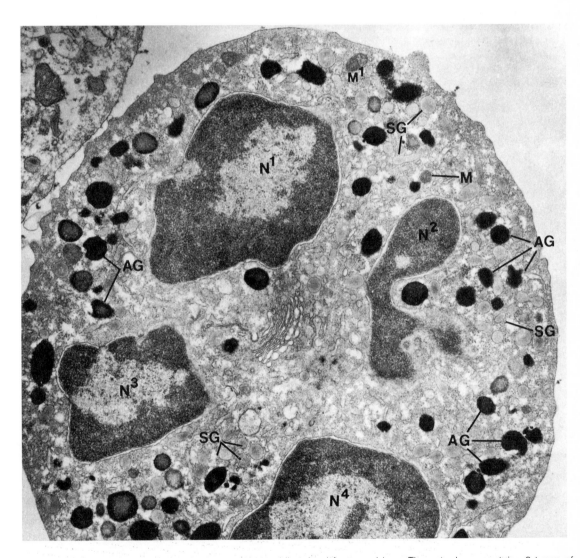

Figure 12–8. Electron micrograph of a human neutrophil stained for peroxidase. The cytoplasm contains 2 types of granules: the small, pale, peroxidase-negative specific granules (SG) and the larger, dense, peroxidase-positive azurophilic granules (AG). The nucleus is lobulated (N^1–N^4), and the Golgi complex (G) is small. Rough endoplasmic reticulum and mitochondria (M) are not abundant since this cell is in the terminal stage of its differentiation. × 27,000. (Reproduced, with permission, from Bainton DF: Selective abnormalities of azurophil and specific granules of human neutrophilic leukocytes. *Fed Proc* 1981;**40:**1443.)

contains a characteristic bilobed nucleus (Fig 12–7). The endoplasmic reticulum, Golgi complex, and mitochondria are poorly developed (Fig 12–9). Glycogen particles are relatively abundant. The main identifying characteristic is the presence of many large, refractile specific granules (about 200 per cell) that are stained by eosin. These granules are 0.5–1.5 μm in length and 0.3–1 μm in width.

Eosinophilic specific granules are surrounded by a unit membrane. A crystalline core **(internum)** lies parallel to the long axis of the granule (see Fig 12–9). It contains a protein with a large number of arginine residues that is called the **major basic protein.** This protein constitutes 50% of the total granule protein and accounts for the eosinophilia of these granules. The major basic protein also seems to function in the killing of parasitic worms such as schistosomes. The

less dense material surrounding the internum is known as the **externum,** or **matrix,** and consists of the enzymes listed in Table 12–3.

An increase in the absolute number of eosinophils in blood **(eosinophilia)** is associated with allergic reactions and helminthic (parasitic) infections. In tissues, eosinophils are found in the connective tissues underlying epithelia of the skin, bronchi, gastrointestinal tract, uterus, and vagina, and surrounding the parasitic worms. In addition, these cells produce substances that modulate inflammation by inactivating the leukotrienes (SRS-A) and histamine produced by other cells.

Corticosteroids (hormones from the adrenal cortex) produce a rapid fall in the number of blood

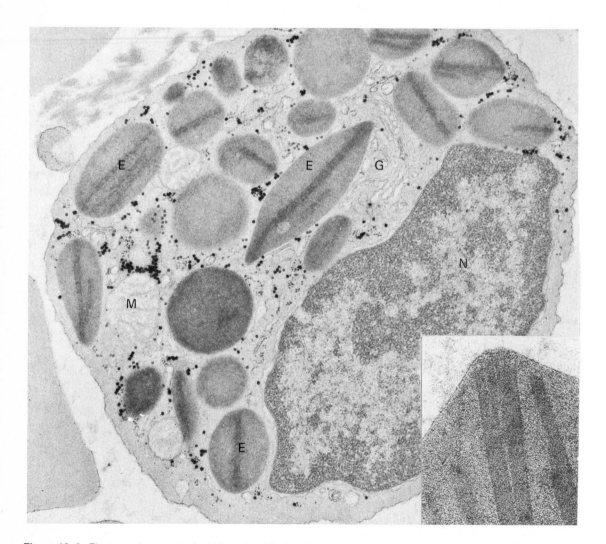

Figure 12–9. Electron micrograph of rabbit eosinophil, showing a nuclear lobe (N), the Golgi complex (G), a mitochondrion (M), and the eosinophil granules (E). × 21,500. The inset, a higher magnification of a specific granule, reveals its crystalloid organization. × 132,000. (Courtesy of DF Bainton and MG Farquhar.)

eosinophils, probably by interfering with the release of granulocytes from the bone marrow into the bloodstream.

Basophils

Basophils make up less than 1% of blood leukocytes and are therefore difficult to locate in smears of normal blood. They are about 12–15 μm in diameter and have a less heterochromatic nucleus than do other granulocytes. The nucleus is divided into irregular lobes, but this is usually obscured by the overlying specific granules.

The specific granules (0.5 μm in diameter) stain metachromatically with the basic dye of the Romanovsky-type mixture (Fig 12–7). This staining is due to the presence of heparin. Specific granules in basophils are fewer and more irregular in size and shape than the granules of the other granulocytes. The granules are also more irregular in size and shape (Fig 12–10). Basophilic specific granules contain heparin and histamine and are capable of generating leukotrienes, which cause slow contraction of smooth muscles. Basophils may supplement the functions of mast cells in immediate hypersensitivity reactions by migrating (under special circumstances) into connective tissues.

There is some similarity between granules of basophils and those of mast cells (see Chapter 5). Both are metachromatic and contain heparin and histamine. Basophils can liberate their granule content in response to certain antigens, as happens with the mast cell (see Chapter 5). Despite the similarities they present, mast cells and basophils are not the same, for even in the same species they have different ultrastructural appearances, and they originate from different stem cells in the bone marrow.

> In the dermatologic disease called **cutaneous basophil hypersensitivity,** basophils are the major cell type at the site of inflammation.

Lymphocytes

Lymphocytes constitute a family of spherical cells with similar morphologic characteristics. They can be

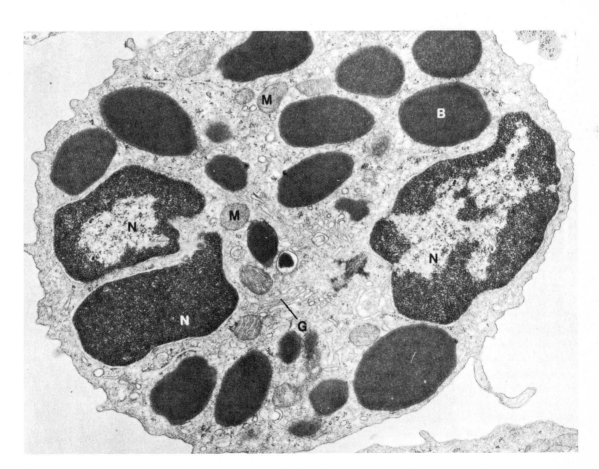

Figure 12–10. Electron micrograph of a rabbit basophil. The lobulated nucleus (N) appears as 3 separated portions. Note the basophilic granules (B), mitochondria (M), and Golgi complex (G). × 16,000. (Reproduced, with permission, from Terry RW, Bainton DF, Farquhar MG: *Lab Invest* 1969;**21**:65.)

classified into several groups according to distinctive surface molecules (markers), which can be distinguished only by immunocytochemistry. They also have diverse functional roles, all related to immune reactions in defending against invading microorganisms, foreign macromolecules, and cancer cells (Table 12–4).

Lymphocytes with diameters of 6–8μm are known as **small lymphocytes** (Fig 12–7). A small number of **medium-sized lymphocytes** and **large lymphocytes** with diameters up to 18 μm are present in the circulating blood. This difference has functional significance in that the larger lymphocytes are thought to be cells activated by specific antigens. These cells will differentiate into effector T or B lymphocytes (see below).

The small lymphocyte, which is predominant in the blood, has a spherical nucleus, sometimes with an indentation. Its chromatin is condensed and appears as coarse clumps, so that the nucleus is intensely stained in the usual preparations, a characteristic that facilitates identification of the lymphocyte (Figs 12–7 and 12–11). In blood smears, the nucleolus of the lymphocyte is not visible, but it can be demonstrated by special staining techniques and with the electron microscope.

The cytoplasm of the small lymphocyte is scanty, and in blood smears it appears as a thin rim around the nucleus. It is slightly basophilic, assuming a light blue color in stained smears (Fig 12–7). It may contain a few azurophilic granules. The cytoplasm of the small lymphocyte has a few mitochondria and a small Golgi complex associated with a pair of centrioles; it contains free polyribosomes (Fig 12–12).

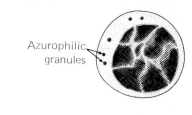

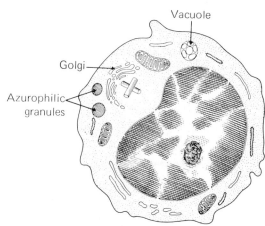

Figure 12–11. A medium lymphocyte as seen with the light microscope **(above)** and the electron microscope **(below).** Cytoplasmic organelles are scanty. Small lymphocytes have even less cytoplasm.

Table 12–4. Summary of lymphocyte types and functions.

Type	Function
B lymphocyte	Carries surface immunoglobulins. When activated by specific antigens, proliferates by mitosis, differentiating into **plasma cells** that secrete large amounts of antibodies; some activated cells originate **memory B Cells.**
T lymphocyte	Carries surface **T cell receptors,** which are not immunoglobulins. Specialized to recognize antigens attached to surfaces of other cells. Four major types of T lymphocytes are **cytotoxic cells, helper cells, suppressor cells,** and **memory T cells.**
Cytotoxic T cell	Destroys transplanted and other foreign cells as well as virus-invaded cells by making holes in their membranes, through which the cell contents leak out.
Helper T cell	Secretes factors that stimulate T and B lymphocytes in their response to some antigens.
Suppressor T cell	Dampens responses to foreign antigens; plays a key role in suppressing responses to self antigens.

Lymphocytes vary in life span; some live only a few days, while others survive in the circulating blood for many years.

A fundamental division of lymphocytes into 2 classes can be made on the basis of their site of differentiation and their possession of distinctive integral membrane proteins. Precursor cells originate in the bone marrow in late fetal life, and slow proliferation of these cells continues during postnatal life. Differentiation into immunocompetent cells occurs in the bone marrow and the thymus (see Chapter 14).

In the early 1960s, experiments using chicken embryos revealed one of the anatomic sites of lymphocyte differentiation. The **bursa of Fabricius** is a mass of lymphoid tissue associated with the cloaca of birds. When this tissue is destroyed in the embryo (either surgically or by the administration of high levels of testosterone), chickens lack the ability to produce immunoglobulins (IgM, IgG, etc) against specific antigens. In other words, **humoral immunity,** a process that requires the presence of immunoglobulins in the blood, is impaired. The number of lymphocytes found in specific areas in the lymph nodes and spleen is profoundly reduced, leading to the designation of these regions as bursa-dependent areas. The affected lymphocytes are known as **B lymphocytes** or **B cells.** In mammals (including humans), it is generally be-

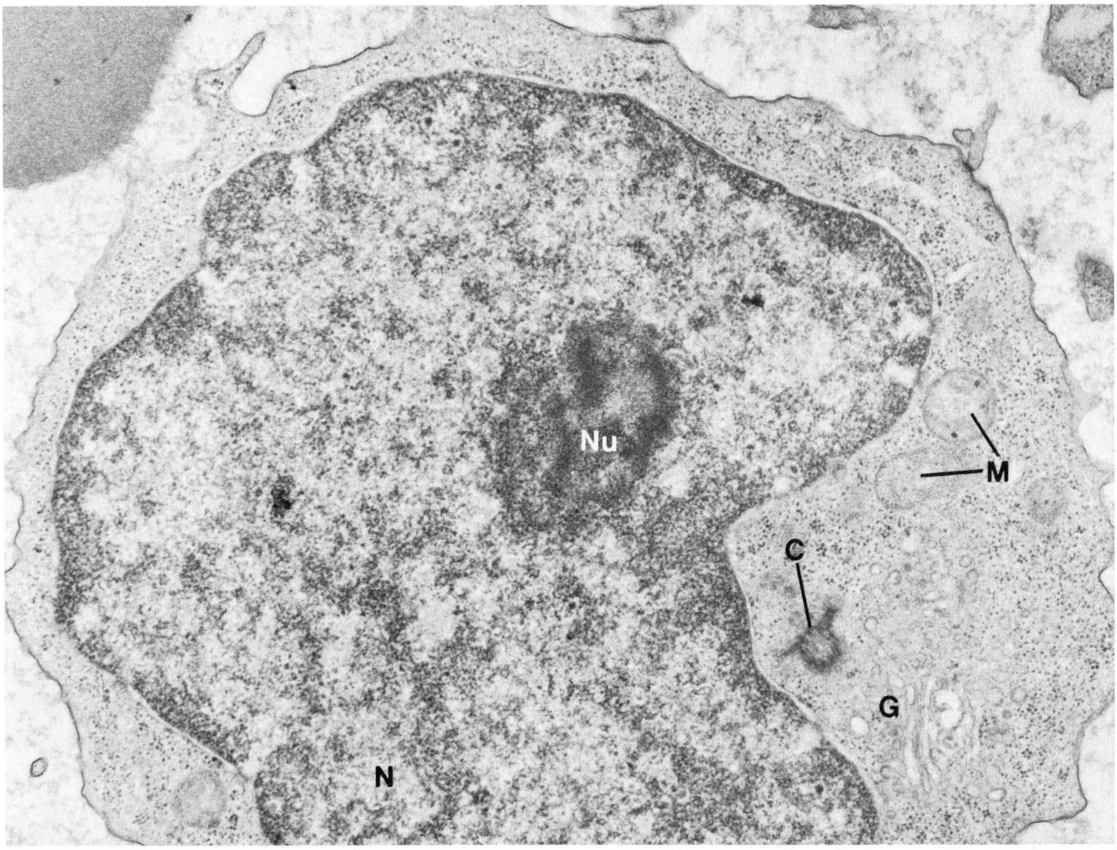

Figure 12–12. Electron micrograph of a human blood lymphocyte. This cell has little rough endoplasmic reticulum but a moderate quantity of free ribosomes. Observe the nucleus (N), the nucleolus (Nu), the centriole (C), the mitochondria (M), and the Golgi complex (G). Reduced from × 22,000. (Courtesy of DF Bainton and MG Farquhar.)

lieved that B lymphocytes acquire their differentiated characters in special microenvironments in the bone marrow.

On the other hand, experiments on newborn mice demonstrated that removal of the **thymus** (see Chapter 14) resulted in profound deficiencies in **cellular immune responses**—responses that require the presence of living cells, in contrast to humoral responses that depend on circulating immunoglobulins (Fig 14–3). An important example of cellular immune response in humans is rejection of transplanted organs, such as skin or kidney. In the thymectomized mice, the lymph nodes and spleen showed depletion of lymphocytes in areas different from those affected by removal of the bursa of Fabricius. These are the thymus-dependent areas; the cells involved are called **T lymphocytes,** or **T cells.**

The thymus and the bursa-equivalent in mammals (bone marrow) are called **primary** or **central lymphoid organs,** and lymphocytes differentiated in these organs colonize **secondary** or **peripheral** areas of the body where lymphoid tissues are found in diffuse, encapsulated, or organ form (see Chapter 14).

In blood, most lymphocytes (∼ 80%) are T cells with a very long life. These cells have several functions. They can regulate the activity of other T cells or B cells both positively (**helper T cells**) and negatively (**supressor T cells).** T cells produce several factors (**lymphokines**) that affect the behavior of macrophages, such as their movement toward inflammatory sites. Some T lymphocytes (**cytotoxic cells**) secrete substances that kill other cells, including tumor cells, virus-infected cells, and foreign grafts. A far smaller percentage of circulating lymphocytes (∼ 15%) are B cells, which, upon appropriate stimulation, divide several times and differentiate into plasma cells in tissues and produce immunoglobulins (see Table 12–4). Specific immunoglobulins (**opsonins**) coat bacteria and other invaders, making them more susceptible to phagocytosis by macrophages. Finally, there are a few lymphocytes in the blood (∼ 5%) that have neither T nor B lymphocyte surface antigens and are called **null cells.** These may be circulating stem cells.

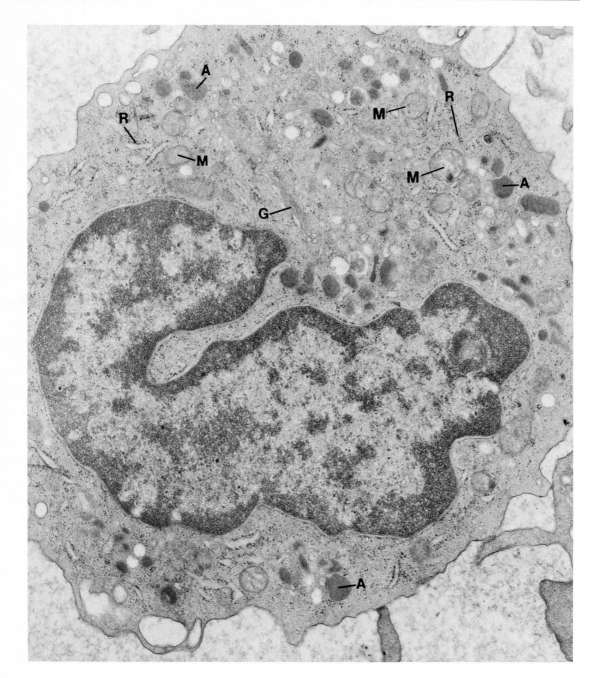

Figure 12–13. Electron micrograph of a human monocyte. Note the Golgi complex (G), the mitochondria (M), and the azurophilic granules (A). Rough endoplasmic reticulum is poorly developed. There are some free ribosomes (R). × 22,000. (Courtesy of DF Bainton and MG Farquhar.)

Both B and T lymphocytes also display the phenomenon of **immunologic memory.** Each lymphocyte is primed to respond to only one antigen. Upon first encountering its specific antigen, the lymphocyte undergoes several cell divisions. Some of the resulting cells differentiate into **effector cells;** eg, a B lymphocyte will differentiate into a plasma cell that will secrete antibodies. Other cells remain inactive **(memory cells)** but are primed to respond more rapidly and to a greater extent upon subsequent exposure to the specific antigen.

Monocytes

These bone-marrow-derived agranulocytes have diameters varying from 12 to 20 μm. The nucleus is oval, horseshoe- or kidney-shaped, and is generally eccentrically placed (Fig 12–7). The chromatin is less condensed and has a more fibrillar arrangement than in the lymphocytes (this is the most constant characteristic of the monocyte; see Fig 12–13). Because of the delicate distribution of this chromatin, the nuclei of monocytes stain more lightly than do those of large lymphocytes.

The cytoplasm of the monocyte is basophilic and frequently contains very fine azurophilic granules, some of which are at the limits of the light microscope's resolution. These granules are distributed through the cytoplasm, giving it a bluish-gray color in stained smears. The azurophilic granules of the monocytes are lysosomes. In the electron microscope, one or 2 nucleoli are seen in the nucleus, and a small quantity of rough endoplasmic reticulum, polyribosomes, and many small elongated mitochondria are observed (Fig 12–3). A Golgi complex involved in the formation of the lysosomal granules is present in the cytoplasm. Many microvilli and pinocytotic vesicles are found at the cell surface.

Monocytes are found in the blood, where they represent the recently formed precursors of the mononuclear phagocyte system (see Chapter 5). After crossing capillary walls and entering connective tissues, monocytes differentiate into macrophages. The half-life of the monocyte in the blood is 12–100 hours, and there is no strong evidence of recirculation after they enter connective tissues. In these tissues they interact with lymphocytes and play an essential role in the recognition and interaction of immunocompetent cells and antigen.

Platelets

Blood platelets **(thrombocytes)** are nonnucleated, disklike cell fragments 2–4 μm in diameter. Platelets originate from the fragmentation of giant polyploid **megakaryocytes** residing in the bone marrow. They promote blood clotting and help repair gaps in the walls of blood vessels, preventing loss of blood. Normal platelet counts range from 200,000 to 400,000 per microliter of blood. Once they enter the bloodstream, platelets have a life span of about 10 days.

In stained blood smears, platelets often appear in clumps. Each platelet has a peripheral light-blue-stained transparent zone, the **hyalomere,** and a central zone containing purple granules, called the **granulomere.**

Platelet ultrastructure is diagrammatically illustrated in Fig 12–14. These corpuscles contain a system of channels, the **open canalicular system,** that connect to invaginations of the platelet plasma membrane (Fig 12–15). It is probable that this arrangement is of functional significance in facilitating liberation of active molecules stored in platelets. Around the periphery of the platelet lies a **marginal bundle** of microtubules; this bundle helps maintain the platelet's ovoid shape. In the hyalomere, there are also a number of electron-dense irregular tubes known as the **dense tubular system.** Actin-containing mi-

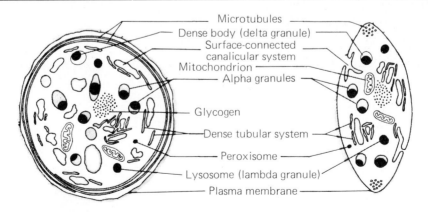

Figure 12–14. Diagrams of a human platelet in horizontal **(left)** and cross **(right)** sections. (Reproduced, with permission, from Bentfeld-Barker ME, Bainton DF: Identification of primary lysosomes in human megakaryocytes and platelets. *Blood* 1982;**59**:472.)

crofilaments in the hyalomere function in the elaboration of filopodia and surface projections during platelet movement and aggregation. A cell coat rich in glycosaminoglycans and glycoproteins, 15–20 nm thick, lies outside the plasmalemma and is involved in platelet adhesion.

The central granulomere possesses a variety of membrane-bound granules and a sparse population of mitochondria and glycogen particles (Figs 12–14 and 12–15). **Dense bodies (delta granules),** 250–300 nm in diameter, contain calcium ions, pyrophosphate, ADP, and ATP. These granules also take up and store serotonin (5-hydroxytryptamine) from the plasma. **Alpha granules** are a little larger (300–500 nm in diameter) and contain fibrinogen, platelet-derived growth factor, and several other platelet-specific proteins. Small vesicles, 175–250 nm in diameter, have been shown to contain only lysosomal enzymes and have been termed **lambda granules.** Most of the azurophilic granules seen with the light microscope

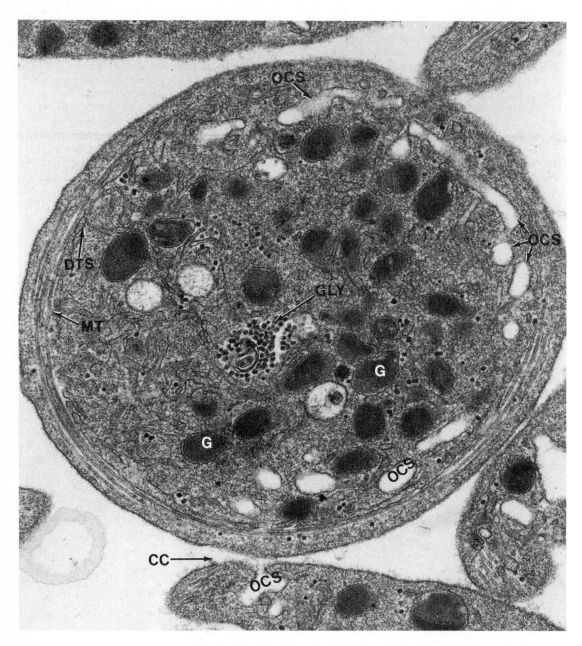

Figure 12–15. Electron micrograph of human platelets. CC, cell coat; OCS, open canalicular system; MT, microtubules; DTS, dense tubular system; G, granules; GLY, glycogen granules. × 40,740. (Courtesy of M Harrison.)

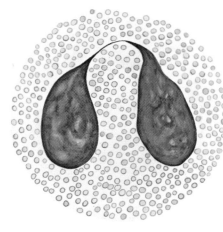

Neutrophilic granulocyte

Eosinophilic granulocyte

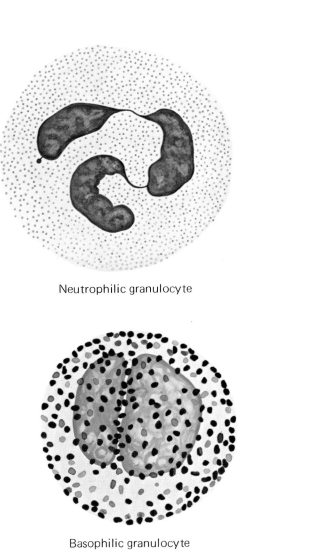

Basophilic granulocyte

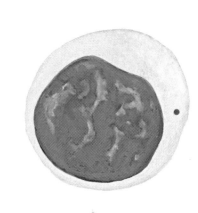

Lymphocyte

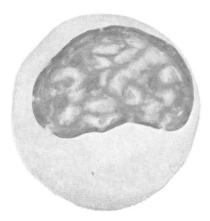

Monocyte

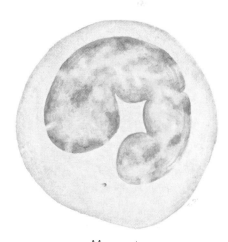

Monocyte

The 5 Types of Human Leukocytes.

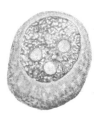

Proerythroblast

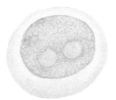

Myeloblast

Basophilic
erythroblast

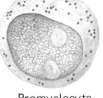

Promyelocyte

Early neutrophilic
myelocyte

Early basophilic
myelocyte

Polychromatophilic
erythroblast

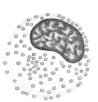

Early eosinophilic
myelocyte

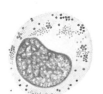

Late neutrophilic
myelocyte

Orthochromatophilic
erythroblast

Late eosinophilic
myelocyte

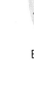

Late basophilic
myelocyte

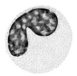

Neutrophilic
metamyelocyte

Reticulocyte

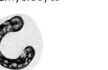

Band cell

Eosinophilic
metamyelocyte

Erythrocyte

Mature neutrophil

Mature eosinophil

Mature basophil

Stages of Development of Erythrocytes and Granulocytes.

in the granulomere of platelets are alpha granules.

Platelet functions. The role of platelets in controlling hemorrhage can be summarized as follows.

1. Primary aggregation–Discontinuities in the endothelium, produced by blood vessel lesions, are followed by absorption of plasma proteins on the subjacent collagen. Platelets immediately aggregate on this damaged tissue, forming a **platelet plug.**

2. Secondary aggregation–Platelets in the plug release the content of their alpha and delta granules. ADP is a potent inducer of platelet aggregation.

3. Blood coagulation–During platelet aggregation, factors from the blood plasma, damaged blood vessels, and platelets promote the sequential interaction (**cascade**) of approximately 13 plasma proteins,

giving rise to a polymer, **fibrin,** that forms a tridimensional network of fibers trapping red cells, leukocytes, and platelets to form a **blood clot,** or **thrombus.**

4. Clot retraction–The clot that initially bulges into the blood vessel lumen contracts because of interaction of platelet actin, myosin, and ATP.

5. Clot removal–Protected by the clot, the vessel wall is restored by new tissue formation. The clot is then removed, mainly by the proteolytic enzyme **plasmin,** formed, through the activation of the plasma proenzyme **plasminogen,** by endothelium-produced **plasminogen activators.** Enzymes released from platelet lambda granules also contribute to clot removal.

REFERENCES

Bainton DF: Sequential degranulation of the 2 types of polymorphonuclear leukocyte granules during phagocytosis of microorganisms. *J Cell Biol* 1973;**58:**249.

Cline MJ: *The White Cell.* Harvard Univ Press, 1975.

Gowans JL: Differentiation of the cells which synthesize the immunoglobulins. *Ann Immunol* (Paris) 1974; **125:**201.

Stites DP, Stobo JD, Wells JV (editors): *Basic & Clinical Immunology,* 6th ed. Appleton & Lange, 1987.

Williams WJ et al: *Hematology,* 4th ed. McGraw-Hill 1990.

Wintrobe MM et al: *Clinical Hematology,* 8th ed. Lea & Febiger, 1981.

Zucker-Franklin D et al: *Atlas of Blood Cells: Function and Pathology.* Vols 1 and 2. Lea & Febiger, 1981.

Hematopoiesis

Mature blood cells have a relatively short life span, and consequently the population must be continuously replaced by the progeny of stem cells produced in the **hematopoietic** (from Greek, *haima,* blood, + *poiesis,* a making) **organs.** In the earliest stages of embryogenesis, blood cells arise from the yolk sac mesoderm. Sometime later, the liver and spleen serve as temporary hematopoietic tissues, but by the second month the clavicle has begun to ossify and begins to develop bone marrow in its core. As the prenatal ossification of the rest of the skeleton accelerates, the bone marrow becomes an increasingly important hematopoietic tissue.

After birth and on into childhood, erythrocytes, granular leukocytes, monocytes, and platelets are derived from stem cells localized in bone marrow. The origin and maturation of these cells are termed, respectively **erythropoiesis** (from Greek, *erythros,* red, + *poiesis*), **granulopoiesis, monocytopoiesis,** and **megakaryocytopoiesis.** The bone marrow also produces cells that migrate to the lymphoid organs producing the various types of lymphocytes that will be discussed in Chapter 14.

Before attaining complete maturity and being released into the circulation, the blood cells go through specific stages of differentiation and maturation. Because these processes are continuous, cells with characteristics that are intermediate between the different stages are frequently encountered in smears of blood or bone marrow.

STEM CELLS, GROWTH FACTORS, & DIFFERENTIATION

Stem cells are defined as undifferentiated cells that can divide continuously and whose daughter cells form specific, irreversibly differentiated cell types. Stem cells play a central role in hematopoiesis and, because of their importance in biomedical research, will be considered in detail in this chapter.

The study of stem cells in bone marrow is possible because of experimental techniques that permit analysis of hematopoiesis **in vivo** and **in vitro.**

In vivo techniques include injecting the bone marrow of normal donor mice into lethally irradiated mice whose hematopoietic cells have been destroyed. In these animals, the transplanted bone marrow cells develop colonies of hematopoietic cells in the spleen.

In vitro investigation of hematopoiesis is made possible through the use of a semisolid tissue culture medium. Made with a layer of cells derived from bone marrow stroma, this medium creates favorable microenvironmental conditions for hematopoiesis.

Data from an extensive series of experiments show that hematopoiesis occurs when suitable microenvironmental conditions and stimulation by growth factors influence the development of the various types of blood cells.

Pluripotential and multipotential stem cells. It is thought that all blood cells arise from a single type of stem cell in the bone marrow. Because this cell can produce all blood cell types, it is called a **pluripotential stem cell.** These cells proliferate and form one cell lineage that will become lymphocytes **(lymphoid cells),** and another lineage that will form the **myeloid cells** that develop in bone marrow (granulocytes, monocytes, erythrocytes, and megakaryocytes). Both these types of stem cells are called **multipotential stem cells** (Fig 13–1). Early in their development, lymphoid cells migrate from the bone marrow to the lymph nodes, spleen, and thymus, where they differentiate into lymphocytes (Fig 13–1; see also Chapter 14).

Progenitor and precursor cells. The proliferating multipotential stem cells form daughter cells with reduced potentiality. These **uni-** or **bipotential progenitor cells** generate **precursor cells (blasts)** in which the morphologic characteristics differentiate for the first time (unlike these cells, stem and progenitor cells cannot be morphologically distinguished and resemble lymphocytes), suggesting the cell types they will become (see Figs 13–1 and 13–6 and color plate). Both pluri- and multipotential stem cells divide at a rate sufficient to maintain their relatively small population (in mouse bone marrow, only 0.1–0.3% of the cells are multipotential cells). Mitotic rate is accelerated in progenitor and precursor cells, producing large numbers of differentiated, mature cells (3×10^9 erythrocytes and 0.85×10^9 granulocytes/kg/day in human bone marrow). While progenitor cells can divide and produce both progenitor and precursor cells, precursor cells produce only mature blood cells.

PHASE	STEM CELLS		PROGENITOR CELLS	PRECURSOR CELLS (BLASTS)	MATURE CELLS
	Pluripotential	Multipotential			
Early morphologic distinctions*	Not morphologically distinguishable; have general aspect of lymphocytes			Beginning of morphologic differentiation	Clear morphologic differentiation
Mitotic activity	Low mitotic activity; self-renewing; scarce in bone marrow	High mitotic activity; self-renewing; common in marrow and lymphoid organs; mono- or bipotential		High mitotic activity; not self-renewing; common in marrow and lymphoid organs; monopotential	No mitotic activity; abundant in blood and hematopoietic organs

*Figure 13-6 (shown in color at the beginning of this chapter) shows the morphologic differentiation of these cells.

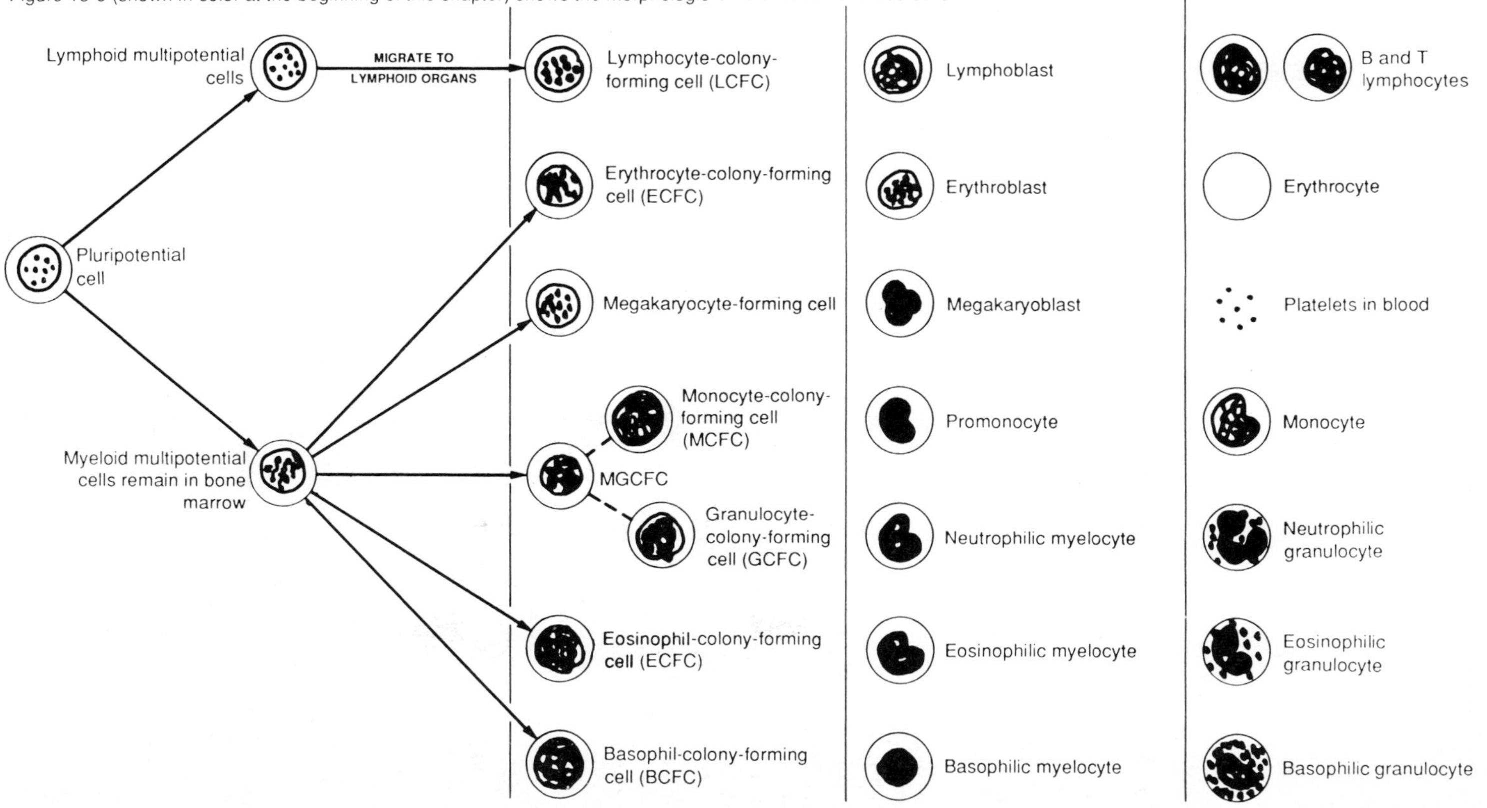

Figure 13–1. Differentiation of pluripotential and multipotential cells during hematopoiesis. See also Fig 13–6 and the corresponding color plate.

Table 13–1. Changes in properties of hematopoietic cells during differentiation.

STEM CELLS	PROGENITOR CELLS	PRECURSOR CELLS (BLASTS)	MATURE CELLS

Potentiality

Mitotic activity

Typical morphologic characteristics

Self-renewing capacity

Influence of growth factors

Differentiated functional activity

Thus hematopoiesis is the result of simultaneous, continuous proliferation and differentiation of cells derived from stem cells that undergo reductions in their potentials as differentiation progresses (Fig 13–1). This process can be observed in the in vivo and in vitro studies previously mentioned, in which colonies of cells derived from stem cells with various potentialities appeared (Table 13–1). Colonies derived from a multipotential myeloid stem cell can produce erythrocytes, granulocytes, monocytes, and megakaryocytes, all in the same colony.

In these experiments, however, some colonies appeared that produced only red blood cells. Other colonies were observed that produced granulocytes and monocytes. Cells forming colonies of specific cell types are called **colony-forming cells** (CFC), or **colony-forming units** (CFU). The convention used in naming these various cell colonies is to use the initial of the cell each colony produces. Thus, MCFC denotes a monocyte-producing colony, ECFC pro-

duces eosinophils, MGCFC produces monocytes and granulocytes, and so on.

Hematopoiesis depends upon the presence of suitable microenvironmental conditions and growth factors. The microenvironmental conditions are furnished by cells of the stroma of hematopoietic organs, which produce an essential extracellular matrix. Once the necessary environmental conditions are present, the development of blood cells depends on factors that affect cell proliferation and differentiation. These substances are called **growth factors, colony-stimulating factors** (CSF), or **hematopoietins** (poietins). Growth factors, which have differing chemical compositions and complex, overlapping functions, act mainly by stimulating proliferation (mitogenic activity) of immature (mostly progenitor and precursor) cells, supporting the differentiation of immature cells as they mature, and enhancing the functions of mature cells.

Table 13–2. Main characteristics of the 5 best-known hematopoetic growth factors (colony-forming substances).

Name	Human Gene Location and Producing Cell	Main Biologic Activity
Granulocyte (G-CSF)	Chromosome 17. Macrophages. Endothelium. Fibroblasts.	Stimulates formation (in vitro and in vivo) of granulocytes. Enhances metabolism of granulocytes. Stimulates malignant (leukemic) cells.
Granulocyte + macrophage (GM-CSF)	Chrososomes 5. T lymphocytes. Endothelium. Fibroblast.	Stimulates in vitro and in vivo production of granulocytes and macrophages.
Macrophage (M-CSF)	Chromosome 5. Macrophages. Endothelium. Fibroblasts.	Stimulates formation of macrophages in vitro. Increases antitumor activity of macrophages.
Interleukin 3(IL3)	Chromosome 5. T Lymphocytes.	Stimulates in vivo and in vitro the production of all myeloid cells.
Erythropoietin (EPO)	Chromosome 7. Renal interstitial cells.	Stimulates red blood cell formation in vivo and in vitro.

These three functions may be present in the same growth factor, but they may be expressed with different intensities in different growth factors. Recently, genes for several growth factors have been isolated and cloned, permitting both the mass production of growth factors and the study of their effects in vivo and in vitro. The main characteristics of the 5 best-characterized growth factors are presented in Table 13–2.

Growth factors have been used clinically to produce an increase in marrow cellularity and blood cell counts in patients. The use of growth factors to stimulate the proliferation of leukocytes is opening broad new applications for clinical therapy. Potential therapeutic uses of growth factors include increasing the numbers of blood cells in diseases or induced conditions (eg, chemotherapy, irradiation) that cause low blood counts; increasing the efficiency of marrow transplants by enhancing cell proliferation; enhancing host defenses in patients with malignancies and infectious and immunodeficient diseases; and enhancing the treatment of parasitic diseases.

Hematopoietic diseases rarely result from malfunctions of hematopoietic organ stroma. They are usually caused by suppression or enhancement of undifferentiated cell production, with a consequent reduction (or overproduction) of hematopoietic cells. In some diseases, however, sequential or simultaneous suppressed and enhanced proliferation of more than one type of stem cell can occur. There are, in such cases, reduced numbers of some cell types (eg, aplastic anemia, a disorder characterized by decreased production of hematopoietic cells) coinciding with increased numbers of others (eg, leukemia, the abnormal proliferation of white blood cells).

The initial experiments transplanting normal bone marrow to lethally irradiated mice established the basis for bone marrow transplantation, now routinely used to treat some hematopoietic-cell-growth disorders.

BONE MARROW

Bone marrow is one of the large organs of the body and the main site of hematopoiesis. Under normal conditions, the production of blood cells by the marrow is perfectly adjusted to the organism's functions. It can adjust rapidly to the body's needs, increasing its activity severalfold in a very short time if required. Bone marrow is found in the medullary canals of long bones and in the cavities of cancellous bones. Two types have been described according to their appearance on gross examination: **red,** or **hematogenous,** whose color is due to the presence of blood and blood-forming cells, and **yellow bone marrow,** whose color is due to the pres-

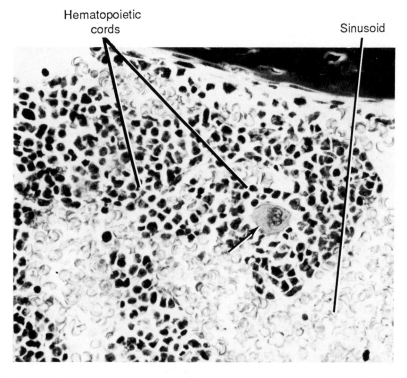

Figure 13–2. Section of active bone marrow showing the cell cords separated by sinusoidal capillaries filled with erythrocytes. The arrow indicates a megakaryocyte. × 140.

ence of a great number of adipose cells. In newborns, all bone marrow is red and is therefore active in the production of blood cells. As the child grows, most of the bone marrow changes gradually into the yellow variety. Under certain conditions, such as severe bleeding or hypoxia, yellow bone marrow converts back into red bone marrow.

Red Bone Marrow

Red bone marrow is composed of a **stroma** (from Greek, bed) **hematopoietic cords,** and **sinusoidal capillaries** (see Fig 13–2). The stroma is a 3-dimensional meshwork of reticular cells with phagocytotic properties and a delicate web of reticular fibers containing hematopoietic cells and macrophages. The matrix of bone marrow, in addition to collagen types I and III, contains fibronectin, laminin, and proteoglycans. Laminin, fibronectin, and another cell-binding substance, **hemonectin,** interact with cell receptors to bind cells to the matrix. The sinusoids are formed by a continuous layer of endothelial cells. Some regions of the endothelium are thin and may be sites for migration of mature cells from the stroma into the sinusoid.

The sinusoidal capillaries are reinforced by an external discontinuous layer of reticular cells and a loose net of reticular fibers. The release of mature bone cells from the marrow is controlled by **releasing factors** produced in response to the needs of the organism. Several substances with releasing activity have been described and include the C3 component of **complement** (a series of immunologically active blood proteins), hormones (glucocorticoids and androgens), and some bacterial toxins. The release

of cells from the marrow is illustrated in Fig 13–3.

The main functions of red bone marrow are the production of blood cells, destruction of red blood cells, and storage (in macrophages) of iron derived from the breakdown of hemoglobin.

MATURATION OF ERYTHROCYTES

A **mature** cell is one that has differentiated to the stage at which it has acquired the capability of carrying out all its specific functions. The basic process in maturation is the synthesis of hemoglobin and the formation of an enucleated, biconcave, small corpuscle, the erythrocyte (see Figs 12–4 and 12–5). During maturation of the erythrocytic series, several major changes occur. Cell volume decreases, and the nucleoli diminish in size until they become invisible under the light microscope. The nuclear diameter decreases, and the chromatin becomes increasingly more dense until the nucleus presents a pyknotic appearance (Fig 13–4) and is finally extruded from the cell. There is a gradual decrease in the number of polyribosomes (basophilia), followed by a simultaneous increase in the amount of hemoglobin (acidophilia) within the cytoplasm, and the mitochondria gradually disappear (Fig 13–5).

There are from 3 to 5 intervening cell divisions between the proerythroblast and the mature erythrocyte. The development of an erythrocyte from the first recognizable cell of the series to the release of reticulocytes into the blood takes approximately 7 days (see Fig 13–5). The hormone erythropoietin and substances such as iron, folic acid, and vitamin B_{12} are essential for the production of erythrocytes.

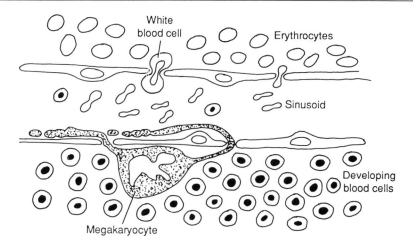

Figure 13–3. Diagram illustrating the passage of erythrocytes, white blood cells, and platelets across a sinusoid in bone marrow. Since immature erythrocytes (unlike the white blood cells) do not have sufficient motility to cross the wall of the sinusoid, it is thought that they enter the sinusoids by a pressure gradient that exists across its wall. White blood cells, after the action of releasing substances (see text), are free to cross the wall of the sinusoid. Megakaryocytes form thin processes that cross the wall of the sinusoid and fragment at their tips, liberating the platelets.

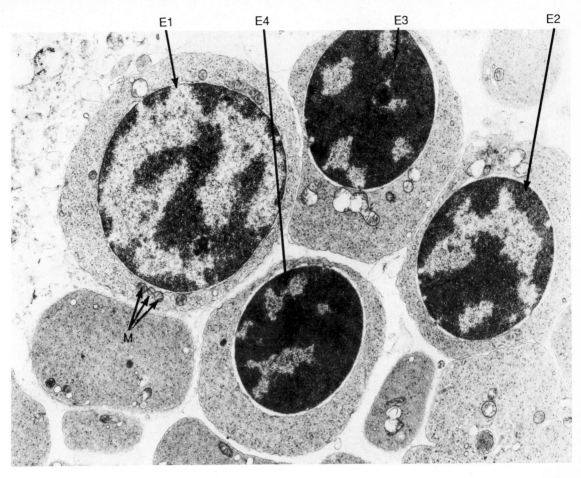

Figure 13–4. Electron micrograph of bone marrow. Four erythroblasts in successive stages of maturation are seen (E1, E2, E3, and E4). As the cell matures, its chromatin becomes gradually condensed, the accumulation of hemoglobin increases the electron density of the cytoplasm, and the mitochondria (M) decrease in number. × 11,000.

Differentiation

The differentiation and maturation of erythrocytes involve the formation (in order) of proerythroblasts, basophilic erythroblasts, polychromatophilic erythroblasts, orthochromatophilic erythroblasts (normoblasts) reticulocytes, and erythrocytes (Fig 13–6 and color plate).

The first recognizable cell in the erythroid series is the **proerythroblast.** It is a large cell with loose, lacy chromatin and clearly visible nucleoli; its cytoplasm is basophilic. The next stage is represented by the *basophilic erythroblast* (*erythros* + Greek, *blastos,* germ), with a strongly basophilic cytoplasm and a condensed nucleus that presents no visible nucleolus. The basophilia of these two cell types is caused by the large number of polyribosomes involved in the synthesis of hemoglobin (Fig 13–7). During the next stage, polyribosomes decrease and areas of the cytoplasm begin to be filled with hemoglobin. Staining at this stage causes several colors to appear in the cell— the **polychromatophilic** (from Greek, *polys,* many,

+ *chroma* + *philein*) **erythroblast.** In the next step, the nucleus continues to condense and no cytoplasmic basophilia is evident, resulting in a uniformly acidophilic cytoplasm—the **orthochromatophilic** (from Greek, *orthos,* correct, + *chroma* + *philein*) **erythroblast.** At a given moment, this cell puts forth a series of cytoplasmic protrusions and expels its nucleus, encased in a thin layer of cytoplasm. The remaining cell still has a small number of polyribosomes that, when treated with the supravital dye brilliant cresyl blue, aggregate to form a stained network. This cell is the **reticulocyte,** which soon loses its polyribosomes and becomes a mature red blood cell (erythrocyte).

MATURATION OF GRANULOCYTES

The **myeloblast is** the most immature recognizable cell in the myeloid series. It has a finely dispersed chromatin, and nucleoli can be seen. In the next stage,

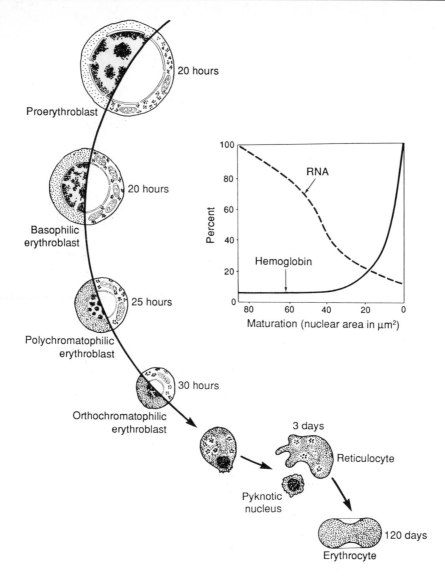

Figure 13–5. Summary of erythrocyte maturation. The stippled part of the cytoplasm (on the left) shows the continuous increase in hemoglobin concentration from proerythroblast to erythrocyte. There is also a gradual decrease in nuclear volume and an increase in chromatin condensation, followed by extrusion of a pyknotic nucleus. In the graph, the highest recorded concentrations of hemoglobin and RNA were considered to be 100%; the times are average life spans.

the **promyelocyte** (from Latin, *pro*, before, + Greek, *myelos*, marrow, + *kytos*) is characterized by its basophilic cytoplasm and azurophilic granules. These granules contain lysosomal enzymes and myeloperoxidase. The promyelocyte gives rise to the 3 known granulocytes. The first sign of differentiation appears in the myelocytes where specific granules gradually increase in quantity and eventually occupy most of the cytoplasm. These **neutrophilic, basophilic,** and **eosinophilic myelocytes** mature with further condensation of the nucleus and a considerable

increase in their specific granule content (Fig 13–8). The neutrophilic granulocyte presents an intermediate stage whose nucleus has the form of a curved rod (band cell; see color plate). This cell appears in quantity in the blood with strong stimulation of hematopoiesis.

The appearance of large numbers of immature neutrophils (band cells) in the blood is called a **shift to the left** and is of clinical significance, usually indicating bacterial infection.

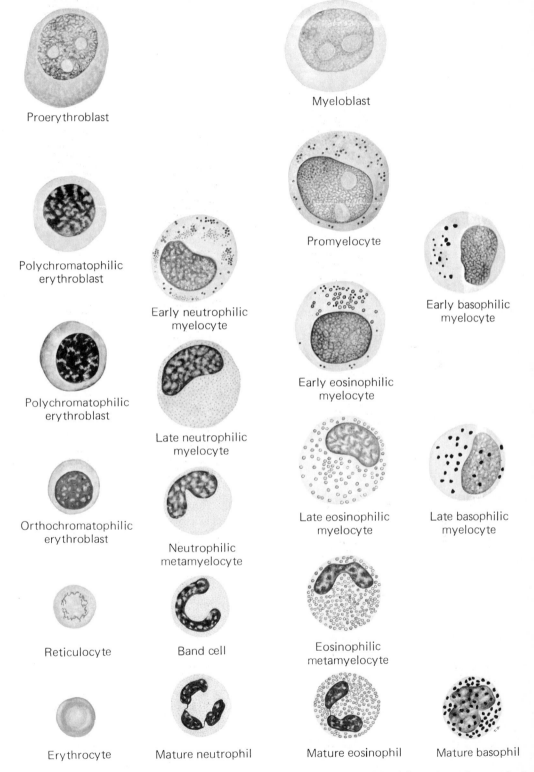

Proerythroblast

Myeloblast

Polychromatophilic
erythroblast

Promyelocyte

Early neutrophilic
myelocyte

Early basophilic
myelocyte

Polychromatophilic
erythroblast

Late neutrophilic
myelocyte

Early eosinophilic
myelocyte

Orthochromatophilic
erythroblast

Neutrophilic
metamyelocyte

Late eosinophilic
myelocyte

Late basophilic
myelocyte

Reticulocyte

Band cell

Eosinophilic
metamyelocyte

Erythrocyte

Mature neutrophil

Mature eosinophil

Mature basophil

Figure 13–6. Maturation of erythrocytic and granulocytic blood cells. Romanovsky staining was used except for the reticulocyte, which was additionally treated with cresyl blue in order to precipitate and stain the RNA found in this cell. The same figure is shown in color on the color plate following page 246. Only the cells in the bottom row are common in normal blood.

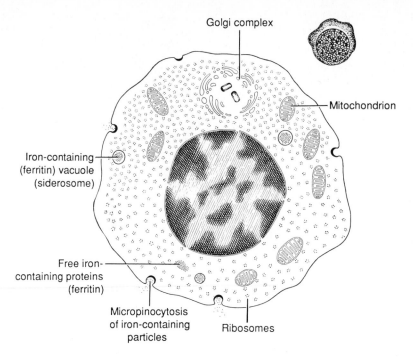

Golgi complex

Mitochondrion

Iron-containing
(ferritin) vacuole
(siderosome)

Free iron-
containing proteins
(ferritin)

Micropinocytosis
of iron-containing
particles

Ribosomes

Figure 13–7. Ultrastructure of a basophilic erythroblast. Its cytoplasm contains many polyribosomes for the synthesis of hemoglobin. The upper-right drawing shows the structure of the same cell as seen in bone marrow smears. The light area near the nucleus contains the Golgi complex and the centrioles.

KINETICS OF NEUTROPHIL PRODUCTION

The total time taken for a myeloblast to emerge as a mature neutrophil in the circulation is about 11 days. Under normal circumstances, 5 mitotic divisions occur in the myeloblast, promyelocyte, and neutrophilic myelocyte stages of development.

Neutrophils pass through several functionally and anatomically defined compartments (Fig 13–9).

The **medullary formation compartment** can be subdivided into a mitotic compartment (~ 3 days) and a maturation compartment (~ 4 days).

A **medullary storage compartment** acts as a buffer system, capable of releasing large numbers of mature neutrophils upon demand. Neutrophils remain in this compartment for about 4 days.

The **circulating compartment** consists of neutrophils suspended in plasma and circulating in blood vessels.

The **marginating compartment** is composed of neutrophils that are present in blood but do not circulate. These neutrophils are in capillaries, temporarily excluded from the circulation by vasoconstriction, or—especially in the lungs—they may be at the periphery of vessels, adhering to the endothelium, and not in the main bloodstream.

The marginating and circulating compartments are of about equal size, and there is a constant interchange of cells between them. The half-life of a neutrophil in these 2 compartments is 6–7 hours. The medullary formation and storage compartments together are about 10 times as large as the circulating and marginating compartments.

Neutrophils and other granulocytes enter the connective tissues by passing through intercellular junctions found between endothelial cells of capillaries and postcapillary venules **(diapedesis).** The connective tissues form a fifth compartment for neutrophils, but its size is not known. Neutrophils reside here for 1–4 days and then die, whether or not they have performed their major function of phagocytosis.

Changes in the number of neutrophils in the peripheral circulation must be evaluated by taking all these compartments into consideration. Thus, **neutrophilia,** an increase in the number of neutrophils in the circulation, does not necessarily imply an increase in neutrophil production. Intense muscular activity or the administration of epinephrine causes neutrophils in the marginating compartment to move into the circulating compartment, causing an apparent neutrophilia even though neutrophil production has not increased.

Neutrophilia may also result from liberation of

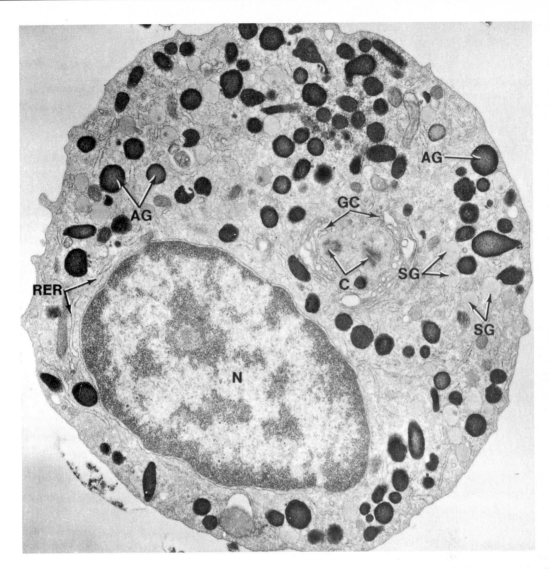

Figure 13–8. Neutrophilic myelocyte from normal human bone marrow treated with peroxidase. At this stage, the cell is smaller than the promyelocyte, and the cytoplasm contains 2 types of granules: large, peroxidase-positive azurophilic granules (AG); and smaller specific granules (SG), which do not stain for peroxidase. Note that the peroxidase reaction product is present only in azurophilic granules and is not seen in the rough endoplasmic reticulum (RER) or Golgi cisternae (GC), which are located around the centriole (C), N, nucleus. × 15,000. (Courtesy of DF Bainton.)

greater numbers of neutrophils from the medullary storage compartment. This type of neutrophilia is transitory and is followed by a recovery period during which no neutrophils are released.

The neutrophilia that occurs during the course of bacterial infections is due to an increase in neutrophil production and a shorter stay of these cells in the medullary storage compartment. In such cases, immature forms such as band cells, neutrophilic metamyelocytes, and even myelocytes may appear in the bloodstream. The neutrophilia that occurs during infection is of longer duration than that which occurs as a result of intense muscular activity.

MATURATION OF LYMPHOCYTES & MONOCYTES

Study of the precursor cells of lymphocytes and monocytes is difficult because these cells do not contain specific cytoplasmic granules or the nuclear lobulation that is present in granulocytes, both of which facilitate the distinction between young and

BONE MARROW

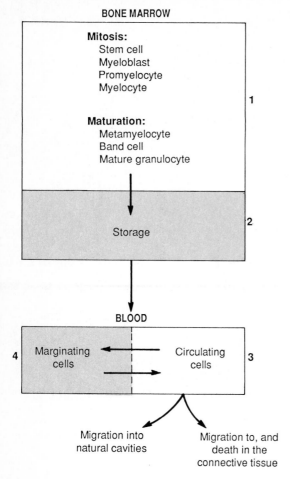

Figure 13–9. Functional compartments of neutrophils. **1:** Medullary formation compartment. **2:** Medullary storage (reserve) compartment. **3:** Circulating compartment. **4:** Marginating compartment. The size of each compartment is roughly proportional to the number of cells.

mature forms. Lymphocytes and monocytes are distinguished mainly on the basis of size, chromatin structure, and the presence of nucleoli in smear preparations. As lymphocyte cells mature, their chromatin becomes more compact, nucleoli become less visible, and the cells decrease in size. In addition, subsets of the lymphocytic series acquire distinctive cell-surface receptors during differentiation that can be detected by immunofluorescence techniques.

Lymphocytes

Circulating lymphocytes originate mainly in the thymus and the peripheral lymphoid organs (spleen, lymph nodes, tonsils, etc). It is now thought, however, that *all* lymphocyte progenitor cells originate in the bone marrow. Some of these relatively undifferentiated lymphocytes migrate to the thymus, where

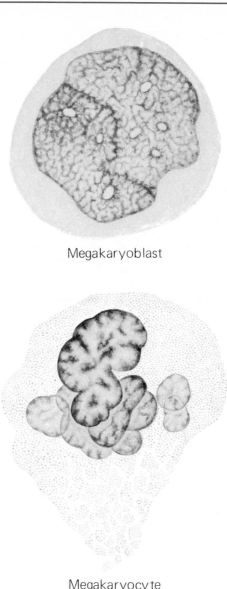

Megakaryoblast

Megakaryocyte

Platelets

Figure 13–10. Cells of the megakaryocytic series shown in a bone marrow smear with Romanovsky-type staining. Observe the formation of platelets at the lower end of the megakaryocyte.

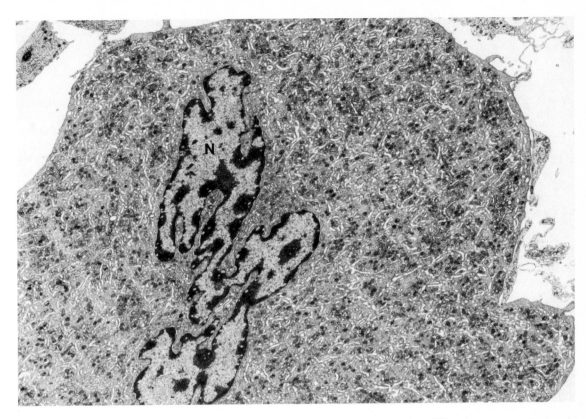

Figure 13–11. Electron micrograph of a megakaryocyte showing the lobulated nucleus (N) and numerous cytoplasmic granules. The demarcation membranes are visible as tubular profiles. × 4900. (Reproduced, with permission, from Junqueira LCU, Salles LMM: *Ultra-Estrutura e Função Celular.* Edgard Blücher, 1975.)

they acquire the attributes of T lymphocytes. Subsequently, T lymphocytes populate specific regions of peripheral lymphoid organs. Other bone marrow lymphocytes remain in the marrow, differentiate into B lymphocytes, and then migrate to peripheral lymphoid organs where they inhabit their own special compartments.

The first identifiable progenitor of lymphoid cells is the **lymphoblast,** a large cell capable of incorporating ^{3}H-thymidine and dividing 2–3 times to form **prolymphocytes.** These latter cells are smaller and have relatively more condensed chromatin but none of the cell-surface antigens that mark prolymphocytes as T or B lymphocytes. In the thymus or bone marrow, these cells synthesize cell-surface receptors characteristic of their lineage, but they are not recognizable as distinct cell types using routine histologic procedures. The distinction is made by using immunocytochemical techniques.

Monocytes

The **monoblast** is a committed progenitor cell that is virtually identical to the **myeloblast** in its morphology. Further differentiation leads to the **promonocyte,** a large cell (up to 18 μm in diameter) with a basophilic cytoplasm and a large, slightly idented nucleus. The chromatin is lacy, and nucleoli are evident. Promonocytes divide twice in the course of their development into **monocytes.** A large amount of rough endoplasmic reticulum is present, as is an extensive Golgi complex in which granule condensation can be seen to be taking place. These granules are **primary lysosomes,** which are observed as fine **azurophilic granules** in blood monocytes. Mature monocytes enter the bloodstream, circulate for about 8 hours, and then enter the connective tissues, where they mature into **macrophages** and function for several months.

Abormal bone marrow can produce diseases based on cells derived from that tissue. **Leukemias** are malignant clones of white blood cell precursors. They occur in lymphoid tissue (**lymphocytic leukemias**) and in bone marrow (**myelogenous** and **monocytic leukemias**). In these diseases, there is usually a release of large numbers of immature cells into the blood. The symptoms of leukemias are a consequence of this shift in cell proliferation, with a lack of some cell types and excessive production of others (which are often abnormal in function). The patient usually exhibits anemia and is prone to infection.

A clinical technique helpful in the study of leukemias and other bone marrow disturbances is **bone marrow aspiration.** A needle is introduced through compact bone (usually the sternum), and a sample of marrow is withdrawn. The sample is spread on a microscope slide and stained. The use of labeled monoclonal antibodies specific to proteins in the membranes of precursor blood cells aids in identifying cell types derived from these stem cells and contributes to a more precise diagnosis of the various possible types of leukemia.

ORIGIN OF PLATELETS

In adults, the platelets originate in the red bone marrow by fragmentation of the cytoplasm of mature **megakaryocytes.** These in turn arise by differentiation of the **megakaryoblasts.**

Megakaryoblasts

The megakaryoblast is 15–50 μm in diameter and has a large ovoid or kidney-shaped nucleus with numerous nucleoli. The nucleus becomes highly polyploid (ie, it contains up to 30 times as much DNA as a normal cell) before cytoplasmic differentiation begins. The cytoplasm of this cell is homogeneous and intensely basophilic (Fig 13–10).

Megakaryocytes

The megakaryocyte is a giant cell (35–150 μm in diameter) with an irregularly lobulated nucleus, coarse chromatin, and no visible nucleoli (Figs 13–10 and 13–11). The cytoplasm contains numerous mitochondria, a well-developed rough endoplasmic reticulum, and an extensive Golgi complex. Alpha granules and vesicles containing lysosomal enzymes (lambda granules) develop from Golgi vesicles and cisternae. With maturation of the megakaryocyte, numerous invaginations of the plasma membrane ramify throughout the cytoplasm, forming the **demarcation membranes.** This system defines areas of the megakaryocyte's cytoplasm that will be shed as platelets after a complex and little-understood process of membrane fusion.

> In certain forms of **thrombocytopenic purpura,** a disease in which the number of blood platelets is reduced, the platelets appear bound to the cytoplasm of the megakaryocytes, indicating a defect in the liberation mechanism of these corpuscles. The life span of these corpuscles was found to be approximately 10 days.

REFERENCES

Becker RP, DeBruyn PP: The transmural passage of blood cells into myeloid sinusoids and the entry of platelets into the sinusoidal circulation. *Am J Anat* 1976;**145:**183.

Berman I: The ulstrastructure of erythroblastic islands and reticular cells in mouse bone marrow. *J Ultrastruct Res* 1967;**17:**291.

Evatt BL, Levine RF, Williams NT: *Megakaryocyte Biology and Precursors: In Vitro Cloning and Cellular Properties.* Elsevier/North-Holland, 1981.

Fleischmann RA et al: Totipotent hematopoietic stem cells: Normal self-renewal and differentiation after transplantation between mouse fetuses. *Cell* 1982;**30:**351.

Pennington DG: The cellular biology of megakaryocytes. *Blood Cells* 1979;**5:**5.

Tavassoli M, Yoffey JM: *Bone Marrow Structure and Function.* Liss, 1983.

Williams WJ et al (editors): *Hematology,* 4th ed. McGraw-Hill, 1990.

The Immune (Lymphoid) System

14

The immune system comprises structures and cells that are distributed throughout the body; their principal function is to protect the organism against invasion and damage by microorganisms and foreign substances. Cells of this system have the ability to distinguish both *self* (the organism's own macromolecules) and *nonself* (foreign substances) and to coordinate the destruction or inactivation of foreign substances. On occasion, the immune system reacts against itself, causing **autoimmune diseases** that can be fatal. The immune system includes both individual structures (eg, lymph nodes, spleen) and free cells (eg, lymphocytes and cells of the mononuclear phagocyte system that are present in the blood, lymph, and connective tissues) that participate in immune reactions.

Structures Involved in Immune Processes

In addition to the free cells, lymphoid organs exhibit a 3-dimensional network of epithelial cells or reticular tissue (see Chapter 5), filled with cells that participate in immune processes. This combination of epithelial cells or reticular tissue and immune cells forms large **lymphoid organs**: the **thymus, spleen,** and **lymph nodes. Lymphoid nodules,** smaller collections of lymphoid tissue, formed mainly of nodular aggregates, are present in the digestive (tonsils, Peyer's patches, and appendix), respiratory, and urinary systems (Fig 14–1). The wide distribution of lymphoid structures and the constant circulation of lymphoid cells in the blood, lymph, and connective tissues provide the body with an elaborate, efficient system of surveillance and defense by immunocompetent cells.

Lymphocytes are the most common cells in the two categories of lymphoid organs. **Central lymphoid organs** include the thymus and bone marrow, where T and B lymphocytes (respectively) originate. Lymphocytes migrate from these organs to the **peripheral lymphoid organs** (spleen, lymphoid nodules, solitary nodules, tonsils, appendix, and Peyer's patches of the ileum) where they proliferate and complete their differentiation.

Basic Types of Immune Reactions

During evolution, 2 different but related systems of immunity developed. The first was **cellular immunity,** in which immunocompetent cells react against and kill microorganisms, foreign cells (from tumors and transplants), and virus-infected cells. This category of immunity is mediated mainly by T lymphocytes, or T cells (see Chapter 12), whose origin and functions are described later in this chapter. The other type of immunity, **humoral immunity,** is related to the presence of circulating glycoproteins called **antibodies** that inactivate or destroy foreign substances. The antibodies are produced by plasma cells derived from B lymphocytes (B cells).

Antigens & Antibodies

The foreign (nonself) substance encountered by the immune system acts as an antigen (from Greek, *anti,* against, + *genin,* to produce), ie, a substance that elicits a response from the host. The response may be cellular, humoral, or (most commonly) both. Antigens may be present in whole cells such as bacteria or tumor cells or in macromolecules, such as proteins, polysaccharides, or nucleoproteins. In any case, the specificity of the immune response is controlled by relatively small molecular domains—**antigenic determinants**—of the antigen. Antigenic determinants for proteins and polysaccharides consist of 4–6 amino acid or monosaccharide units. A complex antigen that has many antigenic determinants (eg, a bacterial cell) will therefore elicit a wide spectrum of humoral and cellular responses.

Antibodies are circulating plasma glycoproteins (they are also called **immunoglobulins**) that interact specifically with the antigenic determinant that elicited their formation. Antibodies are secreted by plasma cells that arise by proliferation and differentiation of B lymphocytes.

Five classes of immunoglobulins are recognized in humans:

IgG, the most abundant class, constitutes 75% of serum immunoglobulins. It also serves as a model for the other classes (as such, it will be described in more detail). IgG consists of 2 identical light chains, and 2 identical heavy chains (Fig 14–2), bound by disulfide bonds and non-covalent forces. When isolated, the 2 carboxy-terminal portions of the heavy chains crystallize easily and are called **Fc** fragments. The Fc regions of several immunoglobulins react with specific receptors of many different cells. The 4 amino-terminal segments (2 formed by light and 2 by heavy chains) constitute the **Fab** (antigen-binding) fragments of the immunoglobulin. The Fab segments are variable in amino acid sequence and are thus responsible for the exquisite specificity of the immune response. IgG is the only immunoglobulin that crosses the placental barrier and is incorporated into the circulatory system of the fetus, protecting the newborn against infection.

IgA is found in small amounts in serum. It is the main immunoglobulin found in tears, colostrum, and saliva; in nasal, bronchial, intestinal and prostatic secretions; and in the vaginal fluid. It is found in secretions as a dimer called **secretory IgA**, which is composed of 2 molecules of monomeric IgA united by a polypeptide chain called **protein J** and combined with another protein, the **secretory**, or **transport, component.** Because it is resistant to several enzymes, secretory IgA provides protection against the proliferation of microorganisms in body secretions. It also aids in defending the body against penetration by foreign molecules. IgA monomers and protein J are secreted by plasma cells in the mucous membranes that line the digestive, respiratory, and urinary passages; the secretory component is synthesized by the mucosal epithelial cells (see Fig 15–2).

IgM constitutes 10% of serum immunoglobulins

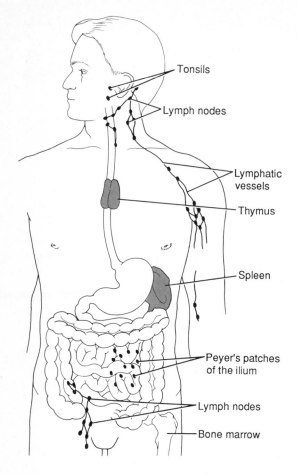

Figure 14–1. Distribution of lymphoid tissue in the body.

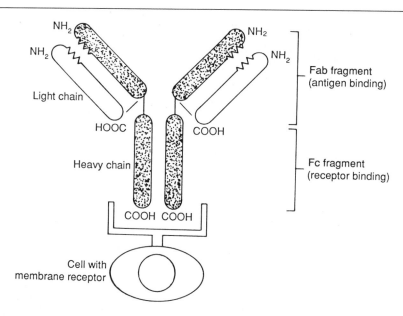

Figure 14–2. Structure and components of an immunoglobulin (antibody) molecule.

and usually exists as a pentamer with a molecular weight of 900,000. It is the dominant immunoglobulin in early immune responses and, together with IgD, is the major immunoglobulin found on the surfaces of B lymphocytes. These 2 classes of immunoglobulins exhibit both membrane-bound and circulating forms. Membrane-bound IgM and IgD serve as receptors for specific antigens. The result of this interaction is the proliferation and further differentiation of B lymphocytes, producing antibody-secreting plasma cells. IgM is also effective in activating the **complement system,** a group of plasma proteins that have the capacity to lyse cells, including bacteria.

IgE usually exists as a monomer. This immunoglobulin has a great affinity for receptors located in the plasma membranes of mast cells and basophils. Immediately after its secretion by plasma cells, IgE attaches to these cells and virtually disappears from the blood plasma. When the antigen that elicited the production of a certain IgE antibody is again encountered, the antigen-antibody complex formed on the surface of a mast cell or basophil triggers the production and liberation of several biologically active substances, such as histamine, heparin, leukotrienes, and ECF-A (eosinophil-chemotactic factor of anaphylaxis). An **allergic reaction** is thus mediated by the activity of IgE and the antigens **(allergens)** that stimulate its production (see discussion of mast cells in Chapter 5).

The properties and activities of **IgD** are not completely understood. It has a molecular weight of 180,000, and its concentration in blood plasma constitutes only 0.2% of the total of immunoglobulins. IgD is found on the plasma membranes of B lymphocytes (together with IgM) and is involved in the differentiation of these cells.

B & T Lymphocytes & Antigen-Presenting Cells

B lymphocytes derive from bone marrow and migrate to non-thymic lymphoid structures where they nest, proliferate when activated, and differentiate into antibody-secreting **plasma cells.** B cells represent 65% of the circulating lymphocytes; each is covered by 150,000 molecules of IgM that can form complexes with specific antigens. Some activated B cells do not become plasma cells; instead they generate **B memory cells,** which react very rapidly to a second exposure to the same antigen (Fig 14–3). **T cells** represent 35% of circulating lymphocytes. They originate in the bone marrow and migrate to the thymus, where they proliferate and produce cells that colonize and mature in non-thymic lymphoid tissues. In these structures, they differentiate further into subpopulations of **helper, suppressor, killer,** and **T memory cells.** Helper cells stimulate the differentiation of B cells into plasma cells. Killer cells (also called cytotoxic lymphocytes, or graft-rejecting cells) act directly by producing proteins **(perforins)** that open holes in foreign cell membranes, with consequent cell

lysis. Helper and suppressor cells are also known collectively as **regulator cells.** Memory T cells react rapidly to the reintroduction of antigen and stimulate production of T killer cells. Suppressor cells regulate both cellular and humoral immunity and inhibit the action of helper and killer cells.

> Helper T cells are killed by the retrovirus that causes the immunodeficiency syndrome known as AIDS, crippling the immunity of infected patients and rendering them susceptible to opportunistic infections—microorganisms that usually do not infect healthy individuals.

B and T cells are not uniformly distributed in the lymphoid system; they occupy special regions in non-thymic lymphoid structures (see Fig 14–20). Although B and T cells are morphologically not distinguishable in either light or electron microscopes, they can be distinguished by immunocytochemical methods. They exhibit different surface proteins (markers) that permit the identification and detection of differentiated subpopulations of these 2 types of cells. When stimulated by antigens, B and T cells produce large basophilic lymphoid cells called **immunoblasts,** whose cytoplasmic basophilia is due to large numbers of polyribosomes. These cells go through several mitotic cycles and may differentiate in several ways. B cells, for example, produce plasma cells whose cytoplasm is specialized for antibody synthesis and export.

Antigen-presenting cells are found in most tissues. They have the capacity to process antigens and retain the product for long periods, presenting them gradually to lymphocytes and thereby activating them. Antigen-presenting cells are derived from the bone marrow and constitute a heterogeneous population of cells that probably belong to the mononuclear phagocyte system (see Chapter 5). They include macrophages, epidermal Langerhans cells, dendritic cells of lymphoid organs, B lymphocytes, and epithelial cells of the thymus. Evidence suggests that antigen-presenting cells, in a process known as antigen processing, ingest foreign proteins, partially digest them in lysosomes, and return selected portions of the lysate to the cell surface. Antigen processing is a necessary preliminary step for the immune reaction since most antigens do not act directly on lymphocytes. These 3 families of cells—T, B, and antigen-presenting—interact continuously among themselves and with other components of the organism, resulting in an extremely efficient and complex immune system.

It is important to remember that several cell types secrete **interleukins,** hormonelike chemical messengers that control the activities of cells involved in immunologic reactions. At least 10 interleukins have been described so far. One of these, interleukin 4, which is produced by T lymphocytes, stimulates the differentiation of B lymphocytes (see Fig 14–3).

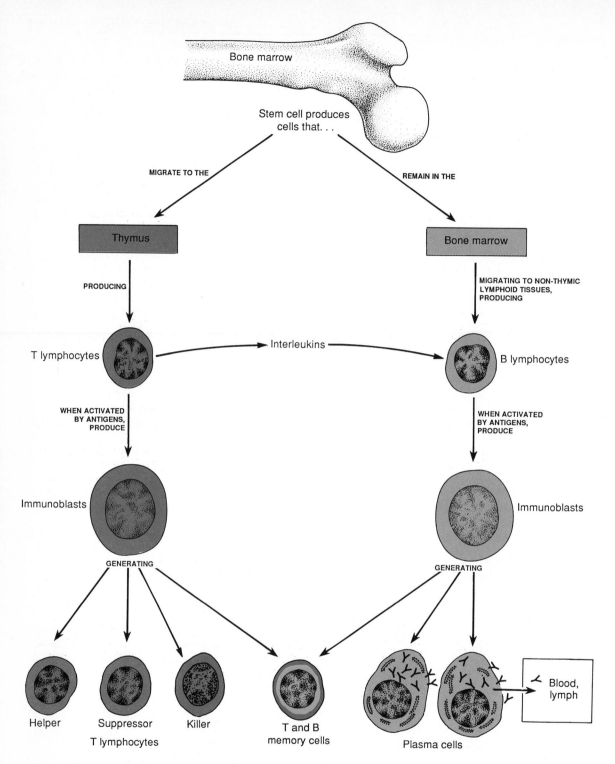

Figure 14–3. All lymphocytes originate from a stem cell, whose morphologic characteristics are not clear. This cell migrates through the blood and invades the thymus, dividing many times to form T lymphocytes (darker color). In birds, the stem cells are conditioned to become B lymphocytes (lighter color) in the bursa of Fabricius, a lymphatic organ located in the cloaca. The mammalian equivalent of the bursa of Fabricius is probably the bone marrow itself. After encountering an antigen, the lymphocyte modulates into a larger cell—the immunoblast—which then proliferates and produces more T lymphocytes or plasma cells. Thymus-dependent antigens promote the transformation of B lymphocytes into plasma cells only when T lymphocytes are also present. This phenomenon is called cooperation between T cells and B cells in antibody production.

The central nervous system also produces peptide hormones for which there are receptors on the surfaces of lymphocytes. This process establishes a poorly understood communication system of chemical messengers between the brain and the immune system, and gives some biochemical support to the empirical observation that the course of some diseases is influenced by the mood of the individuals involved.

THYMUS

The thymus is a lymphoepithelial organ located in the mediastinum; it attains its peak development during youth. While non-thymic lymphoid organs originate exclusively from mesenchyme (mesoderm), the thymus has a dual embryonic origin. Its lymphocytes arise from mesenchymal cells that invade an epithelial primordium that has developed from the endoderm of the third and fourth pharyngeal pouches.

The thymus has a connective tissue capsule that penetrates into the parenchyma and divides it into lobules. Each lobule has a peripheral dark zone known as the **cortex** and a central light zone, called the **medulla** (from Latin, *medius,* middle; see Fig 14–4).

Cortex

The cortex is composed of an extensive population of T lymphocytes, dispersed epithelial reticular cells, a few macrophages, and large lymphocytes. The epithelial reticular cells are stellate cells with lightly staining oval nuclei. They are joined to similar adjacent cells by desmosomes (Fig 14–5). Bundles of cytokeratin fibrils (tonofilaments) in their cytoplasm are evidence of the epithelial origin of these cells (Fig 14–6).

The intense proliferation of lymphocytes that takes place in the thymus during embryonic and prepubertal development pushes the epithelial cells apart. Since these cells are bound together by desmosomes, they remain attached to each other at the ends of their processes, creating an extensive network of epithelial reticular cells.

Because of the proliferation of large lymphocytes in the cortex, immature T lymphocytes are produced in quantity and accumulate in this region. Although most of these lymphocytes die in the cortex and are removed by macrophages, a small number migrate to the medulla and enter the blood stream there through the wall of venules. These cells migrate to non-thymic lymphoid structures and accumulate in specific sites as T lymphocytes (Fig 14–20).

Medulla

The medulla contains a large number of epithelial reticular cells and large and medium-sized lymphocytes; these cause it to stain more lightly than the cortex. The medulla also contains **Hassall's corpuscles,** which are characteristic of this region (Fig 14–7). These structures are concentrically arranged, flattened epithelial reticular cells that degenerate and become filled with keratohyalin granules and cyto-

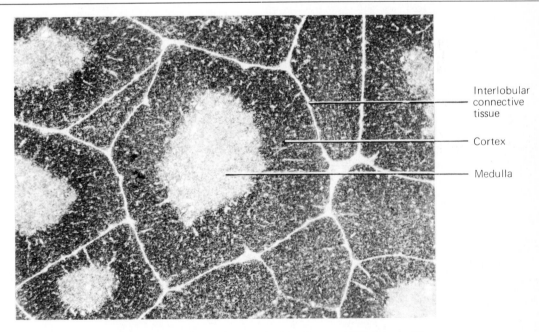

Figure 14–4. Photomicrograph of the thymus. H&E stain, × 32.

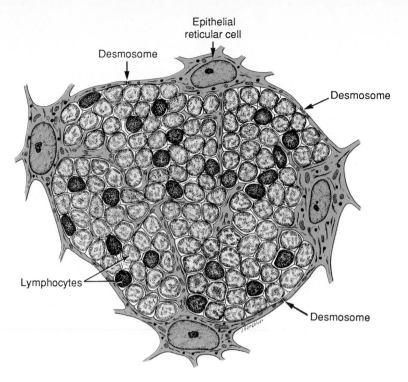

Figure 14–5. The relationship between epithelial reticular cells (shown in color) and thymic lymphocytes. Observe desmosomes and the long processes of epithelial reticular cells extending among the lymphocytes. Note also the absence of reticular fibers.

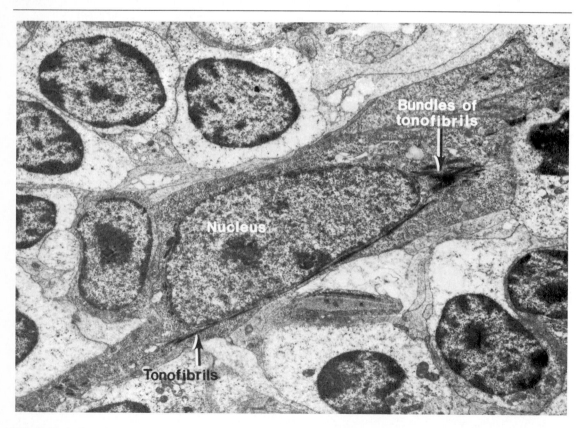

Figure 14–6. Thymic medulla seen under the electron microscope. An epithelial reticular cell runs diagonally across the figure. The nucleus has fine chromatin, and cytokeratin fibrils (tonofilament bundles) are present in the cytoplasm. × 7100.

266

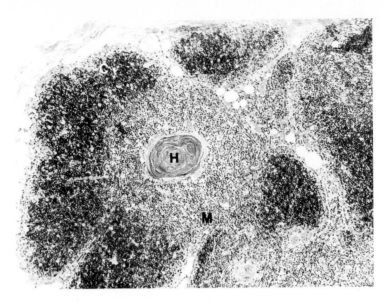

Figure 14–7. Photomicrograph of a human thymus, showing the dense cortical (C) and lighter medullary (M) zones. Near the center, one Hassall's corpuscle (H) appears in the medulla. Connective tissue septa form incomplete lobules. H&E stain, × 118.

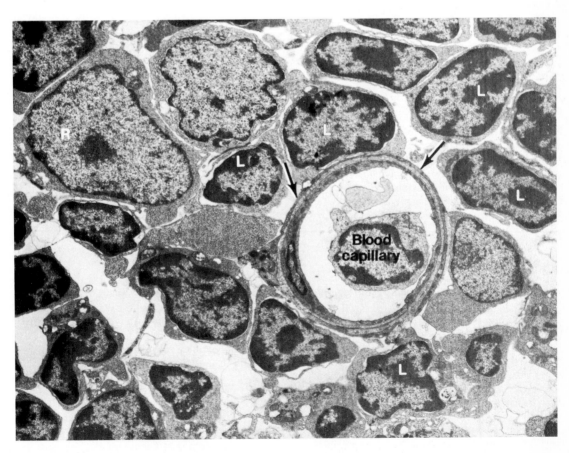

Figure 14–8. Electron micrograph of the thymic cortex. There is a blood capillary showing a thick basement membrane. Arrows point to the epithelial reticular cells covering it. These components that surround the capillary are responsible for the blood-thymus barrier. Note the lymphocytes (L) and the reticular cell (R). × 28,500.

keratin filaments. Hassall's corpuscles vary in size, according to the stage of development; their function is unknown.

Vascularization

Arteries enter the thymus through the capsule; they branch and penetrate the organ more deeply, following the septa of connective tissue. Arterioles leave the septa to penetrate the parenchyma along the border between the cortical and medullary zones. These arterioles give off capillaries that penetrate the cortex in an arched course; they finally reach the medulla, where they drain into venules. The medulla is supplied with capillary branches of the arterioles in the medullary-cortical border. The capillaries of the medulla drain into venules; the latter also receive capillaries returning from the cortical zone.

Thymic capillaries have a nonfenestrated endothelium and a very thick basal lamina. Endothelial cells have thin processes that perforate the basal lamina and may come in contact with epithelial reticular cells. Small vessels of the cortical parenchyma are surrounded by a sheath of epithelial reticular cells that form a **blood-thymus barrier.** This consists of pericytes, the capillary basal lamina, the basal lamina of the epithelial reticular cell, cells of the nonfenestrated endothelium, and the epithelial reticular cells themselves. This system prevents circulating antigens from reaching the thymic cortex where T lymphocytes are being formed (Fig 14–8).

Medullary veins penetrate the connective tissue septa and leave the thymus through its capsule. There is no blood-thymus barrier in the medulla.

The thymus has no afferent lymphatic vessels and does not constitute a filter for the lymph as do lymph nodes. The few lymphatic vessels encountered in the thymus are all efferent; they are localized in the walls of blood vessels and in the connective tissue of the septa and the capsule.

Histophysiology

The thymus shows its maximum development in relation to body weight immediately after birth; it undergoes involution after puberty. It is continually repopulated by cells derived from the bone marrow. These cells begin their differentiation into T cells, but leave the thymus (through blood vessels in the medulla) as immature T lymphocytes. These cells migrate, nest, and mature in thymus-dependent areas of non-thymic lymphoid organs. In mammals, the main thymus-dependent areas are the paracortical zones of lymph nodes, some parts of Peyer's patches, and the periarterial sheaths in the white pulp of the spleen. B lymphocytes, on the other hand, are found in lymphatic nodules of the spleen and lymph nodes as well as in Peyer's patches in the small intestine (see Fig 14–20).

In the congenital disorder **DiGeorge's Syndrome,** the thymus is either absent or atrophic, and afflicted individuals have low blood levels of lymphocytes (reduced B and no T). These individuals have abnormalities in their B cell immunity and no T cell immunity. The requirement for collaboration between T and B cells to provide normal immunologic reactions is thus not met in this defect in thymic development, which is responsible for early death from severe infections.

The thymus produces several protein growth factors that stimulate T lymphocyte proliferation and differentiation. Four of these factors have been identified: thymosin alpha, thymopoetin, thymolin, and thymic humoral factor. The thymus is also subject to the effects of several hormones. Injections of some adrenocorticosteroids cause a reduction in lymphocyte number and mitotic rate and atrophy of the cortical layer of the thymus. Adrenocorticotropic hormone (ACTH) produced by the anterior pituitary achieves the same effect by stimulating the activity of the adrenal cortex. Male and female sex hormones also accelerate thymic involution, while castration has the opposite effect.

Pituitary growth hormone (somatotropin) stimulates thymic development in a nonspecific way; it has a general effect on overall body growth.

ORGAN TRANSPLANTATION

Transplants are classified as **autografts** when the transplanted tissues or organs are taken from different sites on the individual receiving them, **isografts** when the tissues or organs are taken from an identical twin, **homografts** when taken from an individual (related or unrelated) of the same species, and **heterografts** when taken from animals of different species.

Autologous and isologous transplants take readily as long as an efficient blood supply is established. There is no rejection in such cases, because the transplanted cells are genetically identical or similar to those of the host and are composed of molecules that the organism recognizes as its own, and no cellular or humoral reactions occur.

Homologous and heterologous transplants, on the other hand, contain cells whose membranes have constituents that are foreign to the host; they are therefore recognized and treated as such. Transplant rejection is due mainly to the activity of **graft-rejection cells** (Fig 14–9). These cells are T lymphocytes that penetrate the transplant and act there to destroy the transplanted cells.

Although homografts are normally rejected, when this type of transplant is carried out between fraternal twins who shared the same placenta, the graft is not rejected. The organism will never form antibodies

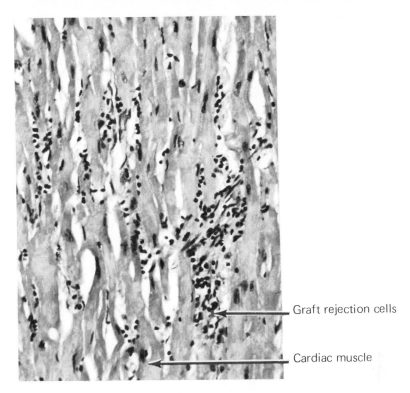

Figure 14–9. Photomicrograph of human myocardium from a transplanted and rejected heart. Among the cardiac muscle fibers that show degenerative changes are many T killer lymphocytes (graft-rejection cells). (Courtesy of T Brito).

against a substance that was present before its immune system started functioning. Only molecules that enter the body after the organism has become **immunocompetent** are recognized as foreign and treated as antigens. In humans, the infant is protected during the first few days of life by antibodies received from the mother through the placenta. This is a passive immunity that protects against infection until the child's own cells begin to produce antibodies; the synthesis of antibodies begins a few days after birth. When the body's cells are modified by disease, they may present foreign substances that generate autoimmune reactions against these modified cells. These **autoimmune diseases** may also be caused by poorly understood changes that occur in lymphoid cells and cause them to become aggressive toward normal (self) macromolecules.

LYMPH NODES

Lymph nodes are encapsulated spherical or kidney-shaped organs composed of lymphoid tissue. They are distributed throughout the body along the course of the lymphatic vessels. The nodes are found in the axilla and groin, along the great vessels of the neck, and in large numbers in the thorax and abdomen,

especially in mesenteries. Lymph nodes constitute a series of in-line filters that are important in the body's defense against microorganisms and the spread of tumor cells. All tissue-fluid-derived lymph is filtered by at least one node before returning to the circulatory system. Lymph nodes have a convex side and a concave depression, the **hilum** (sometimes spelled **hilus**), through which arteries and nerves enter and veins and lymphatic vessels leave the organ. The shape and internal structure of lymph nodes vary greatly, but all have the basic pattern of organization illustrated in Figs 14–10 and 14–11.

The connective tissue **capsule** that surrounds each lymph node sends trabeculae into its interior. Each node contains an **outer** and **inner cortex** and a **medulla** (see Fig 14–10).

Cortices

A. Outer Cortex: At the surface of the outer cortex is the **subcapsular sinus** (from Latin, a hollow), which is limited on its outer boundary by the capsule and on its inner boundary by the outer cortex. It is formed by a loose network of macrophages and reticular cells and fibers. The subcapsular sinus communicates with the medullary sinuses through **intermediate sinuses** that run parallel to the capsular trabeculae. The **outer cortex** is formed by lymphoid

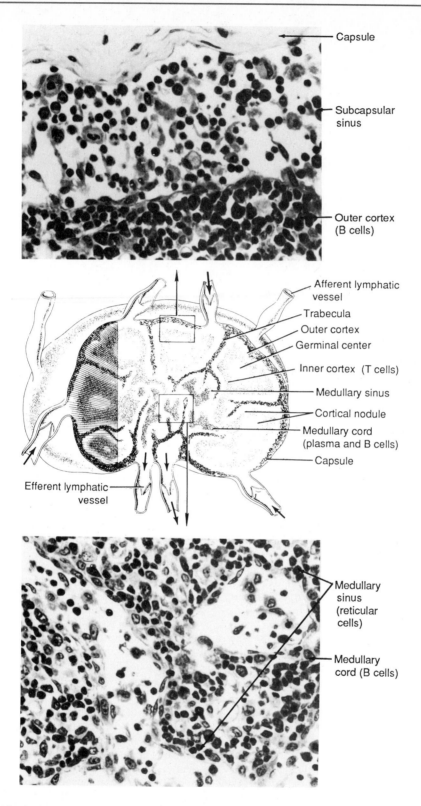

Figure 14–10. Histologic structure of a lymph node. The rectangular areas in the center drawing are magnified in the upper and lower photographs. The cortical layer is composed mainly of lymphoid nodules, whose germinal centers (lightly stained core of each nodule) are clearly seen in the center drawing.

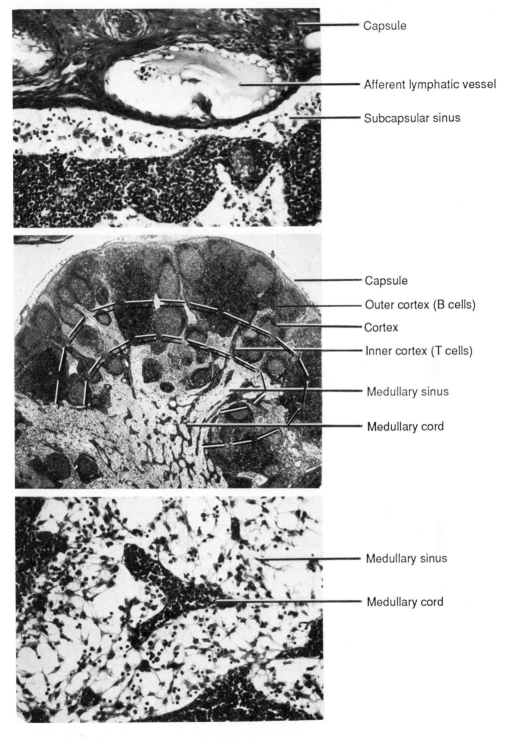

Capsule

Afferent lymphatic vessel

Subcapsular sinus

Capsule

Outer cortex (B cells)

Cortex

Inner cortex (T cells)

Medullary sinus

Medullary cord

Medullary sinus

Medullary cord

Figure 14–11. Photomicrographs of lymph nodes, reduced from × 30 (middle) and × 200 (top and bottom) magnification. H&E stain.

tissue consisting of a network of reticular cells and fibers whose meshwork is populated by lymphoid cells. Within the cortical lymphoid tissue are spherical structures called **lymphoid nodules.**

B. Inner Cortex: The inner cortex is a continuation of the outer cortex and contains few, if any, nodules.

Medulla

The medulla is composed of the **medullary cords,** cordlike, branched extensions of the lymphoid tissue of the inner cortex, which are separated by dilated, capillarylike structures called **medullary lymphoid sinuses** (see Figs 14–10 and 14–11). These are irregular spaces containing lymph; like the subcapsular and intermediate sinuses, they are partially lined by reticular cells and macrophages. Reticular cells and fibers frequently bridge the sinus with a loose network. Large branched **dendritic (follicular) cells** are found in the lymph nodes and function as antigen-presenting cells.

Circulation

Afferent lymphatic vessels cross the capsule of each node and pour lymph into the subcapsular sinus. From there, lymph passes through intermediate sinuses that run parallel to the trabeculae of the capsule and into the interior of the node, where they reach the medullary sinuses. The complex architecture of both the subcapsular and medullary sinuses slows the flow of lymph through the node, facilitating the uptake and digestion of foreign materials by macrophages. Lymph also infiltrates lymphoid tissue and flows slowly from cortex to medulla and is collected by **efferent lymphatic vessels** (Fig 14–10) at the hilum of each node. Valves in both the afferent and efferent vessels aid the unidirectional flow of lymph.

Penetration of blood vessels into lymph nodes is limited to small arteries that enter at the hilum and form capillaries in the lymphoid nodules. In the nodules, small veins originate and exit at the hilum.

Histophysiology

Lymph flows through the lymph nodes to be cleared of foreign particles before its return to the blood circulatory system. Because the nodes are distributed throughout the body, lymph formed in tissues must cross at least one node before entering the bloodstream.

Each node receives lymph from, and is said to be a **satellite node** of, a limited region of the body. Malignant tumors often metastasize via these nodes.

As lymph flows through the sinuses, 99% or more of the antigens and other debris are removed by phagocytotic activity of the macrophages that span the sinuses. Infection and antigenic stimulation cause the affected lymph nodes to enlarge and form multiple germinal centers with active cell proliferation. While plasma cells constitute 1–3% of the cell population in resting nodes, their numbers increase greatly in stimulated lymph nodes and partially account for the enlargement of those structures.

Lymphoid nodules can be classified as **primary** and **secondary** nodules based on their morphologic characteristics. Primary nodules are spherical accumulations of lymphocytes with no clear central regions. These nodules appear in lymph nodes that have not been exposed to antigens, such as those of newborns or animals kept under sterile conditions. The secondary nodule presents a clear zone—a **germinal center**—in its interior (see Figs 14–10 and 14–11). This is a collection of activated, cytoplasm-rich lymphocytes (immunoblasts) that appears only after birth in response to antigen exposure, which stimulates proliferation of B lymphocytes in non-thymic lymphoid tissue.

Recirculation of Lymphocytes:
A Communication System

Lymphocytes leave the lymphoid nodes by efferent lymphatic vessels and eventually reach the blood stream—all lymph formed in the body drains back into the blood. Lymphocytes return to the lymph nodes by leaving the blood through specific blood vessels, the **postcapillary,** or **high endothelial, venules.** These venules have an unusual endothelial lining of tall cuboidal cells, and the lymphocytes are capable of traveling between them. Some lymphocytes are long-living cells and can recirculate many times in this way. High endothelial venules are also present in other lymphoid organs such as the spleen, tonsils, and Peyer's patches. While recirculation of lymphocytes also occurs here, it is most prominent in the lymph nodes.

This homing behavior is due to complementary molecules on the surface of lymphocytes and the tall endothelial cells of postcapillary venules. It seems that through recirculation, locally stimulated lymphocytes (eg, in an infected finger) from satellite lymph nodes will inform other lymphoid organs, and prepare the organism for a generalized immune response against the infection. The continuous recirculation of lymphocytes results in a constant monitoring of all parts of the body by cells that inform the immune system of the presence of foreign antigens.

SPLEEN

The spleen is the largest accumulation of lymphoid tissues in the organism; it is the largest lymphoid organ in the human circulatory system. Because of its abundance of phagocytotic cells and the close contact between circulating blood and these cells, the spleen

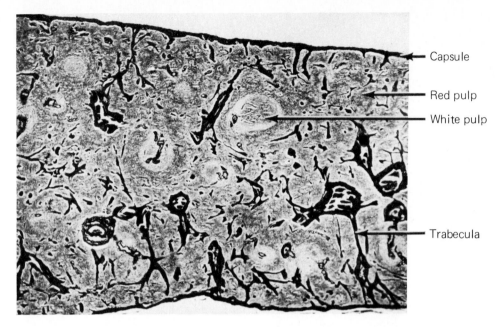

Figure 14–12. Photomicrograph of a silver-stained spleen section, showing the general architecture of the organ. × 30.

represents an important defense against any microorganisms that penetrate the circulation. It is also the site of destruction of many red cells. As is true of all other lymphoid organs, the spleen is a formation site for activated lymphocytes, which pass into the blood. The spleen reacts promptly to antigens carried in the blood and is an important immunologic filter and antibody-forming organ.

General Structure

The spleen is surrounded by a capsule of dense connective tissue that sends out trabeculae that divide the **parenchyma,** or **splenic pulp,** into incomplete compartments (Fig 14–12). At the hilum on the medial surface of the spleen, the capsule gives rise to a number of trabeculae that carry nerves and arteries into the splenic pulp. Veins derived from the parenchyma and lymphatic vessels that originate in the trabeculae leave through the hilum. The splenic pulp has no lymphatic vessels.

In humans, the connective tissue of the capsule and trabeculae contains only a few smooth muscle cells. The spleen, like other lymphoid structures, is formed by a network of reticular tissue that contains lymphoid cells, macrophages, and antigen-presenting cells (Fig 14–16).

Splenic Pulp

On the surface of a cut through an unfixed spleen, one can observe white spots in the parenchyma. These are lymphoid nodules and are part of the **white pulp.**

The nodules appear within the **red pulp,** a dark red tissue that is rich in blood (Figs 14–12, 14–13 and 14–15). Examination under a low-power microscope reveals that the red pulp is composed of elongated structures, the splenic cords **(Billroth's cords),** that lie between the sinusoids (Fig 14–13). The sinusoidal endothelium is formed by fenestrated flattened cells (Fig 14–14) that permit easy communication between its interior and the red pulp.

Blood Circulation

The splenic artery divides as it penetrates the hilum, branching into **trabecular arteries,** vessels of various sizes that follow the course of the connective tissue trabeculae. When they leave the trabeculae to enter the parenchyma, the arteries are immediately enveloped by a sheath of lymphocytes (the **periarterial lymphatic sheath [PALS]**). These vessels are known as **central arteries** or **white pulp arteries.** Although the lymphocytic sheath (white pulp) thickens along its course to form a number of lymphoid nodules in which the vessel occupies an eccentric position (Figs 14–17 and 14–18), the vessel is still called the central artery. During its course through the white pulp, the artery also divides into numerous radial branches that supply the surrounding lymphoid tissue.

After leaving the white pulp, the central artery subdivides to form straight **penicillar arterioles** with an outside diameter of approximately 24 μm. Near their termination, some of the penicillar arterioles are sur-

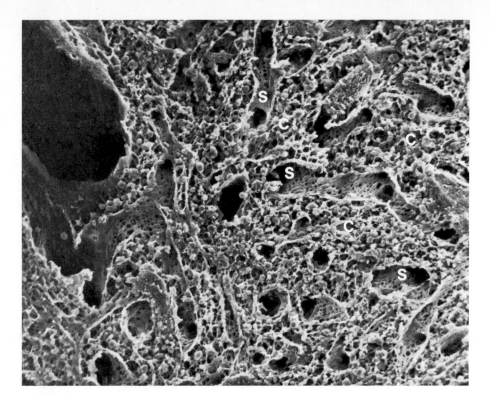

Figure 14–13. General view of splenic red pulp with a scanning electron microscope. Note the sinusoids (S) and the splenic cords (C). × 360. (Reproduced, with permission, from Miyoshi M, Fujita T: Stereo-fine structure of the splenic red pulp: A combined scanning and transmission electron microscope study on dog and rat spleen. *Arch Histol Jpn* 1971;**33**:225.)

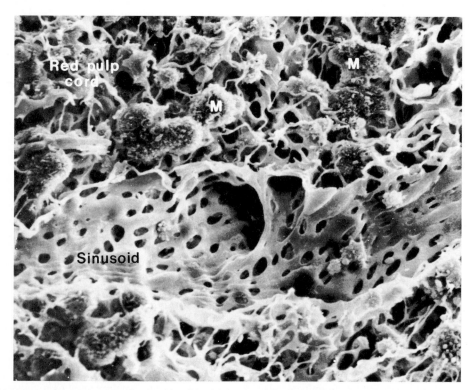

Figure 14–14. Scanning electron micrograph of the red pulp of the spleen showing sinusoids, red pulp cords, and macrophages (M). Observe the multiple fenestrations in the endothelial cells of the sinusoids. × 1600. (Reproduced, with permission, from Miyoshi M, Fujita T: Stereo-fine structure of the splenic red pulp. A combined scanning and transmission electron microscope study on dog and rat spleen. *Arch Histol Jpn* 1971;**33**:225.)

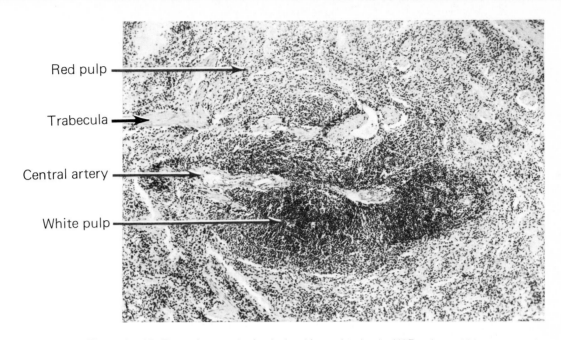

Red pulp

Trabecula

Central artery

White pulp

Figure 14–15. Photomicrograph of splenic white and red pulp. H&E stain, × 100.

rounded by a sheath of reticular cells, lymphoid cells, and macrophages.

Beyond the sheath, the vessels continue as simple arterial capillaries that carry blood to the sinusoids (red pulp sinuses). These sinusoids occupy the area between the red pulp cords (Figs 14–13 and 14–17). The manner in which blood flows from the arterial capillaries of the red pulp to the interior of the sinusoids has not yet been completely explained. Some investigators suggest that the capillaries open directly into the sinusoids, while others maintain that the blood passes through the spaces between the red pulp cord cells and then moves on to be collected by the sinusoids (Figs 14–17 and 14–19). In the first instance, this would mean a closed circulation; ie, the blood always remains inside the vessels. In the second case, the circulation would open into the parenchyma of the red pulp (Billroths's cords), and the blood would pass through the area between the cells in order to reach the sinusoids (open circulation).

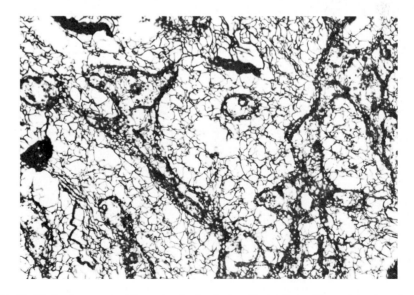

Figure 14–16. Photomicrograph of the network of splenic reticular fibers. Silver-stained section, × 200.

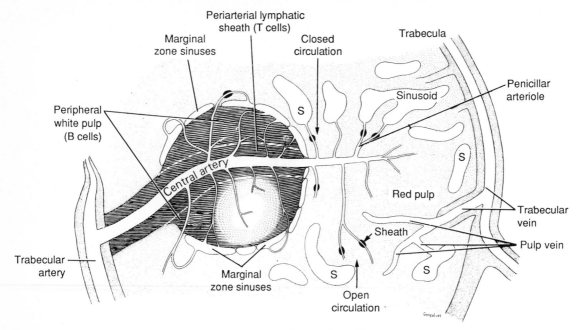

Figure 14–17. Schematic view of the blood circulation of the spleen. Theories of open and closed circulation are represented in this drawing. Splenic sinuses (S) are indicated. (Redrawn and reproduced, with permission, from Greep RO, Weiss L: *Histology*, 3rd ed. McGraw-Hill, 1973.)

Current evidence suggests that blood circulation in the human spleen is of the open type.

From the sinusoids, blood proceeds to the red pulp veins that join together and enter the trabeculae, forming the **trabecular veins** (Fig 14–17). The splenic vein originates from these vessels and emerges from the hilum of the spleen. The trabecular veins do not have individual muscle walls; ie, their walls are composed of trabecular tissue. They can be considered

channels hollowed out in the trabecular connective tissue and lined by endothelium.

White Pulp

White pulp consists of lymphoid tissue that ensheathes both the central arteries and the lymphoid nodules appended to the sheaths. The lymphoid cells surrounding the central arteries are mainly T lymphocytes and form the periarterial lymphatic sheaths (Fig

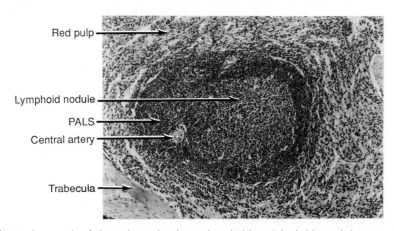

Figure 14–18. Photomicrograph of the spleen showing a lymphoid nodule (white pulp) surrounded by red pulp. × 150.

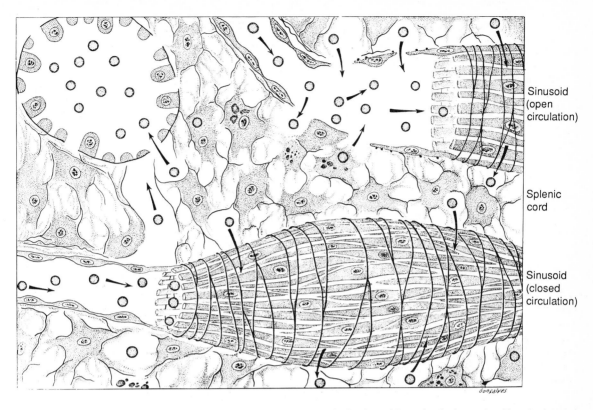

Figure 14–19. Structure of the red pulp of the spleen, showing splenic sinusoids and splenic cords with reticular and phagocytic cells (some with ingested material). The disposition of the reticular fibers in the red pulp is illustrated. In the splenic cords they form a 3-dimensional network; in the sinusoids they are mainly perpendicular to the long axis of the sinusoid. The figure illustrates both the open and closed theories of circulation.

14–17). Lymphoid nodules consist of a preponderance of B lymphocytes.

Between the white pulp and the red pulp lies a **marginal zone** consisting of many sinuses and of loose lymphoid tissue. There are few lymphocytes but many active macrophages here. The marginal zone contains an abundance of blood antigens and thus plays a major role in the immunologic activities of the spleen. Many of the pulp arterioles derived from the central artery extend out and away from the white pulp but then turn back and empty into sinuses of the marginal zone that encircles the nodules. As a consequence of this drainage, which includes the added blood flow from vessels within the white pulp that also terminate in the marginal zone, this area plays a significant role in filtering the blood and initiating an immune response. In addition, large numbers of macrophages remove antigenic debris.

Interdigitating dendritic cells in the marginal zone trap and present antigens to immunologically competent cells. The marginal zone removes not only antigens but also T and B lymphocytes from the blood. As lymphocytes leave the systemic circula-

tion to penetrate the white pulp, they pass dendritic cells. If the appropriate B cells, T cells, and antigen are present, an immune response will be initiated. Activated B cells migrate to the center of the white pulp nodule and give rise to plasma cells and memory B cells. Plasma cells migrate to the splenic cords and release antibodies into the blood in the sinuses.

The lymphocytes of the central portion of the periarterial lymphatic sheaths are **thymus-dependent,** while the marginal zones and the nodules—the **peripheral white pulp**—are populated by B lymphocytes. As a result, B and T lymphocytes are segregated in 2 different sites in the splenic white pulp (Fig 14–20).

Red Pulp

The red pulp is a reticular tissue with a special characteristic, the splenic cords. These structures, which include all cells between the sinusoids, are continuous; the thickness varies according to the local distention of the sinusoids. In addition to reticular cells and fibers, the splenic cords contain macrophages, lymphocytes, plasma cells, and many

LYMPH NODE

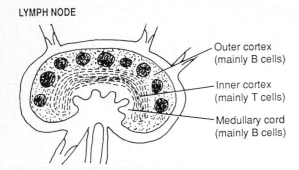

Outer cortex (mainly B cells)

Inner cortex (mainly T cells)

Medullary cord (mainly B cells)

SPLEEN

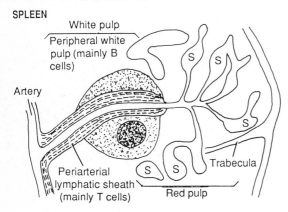

White pulp

Peripheral white pulp (mainly B cells)

Artery

Periarterial lymphatic sheath (mainly T cells)

Red pulp

Trabecula

Figure 14–20. Distribution of B and T cells in lymph nodes and spleen. S, sinusoid.

blood elements (erythrocytes, platelets, and granulocytes).

The sinusoids of the spleen contain elongated endothelial cells with long axes parallel to the long axes of the sinusoids. These cells are enveloped in reticular fibers set mainly in a transverse direction, similar to the hoops on a barrel. The transverse and longitudinal fibers join to form a network enveloping the sinusoid cells and macrophages that occupy the spaces between neighboring endothelial cells (Fig 14–19). Like liver sinusoids, macrophages present in these structures are for phagocytotic activity.

The spaces between cells of the splenic sinusoids are 2–3 μm in diameter or smaller (Fig 14–14), so that only flexible cells are able to pass easily from the red pulp cords to the lumen of the sinusoids.

> Sickle cell disease is a molecular disease in which a glutamic acid residue in the B chain of normal hemoglobin is replaced by a valine residue. This causes profound changes in the conformation of hemoglobin molecules when they are exposed to hypoxic environments, as in the spleen. Under these conditions, hemoglobin crystallizes and forms long aggregates that deform the red blood cell into a characteristic

sickle shape (Fig 12–6). These cells, because of their increased rigidity, cannot pass between the endothelial cells lining the splenic sinusoids. The cells are destroyed here, and anemia results.

As already stated, the non-thymic lymphoid structures have regions that are populated by cells of the T or B family. Fig 14–20 gives a general idea of their distribution in the lymph nodes and spleen.

Histophysiology

The spleen is a lymphoid organ with special characteristics. Its best-known functions are the formation of lymphocytes, destruction of erythrocytes, defense of the organism against foreign particles that enter the bloodstream, and storage of blood.

A. Production of Lymphocytes: The white pulp of the spleen produces lymphocytes that migrate to the red pulp and reach the lumens of the sinusoids, where they are incorporated into the blood.

> In certain pathologic conditions (eg, leukemia), the spleen may reinitiate the production of granulocytes and erythrocytes present during fetal life, undergoing a process known as **myeloid metaplasia** (the occurrence of myeloid tissues in extramedullary sites; a syndrome characterized by splenomegaly (enlarged spleen), anemia, and the presence of immature granulocytes and nucleated erythrocytes).

B. Destruction of Erythrocytes: Red blood cells have an average life span of 120 days, after which they are destroyed, mainly in the spleen. The removal of degenerating erythrocytes also occurs in the bone marrow.

Macrophages in the splenic cords engulf and digest entire pieces of erythrocytes that frequently fragment in the extracellular spaces. The hemoglobin they contain is broken down into several parts. The protein, globin, is hydrolyzed to amino acids that are reused in protein synthesis. Iron is released from heme and transported in blood, in combination with transferrin, to the bone marrow where it is reused in erythropoiesis. Iron-free heme is metabolized to **bilirubin,** which is excreted in the bile by liver cells.

C. Defense of the Organism: Since it contains both B and T lymphocytes as well as antigen-presenting cells and macrophages, the spleen is important in body defense. In the same way that lymph nodes are a filter for the lymph, the spleen is considered a filter for the blood. Of all the phagocytotic cells of the organism, those of the spleen are most active in the phagocytosis of living (bacteria and viruses) and inert particles that find their way into the bloodstream.

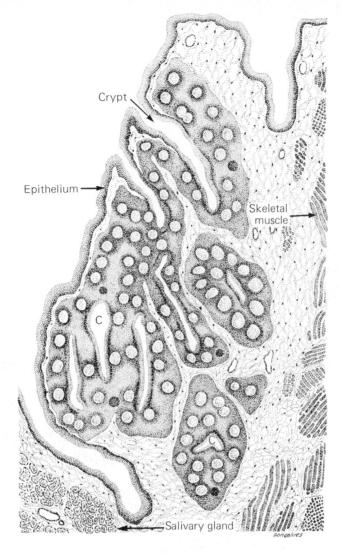

Figure 14–21. Palatine tonsil. There are numerous lymphatic nodules near the stratified squamous epithelium of the oropharynx. The light areas in the lymphoid tissue are germinal centers. Note the sections through the epithelial crypts (C).

UNENCAPSULATED LYMPHOID TISSUE

Lymphoid, or **lymphatic, nodules** also called **lymphatic follicles,** can be found isolated or aggregated in the loose connective tissues of several organs—mainly in the lamina propria of the digestive tract, upper respiratory tract, and urinary passages. Unencapsulated nodules have the same microscopic structure as do nodules in the cortex of a lymph node. They are composed of densely packed lymphocytes (mainly B lymphocytes) that differentiate into plasma cells upon appropriate antigenic stimulation.

Peyer's patches are aggregates of unencapsulated nodules found in the lamina propria of the ileum. They are discussed more extensively in Chapter 15.

TONSILS

Tonsils are organs composed of aggregates of incompletely encapsulated lymphoid tissues that lie beneath, but in contact with, the epithelium of the initial portion of the digestive tract. According to their location, tonsils in the mouth and pharynx are called **palatine, pharyngeal,** or **lingual tonsils.** Tonsils produce lymphocytes, many of which infiltrate the epithelium.

Epithelium with
some infiltration

Heavily infiltrated
epithelium

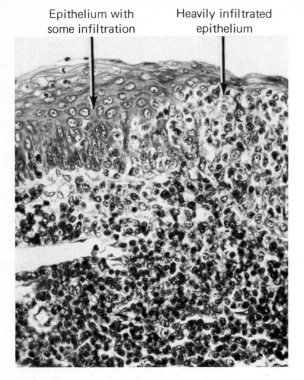

Figure 14–22. Photomicrograph of a palatine tonsil. The stratified squamous epithelium is infiltrated by lymphocytes. H&E stain, × 400.

Palatine Tonsils

The 2 palatine tonsils are located in the lateral walls of the oral part of the pharynx. The dense lymphoid tissue present in these tonsils forms, under the squamous stratified epithelium, a band that contains lymphoid nodules, generally with germinal centers. Each tonsil has 10–20 epithelial invaginations that penetrate the parenchyma deeply, forming **crypts,** whose lumens contain desquamated epithelial cells, live and dead lymphocytes, and bacteria (Figs 14–21 and 14–22). They may appear as purulent spots in tonsilitis. Separating the lymphoid tissue from subjacent structures is a band of dense connective tissue, the **capsule** of the tonsil. This capsule usually acts as a barrier against spreading tonsillar infections.

Pharyngeal Tonsil

This is a single tonsil situated in the superoposterior portion of the pharyx. It is covered by ciliated pseudostratified columnar epithelium typical of the respiratory tract, and areas of stratified epithelium can also be observed.

The pharyngeal tonsil is composed of pleats of mucosa and shows diffuse lymphoid tissue and lymphatic nodules. It has no crypts, and its capsule is thinner than those of the palatine tonsils.

Lingual Tonsils

The lingual tonsils are smaller and more numerous than the others. They are situated at the base of the tongue (Fig 15–3) and are covered by stratified squamous epithelium. Each has a single crypt.

REFERENCES

Alberts B et al: The immune system. In: *Molecular Biology of the Cell,* 2nd ed. Garland, 1989.

Balfour BM et al: Antigen-presenting cells, including Langerhans cells, veiled cells, and interdigitating cells. *Ciba Found Symp* 1981;**84**:281.

Darnell J, Lodish H, Baltimore D: Immunity. In: *Molecular Cell Biology,* 2nd ed. Scientific American Books, 1990.

Douglas SD: Development and structure of cells in the immune system. In: *Basic & Clinical Immunology,* 4th ed. Stites DP et al (editors). Lange, 1982.

Hoefsmit ECM: Macrophages, Langerhans cells, interdigitating and dendritic accessory cells: A summary. *Adv Exp Med Biol* 1982;**149**:463.

Raviola E, Karnovsky MJ: Evidence for a blood-thymus barrier using electron opaque tracers. *J Exp Med* 1972;**136**:466.

Stevens SK, Weissman IL, Butcher EC: Differences in the migration of B and T lymphocytes: Organ-selective localization in vivo and the role of lymphocyte-endothelial cell recognition. *J Immunol* 1982;**128**:844.

Volk P, Meyer LM: The histology of reactive lymph nodes. *Am J Surg Pathol* 1987;**11**:866.

Weiss L: *The Cells and Tissues of the Immune System.* Prentice-Hall, 1972.

Weigent DA, Blalock JE: Interactions between the neuroendocrine and immune systems: Common hormones and receptors. *Immunol Rev* 1987;**100**:79.

Digestive Tract

15

The digestive system consists of the digestive tract—oral cavity, mouth, esophagus, stomach, small and large intestines, rectum, and anus—and its associated glands—salivary glands, liver, and pancreas. Its function is to obtain from ingested food the metabolites necessary for the growth and energy needs of the body. Food is digested and transformed into small molecules that can be easily absorbed through the lining of the digestive tract. Nonetheless, a barrier between the environment and the internal milieu of the body must still be maintained.

The first step in the complex process known as digestion occurs in the mouth, where food is ground by the teeth into smaller pieces and moistened by saliva, which also initiates the digestion of carbohydrates. Digestion continues in the stomach and small intestine, where the food—transformed into its basic components (amino acids, monosaccharides, free fatty acids, monoglycerides, etc)—is absorbed. Water absorption occurs in the large intestine, causing the undigested contents to become semisolid.

GENERAL STRUCTURE OF THE DIGESTIVE TRACT

The entire gastrointestinal tract presents certain common structural characteristics. The digestive tract is a hollow tube composed of a lumen of variable diameter surrounded by a wall made up of 4 principal layers: the **mucosa, submucosa, muscularis,** and **serosa.** The structure of these layers is summarized below and illustrated in Fig 15–1.

The **mucosa** comprises an **epithelial lining;** a **lamina propria** of loose connective tissue rich in blood and lymph vessels and smooth muscle cells, sometimes also containing glands and lymphoid tissue; and the **muscularis mucosae,** usually consisting of a thin inner circular layer and an outer longitudinal layer of smooth muscle cells separating the mucosa from the submucosa. The mucosa is frequently called a **mucous membrane.**

The **submucosa** is composed of loose connective tissue with many blood and lymph vessels and a **submucosal** (also called **Meissner's**) **nerve plexus.** It may also contain glands and lymphoid tissue.

The **muscularis** contains smooth muscle cells that are spirally oriented and divided into 2 sublayers according to the main direction the muscle cells follow. In the internal sublayer (close to the lumen), the orientation is generally circular; in the external sublayer, it is mostly longitudinal. It also contains the **myenteric** (or **Auerbach's**) **nerve plexus,** which lies between the 2 muscle sublayers; and blood and lymph vessels in the connective tissue between the muscle sublayers.

The **serosa** is a thin layer of loose connective tissue, rich in blood and lymph vessels and adipose tissue, and a simple squamous covering epithelium (mesothelium).

The main functions of the epithelial lining of the digestive tract are to provide a selectively permeable barrier between the contents of the tract and the tissues of the body; to facilitate the transport and digestion of food; to promote the absorption of the products of this digestion; and to produce hormones that affect the activity of the digestive system. Cells in this layer either produce mucus or are involved in digestion or absorption of food.

The abundant lymphoid nodules in the lamina propria and the submucosal layer protect the organism (in association with the epithelium) from bacterial invasion. The necessity for this immunologic support is obvious since the entire digestive tract—with the exception of the oral cavity, esophagus, and anal canal—is lined by a simple thin and vulnerable epithelium. Careful study of the lamina propria has demonstrated that just below the epithelium is a zone rich in macrophages and lymphoid cells, some of which actively produce antibodies. These antibodies are mainly immunoglobulin A (IgA) and are bound to a secretory protein produced by the epithelial cells of the intestinal lining and secreted into the intestinal lumen (Fig 15–2). This complex is thought to provide a protective activity against viral and bacterial invasion. It is significant that there are 20–30 IgA-secreting cells for every IgG-producing cell in the submucosa and that IgM-secreting cells are 5 times more numerous than IgG cells.

As discussed in Chapter 14, the IgA present in the respiratory, digestive, and urinary tracts is resistant to proteolytic enzymes. It is therefore more active than IgG (which does not have this resistance), providing

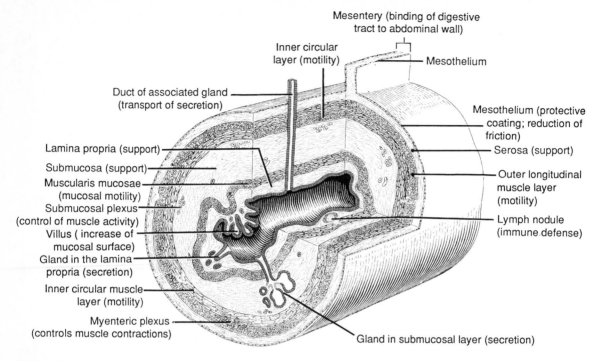

Figure 15–1. Schematic structure of a portion of the digestive tract with various components and their functions. (Redrawn and reproduced, with permission, from Bevelander G: *Outline of Histology,* 7th ed. Mosby, 1971.)

an antibody that can coexist with the proteases present in the intestinal lumen.

The muscularis mucosae promotes the movement of the mucosa independent of other movements of the digestive tract, increasing its contact with the food. The contractions of the muscularis, generated and coordinated by nerve plexuses, propel and mix the food in the digestive tract. These plexuses are composed mainly of nerve cell aggregates (multipolar visceral neurons) that form small parasympathetic ganglia. A rich network of pre- and postganglionic fibers of the autonomic nervous system and some visceral sensory fibers in these ganglia permit communication between them. The number of these ganglia along the digestive tract is variable. They are more numerous in regions of greatest motility.

In certain diseases, such as **Hirschsprung's disease** or **Trypanosoma cruzi** infection (**Chagas disease**), the digestive tract plexuses are severely injured and most of their neurons are destroyed. This results in disturbances of digestive tract motility with frequent dilatations in some areas. The fact that the digestive tract receives abundant innervation from the autonomic nervous system provides an anatomic explanation of the widely observed action of emotional disturbances on the digestive tract—a phenomenon of importance in psychosomatic medicine.

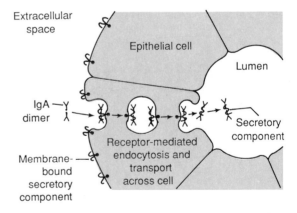

Figure 15–2. The mechanism by which the secretory component mediates the transport of a dimeric IgA molecule across an epithelial cell. The IgA dimer is synthesized by lymphocytes of the lamina propria. The secretory component is synthesized by the epithelial cell as a transmembrane glycoprotein and serves as a receptor on its basolateral surface for binding the IgA dimer. The secretory-component-IgA complex enters the cell and is exocytosed at the apical surface. The part of the secretory component that is bound to the IgA dimer is then cleaved from its transmembrane tail (black dot), releasing the complex into the lumen. (Reproduced, with permission, from Alberts B et al: *Molecular Biology of the Cell,* Garland, 1983.)

THE ORAL CAVITY

The oral cavity is lined with nonkeratinized stratified squamous epithelium. Its superficial cells are nucleated, with scanty granules of keratin in their interiors. In the lips, a transition from nonkeratinized to keratinized epithelium can be observed. The lamina propria has papillae, similar to those in the dermis of the skin, and is continuous with a submucosa containing diffuse small salivary glands.

The roof of the mouth consists of the hard and soft palates, both covered with the same type of stratified squamous epithelium. In the hard palate, the mucous membrane rests on bony tissue. The soft palate has a core of skeletal muscle and numerous mucous glands in its submucosa.

The palatine **uvula** is a small conical process that extends downward from the center of the lower border of the soft palate. It has a core of muscle and areolar connective tissue covered by typical oral mucosa.

1. TONGUE

The tongue is a mass of striated muscle covered by a mucous membrane whose structure varies according to the region. The muscle fibers cross one another in 3 planes; they are grouped in bundles, usually separated by connective tissue. Because the connective tissue of the lamina propria penetrates the spaces between the muscular bundles, the mucous membrane

is strongly adherent to the muscle. The mucous membrane is smooth on the lower surface of the tongue. The tongue's dorsal surface is irregular, covered anteriorly by a great number of small eminences called **papillae.** The posterior one-third of the dorsal surface of the tongue is separated from the anterior two-thirds by a V-shaped boundary. Behind this boundary, the surface of the tongue shows small bulges composed mainly of 2 types of small lymphoid aggregations: small collections of lymphoid nodules; and the lingual tonsils, where lymphoid nodules aggregate around invaginations (crypts) of the mucous membrane (Fig 15–3).

Papillae

Papillae are elevations of the oral epithelium and lamina propria that assume different forms and functions. There are 4 types:

A. Filiform Papillae: These papillae have an elongated conical shape; they are quite numerous and are present over the entire surface of the tongue. Their epithelium, which does not contain taste buds, is frequently partly keratinized (Fig 15–3).

B. Fungiform Papillae: These resemble mushrooms in that they have a narrow stall and a smooth-surfaced, dilated upper part (Fig 15–3). These papillae, which contain scattered taste buds on their upper surfaces, are irregularly interspersed among the filiform papillae.

C. Foliate Papillae: These papillae are poorly developed in humans. They consist of 2 or more parallel ridges and furrows on the dorsolateral surface of the

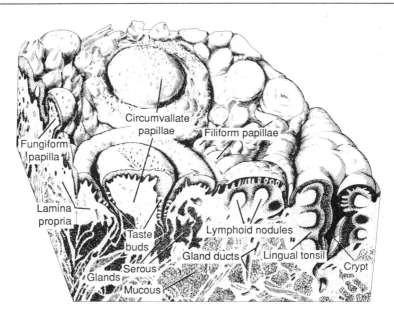

Figure 15–3. Surface of tongue on the region close to its V-shaped boundary between the anterior and posterior portions. Observe the lymphoid nodules, lingual tonsils, glands, and papillae.

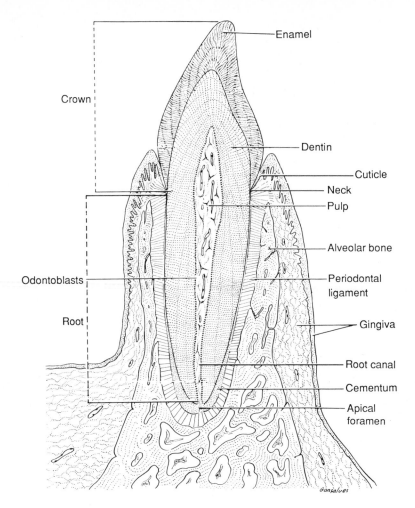

Figure 15–4. Diagram of a sagittal section from an incisor tooth in position in the mandibular bone. (Redrawn and reproduced, with permission, from Leeson TS, Leeson CR: *Histology,* 2nd ed. Saunders, 1970.)

tongue. Ducts from serous glands drain into the bases of the furrows.

D. Circumvallate Papillae: These are extremely large circular papillae whose flattened surfaces extend above the other papillae (Fig 15–3). The 7–12 circumvallate papillae are distributed in the *V* region in the posterior portion of the tongue. Numerous serous (von Ebner) glands drain their contents into the deep groove that encircles the periphery of each papilla. This moatlike arrangement provides a continuous flow of fluid over the great number of taste buds present along the sides of this papilla. The glands also secret a lipase that probably prevents the formation of a hydrophobic layer over the taste buds that would hinder their function. This flow of secretions is important in removing food particles from the vicinity of the taste buds so that they can receive and process new gustatory stimuli. In addition to the serous glands

associated with this type of papilla, other small mucous and serous glands dispersed throughout the lining of the oral cavity act in the same way to prepare the taste buds in other parts of the oral cavity—epiglottis, pharynx, palate, etc—to respond to taste stimuli (see Chapter 24).

2. PHARYNX

The pharynx represents a transitional space between the oral cavity and the respiratory and digestive systems. It forms an area of communication between the nasal region and the larynx. The pharynx is lined by stratified squamous epithelium of the mucous type, except in those regions of the respiratory portions that are not subject to abrasion. These latter areas have a ciliated pseudostratified columnar epithelium with goblet cells.

The pharynx contains the tonsils (described in Chapter 14). The mucosa of the pharynx also has many small mucous glands in its dense connective tissue layer. The constrictor and longitudinal muscles of the pharynx are located outside this layer.

3. TEETH & ASSOCIATED STRUCTURES

In adult humans, the 32 **permanent teeth** are disposed in 2 bilaterally symmetric arches in the maxillary and mandibular bones. There are 8 teeth in each quadrant: 2 incisors, 1 canine, 2 premolars, and 3 molars. The permanent teeth are preceded by 20 **deciduous (baby) teeth;** there are no deciduous precursors of the 12 permanent molar teeth.

Each tooth is composed of a portion that projects above the **gingiva (gum)**—the **crown**—and one or more **roots** below the gingiva that hold the teeth in bony sockets called **alveoli,** one for each tooth (Fig 15–4). The crown is covered by the extremely hard **enamel,** while the roots are covered by **cementum.** These 2 coverings meet at the **neck (cervix)** of the tooth. The interior of a tooth contains another calcified material, **dentin,** which surrounds a tissue-filled space known as the **pulp cavity** (Fig 15–4). The pulp cavity extends to the apex of the root (the root canal), where an orifice **(apical foramen)** permits the entrance and exit of blood vessels, lymphatics, and nerves of the pulp cavity. The **periodontal ligament (or membrane)** is a collagenous, fibrous structure in the cementum that serves to fix the tooth firmly in its bony socket (alveolus).

Dentin

Dentin is a calcified tissue similar to bone but harder because of its higher content of calcium salts. It is composed mainly of type I collagen fibrils, glycosaminoglycans, and calcium salts (70% of dry weight) in the form of **hydroxyapatite** crystals. The organic matrix of dentin is secreted by **odontoblasts,** cells that line the internal surface of the tooth, separating it from the pulp cavity (Figs 15–5 and 15–7). The odontoblast is a slender polarized cell, that produces organic matrix only at the dentinal surface. The cytoplasm of each of these cells contains a nucleus at its base. These cells have the structure of polarized protein-secreting cells with secretion granules containing procollagen. Odontoblasts have slender, branched cytoplasmic extensions that penetrate perpendicularly through the width of the dentin—the **odontoblast processes** (Tomes' fibers). These processes gradually become longer as the dentin becomes thicker, running in small canals called **dentinal tubules** that are extensively branched near the junction between dentin and enamel (Fig 15–6). Odontoblast processes have

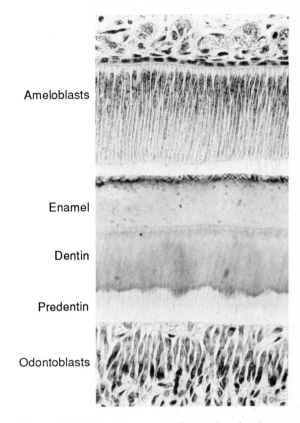

Figure 15–5. Photomicrograph of a section of an immature tooth, showing predentin, dentin, and enamel. The ameloblasts and odontoblasts are both disposed as palisades. Masson's stain, × 350.

(Labels on figure: Ameloblasts, Enamel, Dentin, Predentin, Odontoblasts)

a diameter of 3–4 μm near the cell body but gradually become thinner at their distal ends.

The matrix produced by odontoblasts is initially unmineralized and is called **predentin** (Fig 15–5). The mineralization of developing dentin begins when membrane-limited vesicles—**matrix vesicles**—appear. They contain fine crystals of hydroxyapatite that grow and serve as nucleation sites for further mineral deposition on the surrounding collagen fibrils.

Unlike bone, dentin persists as a mineralized tissue long after destruction of the odontoblasts. It is therefore possible to maintain teeth whose pulp and odontoblasts have been destroyed by infection. In adult teeth, destruction of the covering enamel by erosion from use or dental caries (tooth decay) usually triggers a reaction in the dentin that causes it to resume the synthesis of its components.

Enamel

Enamel is the hardest component of the human body and the richest in calcium. It consists of about 95% calcium salts (mainly hydroxyapatite), 0.5% organic material, and water as the remainder. Enamel is

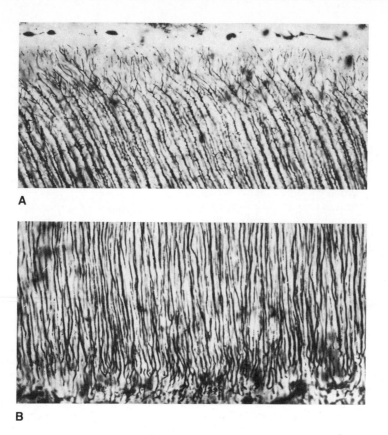

A

B

Figure 15–6. Photomicrograph of a section of a tooth, showing the odontoblast processes of the dentin. **A:** Initial portion. **B:** Terminal portion. These processes gradually get thinner and terminate by branching into delicate extensions. × 400.

produced by cells of ectodermal origin, whereas most of the other structures of teeth derive from mesodermal or neural crest cells. The organic enamel matrix is not composed of collagen fibrils but of at least 2 heterogeneous classes of proteins called **amelogenins** and **enamelins.** The roles of these proteins in the organization of the mineral component of enamel are under intensive investigation.

Enamel consists of elongated rods or columns of hydroxyapatite crystals called **enamel rods (prisms)** that are bound together by **interrod enamel.** Both interrod enamel and enamel rods are formed of hydroxyapatite crystals; they differ only in the orientation of the crystals. Each rod extends through the entire thickness of the enamel layer.

Enamel matrix is secreted by cells called **ameloblasts** (Fig 15–5). These tall columnar cells possess numerous mitochondria in the region below the nucleus. Many profiles of rough endoplasmic reticulum and a well-developed Golgi complex are found above the nucleus. Each ameloblast has an apical extension, known as a **Tomes' process,** containing numerous secretory granules. These granules contain the proteins that make up the enamel matrix.

Pulp

Tooth pulp consists of a loose connective tissue. Its main components are odontoblasts, fibroblasts, thin collagen fibrils, and a ground substance containing glycosaminoglycans (Fig 15–7).

Pulp is a highly innervated and vascularized tissue. Blood vessels and myelinated nerve fibers enter the apical foramen and divide into numerous branches. Some nerve fibers lose their myelin sheaths and extend for a short distance into the dentinal tubules. These fibers are sensitive to pain, the only sensory modality recognized in teeth.

Associated Structures

The structures responsible for maintaining the teeth in the maxillary and mandibular bone consist of the **cementum, periodontal ligament, alveolar bone,** and **gingiva.**

A. Cementum: This tissue covers the dentin of the root and is similar in composition to bone, although haversian systems and blood vessels are absent. It is thicker in the apical region of the root, where there are **cementocytes,** cells with the appearance of osteocytes. Like osteocytes, they are encased

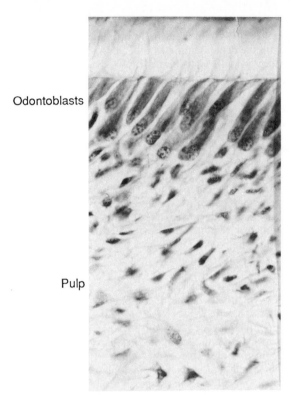

Odontoblasts

Pulp

Figure 15–7. Photomicrograph of dental pulp. Fibroblasts are abundant. In the upper region are the odontoblasts, from which the odontoblast processes derive. H&E stain, × 400.

in lacunae that communicate through canaliculi. Like bone tissue, cementum is labile and reacts by resorption of old or production of new tissue, according to the stresses to which it is subjected. When the periodontal ligament is destroyed, cementum undergoes necrosis and may be resorbed. Continuous production of cementum compensates for the normal growth that teeth undergo. This process maintains close contact between the roots of the teeth and their sockets.

B. Periodontal Ligament: The periodontal ligament is composed of a special type of dense connective tissue whose fibers penetrate the cementum of the tooth and bind it to the bony walls of its socket while permitting limited movement of the tooth. It serves as the periosteum of the alveolar bone. Its fibers are organized so as to support the pressures exerted during mastication. This avoids transmission of pressure directly to the bone—a process that would cause its localized resorption.

Collagen of the periodontal ligament has characteristics that resemble those of immature tissue. It has a high protein turnover rate (as demonstrated by radioautography) and a large soluble collagen content. The space between its fibers is filled with glycosaminoglycans.

This high rate of collagen renewal in the periodontal ligament allows processes affecting protein or collagen synthesis—eg, protein or vitamin C deficiency (**scurvy**)—to cause atrophy of this ligament. As a consequence, teeth become loose in their sockets; in extreme cases they fall out. This relative plasticity of the periodontal ligament is important because it allows orthodontic intervention, which can produce extensive changes in the disposition of teeth in the mouth.

C. Alveolar Bone: This portion of bone is in immediate contact with the periodontal ligament. It is an immature type of bone (woven bone) in which the collagen fibers are not arranged in the typical lamellar pattern of adult bone. Many of the collagen fibers of the periodontal ligament are arranged in bundles that penetrate this bone and the cementum, forming a connecting bridge between these structures. The bone closest to the roots of the teeth forms the socket. Vessels and nerves run through this alveolar bone to the apical foramen of the root to enter the pulp.

D. Gingiva: The gingiva is a mucous membrane firmly bound to the periosteum of the maxillary and mandibular bones. It is composed of stratified squamous epithelium and numerous connective tissue papillae. This epithelium is bound to the tooth enamel by means of a cuticle that resembles a thick basal lamina and forms the **epithelial attachment of Gottlieb.** The epithelial cells are attached to the cuticle by hemidesmosomes. Between the enamel and the epithelium is the **gingival crevice**—a small deepening surrounding the crown.

Development of Teeth

At about 6 weeks of gestation, the basal layer of the oral epithelium (ectoderm) proliferates and bulges into the underlying **ectomesenchyme** derived from the neural crest (Fig 15–8A). A horse-shoe-shaped band known as the **dental lamina** is formed in each jaw. A little later, 10 regions of intensified mitotic activity are noted in each dental lamina. These ectodermal outgrowths form caps over clumps of ectomesenchyme, and each collection of cells (tooth bud) will develop into a deciduous tooth. The ectomesenchyme is formed by mesenchymal cells (see Chapter 5) associated with neural crest cells that originate from the ectoderm. The intervening ectodermal cells later degenerate and disappear. The ectodermal component of a tooth bud forms the **enamel organ** responsible for the secretion of **enamel** (Fig 15–8B and C). The ectomesenchymal component forms the **dental papilla** from which will differentiate odontoblasts (cells that secrete dentin) and other structures of the dental pulp (Fig 15–8D). Mesenchyme also condenses around the enamel organ and will eventually differentiate into **cementoblasts** (cells that form cementum) and the periodontal ligament.

The enamel organ continues to enlarge and assumes

A. Bud stage

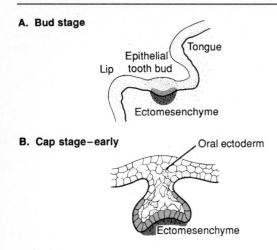

B. Cap stage–early

C. Cap stage–late

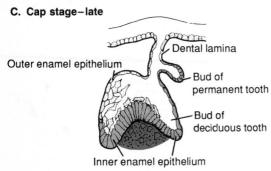

D. Bell stage

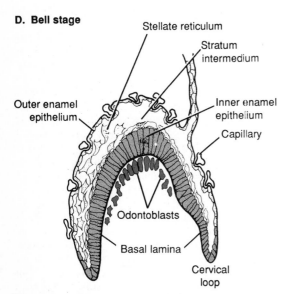

Figure 15–8. The epithelium (lighter color) of a tooth bud **(A)** proliferates and invades the underlying mesenchyme to form a cap-shaped structure **(B)** and **(C).** In the cap stage, the epithelium differentiates into the inner enamel epithelium, which will give rise to ameloblasts. In the bell stage **(D),** neural-crest-derived cells (darker color) differentiate into odontoblasts. (Modified and reproduced, with permission, from Warshawsky H: The teeth. In: *Histology: Cell and Tissue Biology,* 5th ed. Weiss L (editor). Elsevier, 1983.)

a bell shape at about 8 weeks of gestation. The **outer (external) enamel epithelium,** which is continuous with the dental lamina, is indented by numerous capillary vessels. Cells immediately adjacent to the dental papilla assume a columnar shape and form the **inner (internal) enamel epithelium.** These cells differentiate into **ameloblasts** (cells that will secrete enamel). Other epithelial cells between the outer and inner layers form the **stellate reticulum** and the **stratum intermedium;** the functions of these layers are not well defined (Fig 15–8D).

It should be noted that a continuous basal lamina separates the outer enamel epithelium from the surrounding connective tissues. This basal lamina then curves around and separates the inner enamel epithelium from ectomesenchymal cells of the dental papilla. The point (a circle in 3 dimensions) where the outer enamel epithelium meets the inner enamel epithelium is termed the **cervical loop** (Fig 15–8D).

Ameloblast differentiation is induced by ectomesenchymal cells of the dental papilla. Before ameloblasts begin to secrete enamel, they cause a superficial layer of cells of the dental papilla to elongate and differentiate into odontoblasts. Odontoblasts begin to secrete predentin, which in turn stimulates the secretion of enamel by ameloblasts. Thus, a wave of reciprocal inductions passes from the future occlusal surface of the crown toward the neck of the tooth.

A. Formation of Dentin: Odontoblasts secrete procollagen, which becomes organized into the collagen fibrils of predentin. These cells also mediate the mineralization of collagen fibrils, leading to the formation of dentin. The cell bodies of odontoblasts retreat into the pulp cavity as dentin accumulates, but their processes remain in dentinal tubules that span the entire thickness of the dentin.

B. Formation of Enamel: Ameloblasts are unusual epithelial cells in that their bases, adjacent to the basal lamina, become their secretory surfaces. Tight junctions are found around both the histologic apex (functional base) and the histologic base (functional apex) of each cell. Rough endoplasmic reticulum and an elaborate Golgi complex are found in the cytoplasm between the nucleus and the functional apex of these cells. Ameloblasts are responsible for the breakdown of the basal lamina that separates these cells from odontoblasts and dentin. Tomes' processes, the short, conical extensions of ameloblasts are the sites of secretion of enamel matrix. The lateral surfaces of these processes secrete the organic matrix of the interrod enamel, while the apical surface is responsible for deposition of the matrix of enamel rods. The role of ameloblasts in mineralization is not clear, but hydroxyapatite crystals are formed on the organic matrix. This matrix is later almost completely removed, probably by the ameloblasts. After enamel formation is completed, the enamel organ consists of a stratified squamous

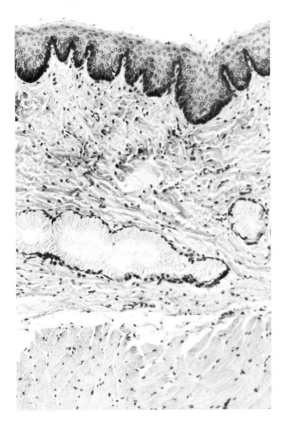

Figure 15–9. Photomicrograph of a section of the upper region of the esophagus. Mucous glands are in the submucosa; striated muscle in the muscularis. H&E stain, × 20.

epithelium that erodes rapidly when the tooth erupts into the oral cavity.

C. Root Development: After crown is completely developed, and just prior to its eruption, the cervical loop grows apically to envelop the dental papilla and forms **Hertwig's root sheath,** which is composed of the fused outer and inner enamel epithelia. The inner layer induces formation of odontoblasts that produce the dentin of the tooth root. When the dentin has been formed, the root sheath breaks up, and the newly formed dentin induces the differentiation of cementoblasts from mesenchymal cells of the surrounding dental sac. Cementoblasts form cementum, the bonelike tissue covering the roots of teeth.

D. Permanent Teeth: On the labial side of each dental lamina, a mass of ectodermal cells pushes out to form the **successional lamina** bud of the permanent tooth; (Fig 15–8C). Here, too, 20 regions of intensified mitotic activity are found, one corresponding to each of the permanent counterparts of the deciduous teeth. In addition, dental lamina cells burrow backward, and the tooth germs of the 3 permanent

molars are budded off in succession. The tooth germs for the second and third molars are not formed until after birth.

ESOPHAGUS

This part of the gastrointestinal tract is a muscular tube whose function is to transport foodstuffs from the mouth to the stomach. It is covered by nonkeratinized stratified squamous epithelium (Fig 15–9). In general, it has the same layers as the rest of the digestive tract. In the submucosa are groups of small mucus-secreting glands, the **esophageal glands.** In the lamina propria of the region near the stomach are groups of glands called **esophageal cardiac glands** that also secrete mucus. At the distal end of the esophagus, the muscular layer consists of only smooth muscle cells; in the mid portion, a mixture of striated and smooth muscle cells; and at the proximal end, only striated muscle cells. Only that portion of the esophagus in the peritoneal cavity is covered by serosa. The rest is covered by a layer of loose connective tissue, the adventitia, which blends into the surrounding tissue.

STOMACH

The stomach is a mixed exocrine-endocrine organ that digests food and secretes hormones. It is a dilated segment of the digestive tract whose main functions are to continue the digestion of carbohydrates initiated in the mouth, add an acidic fluid to the ingested food, transform it by muscular activity into a viscous mass **(chyme),** and promote the initial digestion of proteins with the enzyme **pepsin.** Gross inspection reveals 4 regions: **cardia, fundus, body,** and **pylorus** (Fig 15–10). Because the fundus and body are identical in microscopic structure, only 3 histologic regions are recognized. The mucosa and submucosa of the undistended stomach lie in longitudinally directed folds known as **rugae.** When the stomach is filled with food, these folds are flattened out.

Mucosa

The gastric mucosa consists of a **surface epithelium** that invaginates to varying extents into the lamina propria, forming **gastric pits.** Emptying into gastric pits are branched, tubular glands (cardiac, gastric, and pyloric) characteristic of each region of the stomach. The **lamina propria** of the stomach is composed of loose connective tissue interspersed with smooth muscle and lymphoid cells. Separating the mucosa from the underlying submucosa is a layer of smooth muscle, the **muscularis mucosae.**

When the luminal surface of the stomach is viewed under low magnification, numerous small circular or ovoid invaginations of the lining epithelium are ob-

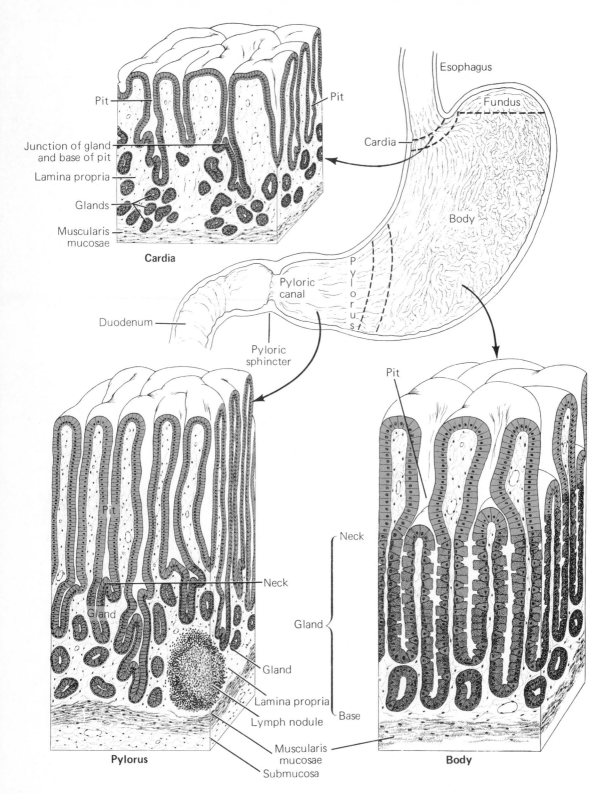

Figure 15–10. Regions of the stomach and their histologic structure.

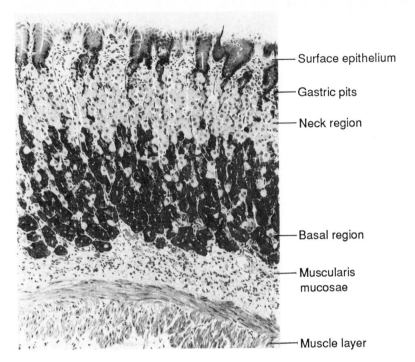

— Surface epithelium

— Gastric pits

— Neck region

— Basal region

— Muscularis mucosae

— Muscle layer

Figure 15–11. Photomicrograph of a section of a gastric gland in the fundus of the stomach. Parietal cells predominate in the upper region of the gland; chief cells (zymogenic cells) predominate in the lower region.

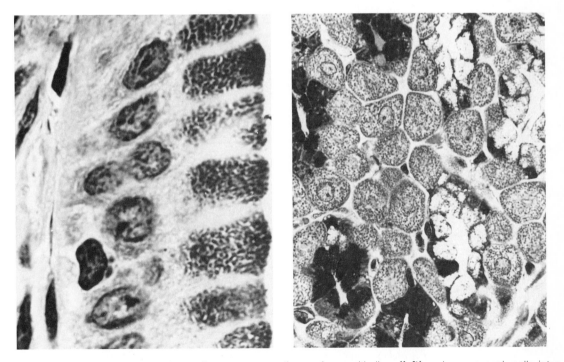

Figure 15–12. Photomicrographs illustrating mucus-secreting surface epithelium **(left)** and mucus neck cells intercalated between parietal cells **(right)**.

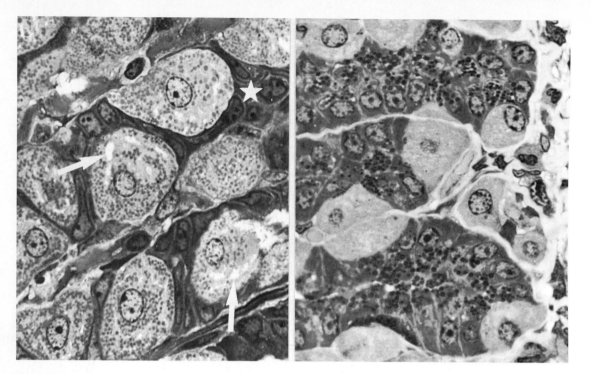

Figure 15–13. Photomicrographs of stomach mucosa in the fundus. **Left:** A section of the neck region showing parietal cells rich in mitochondria and their characteristic intracellular canaliculi (arrows). The asterisk marks undifferentiated cells. **Right:** The basal portion of the gland contains chief cells (characterized by basophilic cytoplasm) and pepsin-containing secretory granules. A few parietal cells are also present. × 900.

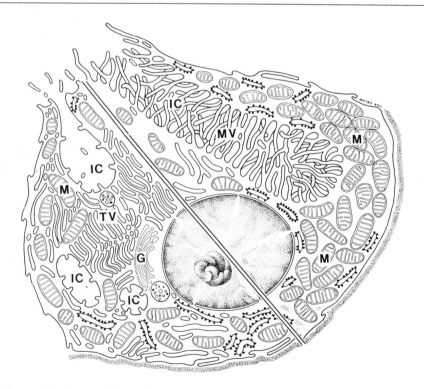

Figure 15–14. Composite diagram of the parietal cell, showing the ultrastructural differences between a resting **(left)** and an active **(right)** cell. Observe that the tubulovesicles (TV) present in the cytoplasm of the resting cell fuse to form microvilli that fill up the intracellular canaliculi (IC). Golgi complex (G), mitochondria (M), microvilli (MV). (Based on the work of S Ito and GC Schofield. *J Cell Biol* 1974;**63**:364.)

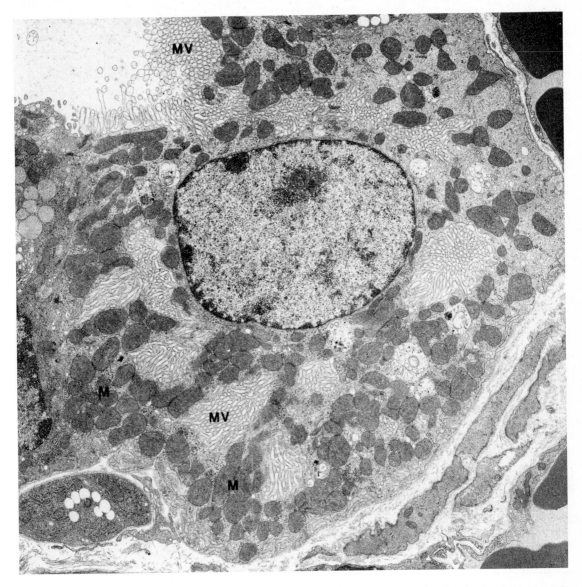

Figure 15–15. Electron micrograph of an active parietal cell. Observe the microvilli (MV) protruding into the intracellular canaliculi and the abundant mitochondria (M). × 10,200. (Courtesy of S Ito.)

served. These are the openings of the gastric pits (Figs 15–10 and 15–11). The epithelium covering the surface and lining the pits is a simple columnar epithelium, and all the cells secrete mucus (Fig 15–12). When released from these cells, the mucus forms a thick layer that protects them from the effects of the strong acid secreted by the stomach.

Recent evidence suggests that tight junctions around surface and pit cells also form a part of the barrier to acid. Stress, psychosomatic factors, or substances (such as aspirin) that cause gastric irritation can disrupt this epithelial layer and lead to ulceration. The initial ulceration may heal, or it may be further aggravated by the local action of pepsin and hydrochloric acid, leading to additional gastric and duodenal ulcers.

Cardiac Region

The cardia is a narrow circular band, 1.5–3 cm in width, at the transition between the esophagus and stomach (Fig 15–10). Its lamina propria contains simple or branched tubular cardiac glands. The terminal portion of these glands is frequently coiled and often has a large lumen. Most of the secretory cells produce mucus and lysozyme, but a few parietal cells (which secrete HCl) can be found. These glands are similar in structure to the cardiac glands of the terminal portion of the esophagus.

Fundus & Body

The lamina propria of these regions is filled with branched, tubular **gastric (fundic) glands,** 3–7 of which open into the bottom of each gastric pit. The distribution of epithelial cells in gastric glands is not uniform (Figs 15–10 and 15–11). The **neck** consists of undifferentiated, parietal, and mucous neck cells (Fig 15–12); the **base** of the glands contains parietal, chief (zymogenic), and enteroendocrine cells.

A. Undifferentiated Cells: Found in the neck region but few in number, these are low columnar cells with oval nuclei near the bases of the cells. Few or no mucous granules are seen in their cytoplasm. These cells have a high rate of mitosis; some of them differentiate and move upward to replace the pit and surface mucous cells, which have a turnover time of 3–7 days. Other undifferentiated cells migrate deeper into the glands and differentiate into mucous neck cells and parietal, chief, and enteroendocrine cells. These cells are replaced much more slowly than are surface mucous cells.

B. Mucous Neck Cells: These cells are present in clusters or as single cells between parietal cells in the necks of gastric glands. Despite being mucous cells, they have morphologic and histochemical characteristics that make their mucous secretion quite different from that of the surface epithelial mucous cells. They are irregular in shape, with their nuclei at the base of the cell. Their ovoid or spherical granules are near the apical surface and are stained intensely with PAS. The function of these cells is not known.

C. Parietal (Oxyntic) Cells: Present mainly in the upper half of gastric glands, parietal cells are scarce in the gland's base. They are rounded or pyramidal cells, with one centrally placed spherical nucleus and intensely eosinophilic cytoplasm (Figs 15–10, 15–11 and 15–13). Upon observation in the electron microscope, the most striking features are a deep, circular invagination of the apical plasma membrane forming the **intracellular canaliculus,** and an abundance of mitochondria (Fig 15–15). In the resting cell, a number of tubulovesicular structures can be seen in the apical region of the cell just below its plasmalemma (Fig 15–14, left side). At this stage, the cell has few microvilli. When stimulated to produce hydrochloric acid, tubulovesicles fuse with the cell membrane and form more microvilli, thus providing a generous increase in the surface of the cell membrane (Fig 15–14, right side). Actin filaments present between tubulovesicles probably play a role in the interaction of these structures. The eosinophilic cytoplasm possesses a great number of mitochondria with abundant cristae, a discrete Golgi complex near the cell base, and no secretory granules (Figs 15–14 and 15–15).

Parietal cells produce the hydrochloric acid present in gastric juice. Parietal cells secrete hydrochloric acid, 0.16 mol/L; potassium chloride, 0.07 mol/L; traces of other electrolytes; and gastric intrinsic factor (see below). There is evidence that the secreted acid originates from chlorides present in the blood plus a cation (H^+) resulting from the action of an enzyme—**carbonic anhydrase.** Carbonic anhydrase acts on CO_2 to produce carbonic acid, which dissociates into bicarbonate and H^+. Both the cation and the chloride ion are actively transported across the cell membrane; water diffuses passively along the osmotic gradient (Fig 15–16). The presence of abundant mitochondria in the parietal cells indicates that their metabolic processes are highly energy consuming. This cell type's histochemical peculiarities characterize it as one of the cells that have the highest observable energy metabolism.

In human disease, the number of parietal cells is correlated with the acid-producing capacity of the stomach. In cases of atrophic gastritis, both parietal and chief cells are much less numerous, and the gastric juice has little or no acid or pepsin activity. Radioautographic studies performed with labeled vitamin B_{12} suggest that the parietal cells are, in humans, the site of production of **intrinsic factor,** a glycoprotein

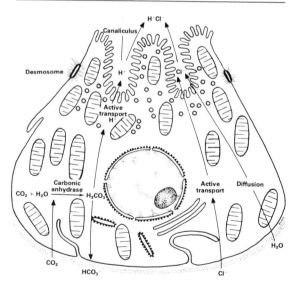

Figure 15–16. Diagram of parietal cell, showing the main steps in the synthesis of hydrochloric acid. Blood CO_2 under the action of carbonic anhydrase produces carbonic acid. This dissociates into a bicarbonate ion and a proton, H^+, which reacts with the chloride ion to produce hydrochloric acid. The tubulovesicles of the cell apex seem to be related to hydrochloric acid secretion, since they decrease in number after parietal cell stimulation. The bicarbonate ion returns to the blood and is responsible for a measurable increase in blood pH during digestion.

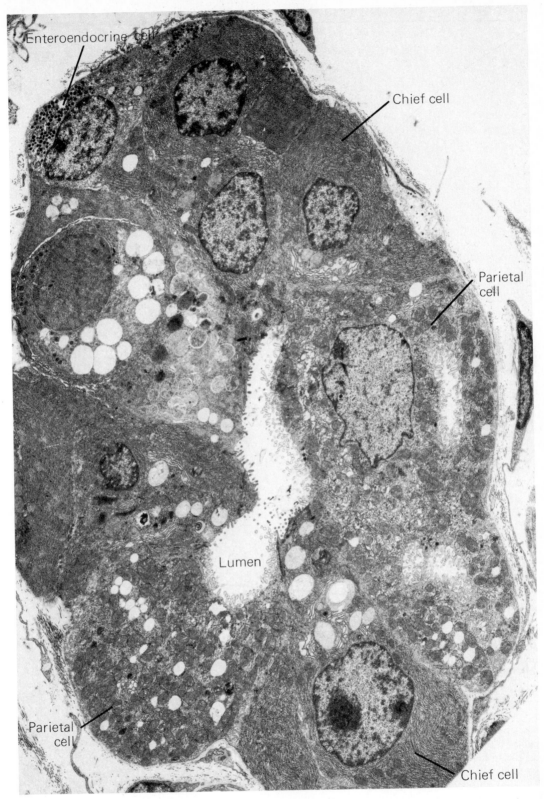

Figure 15–17. Electron micrograph of a section of gastric gland in the fundus of the stomach. Note the lumen and the parietal cells, containing abundant mitochondria; chief cells, with extensive rough endoplasmic reticulum; and entero-endocrine cells, with secretory granules. × 5300.

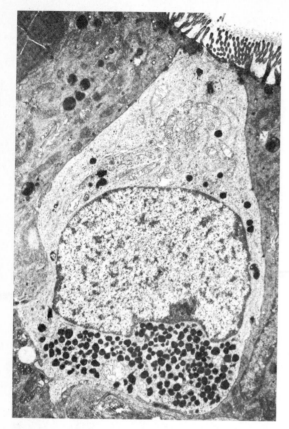

Figure 15–18. Electron micrograph of an enteroendocrine cell of the human duodenum. × 6900. (Courtesy of AGE Pearse.)

that binds avidly to vitamin B_{12}. In other species, however, this substance may be present in other cells.

The presence of intrinsic factor is normally required for vitamin B_{12} absorption, which binds strongly to intrinsic factor in the lumen of the stomach. This complex is absorbed by pinocytosis into the cells in the ileum. This explains why a lack of intrinsic factor can lead to vitamin B_{12} deficiency. This condition results in a disorder of the red blood cell-forming mechanism known as **pernicious anemia;** it is usually caused by **atrophic gastritis.** In a certain percentage of cases, pernicious anemia seems to be an autoimmune disease, since antibodies against parietal cell proteins are often detected in the blood of patients with the disease.

The secretory activity of parietal cells is instigated by different mechanisms. One is through cholinergic nerve endings. Histamine and a polypeptide called **gastrin,** both secreted in the gastric mucosa, act

strongly to stimulate the production of hydrochloric acid.

D. Chief (Zymogenic) Cells: Chief cells (Fig 15–17) predominate in the lower region of the tubular glands and have all the characteristics of a protein-synthesizing and exporting cell. The granules present in their cytoplasm contain the inactive enzyme pepsinogen. Their basophilia is due to the abundant rough endoplasmic reticulum (see Chapter 4). In humans, these cells produce the enzymes pepsin and lipase. When inactive pepsinogen is released into the acid environment of the stomach, the proenzyme is converted into the highly active proteolytic enzyme **pepsin.**

E. Enteroendocrine Cells: These cells, discussed more extensively on page 302, are found near the bases of gastric glands (Figs 15–17 and 15–18).

In the fundus of the stomach, **5-hydroxytryptamine** (serotonin) has been shown to be one of the principal secretory products. Tumors called **carcinoids,** which arise from these cells, are responsible for the clinical symptoms caused by overproduction of serotonin.

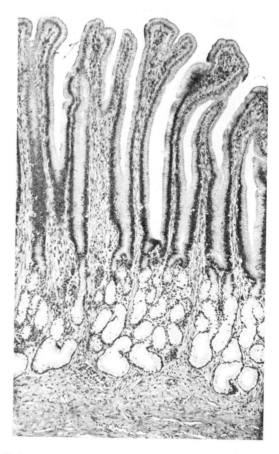

Figure 15–19. Photomicrograph of a section of the pyloric region of the stomach. Observe the deep gastric pits with short pyloric glands in the lamina propria. H&E stain, × 40.

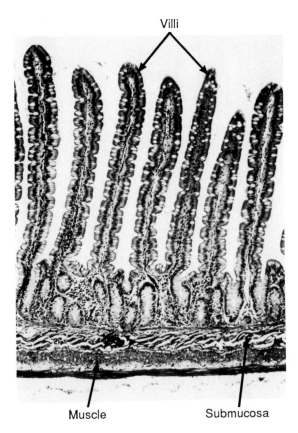

Villi

Muscle   Submucosa

Figure 15–20. Photomicrograph of the small intestine. Observe the villi, intestinal glands, submucosa, and the external and internal muscle layers. H&E stain, × 40.

Pylorus

The pylorus (from Latin, a gatekeeper) has deep gastric pits into which the branched, tubular **pyloric glands** open. These glands are similar to the glands of the cardiac region. In the pyloric region, however, long pits and short coiled glands are found—the reverse of the situation in the cardiac region (Fig 15–19). These glands secrete mucus as well as appreciable amounts of the enzyme lysozyme. **Gastrin (G) cells,** (which release **gastrin**) are intercalated among the mucous cells of pyloric glands. Gastrin stimulates the secretion of acid by the parietal cells of gastric glands. Other enteroendocrine cells (**D cells**) secrete **somatostatin** (*soma* + *stasis*, which inhibits the release of other hormones, including gastrin.

Other Layers of the Stomach

The **submucosa** is composed of loose connective tissue and blood and lymph vessels; it is infiltrated by lymphoid cells, macrophages, and mast cells. The **muscularis** is composed of smooth muscle fibers oriented in 3 main directions. The external layer is longitudinal, the middle layer is circular, and the internal

layer is oblique. At the pylorus, the middle layer is greatly thickened to form the **pyloric sphincter.** The **serosa** is thin and covered by mesothelium.

SMALL INTESTINE

The small intestine is the site of terminal food digestion, metabolite absorption, and endocrine secretion.

The processes of digestion are completed in the small intestine, and the products of digestion are absorbed. The small intestine is relatively long—approximately 5 m—permitting prolonged contact between food and digestive enzymes, as well as between the digested products and the absorptive cells of the epithelial lining. The small intestine consists of 3 segments: **duodenum, jejunum,** and **ileum,** which have many characteristics in common and will be discussed together.

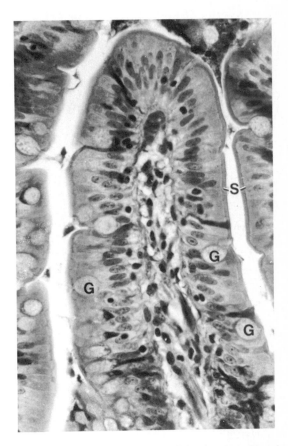

Figure 15–21. Photomicrograph of the tip of a villus of the human ileum. Observe the connective tissue core with blood and lymphatic vessels surrounded by the epithelial layer, in which goblet cells (G) frequently occur. At right, the striated border (S) formed by microvilli on the surface of the cell is clearly visible. H&E stain, × 450.

Mitochondria   Microvilli   Nucleus

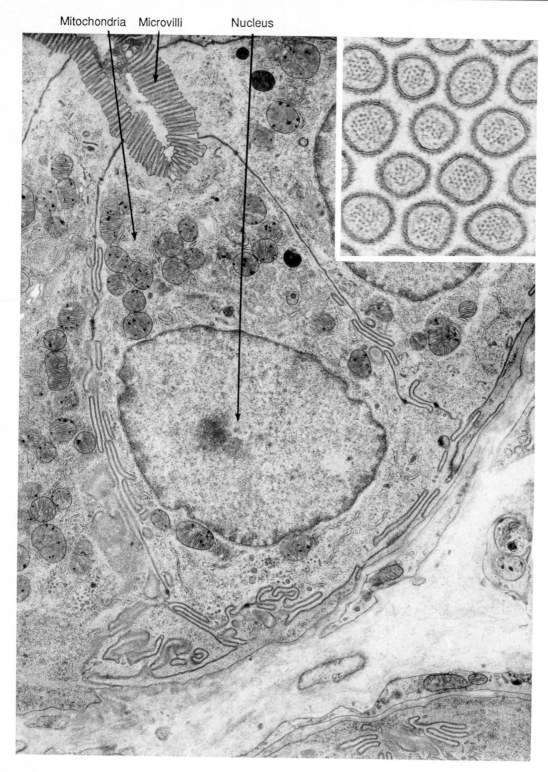

Figure 15–22. Electron micrograph of an absorptive epithelial cell of the small intestine. Observe the accumulation of mitochondria in their apexes. The luminal surface is covered with microvilli (shown in transverse section in the inset). Actin filaments, sectioned transversely, constitute the principal structural feature in the core of the microvilli. × 6300. (Courtesy of KR Porter.)

Mucous Membrane

Viewed with the naked eye, the lining of the small intestine shows a series of permanent folds, **plicae circulares (Kerckring's valves),** consisting of mucosa and submucosa and having a semilunar, circular, or spiral form. The plicae are most developed in, and consequently a characteristic of, the jejunum. Although frequently present, they do not constitute a significant feature of the duodenum and ileum. Under magnification, **intestinal villi** are seen. These structures, 0.5–1.5 mm long, are outgrowths of the mucosa (epithelium plus lamina propria) projecting into the lumen of the small intestine. In the duodenum they are leaf-shaped, gradually assuming the form of a finger as the ileum is reached (Figs 15–20 and 15–24).

Between the villi are small openings of simple tubular glands called **intestinal glands (crypts,** or **glands of Lieberkühn)** (Figs 15–20 and 15–24).

The epithelium of the villi is continuous with that of the glands. In the intestinal glands one finds mainly undifferentiated cells, some absorptive cells, goblet cells, Paneth cells, and enteroendocrine cells. The undifferentiated cells of the crypts give rise to the columnar absorptive cells and the mucus-secreting goblet cells of the villus epithelium.

Absorptive cells are tall columnar cells, each with an oval nucleus in the basal half of the cell. At the apex of each cell is a homogeneous layer called the **striated (brush) border** (Fig 15–21). With the aid of the electron microscope, the striated border is seen to be a layer of densely packed **microvilli** (Figs 15–22 and 15–23). Each microvillus is a cylindrical protrusion of the apical cytoplasm and consists of a cell membrane enclosing a core of actin filaments. Each microvillus is approximately 1 μm tall × 0.1 μm in diameter. It is estimated that each absorptive cell has an average of about 3000 microvilli and that 1 mm² of mucosa contains about 200 million of these structures. Microvilli have the important physiologic function of considerably increasing the area of contact between the intestinal surface and food. Studies performed by isolating the striated border of these cells by differential centrifugation and then applying immunofluorescence techniques suggest that the striated border is the site of activity of the disaccharidases and dipeptidases of the small intestine. These enzymes, bound to microvilli, hydrolyze the disaccharides and dipeptides into monosaccharides and amino acids that are easily absorbed.

Deficiencies of these disaccharidases have been described in human diseases characterized by digestive disturbances. Some of these enzymatic deficiencies seem to be of genetic origin.

A more important function of the columnar intestinal cells is to absorb the metabolites that result from the digestive process. This is discussed further below.

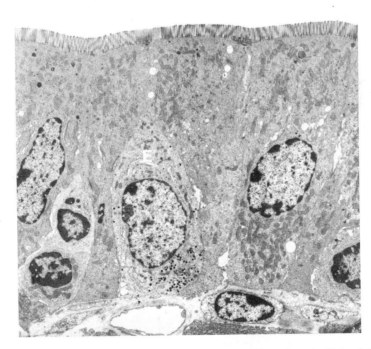

Figure 15–23. Electron micrograph of epithelium of the small intestine. When viewed with the light microscope, abundant microvilli at the cell apex can be seen to form the striated border. At left are 2 lymphocytes migrating in the epithelium. In the center is an enteroendocrine cell (E) with its basal secretory granules. × 1850.

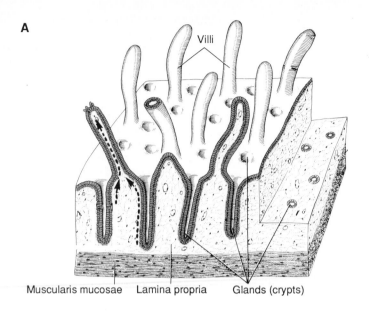

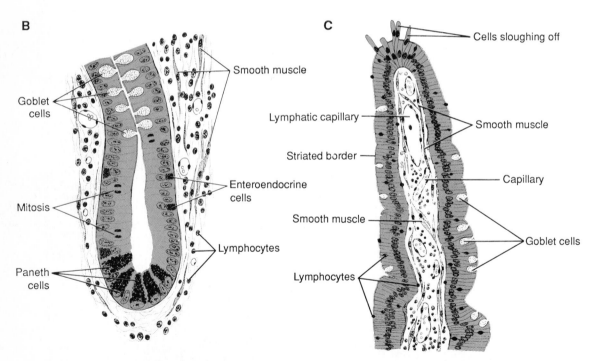

Figure 15–24. Schematic diagrams illustrating the structure of the small intestine. **A:** The small intestine under low magnification. In the villus to the left, observe the desquamation of epithelial cells. Because of constant mitotic activity of the cells from the blind end of the glands and the upward migration of these cells (dashed arrows), the intestinal epithelium is continuously renewed. Observe the intestinal glands (of Lieberkühn). **B:** The intestinal glands have a lining of intestinal epithelium and goblet cells (upper portion). At a lower level, the immature epithelial cells are frequently seen in mitosis; note also the presence of Paneth and enteroendocrine cells. As the immature cells progress upward, they differentiate and develop microvilli, seen as a striated border in the light microscope. Cell proliferation and cell differentiation occur simultaneously in the blind end of these glands. **C:** A villus tip showing the columnar covering epithelium with its striated border and a moderate number of goblet cells. Capillaries, a lymphatic capillary, smooth muscle cells, and leukocytes can be seen in the connective tissue core of the villus. Lymphocytes are in the epithelial layer in great numbers. Cells are sloughing off at the apex of the villus. (Redrawn and reproduced, with permission, from Ham AW: *Histology*, 6th ed. Lippincott, 1969.)

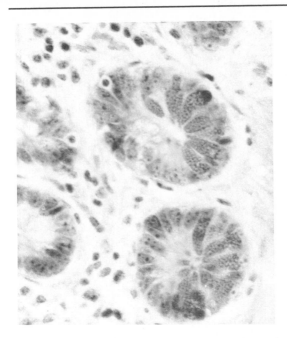

Figure 15–25. Section of the basal portion of the intestinal glands showing the Paneth cells with their typical large secretory granules. × 600.

Goblet cells are interspersed between the absorptive cells (Figs 15–21 and 15–24). They are less abundant in the duodenum and increase in number as the ileum is approached. These cells produce acid glycoproteins whose main function is to protect and lubricate the lining of the intestine.

Paneth cells in the basal portion of the intestinal glands are exocrine serous cells that synthesize a complex of protein and polysaccharide. Researchers using immunocytochemical methods have detected lysozyme—an enzyme that digests the cell wall of some bacteria—in the large, eosinophilic secretory granules of these cells (Figs 15–24, 15–25, and 15–26). Lysozyme possesses antibacterial activity and may play a role in controlling the intestinal flora.

M (membranous epithelial) cells are specialized epithelial cells overlying the lymphoid follicles of Peyer's patches. These cells are characterized by the presence of numerous membrane invaginations forming pits at their apical and lateral surfaces that contain intraepithelial lymphocytes. M cells can endocytose antigens and transport them to the underlying lymphoid cells that then migrate to the lymphoid system (nodes), where immune responses to foreign antigens are initiated. M cells represent

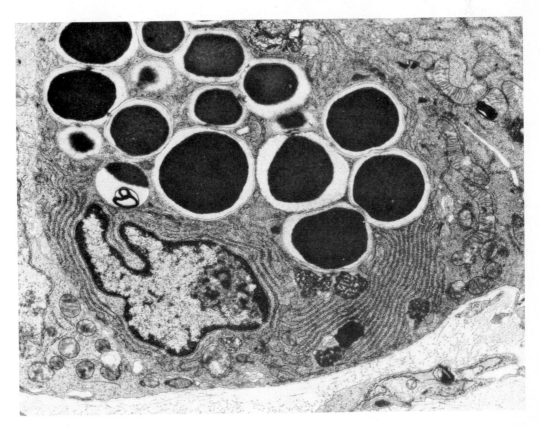

Figure 15–26. Electron micrograph of a Paneth cell. Observe basal nucleus with prominent nucleolus, abundant rough endoplasmic reticulum, and large secretory granules with a protein core surrounded by a halo of polysaccharide-rich material. These granules contain lysozyme, a lytic enzyme involved in the regulation of intestinal bacteria. × 3000.

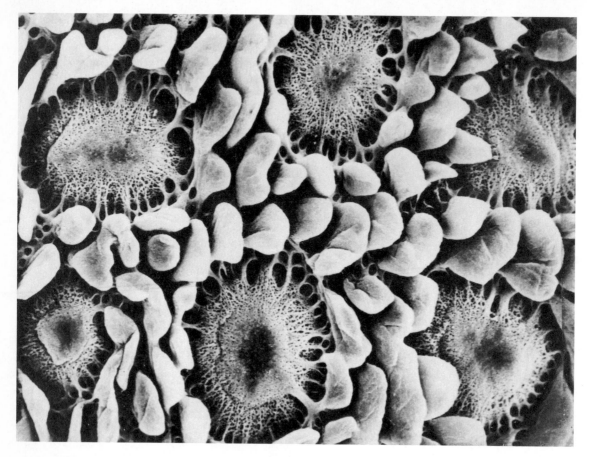

Figure 15–27. Scanning electron micrograph of the intestinal surface following removal of the mucosal epithelium, showing the basement membrane. Observe that this layer is continuous when covering the remnants of the intestinal villi, but assumes the structure of a sieve when covering the lymphoid follicles above Peyer's patches. This configuration permits an easier means for immunogenic materials to reach underlying lymphoid tissues. (Courtesy of S McClugage.)

an important link in the intestinal immunological system (Fig 15–28). The basement membrane is discontinuous under M cells, facilitating transit between the lamina propria and M cells (Fig 15-27).

Endocrine Cells of the Gastrointestinal Tract

In addition to the cells discussed above, the gastrointestinal tract contains a series of widely distributed cells with characteristics of the **diffuse neuroendocrine system** (see Chapter 4). The main results obtained so far are summarized in Fig 15–29 and Table 15–1. Analysis of the figure shows that the distribution of these cells in the digestive tract is not uniform.

Polypeptide-secreting cells of the digestive tube fall into 2 classes: the **open type,** in which the apex of the cell presents microvilli and contacts the lumen of the organ (Fig15-18); and the **closed type,** in which the cellular apex is covered by other epithelial cells (Fig 15-17). It has been suggested that in the open type,

the chemical contents of the digestive tube might act on its microvilli and thereby influence secretion of these cells. Although the picture of gastrointestinal endocrinology is still incomplete, it is clear that the activity of the digestive system is controlled by the nervous system and modulated by a complex and efficient system of peptide hormones locally produced.

Lamina Propria Through Serosa

The lamina propria of the small intestine is composed of loose connective tissue with blood and lymph vessels, nerve fibers, and smooth muscle cells. Just below the basal lamina is a layer of antibody-producing lymphoid cells and macrophages, forming an immunologic barrier at this region.

The lamina propria penetrates the core of the intestinal villi, taking along blood and lymph vessels, nerves, connective tissue, and smooth muscle cells. The smooth muscle cells are responsible for the rhythmic movements of the villi, which are important for absorption (see Fig 15–24).

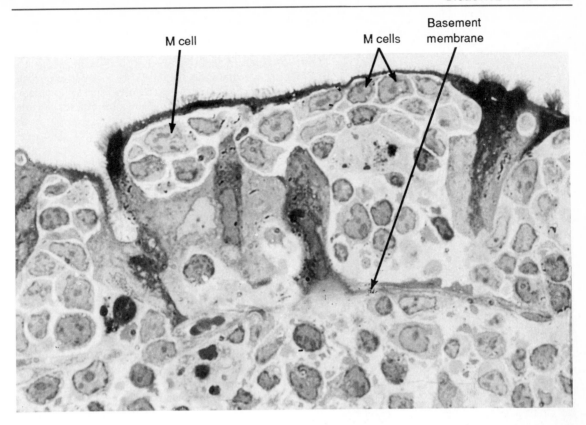

Figure 15–28. Micrograph from a region of intestine where a lymphoid nodule is covered by the intestinal mucosa. Observe the presence of M cells interspersed through lymphoid cells. (Courtesy of M Neutra.)

The muscularis mucosae does not present any peculiarities in this organ. The **submucosa** contains, in the initial portion of the duodenum, clusters of ramified, coiled tubular glands that open into the intestinal glands. These are the **duodenal** (or **Brunner's**) **glands** (Figs 15–30). Their cells are of the mucous type. The product of secretion of the glands is distinctly alkaline (pH 8.1–9.3). It acts to protect the duodenal mucous membrane against the effects of the acid gastric juice and to bring the intestinal contents to the optimum pH for pancreatic enzyme action.

The lamina propria and the submucosa of the small intestine contain aggregates of lymphoid nodules known as Peyer's patches. Each patch consists of

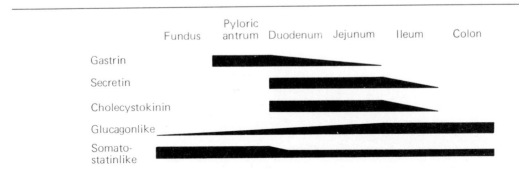

Figure 15–29. Distribution of gastrointestinal endocrine-cell secretions along the digestive tract. (Based on Grossman MI: Distribution of gastrointestinal APUD cells along the digestive tract. *Proc Int Cong Endocrinol* 1976;**2**:1.)

Table 15-1. Principal enteroendocrine cells in the gastrointestinal tract.

Cell Type and Location	Hormone Produced	Major Action
A–stomach	Glucagon	Hepatic glycogenolysis
G–pylorus	Gastrin	Stimulation of gastric acid secretion
S–small intestine	Secretin	Pancreatic and biliary bicarbonate and water secretion
K–small intestine	Gastric inhibitory polypeptide (GIP)	Inhibition of gastric acid secretion
L–small intestine	Glucagonlike substance (glicentin)	Hepatic glycogenolysis
I–small intestine	Cholecystokinin	Pancreatic enzyme secretion, gallbladder contraction
D–pylorus, duodenum	Somatostatin	Local inhibition of other endocrine cells
Mo–small intestine	Motilin	Increased gut motility
EC–digestive tract	Serotonin, substance P	Increased gut motility
D$_1$–digestive tract	Vasoactive intestinal polypeptide (VIP)	Ion and water secretion, increased gut motility

10–200 nodules and is visible to the naked eye as an oval area on the antimesenteric side of the intestine. There are about 30 patches in the human, most of them found in the ileum. When viewed from the luminal surface, each Peyer's patch appears as a dome-shaped area devoid of villi. Instead its covering epithelium consists of **M cells.**

Vessels & Nerves

The blood vessels that nourish the intestine and remove absorbed products of digestion penetrate the muscularis and form a large plexus in the submucosa (Fig 15–31). From the submucosa, branches extend through the muscularis mucosae and lamina propria and into the villi. Each villus receives, according to its size, one or more branches that form a capillary network just below its epithelium. At the tips of the villi, one or more venules arise from these capillaries and run in the opposite direction, reaching the veins of the submucosal plexus. The lymph vessels of the intestine begin as blind tubes in the core of the villi. These structures, despite being larger than the blood capillaries, are difficult to observe because their walls are usually collapsed. These vessels (**lacteals**) run to the region of lamina propria above the muscularis mucosae, where they form a plexus. From there they are directed to the submucosa, where they surround lymphoid nodules. These vessels anastomose repeatedly and leave the intestine along with the blood vessels.

The innervation of the intestines is formed by an **intrinsic** and an **extrinsic component.** The intrinsic component is constituted by groups of neurons that form the myenteric (Auerbach's) nerve plexus (Fig

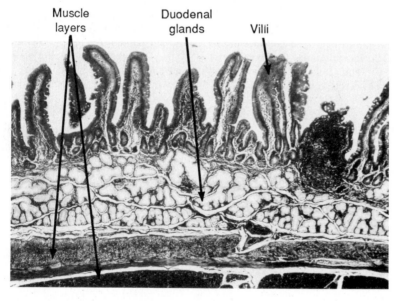

Figure 15-30. Photomicrograph of the duodenum, showing villi and duodenal glands in the submucosa. The dark structure at the right is a lymphoid nodule; at the bottom are 2 smooth muscle layers of the muscularis. H&E stain, × 30.

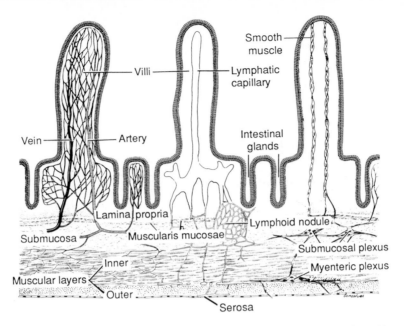

Figure 15–31. Diagram showing the blood circulation **(left)**, lymphatic circulation **(center)**, and innervation **(right)** of the small intestine. The smooth muscle system for contracting the villi is illustrated in the villus on the right.

15–32) between the outer longitudinal and the inner circular layers of the muscularis and the **submucosal (Meissner's) plexus** in the submucosa. The plexuses contain some sensory neurons that receive information from nerve endings near the epithelial layer and in the smooth muscle layer regarding the composition of the intestinal content (chemoreceptors) and the degree of expansion of the intestinal wall (mechanoreceptors). The other nerve cells are effectors and innervate the muscle layers and hormone-secreting cells. The intrinsic innervation formed by these plexuses is responsible for the intestinal contractions that occur in the total absence of the extrinsic innervation. The extrinsic innervation is formed by parasympathetic cholinergic nerve fibers that stimulate the activity of the intestinal smooth muscle and by sympathetic adrenergic nerve fibers that depress intestinal smooth muscle activity.

Histophysiology

The presence of plicae, villi, and microvilli greatly increases the surface of the intestinal lining—an important characteristic in an organ where absorption occurs so intensely. It has been calculated that the presence of plicae increases the intestinal surface 3-fold, the villi increase it 10-fold, and the microvilli increase it 20-fold. Together these processes are thus responsible for a 600-fold increase in the intestinal surface, resulting in a total area of 200 m^2.

The digestive process is completed and its products are absorbed in the small intestine. Lipid digestion occurs mainly as a result of the action of pancreatic

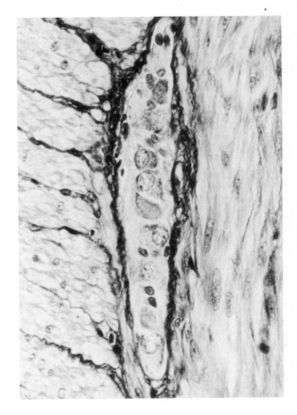

Figure 15–32. Photomicrograph of a group of neurons and satellite cells constituting a component of the myenteric plexus between 2 smooth muscle layers.

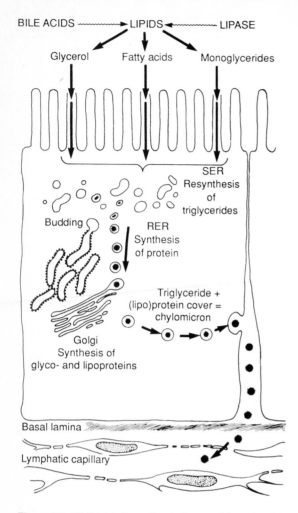

Figure 15–33. Lipid absorption in the small intestine. Lipase promotes the hydrolysis of lipids to monoglycerides and fatty acids in the intestinal lumen. These compounds are stabilized in an emulsion by the action of bile acids. The products of hydrolysis cross the microvilli membranes passively and are collected in the cisternae of the smooth endoplasmic reticulum, where they are resynthesized to triglycerides. These triglycerides are surrounded by a thin layer of proteins that form particles called chylomicrons (0.2–1 μm in diameter). Chylomicrons are transferred to the Golgi complex, from where they migrate to the lateral membrane, cross it by a process of membrane fusion (exocytosis), and flow into the extracellular space in the direction of the blood and lymph vessels. Most chylomicrons go to the lymph; a few go to the blood vessels. The long-chain lipids ($>C_{12}$) go mainly to the lymph vessels. Fatty acids of fewer than 10–12 carbon atoms are not reesterified to triglycerides but leave the cell directly and enter the blood vessels. RER, rough endoplasmic reticulum; SER, smooth endoplasmic reticulum. (Based on results published by HI Friedman and RR Cardell Jr in *Anat Rec* 1977;**188**:77.)

lipase and bile. In humans, most of the lipid absorption occurs in the duodenum and upper jejunum. Figs 15–33 and 15–34 illustrate present concepts of this process of absorption.

The amino acids and monosaccharides derived from digestion of proteins and carbohydrates are absorbed by the epithelial cells by active transport. In newborn animals, but apparently not in humans, transfer of undigested proteins from colostrum can be clearly observed as a result of pinocytotic processes in the cell apex. In this way, antibodies secreted into the colostrum can be transferred to the young animal—an important aspect of the immune defense mechanism. This capacity to transfer proteins is almost completely lost after a few days and is minimal in adults.

> In diseases marked by severe damage to epithelial cells, the transfer of undigested proteins to the blood increases considerably.
>
> The absorption of metabolites is greatly hindered in disorders marked by atrophy of the intestinal mucosa caused by infections or nutritional deficiencies, producing the **malabsorption syndrome.**

Another process that is probably important for intestinal function is the rhythmic movement of the villi. This is the result of the contraction of smooth muscle cells running vertically between the muscularis mucosae and the tip of the villi (see villus at right in Fig 15–31). These movements occur at the rate of several strokes per minute. During digestion, their rate increases; in fasting animals, the rate is much lower. These contractions also tend to empty the lymph vessels and propel the lymph and absorbed metabolites to the mesenteric lymphatics.

The microfilaments found in the microvilli (Figs 15–22 and 15–35) are composed of actin. Movement of the microvilli is thought to play an important role in mixing the microenvironment—an important event in the process of metabolite absorption.

Lymphocytes are frequently seen between the intestinal epithelial cells. They are believed not to migrate to the intestinal lumen but to move to the lamina propria and from there to the lymph vessels. During this migration, it is probable that these lymphocytes are stimulated by external antigens and thus play a role in the immunologic defense provided by the intestines.

LARGE INTESTINE

The large intestine consists of a mucosal membrane with no folds except in its distal (rectal) portion. No villi are present in this portion of the intestine (Fig 15–36). The intestinal glands are long and characterized by a great abundance of goblet and absorptive cells and a small number of enteroendocrine cells

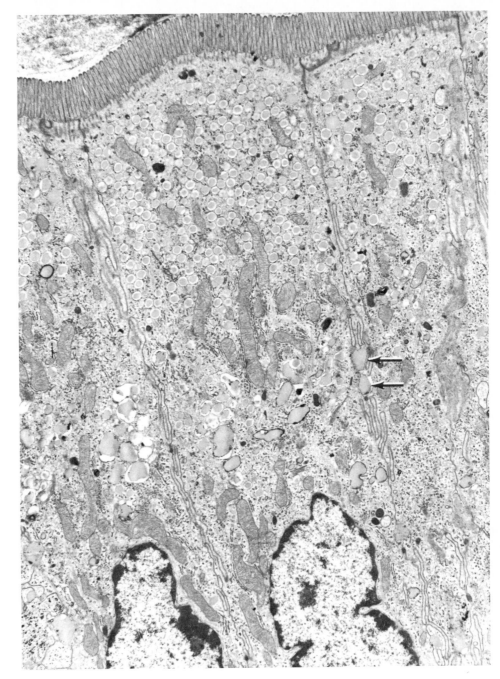

Figure 15–34. Electron micrograph of intestinal epithelium in the lipid-absorption phase. Observe the accumulation of lipid droplets in vesicles of the smooth endoplasmic reticulum. (Compare with Fig 15–22.) These vesicles fuse near the nucleus, forming larger lipid droplets that migrate laterally and cross the cell membranes to the extracellular space (arrows). × 5000. (Courtesy of HI Friedman.)

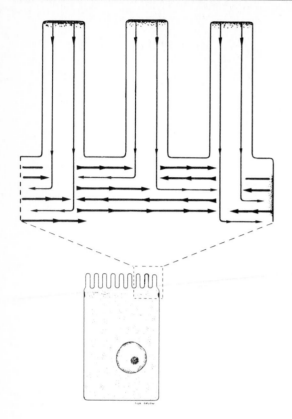

Figure 15–35. Diagram explaining the movement of microvilli. The upper drawing is an enlargement of part of the surface of an intestinal cell. The microvilli contain actin filaments (thin arrows) that interact with myosin filaments (thick arrows) in the cell apex. The dense regions in the tips of the microvilli are the probable sites of insertion of the actin filaments. The location of these proteins was identified through immunofluorescence cytochemistry. Compare this figure with Fig 4–9. (Based on studies by R Rodewald, SB Newman, and MJ Karnovsky in *J Cell Biol* 1976;**70**:541.)

(Figs 15–36, 15–37, and 15–38). The absorptive cells are columnar and have short, irregular microvilli (Fig 15–37). This organ is well suited to its main functions: absorption of water and formation of the fecal mass plus production of mucus. This last is a highly hydrated gel that not only lubricates the intestinal surface but also covers bacteria and particulate matter. The absorption of water is passive, following the active transport of sodium out of the basal surfaces of these epithelial cells.

The lamina propria is rich in lymphoid cells and nodules. The nodules frequently extend into the submucosa. This richness in lymphoid tissue is probably the result of the extremely abundant bacterial population present in the large intestine. The muscularis comprises longitudinal and circular strands. This layer differs here from that of the small intestine,

since fibers of the outer longitudinal layer congregate in 3 thick longitudinal bands called **teniae coli.** In the intraperitoneal portions of the colon, the serous layer is characterized by small, pendulous protruberances composed of adipose tissue—the **appendices epiploicae** (Fig 15–39).

In the anal region, the mucous membrane forms a series of longitudinal folds, the **rectal columns of Morgagni.** About 2 cm above the anal opening, the intestinal mucosa is replaced by stratified squamous epithelium. In this region, the lamina propria contains a plexus of large veins that, when excessively dilated and varicose, produce hemorrhoids.

Cell Renewal in the Gastrointestinal Tract

The epithelial cells of the entire gastrointestinal tract respond to certain stimuli (hormones, cholinergic neural activity) by producing new cells. Cells of the basal layer of the esophageal epithelium, the neck of gastric glands, the lower half of the intestinal glands, and the lower third of the crypts of the large intestine are rapidly labeled with ^{3}H-thymidine and consequently identified as proliferating cells. From this proliferative zone in each region, cells move to

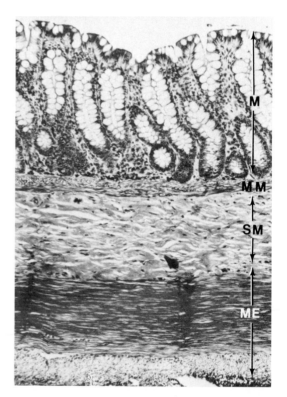

Figure 15–36. Photomicrograph of a section of large intestine with its various layers. Observe the absence of villi. M, mucosa; MM, muscularis mucosae; SM, submucosa; ME, muscularis externa. H&E stain, × 30.

Golgi

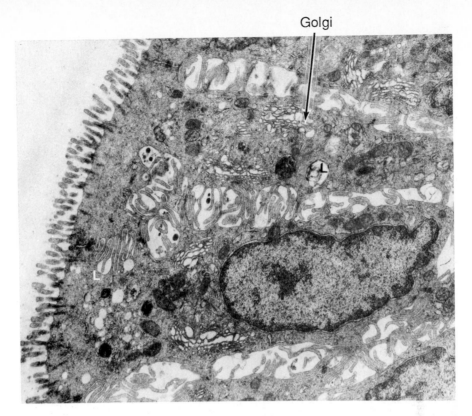

Figure 15–37. Electron micrograph of epithelial cells of the large intestine. Observe the microvilli at the luminal surface, the well-developed Golgi complex, and dilated intercellular spaces filled by interdigitating membrane leaflets, a sign of active water transport. × 3900.

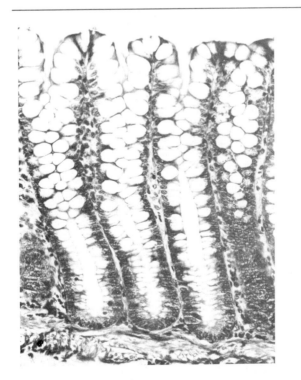

Figure 15–38. Photomicrograph of a section of large intestine. Observe the intestinal glands with abundant goblet cells. H&E stain, × 95.

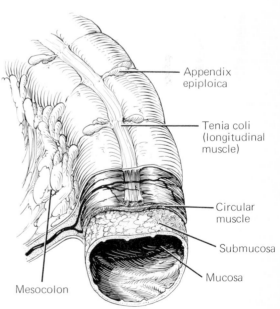

Appendix epiploica

Tenia coli (longitudinal muscle)

Circular muscle

Submucosa

Mucosa

Mesocolon

Figure 15–39. Cross section of colon. (Reproduced, with permission, from Way LW [editor]: *Current Surgical Diagnosis & Treatment*, 8th ed. Appleton & Lange, 1988.)

the maturation area where they undergo structural and enzymatic maturation, providing the functional cell population of each region.

In humans, replacement of the esophageal epithelium occurs every 2–3 days. In the gastric epithelium, mitotic activity is found only in the undifferentiated cells of the neck region of gastric glands. Most of the new cells migrate upward to form pit and surface mucous cells. These cells live only 4–6 days before they are sloughed off. Other new cells differentiate into mucous neck, parietal, chief, or enteroendocrine cells. These cells turn over at a much slower rate.

The lower half of the intestinal gland is the site of undifferentiated cell proliferation in the small intestine (Fig 15–24). Most of these cells migrate upward and differentiate into absorptive cells. Others become goblet cells or enteroendocrine cells. All 3 cell types live only 3–6 days.

Epithelial cells of the large intestine are replaced about every 6 days by the proliferation and differentiation of cells in the lower third of the glands.

This high replacement rate explains why the intestine is promptly affected by the administration of antimitotic drugs, as in cancer chemotherapy. The epithelial cells continue to be lost at the tips of villi, but the drugs inhibit cell proliferation. This promotes atrophy of the epithelium, which results in defective absorption of nutrients, excessive fluid loss, and diarrhea. Paneth cells of the crypts turn over much more slowly, living about 30 days before being replaced.

APPENDIX

The appendix is an evagination of the cecum; it is characterized by a relatively small, narrow, and irregular lumen that is caused by the presence of abundant lymphoid follicles in its wall. Although its general structure is similar to that of the large intestine, it contains fewer and shorter intestinal glands and has no teniae coli (Fig 15–40).

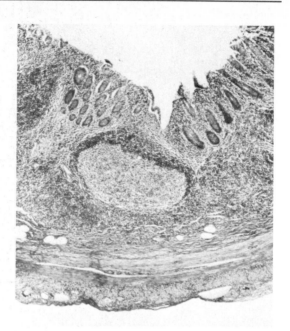

Figure 15–40. Photomicrograph of a section of appendix. There are a few glands and numerous lymphoid nodules. H&E stain, × 20.

Because the appendix is a blind-ended invagination, its contents are not renewed rapidly and it frequently becomes a site of inflammation (**appendicitis**). This inflammation can progress to the point of destruction of this structure with consequent infection of the peritoneal cavity.

Cancer of the Digestive Tract

Approximately 90–95% of malignant tumors of the digestive system are derived from intestinal or gastric epithelial cells. Malignant tumors of the large bowel are derived almost exclusively from its glandular epithelium (**adenocarcinomas**) and are the second most common cause of cancer deaths in the United States.

REFERENCES

Cheng H, Leblond CP: Origin, differentiation and renewal of the four main epithelial cell types in the mouse small intestine. 5. Unitarian theory of the origin of the four epithelial cell types. *Am J Anat* 1974;**141**:537.

Forte JG: Mechanism of gastric H⁺ and Cl⁻ transport. *Annu Rev Physiol* 1980;**42**:111.

Friedman Hl, Cardell RR Jr: Alterations in the endoplasmic reticulum and Golgi complex of intestinal epithelial cells during fat absorption and after termination of this process: A morphological and morphometric study. *Anat Rec* 1977;**188**:77.

Gabella G: Innervation of the gastrointestinal tract. *Int Rev Cytol* 1979;**59**:130.

Grube D: The endocrine cells of the digestive system: Amines, peptides and modes of action. *Anat Embryol (Berl)* 1986;**175**:151.

Hoedemseker PJ et al: Further investigations about the site

of production of Castle's gastric intrinsic factor. *Lab Invest* 1966;**15**:1163.

Ito S: Functional gastric morphology. In: *Physiology of the Gastrointestinal Tract.* Vol 1. Johnson LR (editor). Raven Press, 1981.

Klockars M, Reitamo S: Tissue distribution of lysozyme in man. *J Histochem Cytochem* 1975;**23**:932.

McClugage SG, Lew FN, Zimmy ML: Porosity of the basement membrane overlying Peyer's patches in rats and monkeys. *Gastroenterology* 1986;**91**:1128

Moog F: The lining of the small intestine. *Sci Am* (Nov) 1981;**245**:154.

Mooseker MS, Tilney LG: Organization of an actin filament-membrane complex: Filament polarity and membrane attachment in the microvilli of intestinal epithelial cells. *J Cell Biol* 1975;**67**:725.

Owen D: Normal histology of the stomach. *Am J Surg Pathol* 1986;**10**:48.

Pabst R: The anatomical basis for the immune function of the gut. *Anat Embryol (Berl)* 1986;**176**:135.

Pfeiffer CJ, Rowden G, Weibel J: *Gastrointestinal Ultrastructure.* Academic Press, 1974.

Glands Associated With the Digestive Tract

The glands associated with the digestive tract include the salivary glands, pancreas, liver, and gallbladder. The functions of the salivary glands are to wet and lubricate the oral cavity and its contents, to initiate the digestion of carbohydrates, and to secrete such substances as IgA, lysozyme, and lactoferrin. The main functions of the pancreas are to produce digestive enzymes that act in the small intestine and to secrete the hormones insulin and glucagon into the bloodstream. The liver produces bile, an important fluid in the digestion of fats. It plays a major role in lipid, carbohydrate, and protein metabolism and inactivates and metabolizes many toxic substances and drugs. The liver also participates in iron metabolism and the synthesis of blood proteins and the factors necessary for blood coagulation. The gallbladder absorbs water from the bile and stores the bile in a concentrated form.

SALIVARY GLANDS

Exocrine glands in the mouth produce saliva, which has digestive, lubricating, and immunologic functions. There are 3 pairs of large salivary glands in addition to the small glands scattered throughout the oral cavity (described in the previous chapter): the **parotid, submandibular (submaxillary),** and **sublingual glands.**

These glands consist of 2 general types of secretory cells—serous and mucous (Fig 16–1).

Serous cells are usually pyramidal in shape with a broad base resting on the basal lamina and a narrow apical surface with short, irregular microvilli facing the lumen (Figs 16–2 and 16–3). They exhibit characteristics of polarized protein-secreting cells (Figs 4–19 and 4–25). Adjacent secretory cells are joined together by junctional complexes consisting of zonulae occludentes (tight junctions), zonulae adherentes (adhering junctions), desmosomes, and gap junctions. Serous cells usually form a spherical mass of cells called an **acinus (alveolus)** with a lumen in the center. This structure can be likened to a grape attached to its stem. The stem corresponds to the duct system (described below).

Mucous cells are usually cuboidal to columnar in shape; their nuclei are oval and pressed toward the bases of the cells. They present the characteristics of mucus-secreting cells (Figs 4–23, 4–25, 16–3, and 16–5). Mucous cells are most often organized as **tubules,** consisting of cylindrical arrays of secretory cells surrounding a lumen.

In the human **submandibular gland,** serous and mucous cells are arranged in a characteristic pattern. The mucous cells form tubules, but their ends are capped by serous cells, which constitute the **serous demilunes** (Figs 16–1 and 16–3).

Myoepithelial cells, described in Chapter 4, are found within the basal lamina of glandular and ductal epithelia of salivery glands. Myoepithelial cells surrounding serous acini are highly branched cells (sometimes called **basket cells**); those associated with mucous tubules and intercalated ducts are spindle-shaped and lie parallel to the length of the duct.

Secretory end-pieces empty into **intercalated ducts** lined by cuboidal epithelial cells. Several of these ducts then join to form another type of **intralobular duct,** the **striated duct** (Fig 16–1).

Striated ducts are characterized by radial striations that extend from the bases of the cells to the level of the nuclei. When viewed in the electron microscope, these striations are seen to consist of infoldings of the basal plasma membrane as well as numerous mitochondria aligned parallel to the infolded membranes characteristic of ion-transporting cells (Figs 4–17; see Chapter 4 for further discussion).

Striated ducts of each lobule converge and drain into ducts in the connective tissue septae separating the lobules. At these points, they become **interlobular ducts** or **excretory ducts.** Their lining epithelium is initially stratified cuboidal, but more distal parts of the excretory ducts are lined by stratified columnar epithelium. The main duct of each major salivary gland ultimately empties into the oral cavity and is lined by nonkeratinized stratified squamous epithelium.

The large salivary glands are not mere collections of epithelial cells but contain other components such as connective tissue, blood and lymph vessels, and

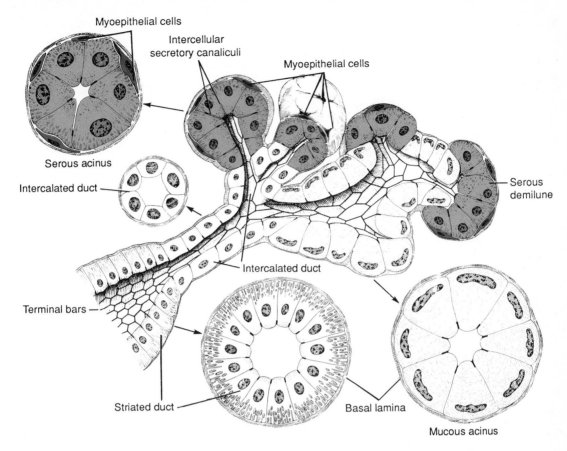

Figure 16–1. The structure of the submandibular (submaxillary) gland. Acini in the secretory portion are composed of pyramidal serous (lighter color) and mucous (stippled) cells and the tubules of mucous cells. The nuclei of serous cells are euchromatic and rounded, and an accumulation of rough endoplasmic reticulum is evident in the basal third of the cell. The apex of the cell is filled with protein-rich secretory granules. The nuclei of mucous cells, flattened with condensed chromatin, are located near the bases of the cells. Mucous cells have little rough endoplasmic reticulum and contain distinct secretory granules. The short intercalated ducts are lined with cuboidal epithelium. The striated ducts are composed of columnar cells with such characteristics of ion-transporting cells (see Chapter 4) as basal membrane invaginations and mitochondrial accumulation. Myoepithelial cells are shown in darker color.

nerves, organized in a definite pattern. These glands are surrounded by a capsule of connective tissue, rich in collagen fibers. From this capsule, septa of connective tissue penetrate the gland, dividing it into lobules. Vessels and nerves enter the gland at the hilum and gradually branch into the lobules. A rich vascular and nervous plexus surrounds the secretory and ductal components of each lobule.

Parotid Glands

The parotid gland is a branched acinar gland. Its secretory portion is composed almost exclusively of serous cells (Fig 16–2). In humans, in addition to having the characteristics of a serous cell, the secretory granules of these cells exhibit a positive periodic acid-Schiff (PAS) reaction that indicates the presence of polysaccharides. The secretory granules are rich in proteins and have a high amylase activity. The other components of this gland are similar. The encapsulating connective tissue contains many plasma cells and lymphocytes. The plasma cells secrete an immunoglobulin, IgA (Fig 15–2), which complexes with a **secretory component** synthesized by the serous acinar, intercalated duct, and striated duct cells. The IgA-secretory-piece complex released into the saliva is resistant to enzymatic digestion and constitutes an immunologic defense mechanism against pathogens that will eventually be present in the oral cavity.

Submandibular (Submaxillary) Glands

The submandibular gland is a branched tubuloacinar gland (Figs 16–3 and 16–4). Its secretory portion contains both mucous and serous cells. The serous

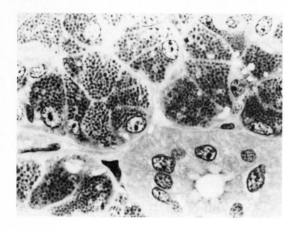

Figure 16–2. Photomicrograph of a human parotid gland, showing serous acini and striated ducts. A connective tissue septum separates the lobules. H&E stain, × 360.

cells contain protein secretory granules that are PAS-positive because of the presence of carbohydrate moieties. The serous cells are the main component and are easily distinguished from pure mucous cells by their rounded nuclei and basophilic cytoplasm. The presence of extensive lateral and basal membrane infoldings toward the vascular bed increases the ion-transporting surface area 60 times, facilitating electrolyte and water transport during primary secretion. As a consequence of these folds, the cell boundaries are indistinct. These cells are responsible for the weak amylolytic activity present in this gland and its saliva. The cells that form the demilunes in both the submandibular and sublingual glands contain and secrete the enzyme **lysozyme,** whose main activity is to hydrolyze the walls of certain bacteria.

Sublingual Gland

The sublingual gland, like the submandibular gland, is a branched tubuloacinar gland formed by serous and mucous cells. It contains no acini formed exclusively by serous cells, however. Mucous cells predominate in the sublingual gland, and its serous cells are present only on demilunes of mucous acini (Fig 16–5).

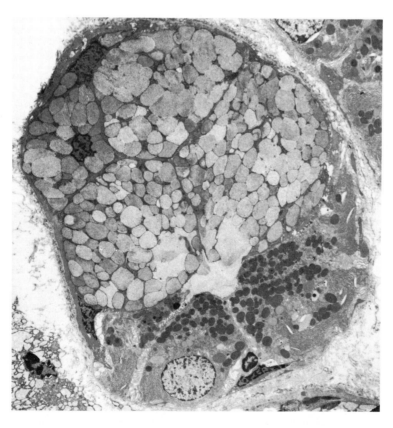

Figure 16–3. Electron micrograph of a mixed acinus from a human submandibular gland. Note the difference between the serous (lower part) and mucous (upper part) secretory granules. × 2500. (EM picture courtesy of JD Harrison.)

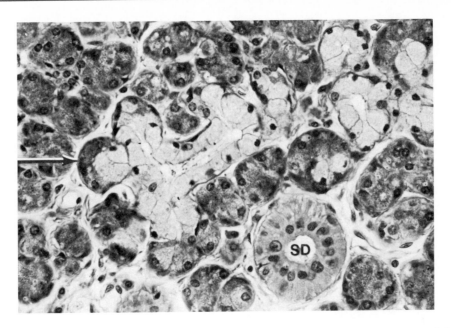

Figure 16–4. Photomicrograph of a section of human submandibular gland. Observe the presence of dense serous cells forming acini and demilunes. The pale-staining mucous cells are grouped along the tubular portion of this tubuloacinar gland. In the lower right region is a striated duct (SD). The arrow indicates a demilune where serous cells are eccentrically displaced, assuming the form of a crescent. H&E stain, × 360.

Histophysiology

Moistening and lubricating functions of the salivary glands are performed by the water and glycoproteins of saliva. The latter are synthesized mainly by the mucous cells and to a lesser degree by the serous cells of the glands. These fluids also provide solvents for substances that stimulate the taste buds. Human saliva consists of secretions from the parotid glands (25%), the submandibular glands (70%), and the sublingual gland (5%).

Another function of these glands is the digestion of carbohydrates. The major part of the hydrolysis of ingested carbohydrates is the result of salivary amylase activity. This digestion, which begins in the mouth, also takes place in the stomach before the gastric juice acidifies the food and thus decreases amylase activity considerably.

As mentioned above, serous acinar, intercalated duct, and striated duct cells synthesize the secretory component necessary for the transport of secretory IgA from the connective tissues, across the acinar and duct cells, and into the saliva. Lactoferrin and lysozyme are also secreted by acinar and intercalated duct cells. Lactoferrin binds iron, a nutrient necessary for bacterial growth, while lysozyme hydrolyzes the cell walls of certain bacteria. Thus, saliva is important in defending the oral cavity against pathogens.

Parasympathetic stimulation of the salivary glands, usually through the smell or taste of food, provokes a

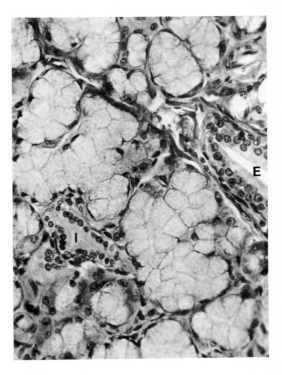

Figure 16–5. Photomicrograph of a human sublingual gland showing the predominance of mucous cells. Examples of an intralobular (I) and connective-tissue-ensheathed interlobular (E) duct are also present. H&E stain, × 600.

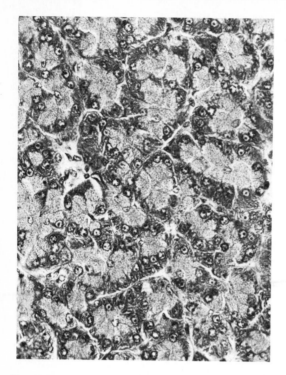

Figure 16–6. Photomicrograph showing the appearance of the acinar portion of the pancreas with its secretory cells. H&E stain, × 400.

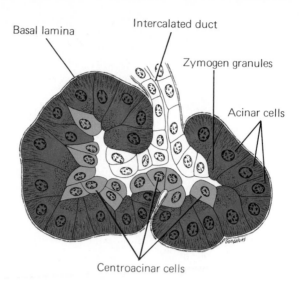

Figure 16–7. Schematic drawing of the structure of pancreatic acini. Acinar cells (darker color) are pyramidal, with granules at their apex and rough endoplasmic reticulum at the cell base. The intercalated duct partly penetrates the acini. These duct cells are known as centroacinar cells (lighter color). Note the absence of myoepithelial cells.

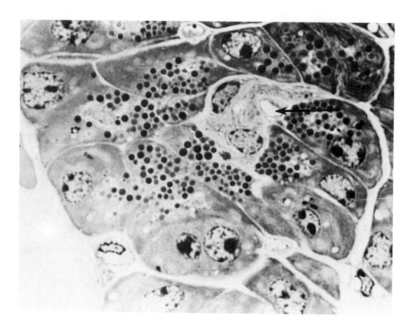

Figure 16–8. Photomicrograph of pancreatic acinus showing secretory granules at the cell apex and 2 centroacinar cells at the margin of a small lumen (arrow).

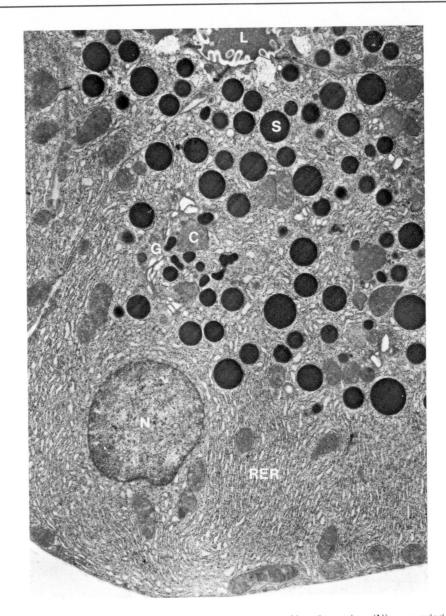

Figure 16–9. Electron micrograph of an acinar cell from a rat pancreas. Note the nucleus (N) surrounded by numerous cisternae of rough endoplasmic reticulum (RER) near the base of the cell. The Golgi complex (G) is situated at the apical pole of the nucleus and is associated with several condensing vacuoles (C) and numerous mature secretory (zymogen) granules (S). The lumen (L) contains proteins recently released from the cell by exocytosis. × 8000.

copious watery secretion with relatively little organic content. Sympathetic nerve stimulation produces small amounts of viscous saliva, rich in organic material.

PANCREAS

The pancreas is a mixed exocrine and endocrine gland that produces digestive enzymes and hor- **mones. The enzymes are stored and released by cells of the exocrine portion. The hormones are synthesized in cells of the endocrine tissue known as *islets of Langerhans* (see Chapter 21).** The exocrine portion of the pancreas is a compound acinar gland (Fig 16–6), similar in structure to the parotid gland. In histologic sections, a distinction can be made based on the absence of striated ducts and the presence of the islets of Langerhans in the pancreas. Another characteristic detail is that the initial portions

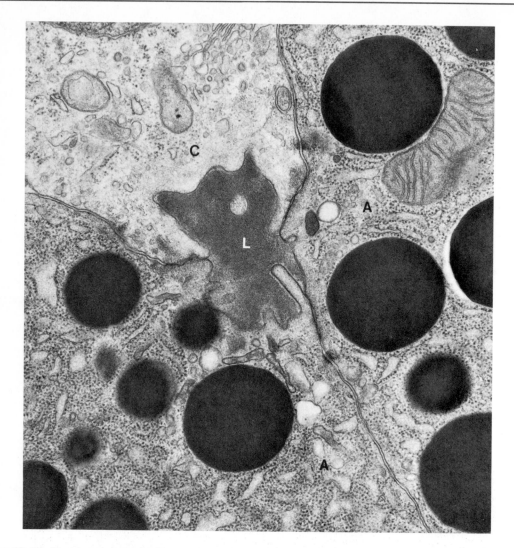

Figure 16–10. Electron micrograph of the apex of 2 pancreatic acinar cells (A) and a centroacinar cell (C) from a rat pancreas. Observe the lack of secretory granules and the very scant rough endoplasmic reticulum in the centroacinar cell as compared with the acinar cell. L, acinar lumen. × 30,000.

of intercalated ducts penetrate the lumens of the acini. Nuclei, surrounded by a pale cytoplasm, belong to **centroacinar cells** that constitute the intra-acinar portion of the intercalated duct (Figs 16–7 and 16–8). Such cells are found only in pancreatic acini. Intercalated ducts are tributaries of larger interlobular ducts lined by columnar epithelium in which goblet cells can be observed. Striated ducts are not present in the pancreatic duct system.

The exocrine pancreatic acinus is composed of several serous cells surrounding a lumen (Figs 16–9 and 16–10). These cells are highly polarized; they have a spherical nucleus and are typical protein-secreting cells. The number of zymogen granules present in each cell is variable and depends on the digestive phase, attaining its maximum in animals that have fasted.

The pancreas is covered by a thin capsule of connective tissue that sends septa into it, separating the pancreatic lobules. The acini are surrounded by a basal lamina that is supported by a delicate sheath of reticular fibers. It has a rich capillary network.

In addition to water and ions, the human exocrine pancreas secretes the following digestive enzymes and proenzymes: **trypsinogen, chymotrypsinogen, carboxypeptidase, ribonuclease, deoxyribonuclease, triacylglycerol lipase, phospholipase A$_2$, elastase,** and **amylase.**

Pancreatic secretion is controlled mainly through 2 hormones—**secretin** and **cholesystokinin** (previ-

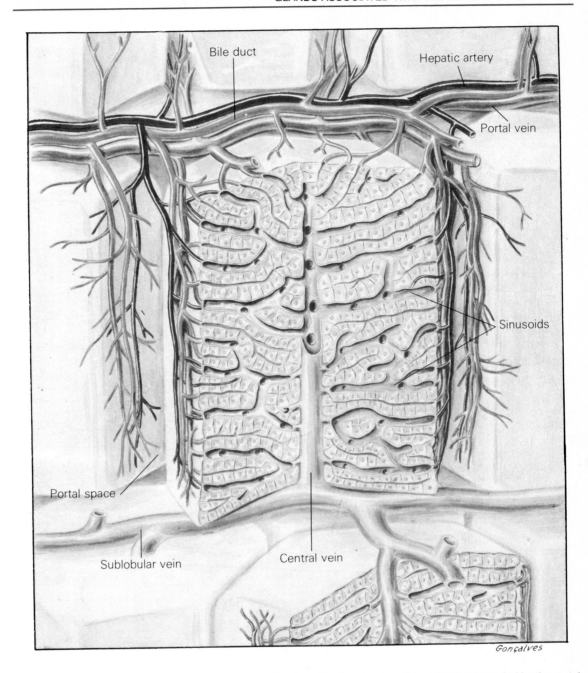

Gonçalves

Figure 16–11. Schematic drawing of the structure of the liver. The liver lobule in the center is surrounded by the portal space (dilated here for the sake of clarity). In the human liver, these spaces are much smaller; in some places, they are nonexistent. Arteries, veins, and bile ducts occupy the portal spaces. Lymphatic vessels, nerves, and connective tissue are also present but are (again for the sake of clarity) not shown in this illustration. Observe in the lobule the radial disposition of the plates formed by liver cells; the sinusoidal capillaries separate the plates. The bile canaliculi can be seen between the liver cells. The sublobular (intercalated) veins drain blood from the lobules. (Redrawn and reproduced, with permission, from Bourne G: *An Introduction to Functional Histology.* Churchill, 1953.)

ously called **pancreozymin**)—that are produced by enteroendocrine cells of the duodenal mucosa. Stimulation of the vagus nerve will also produce pancreatic secretion.

Secretin promotes secretion of an abundant fluid, poor in enzyme activity and rich in bicarbonate. It is probably secreted by the duct cells, not in the acinar cells. This secretion serves to neutralize the acidic **chyme** (partially digested food) so that pancreatic enzymes can function at their optimal neutral pH range. Cholecystokinin promotes secretion of a less abundant but enzyme-rich fluid. This hormone acts mainly in the extrusion of zymogen granules. The integrated action of both these hormones provides for a heavy secretion of enzyme-rich pancreatic juices.

In conditions of extreme malnutrition such as **kwashiorkor,** pancreatic acinar cells and other active protein-secreting cells undergo atrophy and lose much of their rough endoplasmic reticulum. The production of digestive enzymes is hindered.

LIVER

The liver is the organ where nutrients absorbed in the digestive tract are processed, and stored for use by other parts of the body. It is thus an interface between the digestive system and the blood.

With the exception of the skin, the liver is both the largest organ of the body and the largest gland, weighing about 1.5 kg. It is situated in the abdominal cavity beneath the diaphragm. Most of its blood (70–80%) comes from the portal vein; the smaller percentage is supplied by the hepatic artery. All the materials absorbed via the intestines reach the liver through the portal vein, except the complex lipids (**chylomicrons),** which are transported mainly by lymph vessels. The position of the liver in the circulatory system is optimal for gathering, transforming, and accumulating metabolites and for neutralizing and eliminating toxic substances. This elimination occurs in the bile, an exocrine secretion of the liver that is important in lipid digestion.

1. STRUCTURE

Stroma

The liver is covered by a thin connective tissue capsule (**Glisson's capsule)** that becomes thicker at the **hilum,** where the portal vein and hepatic artery enter the liver and the right and left hepatic ducts and lymphatics exit. These vessels and ducts are surrounded by connective tissue all the way to their termination (or origin) in the portal spaces between classic liver lobules. At this point, a delicate retic-

ular fiber network is formed that supports the hepatocytes and sinusoidal endothelial cells of the liver lobules.

The Liver Lobule

The basic structural component of the liver is the liver cell, or **hepatocyte** (from Greek, *hepar,* liver, + *kytos*). These epithelial cells are grouped in interconnected plates. In light microscope sections, structural units called **classic liver lobules** can be seen (Fig 16–11). The liver lobule is formed of a polygonal mass of tissue about 0.7×2 mm in size (Figs 16–11 and 16–12). In certain animals (eg, the pig), lobules are separated from each other by a layer of connective tissue. This does not occur in humans, where the lobules are in close contact along most of their extent, making it difficult to establish the exact limits between different lobules. In some regions, the lobules are demarcated by connective tissue containing bile ducts, lymphatics, nerves, and blood vessels. These regions, the **portal spaces,** are present at the corners of the lobules and are occupied by the **portal triads.** The human liver contains 3–6 portal triads per lobule, each with a venule (a branch of the portal vein); an arteriole (a branch of the hepatic artery); a duct (part of the bile duct system); and lymphatic vessels. The venule is usually the largest of these structures, containing blood from the superior and inferior mesenteric and splenic veins. The arteriole contains blood from the celiac trunk of the abdominal aorta. The duct, lined by cuboidal epithelium, carries bile from the parenchymal cells (hepatocytes) and eventually empties into the hepatic duct. One or more lymphatics carry lymph, which eventually enters the blood circulation. All these structures are embedded in a sheath of connective tissue (Fig 16–13).

The hepatocytes are radially disposed in the liver lobule. They form a layer 1 or 2 cells thick in a fashion similar to the bricks of a wall. These cellular plates are directed from the periphery of the lobule to its center and anastomose freely, forming a labyrinthine and spongelike structure (Fig 16–12). The space between these plates contains capillaries, the **liver sinusoids** (Figs 16–11, 16–12, and 16–13). As discussed in Chapter 11, sinusoids are irregularly dilated vessels composed solely of a discontinuous layer of fenestrated endothelial cells. The fenestrae are about 100 nm in diameter and are grouped in clusters that form "sieve plates" (Fig 16–14).

The endothelial cells are separated from the underlying hepatocytes by a subendothelial space known as the **space of Disse,** which contains some reticular fibers and microvilli of the hepatocytes (Figs 16–18 and 16–21). Consequently, blood fluids readily percolate through the endothelial wall and make intimate contact with the hepatocyte surface, permitting an easy exchange of macromole-

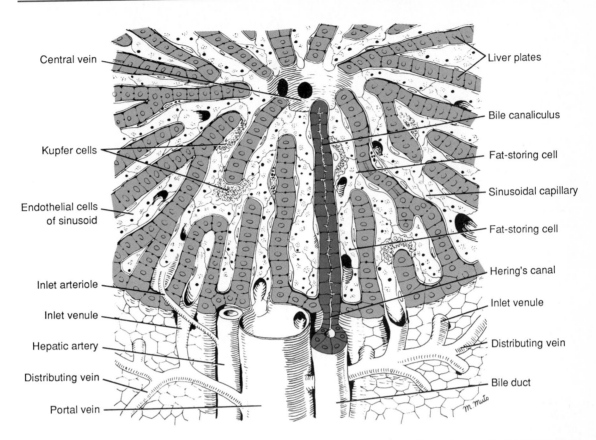

Figure 16–12. Three-dimensional aspect of the normal liver. In the upper center is the central vein; in the lower center, the portal vein. Observe the bile canaliculus (darker color), liver plates (lighter color), Hering's canal, Kupffer cells, sinusoid, fat-storing cell, and sinusoid endothelial cell. (Courtesy of M Muto.)

cules from the sinusoidal lumen to the liver cell and vice versa. This is physiologically important not only because of the large number of macromolecules (eg, lipoproteins, albumin, fibrinogen) secreted into the blood by hepatocytes but because the liver also takes up and catabolizes many of these large molecules. The sinusoid is surrounded and supported by a delicate sheath of reticular fibers. In addition to the endothelial cells, the sinusoids also contain phagocytotic cells of the mononuclear phagocyte series known as **Kupffer cells.** These cells are found on the luminal surface of the endothelial cells. Kupffer cells are typical macrophages. Their main functions are to metabolize aged erythrocytes, digest hemoglobin, and secrete proteins related to immunologic processes. The **fat-storing cells (Ito cells)** (Fig 16–12) are stellate cells located in the spaces of Disse. They have the capacity to accumulate exogenously administered vitamin A as retinyl esters in lipid droplets, but the role of these cells in vitamin A metabolism and transport remains obscure.

The sinusoids arise in the periphery of the lobule,

fed by the inlet venules, terminal branches of the portal veins, and hepatic arterioles. They run in the direction of its center, where they drain into the central vein (Figs 16–11 and 16–12).

Blood Supply

The liver is unusual in that it receives blood from 2 sources: the **portal vein** that carries oxygen-poor nutrient-rich blood from the abdominal viscera; and the **hepatic artery** that supplies oxygen-rich blood (Figs 16–11 and 16–12).

A. Portal Vein System: The portal vein branches repeatedly and sends small venules, the **portal venules,** to the portal triads. The portal venules, sometimes called the **interlobular branches,** branch into the **distributing veins** that run around the periphery of the lobule. From the distributing veins, small **inlet venules** empty into the **sinusoids.** The sinusoids run radially, converging in the center of the lobule to form the **central,** or **centrolobular, vein.** This vessel has thin walls consisting only of endothelial cells supported by a sparse population of collagen fibers. As the central vein progresses along

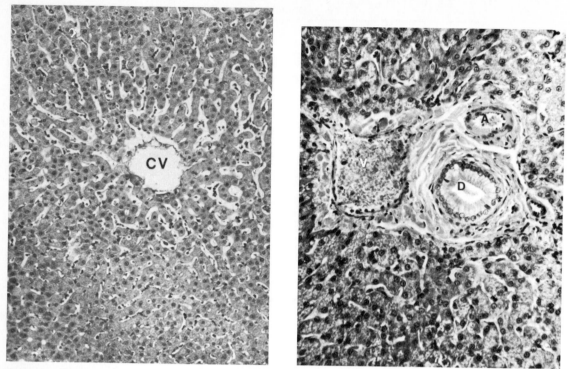

Figure 16–13. Photomicrograph of the liver. **Left:** A central vein (CV). Observe the liver plates that anastomose freely, limiting the space occupied by the sinusoids. H&E stain, × 200. **Right:** A portal space with its characteristic artery (A), vein (V), and bile duct (D) surrounded by connective tissue. Masson's stain, × 300.

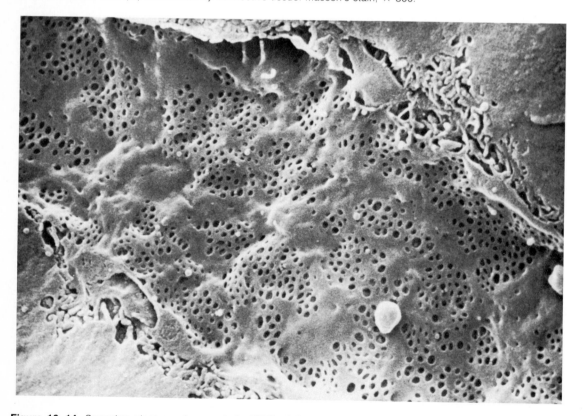

Figure 16–14. Scanning electron micrograph (× 6500) of the endothelial lining of a sinusoidal capillary in rat liver showing the grouped fenestrations in its wall. At the borders, edges of cut hepatocytes are present with their villi protruding into spaces of Disse. (SEM picture courtesy of E Wisse.)

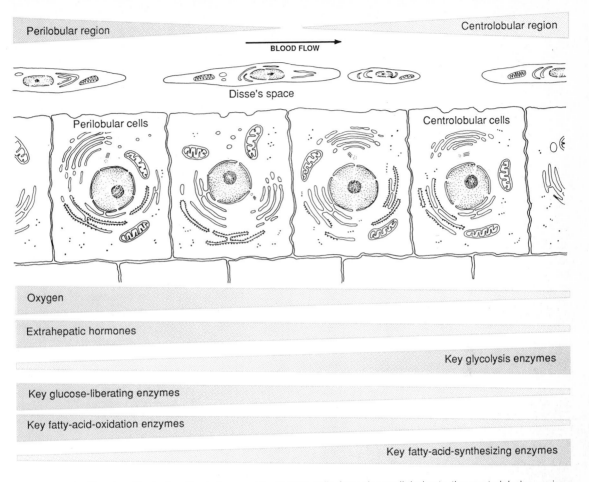

Figure 16–15. Drawing illustrating the heterogeneity of liver cells from the perilobular to the centrolobular regions. (Courtesy of A Brecht.)

the lobule, it receives more and more sinusoids and gradually increases in diameter. At its end, it leaves the lobule at its base by merging with the larger **sublobular vein** (Fig 16–11). The sublobular veins gradually converge and fuse, forming the 2 or more large **hepatic veins** that empty into the inferior vena cava.

B. Arterial System: The hepatic artery branches repeatedly and forms the **interlobular arteries.** Some irrigate the structures of the portal canals and others form arterioles (inlet arterioles; see Fig 16–12) that end directly in the sinusoids at varying distances from the portal spaces, thus providing a mixture of arterial and portal venous blood in the sinusoids.

Blood flows from the periphery to the center of the **classic hepatic lobule.** Consequently, oxygen and metabolites, as well as all other toxic or nontoxic substances absorbed in the intestines, reach first the peripheral cells and then the central cells of the lobule. This partly explains why the behavior of the perilobular cells is different from that of the centrolobular cells (Fig 16–15).

> This duality of behavior of the hepatocyte is particularly evident in pathologic specimens, where certain changes occur in either the central or the peripheral cells of the lobule.

This description of the liver lobule with its blood supply corresponds to the classic concept of this subject in which the centrolobular vein constitutes the axis of the lobule. Fig 16–16 illustrates the hexagons limited by portal spaces (PS) with the central vein (CV) in the center.

Other points of reference can be used in analyzing possible functional units of the liver's structure. Another unit can be visualized—the **portal lobule**—which has at its center the portal triad and at its periphery the regions of adjoining hepatic lobules, all of which drain bile into the bile duct of the cen-

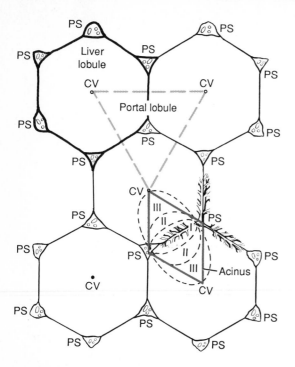

Figure 16–16. Schematic drawing illustrating the territories of the classic liver lobules, hepatic acini, and portal lobules. The classic lobule has a central vein (CV) and is outlined by the solid lines that connect the portal spaces (PS). The portal lobules (lighter color) have their centers in the portal spaces; they are outlined by lines that connect the central veins (upper triangle). The portal lobules constitute the portion of the liver from which bile flows to a portal space. The hepatic acinus (darker color) is the region irrigated by a single distributing vein (diamond-shaped figure). Zones of the hepatic acinus are indicated by I, II, and III. (Redrawn and reproduced, with permission, from Leeson TS, Leeson CR: *Histology,* 2nd ed. Saunders, 1970.)

Based on their proximity to the distributing veins, cells in the hepatic acinus can be subdivided into zones (Fig 16–16). Cells in zone I would be those closest to the vessel and consequently the first to alter or be affected by the incoming blood. Cells in zone II would be second to respond to the blood, and those in zone III would see portal vein blood that had already been altered by cells in zones I and II. For example, after feeding, cells in zone I would be the first to receive incoming glucose and to store it as glycogen. Any glucose passing the cells in zone I would likely be picked up by cells in zone II. In the event of fasting, cells in zone I would be the first to respond to glucose-poor blood by breaking down glycogen and releasing it as glucose. In this event, the cells in zones II and III would not respond to the fasting condition until the glycogen in zone I cells was depleted.

This zonal arrangement would account for some of the differences in the selective damage of hepatocytes by various noxious agents or various disease conditions.

The Hepatocyte

Liver cells are polyhedral, with 6 or more surfaces, and have a diameter of 20–30 μm. In sections stained with hematoxylin and eosin, the cytoplasm of the hepatocyte is eosinophilic, mainly because of the presence of large numbers of mitochondria and some smooth endoplasmic reticulum. Hepatocytes located at different distances from the portal triads show variations in structural, histochemical, and biochemical characteristics. The surface of each liver cell is in contact with the wall of the sinusoids, through the space of Disse, and with the surfaces of other hepatocytes. Wherever 2 hepatocytes abut, they delimit a tubular space between them known as the **bile canaliculus** (Figs 16–12, 16–17, 16–18, and 16–19).

The canaliculi, the first portions of the bile duct system, are tubular spaces 1–2 μm in diameter. They are limited only by the plasma membranes of 2 hepatocytes and have a small number of microvilli in their interiors (Figs 16–18 and 16–19). The cell membranes near these canaliculi are firmly joined by tight junctions (described in Chapter 4). Gap junctions are frequent between hepatocytes and are sites of intercellular communication, an important process in the coordination of these cells' physiologic activities. The bile canaliculi form a complex anastomosing network progressing along the plates of the liver lobule and terminating in the region of the portal spaces (Fig 16–12). The bile flow therefore progresses in a direction opposite to that of the blood, ie, from the center of the classic lobule to its periphery. At the periphery, bile enters the **bile**

tral portal triad. A portal lobule would be triangular, as opposed to the polygonal appearance of the classic liver lobule. It would have a central vein at the tip of each of its angles, and it would contain parts of 3 adjoining liver lobules. See the dashed triangle in Fig 16–16 with the portal space (PS) at its center.

Another way of subdividing the liver into functional lobules is to regard as a unit of liver parenchyma that region which is irrigated by a terminal branch of the distributing veins. This unit, called the **hepatic acinus** (of Rappaport), appears diamond-shaped in section (area CV-PS-CV-PS in Fig 16–16). In addition to the terminal branches of the portal vein, an arterial branch and a bile ductule are in the center of this subdivision of hepatic parenchyma, which is situated in adjacent areas of 2 different classic hepatic lobules (Fig 16–16).

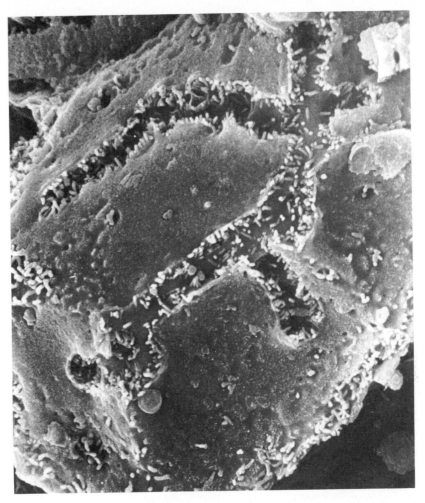

Figure 16–17. Branching bile canaliculi observed in the liver by scanning electron microscopy. Observe the microvilli lining the internal surface. (Reproduced, with permission, from Motta P, Muto M, Fujita T: *the Liver: An Atlas of Scanning Electron Microscopy.* Igaku-Shoin, 1978.)

ductules, or **Hering's canals** (Figs 16–12 and 16–20). These are composed of cuboidal cells with a clear cytoplasm and few organelles. After a short distance, the ductules cross the limiting hepatocytes of the lobule and end in the **bile ducts** in the portal triads (Figs 16–11 and 16–20). Bile ducts are lined by cuboidal or columnar epithelium and have a distinct connective tissue sheath. They gradually enlarge and fuse, forming the right and left **hepatic ducts** that subsequently leave the liver.

The surface of the hepatocyte that faces the space of Disse bears many microvilli protruding in that space, but there is always a space between them and the cells of the sinusoidal wall (Figs 16–18 and 16–21). The liver cell has 1 or 2 rounded nuclei with 1 or 2 typical nucleoli. Some of the nuclei are polyploid; ie, they contain some even multiples of the haploid number of chromosomes. Polyploid nuclei are characterized by their greater size, which is proportional to their ploidy. The hepatocyte has an abundant endoplasmic reticulum—both smooth and rough (Figs 16–18 and 16–22). In the hepatocyte, the rough endoplasmic reticulum forms aggregates dispersed in the cytoplasm; these are called **basophilic bodies** by classic microscopists. Several proteins (eg, blood albumin, fibrinogen) are synthesized on polyribosomes in these structures. Various important processes occur in the smooth endoplasmic reticulum that is distributed diffusely throughout the cytoplasm. This organelle is responsible for the processes of oxidation, methylation, and conjugation required for inactivation or detoxification of various substances before their excretion from the body. The smooth endoplasmic reticulum of the hepatocyte is a labile system that reacts promptly to changes in the environment.

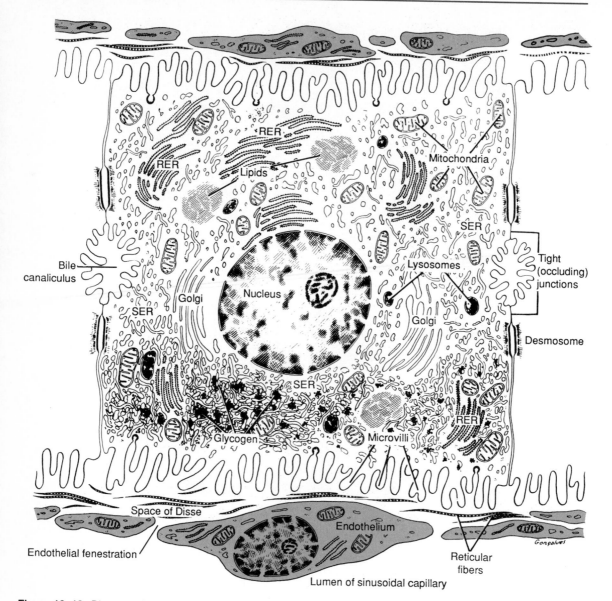

Figure 16–18. Diagram of the ultrastructure of a hepatocyte. RER, rough endoplasmic reticulum; SER, smooth endoplasmic reticulum. Cells of the sinusoidal capillary are shown in color. × 10,000.

One of the main processes occurring in the smooth endoplasmic reticulum is the conjugation of hydrophobic toxic bilirubin by glucuronyltransferase to form a water-soluble nontoxic bilirubin glucuronide. This conjugate is excreted by hepatocytes into the bile. When bilirubin or bilirubin glucuronide is not excreted, several diseases characterized by jaundice can occur (Fig 16–25). One of the frequent causes of jaundice in newborns is the often underdeveloped state of the smooth endoplasmic reticulum in their hepatocytes (**neonatal hyperbilirubinemia**; *hyper* + Latin, *bilis*, bile, + *ruber*, red, + Greek, *haima*). The current treatment for these cases is exposure to blue light from ordinary fluorescent tubes; this transforms unconjugated bilirubin to a water-soluble photoisomer that can be excreted by the kidneys.

The liver cell frequently contains glycogen. This polysaccharide appears in the electron microscope as coarse, electron-dense granules that frequently collect within accumulations of smooth endoplasmic

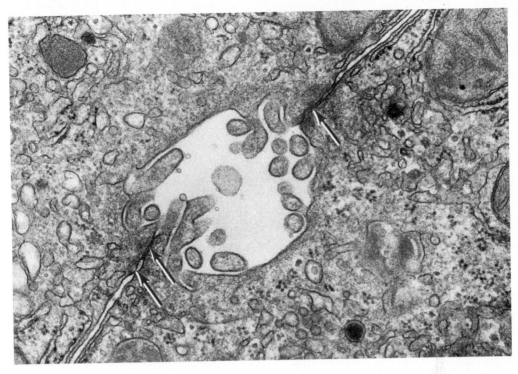

Figure 16–19. Electron micrograph of a rat liver bile canaliculus showing the microvilli in its lumen and the junctional complexes (arrows) that seal off this space from the remaining extracellular space. × 54,000. (Courtesy of SL Wissig.)

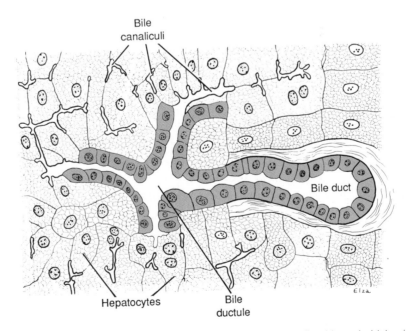

Figure 16–20. The confluence of bile canaliculi and bile ductules, which are lined by cuboidal epithelium (shown in color). These ductules merge with bile ducts in the portal spaces.

Sinusoid

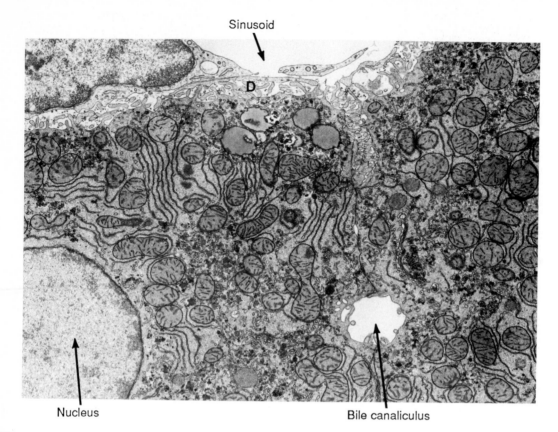

Nucleus

Bile canaliculus

Figure 16–21. Electron micrograph of the liver of a rat. Note the 2 adjacent hepatocytes with a bile canaliculus between them. The hepatocytes contain numerous mitochondria (M) and smooth (SER) and rough (RER) endoplasmic reticula. A prominent Golgi complex (G) is near the bile canaliculus. The sinusoid is lined by endothelial cells with large open fenestrae. The space of Disse (D) is occupied by numerous microvilli projecting from the hepatocytes. L, lipid droplet. × 9200. (Courtesy of D Schmucker.)

reticulum (Figs 16–18 and 16–23). The amount of glycogen present in the liver conforms to a diurnal rhythm; it also depends upon the nutritional state of the animal. Liver glycogen is a depot for glucose and is mobilized if the blood glucose level falls below normal. In this way, hepatocytes maintain a steady level of blood glucose, one of the main sources of energy for use by the body.

Each liver cell has approximately 2000 mitochondria. Another common cellular component is the lipid droplet, whose numbers vary greatly (Fig 16–21). Hepatocyte lysosomes are important in the turnover and degradation of intracellular organelles. They also play a fundamental role in the receptor-mediated endocytosis of many macromolecular ligands. These macromolecules are first transported to endosomes that later fuse with lysosomes. Catabolism of macromolecules occurs in these secondary lysosomes. Peroxisomes are abundant in hepatocytes. Golgi complexes in the liver are numerous—up to 50 per cell. Each complex consists of flattened cisternae,

small vesicles, and larger vacuoles lying near the bile canaliculi. The functions of this organelle include the formation of lysosomes and secretion of plasma proteins (eg, albumin), glycoproteins (eg, transferrin), and lipoproteins (eg, very low density lipoproteins [VLDL]).

2. FUNCTIONS

The liver cell probably is the most versatile cell in the body. It is a cell with both endocrine and exocrine functions; it also synthesizes and accumulates certain substances, detoxifies others, and transports still others.

Protein Synthesis

In addition to synthesizing proteins for its own maintenance, the liver cell produces various plasma

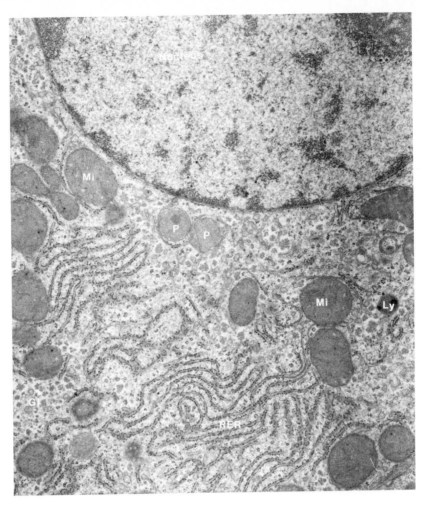

Figure 16–22. Electron micrograph of a hepatocyte. In the cytoplasm, below the nucleus, are mitochondria (Mi), rough endoplasmic reticulum (RER), glycogen (Gl), lysosomes (Ly), and peroxisomes (P). × 6600.

proteins for export—among them albumin, prothrombin, fibrinogen, and lipoproteins. These proteins are synthesized on polyribosomes attached to the rough endoplasmic reticulum. Contrary to what is observed in other glandular cells, the hepatocyte does not store proteins in its cytoplasm as secretory granules but continuously releases them into the bloodstream, thus functioning as an endocrine gland (Fig 16–23). About 5% of the protein exported by the liver is produced by the cells of the macrophage system (Kupffer cells); the remainder is synthesized in the hepatocytes.

Bile Secretion

Bile production is an exocrine function in the sense that the hepatocytes promote the uptake, transformation, and excretion of blood components into the bile canaliculi. Bile has several other essential components in addition to water and electrolytes: bile acids, phospholipids, cholesterol, and bilirubin. The secretion of bile acids is illustrated in Fig 16–24. About 90% of these substances are derived by absorption from the distal intestinal epithelium and are transported as such by the hepatocyte from the blood to bile canaliculi (enterohepatic recirculation). About 10% of these compounds are synthesized in the smooth endoplasmic reticulum of the hepatocyte by conjugation of cholic acid (synthesized by the liver from cholesterol) with the amino acid glycine or taurine, producing glycocholic and taurocholic acids. Bile acids have an important function in emulsifying the lipids in the digestive tract, promoting easier digestion by lipase and subsequent absorption. Bile acids, along with biliary phospholipids, serve to

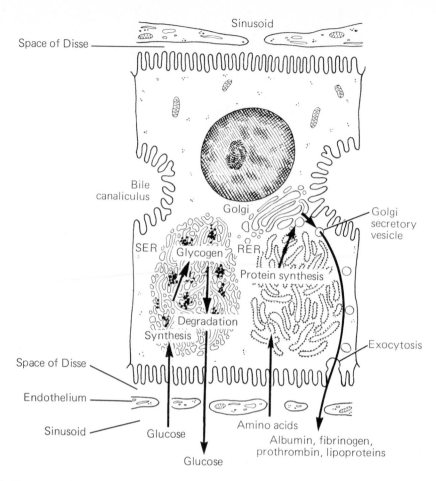

Figure 16–23. Protein synthesis and carbohydrate storage in the liver. Protein synthesis occurs in the rough endoplasmic reticulum, which explains why liver-cell lesions or starvation lead to a decrease in the amounts of albumin fibrinogen, and prothrombin in a patient's blood. In several diseases, glycogen degradation is depressed, with abnormal intracellular accumulation of this compound. SER, smooth endoplastic reticulum; RER, rough endoplastic reticulum.

solubilize cholesterol and facilitate its excretion from the body.

Abnormal proportions of these constituents may lead to the formation of gallstones (cholelithiasis). Gallstones can block bile flow and cause jaundice—bile pigments in blood—from the rupture of tight junctions around the bile canaliculi.

Bilirubin, most of which results from the breakdown of hemoglobin, is formed in the mononuclear phagocyte system (this includes the Kupffer cells of the liver sinusoids) and is transported to the hepatocytes. In the smooth endoplasmic reticulum of the hepatocyte, hydrophobic (water-insoluble) bilirubin is conjugated to glucuronic acid, forming water-soluble **bilirubin glucuronide** (Fig 16–25). In a further step, bilirubin glucuronide is secreted into the bile canaliculi.

The hepatocyte also has the ability to transport several dyes actively. This ability to eliminate dyes is used as a test of liver function. One of the dyes most often used for this purpose is sulfobromophthalein.

Metabolite Storage

Lipids and carbohydrates are stored in the liver in the form of triglycerides and glycogen (Figs 16–21 and 16–23). This capacity to store metabolites is important because it supplies the body with energy between meals. Fig 16–23 shows how this is done for the carbohydrates. The liver also serves as the

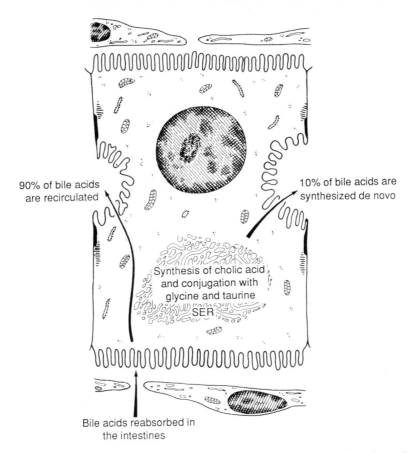

90% of bile acids
are recirculated

10% of bile acids are
synthesized de novo

Synthesis of cholic acid
and conjugation with
glycine and taurine
SER

Bile acids reabsorbed in
the intestines

Figure 16–24. Mechanism of secretion of bile acids. About 90% of these compounds derive from bile acids absorbed in the intestinal epithelium and recirculated to the liver. The remainder are synthesized in the liver by conjugating cholic acid with the amino acids glycine and taurine. This process occurs in the smooth endoplasmic reticulum (SER).

major storage compartment for vitamins, especially vitamin A.

Metabolic Functions

The hepatocyte is responsible for converting lipids and amino acids into glucose by means of a complex enzymatic process called **gluconeogenesis** (from Greek, *glykys*, sweet, + *neos* + *genesis*, production). It is also the main site of amino acid deamination, resulting in the production of urea. This compound is transported in the blood to the kidney and excreted by that organ.

Detoxification & Inactivation

Various drugs and substances can be inactivated by oxidation, methylation, or conjugation. The enzymes participating in these processes are located mainly in the smooth endoplasmic reticulum. Glucuronyltransferase, an enzyme that conjugates glucuronic acid to bilirubin, also causes conjugation of several other compounds such as steroids, barbiturates, antihistamines, and anticonvulsants.

The observation that the administration of barbiturates to laboratory animals resulted in rapid development of smooth endoplasmic reticulum in hepatocytes led to further studies. These showed that barbiturates can also increase synthesis of glucuronyltransferase and led to the use of barbiturates in the treatment of glucuronyltransferase deficiencies. This is a typical example of the clinical use—and value—of data from experimental research in cell biology.

Liver Regeneration

Despite being an organ whose cells are renewed at a slow rate, the liver has an extraordinary capacity for regeneration. The loss of hepatic tissue by surgical removal or from the action of toxic substances triggers a mechanism by which liver cells begin to divide, continuing until the original mass of tissue is restored. In rats, the liver can regenerate a loss of 75% of its weight in 1 month. In humans, this capac-

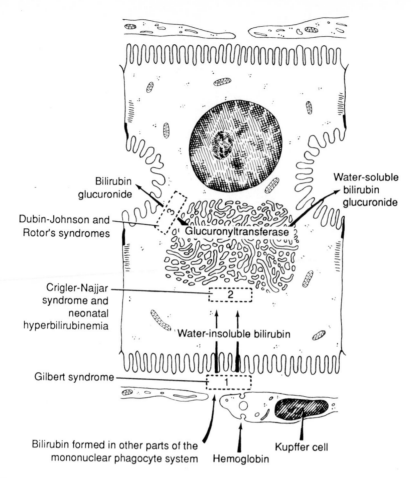

Figure 16–25. The secretion of bilirubin. This water-insoluble compound is derived from the metabolism of hemoglobin in macrophages of the mononuclear phagocyte system. Glucuronyltransferase activity in the hepatocytes causes bilirubin to be conjugated with glucuronide in the smooth endoplasmic reticulum, forming a water-soluble compound. When bile secretion is blocked, the yellow bilirubin or bilirubin glucuronide is not excreted; it accumulates in the blood, and jaundice results. Several defective processes in the hepatocytes can cause diseases that produce jaundice: a defect in the capacity of the cell to trap and absorb bilirubin (rectangle 1); the inability of the cell to conjugate bilirubin because of a deficiency in glucuronyltransferase (rectangle 2); or problems in the transfer and excretion of bilirubin glucuronide into the biliary canaliculi (rectangle 3). One of the most frequent causes of jaundice, however—unrelated to hepatocyte activity—is the obstruction of bile flow as a result of gallstones or tumors of the pancreas.

ity is considerably restricted. The process of regeneration is probably controlled by circulating substances called **chalones,** which inhibit the mitotic division of certain cell types.

When a tissue is injured or partially removed, the amount of chalones it produces decreases; consequently, a burst of mitotic activity occurs in this tissue. As regeneration proceeds, the amount of chalones produced is increased and mitotic activity decreases. This process is self-regulating.

The regenerated liver tissue is usually similar to the removed tissue. If there is continuous or repeated damage to this organ, however, liver cell regeneration and an abundant production of connective tissue occur simultaneously. This excess of connective tissue results in disorganization of the liver structure, a condition known as **cirrhosis.** Liver function is impaired in this condition, since scar tissue (collagen) not only replaces functional hepatocytes but also disorganizes the liver, vascular, and bile duct systems.

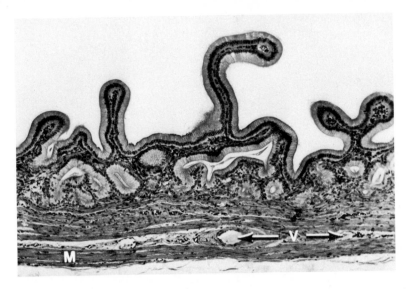

Figure 16–26. Photomicrograph of a section of gallbladder. Observe the lining columnar epithelium, the smooth muscle layer (M), and the blood vessels (V). H&E stain, × 30.

BILIARY TRACT

The bile produced by the liver cell flows through the **bile canaliculi, bile ductules,** and **bile ducts.** These structures gradually merge, forming a network that converges to form the **hepatic duct.** The hepatic duct, after receiving the **cystic duct** from the gallbladder, continues to the duodenum as the **common bile duct (ductus choledochus).**

The hepatic, cystic, and common bile ducts are lined by a mucous membrane of simple columnar epithelium. The lamina propria is thin and surrounded by an inconspicuous layer of smooth muscle. This muscle layer becomes thicker near the duodenum and finally forms, in the intramural portion, a sphincter that regulates bile flow (sphincter of Oddi).

GALLBLADDER

The gallbladder is a hollow, pear-shaped organ attached to the lower surface of the liver. It can store 30–50 mL of bile and communicates with the hepatic duct through the cystic duct. The wall of the gallbladder consists of the following layers (Fig 16–26): a mucosa composed of simple columnar epithelium and lamina propria, a layer of smooth muscle, a well-developed perimuscular connective tissue layer, and a serous membrane.

The mucosa has abundant folds that are particularly evident in the empty bladder. The epithelial cells are rich in mitochondria and have their nuclei in their basal third (Fig 16–27). All these cells are capable of secreting small amounts of mucus. Microvilli are fre-

quent at the apical surface. Near the cystic duct, the epithelium invaginates into the lamina propria, forming tubuloacinar glands with wide lumens. Cells of these glands have characteristics of mucus-secreting cells and are responsible for the production of most of the mucus present in bile.

The muscular layer is thin, with most of the smooth muscle cells oriented around the circumference of the gallbladder. A thick connective tissue layer binds the superior surface of the gallbladder to the liver. The opposite surface is covered by a typical serous layer, the peritoneum.

The main function of the gallbladder is to store bile, concentrate it by absorbing its water, and release it when necessary into the digestive tract. This process depends upon an active sodium-transporting mechanism in the gallbladder's epithelium. Water absorption is an osmotic consequence of the sodium pump. Contraction of the smooth muscle of the gallbladder is induced by **cholecystokinin,** a hormone produced by enteroendocrine cells (I-cells) located in the epithelial lining of the small intestine. Release of cholecystokinin is, in turn, stimulated by the presence of dietary fats in the small intestine.

Tumors of the Digestive Glands

The majority of malignant tumors of the liver derive from hepatic parenchyma or epithelial cells of the bile duct. Liver carcinomas are often preceded by connective tissue proliferation (cirrhosis). Most tumors of the exocrine pancreas arise from ductal epithelial cells; the mortality rate is high.

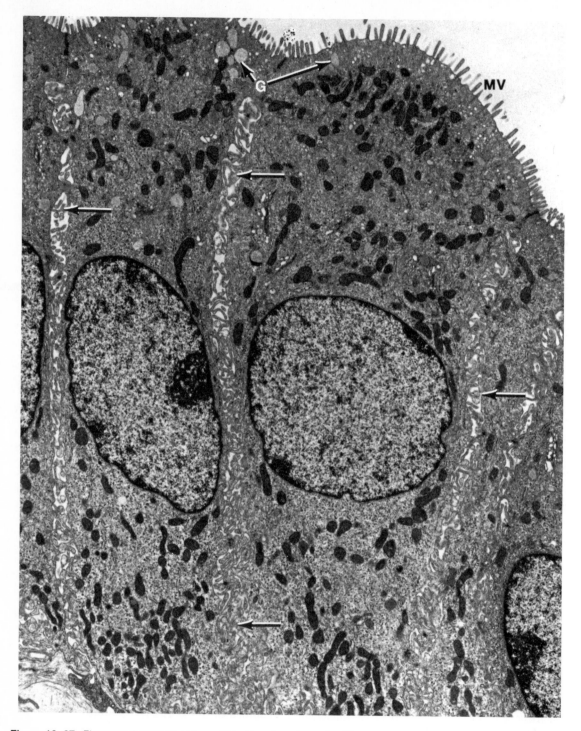

Figure 16–27. Electron micrograph of the gallbladder of a guinea pig. Observe the microvilli (MV) on the surface of the cell and the secretory granules (G) containing mucus. Arrows indicate the intercellular spaces. These cells transport sodium chloride from the lumen to the subjacent connective tissue. Water follows passively, causing the bile to become concentrated. × 5600.

REFERENCES

Pancreas & Salivary Glands

Mason DK, Chisholm DM: *Salivary Glands in Health and Disease.* Saunders, 1975.

Young JA, Van Lennep DW: *The Morphology of Salivary Glands.* Academic Press, 1978.

Young JA et al: A microperfusion investigation of sodium resorption and potassium secretion by the main excretory duct of the rat submaxillary gland. *Pfluegers Arch* 1967;**295**:157.

Liver & Biliary Tract

Gerber MA, Swan NT: Histology of the liver. *Am J Surg Pathol* 1987;**11**:709.

Ito T, Shibasaki S: Electron microscopic study on the hepatic sinusoidal wall and the fat-storing cells in the human normal liver. *Arch Histol Jpn* 1968;**29**:137.

Jones AL, Fawcett CW: Hypertrophy of the agranular endoplasmic reticulum in hamster liver induced by phenobarbital. *J Histochem Cytochem* 1966;**14**:215.

Rouiller C (editor): *The Liver: Morphology, Biochemistry, Physiology.* 2 vols. Academic Press, 1963, 1964.

The respiratory system includes the **lungs** and a system of tubes that link the sites of gas exchange with the external environment. There is also a **ventilation mechanism,** consisting of the thoracic cage, intercostal muscles, diaphragm, and elastic and collagen components of the lungs, that is important in the movement of air through the conducting and respiratory parts of the lungs. It is customary to divide the respiratory system into 2 principal regions (Fig 17–1): a **conducting portion,** consisting of the nasal cavity, nasopharynx, larynx, trachea, bronchi (from Greek, *bronchos,* windpipe), bronchioles, and terminal bronchioles; and a **respiratory portion** (where gas exchange takes place), consisting of respiratory bronchioles, alveolar ducts, and alveoli. **Alveoli** are specialized saclike structures that make up the greater part of the lungs. They are the main sites for the exchange of oxygen and carbon dioxide between inspired air and blood—the principal function of the lungs.

The conducting portion serves 2 main functions: to provide a conduit through which air can travel to and from the lungs; and to condition the inspired air. In order to ensure an uninterrupted supply of air, a combination of cartilage, elastic and collagen fibers, and smooth muscle provides the conducting portion with rigid structural support and the necessary flexibility and extensibility. The cartilages, primarily hyaline (with some elastic cartilage in the larynx), are found in the periphery of the lamina propria. They have various forms, ranging from small plaques to irregular rings and, in the trachea, C-shaped cartilages. The cartilages generally serve to support the walls of the conducting portion, preventing collapse of the lumen and thereby ensuring continuous access of air to the lungs. Both the conducting and respiratory portions are richly endowed with elastic fibers that provide these structures with flexibility and allow them to spring back after distention. In the conducting portion, the elastic fibers are found in the lamina propria; their orientation is mainly longitudinal. Elastic fiber concentration is inversely proportionate to the diameter of the conducting tubule (ie, the smallest bronchioles have the highest proportion of elastic fibers). Bundles of smooth muscle are found encircling the tubes from the trachea to the alveolar ducts (a subdivision of the respiratory portion). Contraction of the

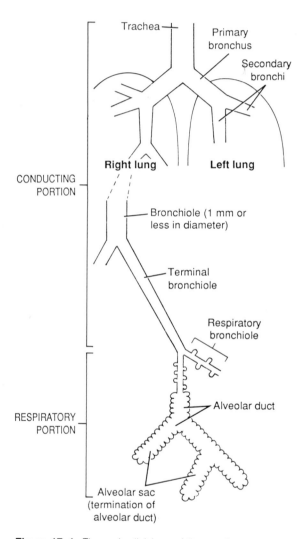

Figure 17–1. The main divisions of the respiratory tract. The natural proportions of these structures have been altered for clarity; the respiratory bronchiole, for example, is in reality a short transitional structure.

smooth muscle reduces the diameter of the conducting tubules and thereby regulates air flow during inspiration and expiration. The conducting portion of the respiratory system is gradually transformed into the respiratory portion. Its content of ciliated epithelium, goblet cells, and cartilage is reduced, while the content of smooth muscle and elastic fibers gradually increases (Table 17–1).

Conditioning of Air

A major function of the conducting portion is to condition the inspired air. Before it enters the lungs, inspired air is cleansed, moistened, and warmed. To carry out these functions, the mucosa of the conducting portions is lined by a specialized **respiratory epithelium,** and there are numerous mucous and serous glands as well as a rich superficial vascular network in the lamina propria.

As the air enters the nose, large **vibrissae** (specialized hairs) remove coarse particles of dust. Once the air reaches the **nasal fossae,** particulate and gaseous impurities are trapped in a layer of mucus. This mucus, in conjunction with serous secretions, also serves to moisten the incoming air, protecting the delicate alveolar lining from desiccation. The incoming air is also warmed by a rich superficial vascular network.

Respiratory Epithelium

Most of the conducting portion is lined by ciliated pseudostratified columnar epithelium that contains a rich population of goblet cells. Deeper in the bronchial tree, this epithelial cell population is modified in a transition to simple squamous epithelium. As the bronchi subdivide into the bronchioles, the pseudostratified organization gives way to a simple columnar epithelium, which is further reduced to a simple

cuboidal layer in the smallest (terminal) bronchioles. The rich goblet cell population tapers off in the smaller bronchi and is totally absent from the epithelium in the terminal bronchioles. It is important to note that ciliated cells, which accompany the goblet cells, continue through the finer bronchioles in the absence of goblet cells. The continuation of the ciliated cells beyond the goblet cells serves to prevent mucus from accumulating in the respiratory portion of the system. The superficial mucus, which traps particulate matter and absorbs water-soluble gases (eg, SO_2 and ozone), floats on a subjacent sol phase secreted by serous glands located in the lamina propria (Fig 17–4). Cilia of these epithelia move the more fluid sol phase, together with the overlying mucous layer, toward the oral cavity. Here, the mucous layer is either swallowed or expectorated.

Typical respiratory epithelium consists of 5 cell types as seen in the electron microscope. **Ciliated columnar cells** constitute the most abundant type. Each cell possesses about 300 cilia on its apical surface (Figs 17–2, 17–3, and 17–4); beneath the cilia, in addition to basal bodies, are numerous small mitochrondia. From experimental studies, it has been demonstrated that adenosine triphosphate (ATP) is required for ciliary beating, an observation that is consistent with the apical localization of mitochondria.

Immotile cilia syndrome (Kartagener's syndrome), a disorder that causes infertility in males and chronic respiratory-tract infections in both sexes, is caused by immobility of cilia and flagella induced by deficiency of **dynein,** a protein normally present in the cilia. This protein is responsible for the sliding of the microtubules, a

Table 17–1. Structural changes in the conducting portions of the respiratory tract.

	Nasal Fossae	Naso-pharynx	Larynx	Trachea	Bronchi Large	Bronchi Small	Bronchioles Regular	Bronchioles Terminal	Bronchioles Respiratory
Epithelium	Ciliated pseudostratified columnar[1,2]						→ Transition →		
							Ciliated pseudo-stratified columnar	Ciliated simple columnar	Ciliated simple cuboidal
Goblet cells	Abundant				Present	Few	Scattered	None	
Glands	Abundant		Present			Few	None		
Cartilage			Complex (hyaline and elastic)	C-shaped rings	Irregular rings	Plates and islands	None		
Smooth muscle	None			Spanning open ends of C-shaped rings	Crisscrossing spiral bundles				
Elastic fibers	None	Present				Abundant			

[1] Stratified squamous in regions of direct air flow or abrasion.
[2] Vestibule of nose shows transition from keratinized stratified squamous to ciliated pseudostratified columnar epithelium.

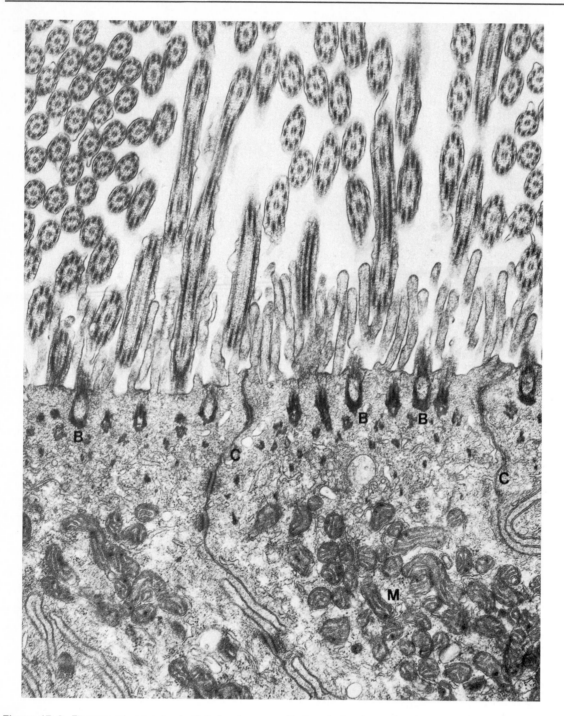

Figure 17–2. Electron micrograph of ciliated columnar epithelium in the lung, showing the ciliary microtubules in transverse and oblique section. In the cell apex are the U-shaped basal bodies (B) that serve as the source of and anchoring sites for the ciliary axonemes. The local accumulation of mitochondria (at M) is related to energy production for ciliary movement. Observe junctional complexes at C, and note the emergence of microvilli between the ciliary roots. × 9200.

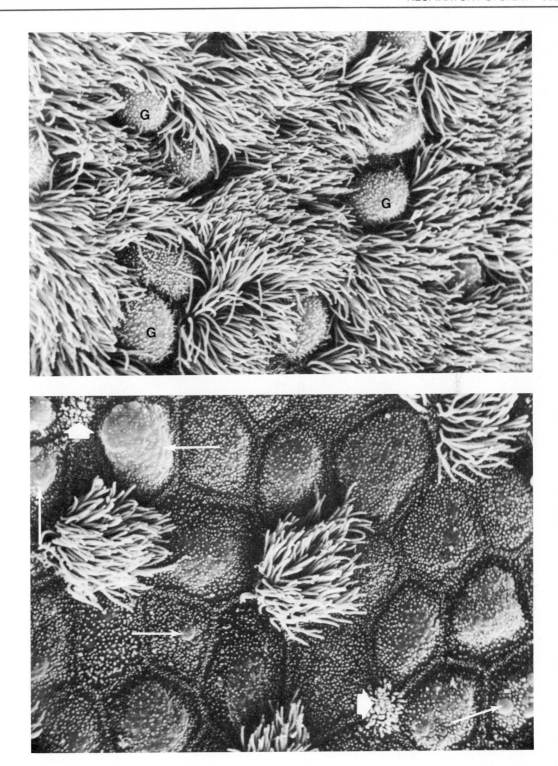

Figure 17–3. Scanning electron micrograph of the surface of rat respiratory mucosa. G, goblet cells. Most of the surface is covered by cilia. In the lower micrograph, subsurface accumulations of mucus are evident in the goblet cells (thin arrows). Examples of brush cells are indicated by the thick arrows. **Top,** × 2500. **Bottom,** × 3000. (Reproduced, with permission, from Andrews P: A scanning electron microscopic study of the extrapulmonary respiratory tract. *Am J Anat* 1974;**139:**421.)

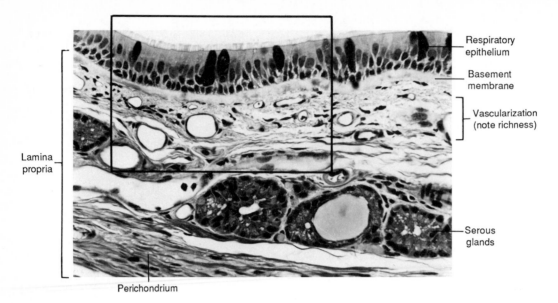

Respiratory epithelium

Basement membrane

Vascularization (note richness)

Lamina propria

Serous glands

Perichondrium

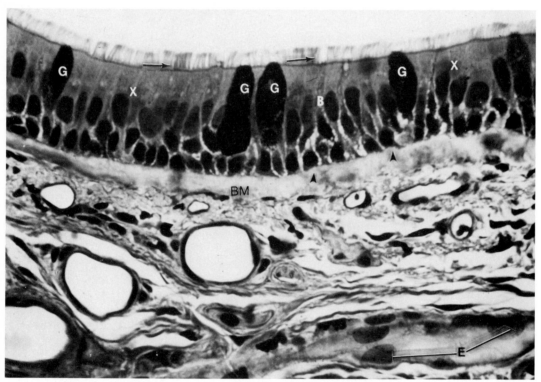

Figure 17–4. Top: Section of monkey trachea showing typical respiratory epithelium, thick basement membrane, richly vascularized connective tissue of the lamina propria, and the presence of glands containing both serous and mucous cells. Beneath the glands lies the dense connective tissue of the perichondrium, which surrounds the supporting hyaline cartilage (not visible). × 200. **Bottom:** Enlargement of the rectangular area shown above. The tracheal lumen is lined by typical ciliated pseudostratified columnar epithelium with goblet cells. This epithelium plays a significant role in conditioning the inspired air. Beneath the unusually thick basement membrane (BM) lies the lamina propria, whose rich vascularity aids in warming the incoming air. G, goblet cells containing mucous secretion; X, ciliated columnar cells; B, nonciliated brush cell; arrowheads, rounded basal cell; small arrows, cilia; E, *en face* view of venule endothelial cells. × 500.

process that is necessary for ciliary movement (see Chapter 3).

The next most abundant cells are the **mucous goblet cells** (Fig 17–4). The apical portion of these cells (described in Chapter 4) contains the polysaccharide-rich mucous droplets. The remaining columnar cells are known as **brush cells** (Figs 17–3 and 17–4) because of the numerous microvilli present on their apical surface. Brush cells have afferent nerve endings on their basal surfaces and are considered to be sensory receptors. **Basal (short) cells** are small rounded cells that lie on the basal lamina but do not extend to the luminal surface of the epithelium. These cells are believed to be generative cells that undergo mitosis and subsequently differentiate into the other cell types. The remaining cell type is the **small granule cell,** which resembles a basal cell except that it possesses numerous granules 100–300 nm in diameter with dense cores. Histochemical studies reveal that these cells constitute a population of cells of the diffuse neuroendocrine system (see Chapter 4). These endocrinelike granule cells may act as effectors in the integration of the mucous and serous secretory processes. All cells of the ciliated pseudostratified columnar epithelium touch the basement membrane (Fig 17–4, bottom).

From the nasal cavity through the larynx, portions of the epithelium are stratified squamous. This type of epithelium is evident in regions exposed to direct air flow or physical abrasion (eg, oropharynx, epiglottis, vocal folds); it provides more protection from attrition than does typical respiratory epithelium. If air-flow currents are altered or new abrasive sites develop, the affected areas can convert from typical ciliated pseudostratified columnar epithelium to stratified squamous epithelium. Similarly, in smokers, the proportion of ciliated cells to goblet cells is altered in order to aid in clearing the increased particulate and gaseous pollutants (eg, CO, SO_2). Although the greater numbers of goblet cells in a smoker's epithelium provide for a more rapid clearance of pollutants, the reduction of ciliated cells caused by excessive CO results in a decrease in the movement of the mucous layer and frequently leads to congestion of the smaller airways. These reversible changes in tissue organization are referred to as metaplasia (see Chapter 4).

NASAL CAVITY

The nasal cavity consists of 2 structures: the external **vestibule** and the internal **nasal fossae;** the latter are separated by the osseous nasal septum.

Vestibule

The vestibule is the most anterior and dilated portion of the nasal cavity. The outer integument of the nose enters the **nares** (nostrils) and continues part way up the vestibule. Around the inner surface of the nares are numerous sebaceous and sweat glands, in addition to the thick short hairs, or **vibrissae,** that filter out large particles from the inspired air. Within the vestibule. the epithelium loses its keratinized nature and undergoes a transition into typical respiratory epithelium before entering the nasal fossae.

Nasal Fossae

Within the skull lie 2 cavernous chambers separated by the **nasal septum.** Extending from each lateral wall are 3 bony shelflike projections known as **conchae.** Of the superior, middle, and inferior conchae, only the middle and inferior projections are covered by respiratory epithelium. The superior conchae are covered by a specialized olfactory epithelium. The structure and function of olfactory epithelium are discussed in Chapter 24. The narrow, ribbonlike passages created by the conchae improve the conditioning of the inspired air by increasing the surface area containing respiratory epithelium and by creating turbulence in the air flow, which results in increased contact between air streams and the mucous layer. Within the lamina propria of the conchae are large venous plexuses known as **swell bodies.** Every 20–30 minutes, the swell bodies on one side of the nasal fossae become engorged with blood, resulting in distention of the conchal mucosa and a concomitant decrease in the flow of air. During this time, most of the air is directed through the other nasal fossa. These periodic intervals of occlusion reduce air flow, so that the respiratory epithelium can recover from desiccation.

Allergic reactions and inflammation can cause abnormal engorgement of swell bodies in both fossae and result in a severely restricted air flow.

In addition to swell bodies, the nasal cavity has a rich and complexly organized vascular system. Large vessels form a close-meshed latticework next to the periosteum, from which arcading branches lead toward the surface. Smaller vessels branch from the arcading vessels and run perpendicular to the surface. These smaller vessels form a rich capillary bed beneath the epithelium. Blood flows forward from the rear to each fossa. In each arcading loop, the flow of blood counters the flow of inspired air. As a result, the incoming air is efficiently warmed by a countercurrent system.

PARANASAL SINUSES

The paranasal sinuses are blind cavities in the frontal, maxillary, ethmoid, and sphenoid bones. They

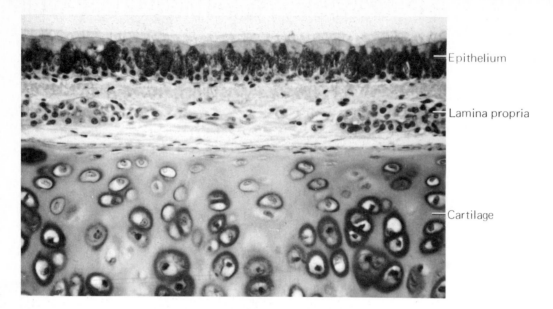

Figure 17–5. Photomicrograph of a section of dog trachea. × 200.

are lined with a thinner respiratory epithelium that contains few goblet cells. The lamina propria contains only a few small glands and is continuous with the underlying periosteum. Communication with the nasal cavity is through small openings. The mucus produced in these cavities drains into the nasal passages as a result of the activity of its ciliated epithelial cells.

Sinusitis is an inflammatory process of the sinus that persists for long periods of time, mainly because of obstruction of drainage orifices. Chronic sinusitis is a component of Kartagener's syndrome, which is characterized by defective ciliary action.

NASOPHARYNX

The nasopharynx is the first part of the pharynx, continuing caudally with the oropharynx, the oral portion of this organ. It is lined with respiratory-type

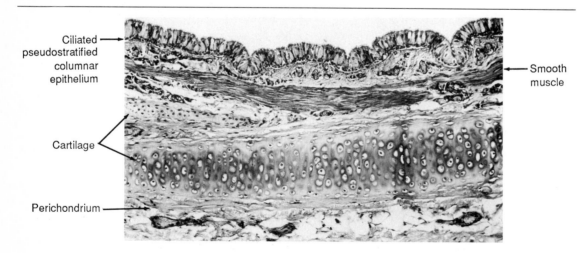

Figure 17–6. Photomicrograph of a large bronchus. Observe the ciliated pseudostratified columnar epithelium with many goblet cells, 2 cartilaginous plates, and smooth muscle. H&E stain, × 180.

epithelium in the portion that is in contact with the soft palate.

LARYNX

The larynx is an irregular tube that connects the pharynx to the trachea. Within the lamina propria lie a number of laryngeal cartilages, structurally the most complex in the respiratory system. The larger cartilages (thyroid, cricoid, and most of the arytenoids) are hyaline, and some are subject to calcification in the elderly. The smaller cartilages (epiglottis, cuneiform, corniculate, and the tips of the arytenoids) are elastic cartilages. Ligaments bind the cartilages together; most are articulated by the intrinsic muscles of the larynx, which are themselves unusual in that they are striated skeletal muscle. In addition to their supporting role (maintenance of an open airway), these cartilages serve as a valve to prevent swallowed food or fluid from entering the trachea. They also participate in producing sounds for phonation.

The **epiglottis,** which projects from the rim of the larynx, extends into the pharynx and has both a lingual and a laryngeal surface. The entire lingual surface and the apical portion of the laryngeal side are covered by stratified squamous epithelium. Toward the base of the epiglottis on the laryngeal side, the epithelium undergoes a transition into ciliated pseudostratified columnar epithelium. Mixed mucous and serous glands are found beneath the epithelium.

Below the epiglottis, the mucosa forms 2 pairs of folds that extend into the lumen of the larynx. The upper pair constitutes the **false vocal cords** (vestibular folds), covered by typical respiratory epithelium beneath which lie numerous serous glands within the lamina propria. The lower pair of folds constitutes the **true vocal cords.** Large bundles of parallel elastic fibers that compose the **vocal ligament** lie within the

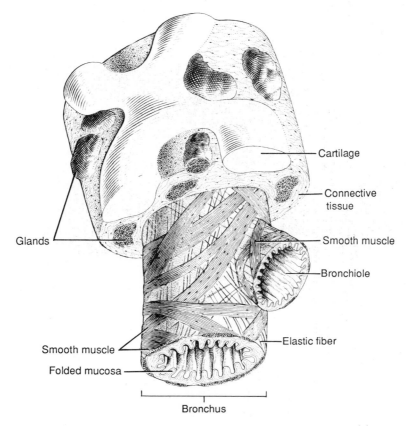

Figure 17–7. Diagram of a bronchus showing its structure. Contraction of this muscle induces folding of the mucosa. Smooth muscle is present in all of the bronchiolar tree, including the respiratory bronchiole. The elastic fibers in the bronchus continue into the bronchiole. An irregular cartilaginous plate sectioned in 2 regions is shown in white. The lower portion of this figure represents a region that had its connective tissue removed to show the presence of elastic fibers and smooth muscle. The adventitia is not shown in this drawing.

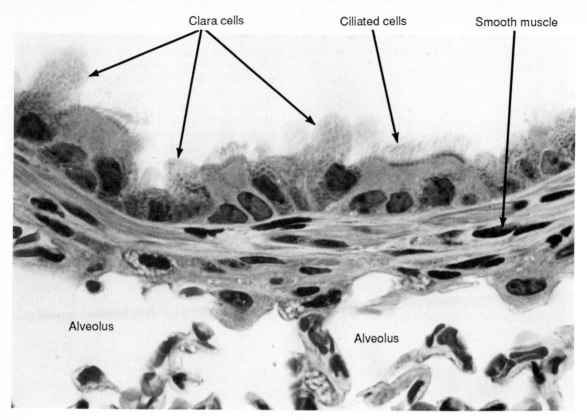

Figure 17–8. Portion of a terminal bronchiole in mouse lung. In addition to the ciliated cuboidal cells, there are larger secretory Clara cells. Bundles of smooth muscle cells lie beneath the epithelium, and alveoli surround the terminal bronchiole. × 800.

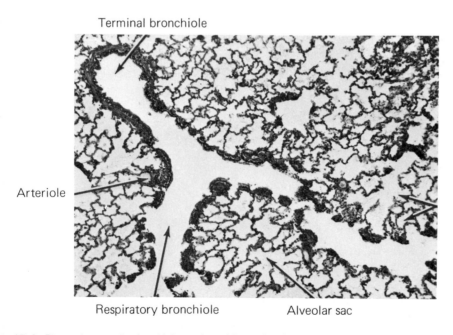

Figure 17–9. Photomicrograph of a thick section of lung showing a terminal bronchiole dividing into 2 respiratory bronchioles in which alveoli appear. The spongelike appearance of the lung is due to the abundance of alveoli and alveolar sacs. H&E stain, × 80.

vocal folds, which are covered by a stratified squamous epithelium. Parallel to the ligaments are bundles of skeletal muscle, the **vocalis muscles,** which regulate the tension of the fold and its ligaments. As air is forced between the folds, these muscles provide for the production of sounds of different frequencies.

TRACHEA

The trachea is a thin-walled tube, about 10 cm long, that extends from the base of the larynx (the cricoid cartilage) to the point at which it bifurcates into the 2 primary bronchi. The trachea is lined with a typical respiratory mucosa (Figs 17–4 and 17–5). In the lamina propria are 16–20 C-shaped rings of hyaline cartilage that serve to keep the tracheal lumen open. The open ends of the C-shaped rings are located on the posterior surface of the trachea. A fibroelastic ligament and bundle of smooth muscle (trachealis muscle) bind to the perichondrium and bridge the open ends of these C-shaped cartilages. The ligament prevents overdistention of the lumen, while the muscle allows regulation of the lumen.

Contraction of the muscle and the resultant narrowing of the tracheal lumen are used in the cough reflex. The smaller bore of the trachea following contraction provides for increased velocity of expired air, which aids in clearing the air passage.

BRONCHIAL TREE

The trachea divides into 2 **primary bronchi** that enter the lungs at the hilum (Fig 17–1). Arteries enter and veins and lymphatic vessels leave the lungs at

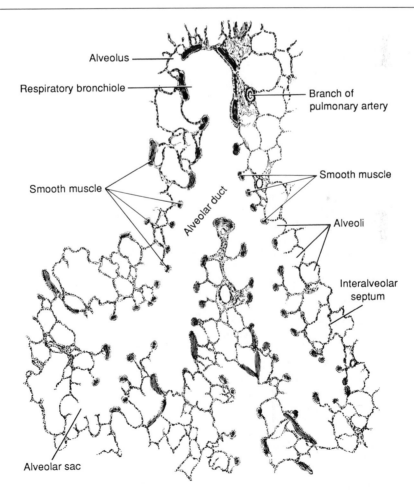

Figure 17–10. Diagram of a portion of the bronchial tree. Observe that the smooth muscle present in the alveolar ducts disappears in the alveoli. (Redrawn from Baltisberger.)

each hilum. These structures are surrounded by dense connective tissue and form a unit called the **pulmonary root.**

After entering the lungs, the primary bronchi course downward and outward, giving rise to 3 bronchi in the right lung and 2 in the left lung, each of which supplies a pulmonary lobe (Fig 17–1). These **lobar bronchi** divide repeatedly, giving rise to smaller bronchi, whose terminal branches are called **bronchioles.** Each bronchiole enters a pulmonary lobule, where it branches to form 5–7 **terminal bronchioles.**

The pulmonary lobules are pyramid-shaped, with the apex directed toward the pulmonary hilum. Each lobule is delineated by a thin connective tissue septum, best seen in the fetus. In adults, these septa are frequently incomplete, resulting in a poor delineation of the lobules.

The primary bronchi generally have the same histologic appearance as the trachea. Proceeding toward the respiratory portion, a simplification of the histologic organization of both the epithelium and underlying lamina propria can be observed. It must be stressed that this simplification is gradual, and no abrupt transition can be observed between the bronchi and bronchioles. For this reason, the division of the bronchial tree into bronchi, bronchioles, etc, is to some extent artificial—despite the fact that it has both pedagogic and practical value.

Bronchi

Each primary bronchus branches dichotomously 9–12 times, with each branch becoming progressively smaller until a diameter of about 5 mm is reached. Except for the organization of cartilage and smooth muscle, the mucosa of the bronchi is structurally similar to that of the mucosa of the trachea (Figs 17–6 and 17–7). The bronchial cartilages are more irregular in shape than those found in the trachea; in the larger portions of the bronchi, the cartilage rings completely encircle the lumen. As bronchial diameter decreases, the cartilage rings are replaced by isolated plates, or islands, of hyaline cartilage. Beneath the epithelium, in the bronchial lamina propria, one can observe the presence of a smooth muscle layer consisting of crisscrossing bundles of spirally arranged smooth muscle (Fig 17–7). Bundles of smooth muscle become a more prominent feature in the walls of the conducting portion nearing the respiratory zone. In histologic sections, this muscle layer appears to be discontinuous. Contraction of this muscle after death is responsible for the folded appearance of the bronchial mucosa observed in histologic section. The lamina propria is rich in elastic fibers; it contains an abundance of mucous and serous glands whose ducts open into the bronchial lumen. Numerous lymphocytes are found both within the lamina propria and among the epithelial cells. Lymphatic nodules are present and

are particularly numerous at the branching points of the bronchial tree.

Bronchioles

Bronchioles, intralobular airways with diameters of 5 mm or less (Fig 17–7), have neither cartilage nor glands in their mucosa; there are only scattered goblet cells within the epithelium of the initial segments. In the larger bronchioles, the epithelium is ciliated pseudostratified columnar, which decreases in height and complexity to become ciliated simply columnar or cuboidal epithelium in the smaller **terminal bronchioles.** The epithelium of terminal bronchioles also contains **Clara cells** (Fig 17–8). These cells, which are devoid of cilia, present secretory granules in their apex and are known to secrete glycosaminoglycans that probably protect the bronchiolar lining.

The lamina propria is composed largely of smooth muscle and elastic fibers. The musculature of both the bronchi and the bronchioles is under the control of the vagus nerve and the sympathetic nervous system. Stimulation of the vagus nerve decreases the diameter of these structures; sympathetic stimulation produces the opposite effect.

> This stimulation explains why epinephrine and other sympathomimetic drugs are frequently employed to relax smooth muscle during asthma attacks. When the thicknesses of the bronchial and bronchiolar walls are compared, it can be seen that the bronchiolar muscle layer is proportionately better developed than that of the bronchi. Increased airway resistance in asthma is believed to be due mainly to contraction of bronchiolar smooth muscle.

Respiratory Bronchioles

Each terminal bronchiole subdivides into 2 or more respiratory bronchioles that serve as regions of transition between the conducting and respiratory portions of the respiratory system (Figs 17–9 and 17–10). The respiratory bronchiolar mucosa is structurally identical to that of the terminal bronchioles except that their walls are interrupted by numerous saccular **alveloi** where gas exchange occurs (Figs 17–1, 17–9, and 17–10). Portions of the respiratory bronchioles are lined with ciliated cuboidal epithelial cells and Clara cells, but at the rim of the alveolar openings the bronchiolar epithelium becomes continuous with the squamous alveolar lining cells (type I alveolar cells). Proceeding distally along these bronchioles, the number of alveoli increases greatly, and the distance between them is markedly reduced. Between alveoli, the bronchiolar epithelium consists of ciliated cuboidal epithelium; however, the cilia may be absent in more distal portions. Smooth muscle and elastic connective tissue lie beneath the epithelium of respiratory bronchioles.

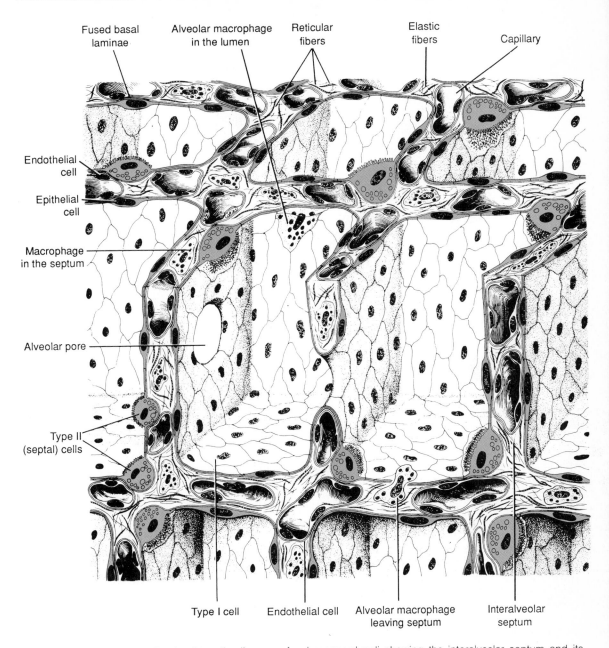

Fused basal laminae

Alveolar macrophage in the lumen

Reticular fibers

Elastic fibers

Capillary

Endothelial cell

Epithelial cell

Macrophage in the septum

Alveolar pore

Type II (septal) cells

Type I cell

Endothelial cell

Alveolar macrophage leaving septum

Interalveolar septum

Figure 17–11. Three-dimensional schematic diagram of pulmonary alveoli showing the interalveolar septum and its structure. Observe the capillaries, connective tissue, and macrophages. These cells can also be seen in—or passing into—the alveolar lumens. Alveolar pores are numerous. Type II cells are identified by their abundant apical microvilli. The alveoli are lined by a continuous epithelial layer of Type I cells.

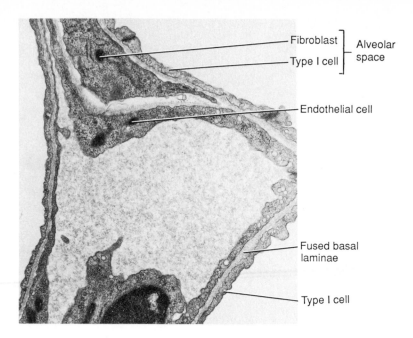

Figure 17–12. Electron micrograph of the alveolar wall. Note the capillary lumen, alveolar spaces, alveolar type I epithelial cells, capillary endothelial cells, fused basal laminae, and a fibroblast. × 30,000. (Courtesy of MC Williams.)

Alveolar Ducts

Proceeding distally along the respiratory bronchioles, the number of alveolar openings into the bronchiolar wall becomes ever greater until the wall consists of nothing else, and the tube is now termed an **alveolar duct** (Fig 17–10). Both the alveolar ducts and alveoli are lined by extremely attenuated squamous alveolar cells. In the lamina propria surrounding the rim of the alveoli is a network of smooth muscle cells. These sphincterlike smooth muscle bundles appear as knobs between adjacent alveoli. Smooth muscle disappears at the distal ends of alveolar ducts. A rich matrix of elastic and collagen fibers provides the only support of the duct and its alveoli.

Alveolar ducts open into **atria** that communicate with **alveolar sacs,** 2 or more of which arise from each atrium. A heavy investment of elastic and reticular fibers forms a complex network encircling the openings of atria, alveolar sacs, and alveoli. The elastic fibers enable the alveoli to expand upon inspiration and to contract passively during expiration. The reticular fibers serve as a support that prevents overdistention and damage to the delicate capillaries and thin alveolar septa.

Alveoli

Alveoli are saclike evaginations, about 200 μm in diameter, of the respiratory bronchioles, alveolar ducts, and alveolar sacs. Alveoli are the terminal portions of the bronchial tree; they are responsible for the spongy structure of the lungs. Structurally, alveoli resemble small pockets that are open on one side, similar to the honeycombs of a beehive. Within these cuplike structures, oxygen and carbon dioxide are exchanged between the air and the blood. The structure of the alveolar walls is specialized for enhancing diffusion between the external and internal environments. Generally, each wall lies between 2 neighboring alveoli and is therefore termed an **interalveolar septum,** or **wall.** An alveolar septum consists of 2 thin squamous epithelial layers between which lie capillaries, fibroblasts, elastic and collagen fibers, and macrophages. The capillaries and connective tissue matrix constitute the **interstitium.** Within the interstitium of the alveolar septum is found the richest capillary network in the body (Fig 17–11).

Air in the alveoli is separated from capillary blood by 3 components referred to collectively as the **blood-air barrier:** the surface lining and cytoplasm of the alveolar cells; the fused basal laminae of the closely apposed alveolar and endothelial cells; and the cytoplasm of the endothelial cells (Figs 17–11, 17–12, and 17–13). The total thickness of these layers varies from 0.1 to 1.5 μm. Within the interalveolar septum, anastomosing pulmonary capillaries are supported by a meshwork of reticular and elastic fibers. These fibers, which are arranged to permit expansion and contraction of alveolar walls, are the primary means of structural support of the alveoli. The basement membrane, leukocytes, macrophages,

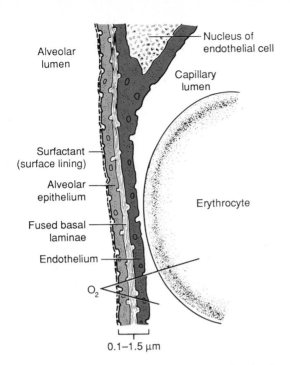

Alveolar lumen

Nucleus of endothelial cell

Capillary lumen

Surfactant (surface lining)

Alveolar epithelium

Erythrocyte

Fused basal laminae

Endothelium

O_2

0.1–1.5 μm

Figure 17–13. Portion of the alveolar septum showing the blood-air barrier. To reach the red cell, O_2 transverses the surface lining, the alveolar epithelial cytoplasm, the basal laminae, the endothelial cell cytoplasm, and the plasma. In some locations, there is loose interstitial tissue between the epithelium and the endothelium. (Approximate magnification × 20,000.) (Modified and reproduced, with permission, from Ganong WF: *Review of Medical Physiology,* 8th ed. Lange, 1977.)

and fibroblasts can also be found within the interstitium of the septum (Fig 17–11). The basement membrane is formed by the fusion of 2 basal laminae produced by the endothelial cells and by the epithelial (alveolar) cells of the alveolar wall.

Oxygen from the alveolar air passes into the capillary blood through these layers (Fig 17–13); CO_2 diffuses in the opposite direction. Liberation of CO_2, from H_2CO_3 is catalyzed by the enzyme **carbonic anhydrase** present in red blood cells. The approximately 300 million alveoli in the lungs considerably increase their internal exchange surface, which has been calculated to be approximately 140 m^2.

The interalveolar septum is composed of 5 main cell types: capillary endothelial cells (30%); type I (squamous) alveolar cells (8%); type II (septal, great alveolar) cells (16%); interstitial cells, including fibroblasts and mast cells (36%); and alveolar macrophages (10%). (See Figs 17–11, 17–12, and 17–14.)

Endothelial cells of the capillaries are extremely thin and can be easily confused with type I alveolar epithelial cells. The endothelial lining of the capillaries is continuous and not fenestrated (Fig 17–12). The clustering of the nuclei and other organelles allows the remaining areas of the cell to become extremely thin in order to increase the efficiency of gas exchange. The most prominent feature of the cytoplasm in the flattened portions of the cell is numerous pinocytotic vesicles.

Type I cells, also called **squamous alveolar cells,** are extremely attenuated cells that line the alveolar surfaces. Type I cells make up 97% of the alveolar surfaces; type II cells make up the remaining 3%. These cells are so thin, sometimes only 25 nm in thickness, that analysis with the electron microscope was needed to prove that all alveoli are covered by an epithelial lining (Figs 17–11 and 17–12). Organelles such as the Golgi complex, endoplasmic reticulum, and mitochondria are grouped around the nucleus, reducing the thickness of the blood-air barrier and leaving large areas of cytoplasm virtually free of organelles (Fig 17–17). The cytoplasm in the thin portion contains abundant pinocytotic vesicles, which may play a role in the turnover of surfactant (described below) and the removal of small particulate contaminants from the outer surface. In addition to desmosomes, all type I epithelial cells have occluding junctions that serve to prevent the leakage of tissue fluid into the alveolar air space (Fig 17–15). The main role of this cell is to provide a barrier of minimal thickness that is readily permeable to gases.

Type II cells, or **great alveolar cells** (also called **septal cells**), are found interspersed among the type I alveolar cells with which they have occluding and desmosomal junctions (Figs 17–11 and 17–16). Type II cells are roughly cuboidal cells that are usually found in groups of 2 or 3 along the alveolar surface at points where the alveolar walls unite and form angles. These cells, which rest on the basement membrane, are part of the epithelium, for they have the same origin as the type I cells that line the alveolar walls. These cells resemble typical secretory cells. They have mitochondria, rough endoplasmic reticulum, a well-developed Golgi complex, and microvilli on their free apical surfaces. In histologic sections, they exhibit a characteristic vesicular or foamy cytoplasm. These vesicles are caused by the presence of **lamellar bodies** (Figs 17–16 and 17–17) that are preserved and evident in tissue prepared for electron microscopy. These structures, which average 1–2 μm in diameter, contain concentric or parallel lamellae limited by a unit membrane. Histochemical studies reveal that these bodies, which contain phospholipids, glycosaminoglycans, and proteins, are continuously synthesized and released at the apical surface of the cell. The lamellar bodies give rise to a material that spreads over the alveolar surfaces, providing an extracellular alveolar coating, **pulmonary surfactant,** that lowers alveolar surface tension. The secretion of pulmonary surfactant by type II cells has been shown

Type II   Type I

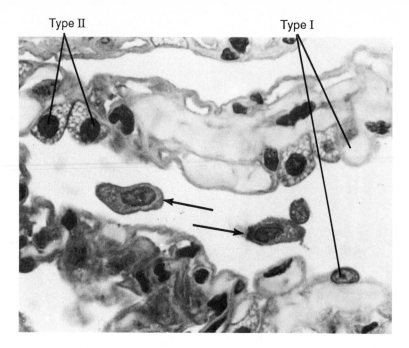

Figure 17–14. Photomicrograph of lung alveolar walls showing type I and II cells, capillaries, and intra-alveolar macrophages (arrows).

with the aid of electron microscopy and radioautography and is summarized in Fig 17–17.

The surfactant layer consists of an aqueous, protein-containing hypophase covered by a monomolecular phospholipid film, primarily composed of **dipalmitoyl lecithin.** Pulmonary surfactant serves several major functions in the economy of the lung. It primarily aids in reducing the surface tension of the alveolar cells. The reduction of surface tension means that less inspiratory force is needed to inflate the alveoli, thus reducing the work of breathing. In addition, without surfactant, alveoli would tend to collapse during expiration. In fetal development, surfactant appears in the last weeks of gestation and coincides with the appearance of lamellar bodies in the type II cells.

In cases of premature birth, infants frequently exhibit the labored breathing that signifies respiratory distress. **Hyaline membrane disease** in such newborns has been shown to be the result of insufficient surfactant production, and the infant has difficulty in expanding the alveoli. Fortunately surfactant synthesis can be induced by administration of glucocorticoids, so that the **respiratory distress syndrome** usually represents a short-term management problem. Recently, surfactant has also been suggested to have a bactericidal effect, aiding in the removal

of potentially dangerous bacteria that reach the alveoli.

The surfactant layer is not static but is constantly being turned over. The lipoproteins are gradually removed from the surface by the pinocytotic vesicles of the squamous epithelial cells, by macrophages, and by type II alveolar cells. These substances therefore undergo a continuous cycle of secretion and absorption.

Alveolar lining fluids are also removed via the conducting passages as a result of ciliary activity. As the secretions pass up through the airways, they combine with bronchial mucus, forming a **bronchoalveolar fluid.** This fluid aids in the removal of particulate and noxious components from the inspired air. Within the fluids are several lytic enzymes (eg, lysozyme, collagenase, β-glucuronidase) that are probably derived from the alveolar macrophages.

Alveolar Septum

The thinnest barrier between blood plasma and inspired air is reduced to an alveolar epithelium, a basement membrane of 2 fused basal luminae, and the capillary endothelium. Alveolar macrophages, also called **dust cells,** are derived from monocytes that originate in bone marrow. They are found in the interior of the alveolar septum and are often seen on the surface of the alveolus. Numerous carbon- and dust-

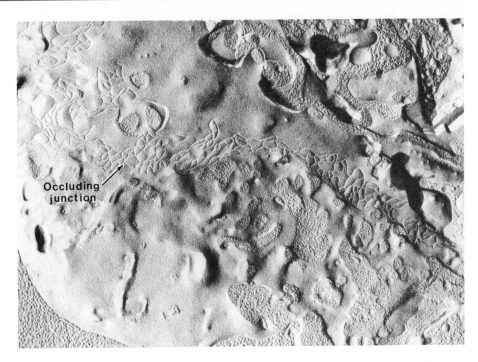

Figure 17–15. Cryofracture preparation showing an occluding junction between 2 type I epithelial cells of the alveolar lining. × 25,000. (Reproduced, with permission, from Schneeberger EE: *Lung Liquids.* Ciba Foundation Symposium No. 38. Elsevier/North-Holland, 1976.)

laden macrophages in the connective tissue around major blood vessels or in the pleura probably represent cells that have never passed through the epithelial lining. The phagocytized debris within these cells was most likely passed from the alveolar lumen into the interstitium by the pinocytotic activity of the type I alveolar cells. The alveolar macrophages that scavenge the outer surface of the epithelium within the surfactant layer are carried to the pharynx, where they are swallowed.

> In congestive heart failure, the lungs become congested with blood, and red blood cells pass into alveoli, where they are phagocytized by alveolar macrophages. In such cases, these macrophages are called **heart failure cells** when present in the lung and sputum; they are identified by a positive histochemical reaction for iron pigment (hemosiderin).

In addition to the cells discussed above, the alveolar septum contains fibroblasts, mast cells, and contractile cells. Interstitial fibroblasts synthesize collagen, elastic fibers, and glycosaminoglycans. Collagen constitutes 15–20% of the parenchymal mass and consists primarily of types I and III collagen. Type III collagen is present mainly in the alveolar reticular fibers (Fig 17–11); type I collagen is

concentrated in the walls of the conducting passages and in the pleura. Increased production of collagen is common, and more than 100 disease entities that lead to respiratory distress are known to be associated with lung fibrosis.

Contractile interstitial cells in the septum are found bound to the basal surface of the alveolar epithelium and not to the endothelial cells. These cells, which react with antiactin and antimyosin antibodies, contract and reduce the volume of the alveolar lumen. In vitro, it has been demonstrated that lung parenchymal tissue contracts when exposed to pharmacologic agents such as epinephrine and histamine.

Alveolar Pores

The interalveolar septum may contain one or more pores, 10–15 μm in diameter, connecting neighboring alveoli (Figs 17–11 and 17–18). They may equalize pressure in the alveoli or enable the collateral circulation of air when a bronchiole is obstructed.

Alveolar-Lining Regeneration

It has been observed that inhalation of NO_2 promotes destruction of most of the cells lining the alveoli (type I and type II cells). The action of this compound or other toxic substances with the same effect is followed by a drastic increase in the mitotic activity of the remaining type II cells. In the second step of alveolar-lining regeneration, most of the type II cells are transformed into type I cells, and the alveolar lining regains its normal appearance. The normal turnover rate of type II cells is estimated to be 1% per day, maintaining a continuous renewal of both its own type and type I cells.

Collagen and elastic fibers are important components that contribute resilience and elasticity, respectively, to the biomechanical properties of the lung. Changes in the content of these fibers by lung tissues lead to a variety of respiratory ailments.

The destruction of the alveolar wall with subsequent reduction of the respiratory portion of the

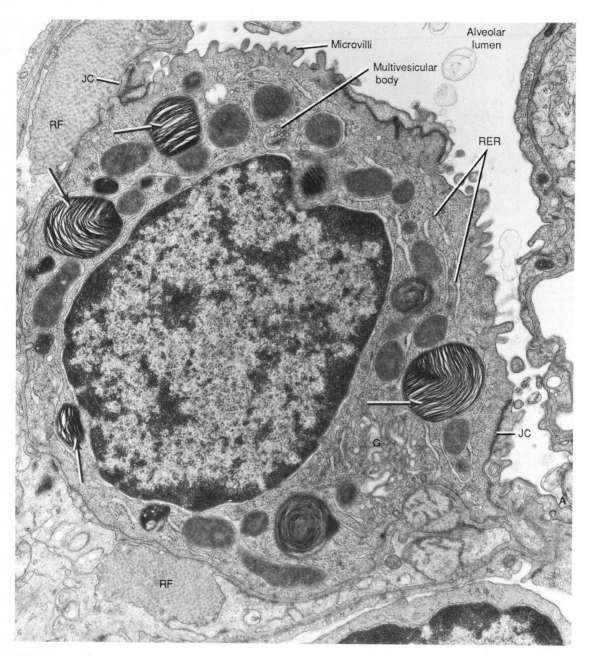

Figure 17–16. Type II cell from rat lung protruding into the alveolar lumen. Arrows point to lamellar bodies containing newly synthesized pulmonary surfactant. RER, rough endoplasmic reticulum; G, Golgi complex; RF, reticular fibers. The cytoplasm of a type I epithelial cell is seen at A. Note the microvilli of the type II cell and the junctional complexes (JC) with the type I epithelial cell. × 17,000. (Courtesy of MC Williams.)

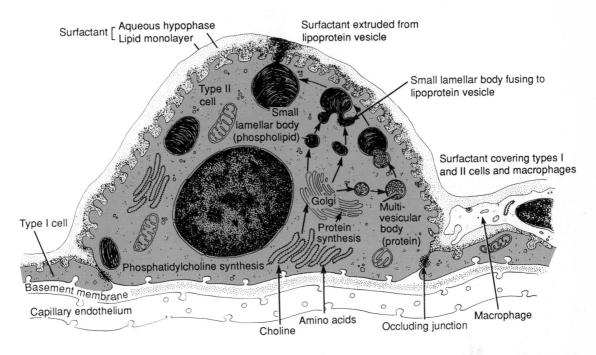

Figure 17–17. Surfactant secretion by the type II cell. The surfactant is a protein-lipid complex synthesized in the rough endoplasmic reticulum and Golgi complex and stored in the lamellar bodies. It is continuously secreted by exocytosis and forms an overlying monomolecular film of lipid covering an underlying aqueous hypophase. When present in the alveolar lumen, macrophages lie outside the epithelium but within the surfactant layer. Occluding junctions around the margins of the epithelial cells prevent leakage of tissue fluid into the alveolar lumen.

lungs is called **emphysema.** It usually develops gradually and results in respiratory insufficiency. Emphysema, a leading cause of death in the industrialized world, is clearly associated with smoking and environmental air pollution.

PULMONARY BLOOD VESSELS

Circulation in the lungs includes both nutrient (systemic) and functional (pulmonary) vessels. The functional circulation is represented by pulmonary arteries and veins. Pulmonary arteries are thin-walled, owing to the low pressures (25 mm Hg systolic, 5 mm Hg diastolic) encountered in the pulmonary circuit. These arteries contain more smooth muscle cells and elastic fibers than do pulmonary veins. The arteries have an internal elastic membrane; this structure is absent in pulmonary veins. Within the lung the pulmonary artery branches, accompanying the bronchial tree (Fig 17–19). Its branches are surrounded by adventitia of the bronchi and bronchioles. At the level of the alveolar duct, the branches of this artery form a capillary network in the interalveolar septum and in close contact with the alveolar epithelium. The lung has the best-developed capillary network in the body. The

capillaries occur between all alveoli, including those in the respiratory bronchioles.

Venules that originate in the capillary network occur singly in the parenchyma, somewhat removed from the airways; they are supported by a thin covering of connective tissue and enter the interlobular septum (Fig 17–19). After veins leave a lobule, they follow the bronchial tree toward the hilum.

Nutrient vessels follow the bronchial tree and distribute blood to most of the lung up to the respiratory bronchioles, at which point they anastomose with small branches of the pulmonary artery.

PULMONARY LYMPHATIC VESSELS

The lymphatic vessels (Fig 17–19) follow the bronchi and the pulmonary vessels; they also occur in the interlobular septum, and all drain into lymph nodes in the region of the hilum. This lymphatic network is called the deep network to distinguish it from the superficial network, which includes lymphatic vessels present in the visceral pleura. The lymphatic vessels of the superficial network drain toward the hilum. They either follow the entire length of the pleura or penetrate the lung tissue via the interlobular septum.

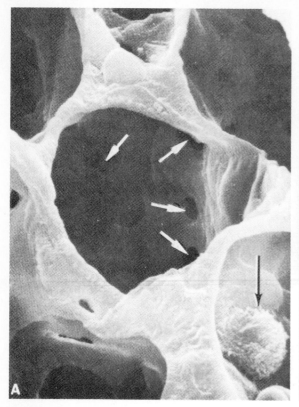 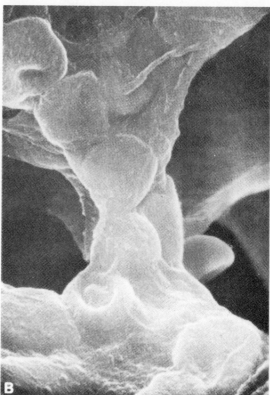

Figure 17–18. Scanning electron micrograph of mouse lung. **A:** Observe the thin septa and an alveolar pore (white arrow). At the black arrow, a macrophage with its typical ruffled membrane is seen. × 3200. **B:** Here, the alveolar wall is so thin that the shape of the red blood cells in a capillary can be seen. × 6700. (Courtesy of Greenwood MF, Holland P: The mammalian respiratory tract surface: A scanning electron microscope study. *Lab Invest* 1972;**27:**296.)

Lymphatic vessels do not occur in the terminal portions of the bronchial tree and beyond the alveolar ducts.

NERVES

Both parasympathetic and sympathetic efferent fibers innervate the lungs; general visceral afferent fibers, carrying poorly localized pain sensations, are also present. Most of the nerves are found in the connective tissues surrounding the larger airways.

> Parasympathetic stimulation, via the vagus nerve, results in bronchial constriction, while sympathetic stimulation causes bronchial dilatation. Drugs that mimic sympathetic neurotransmitters, such as isoproterenol, are used to cause bronchial dilatation during asthma attacks.

PLEURA

The pleura (Fig 17–19) is the serous membrane covering the lung. It consists of 2 layers, parietal and visceral, that are continuous in the region of the hilum. Both membranes are composed of mesothelial cells resting on a fine connective tissue layer containing collagen and elastic fibers. The elastic fibers of the visceral pleura are continuous with those of the pulmonary parenchyma.

These 2 layers define a cavity entirely lined by squamous mesothelial cells. Under normal conditions, this pleural cavity contains only a film of liquid that acts as a lubricating agent, permitting the smooth sliding of one surface over the other during respiratory movements.

> In certain pathologic states, the pleural cavity can become a real cavity, containing liquid or air in its interior. The walls of the pleural cavity, like all serosal cavities (peritoneal and pericardial), are quite permeable to water and other substances—thus the high frequency of fluid accumulation (pleural effusion) in this cavity in pathologic conditions. This fluid is derived from the blood plasma by exudation. Conversely, under certain conditions, liquids or gases present in the pleural cavity can be rapidly absorbed.

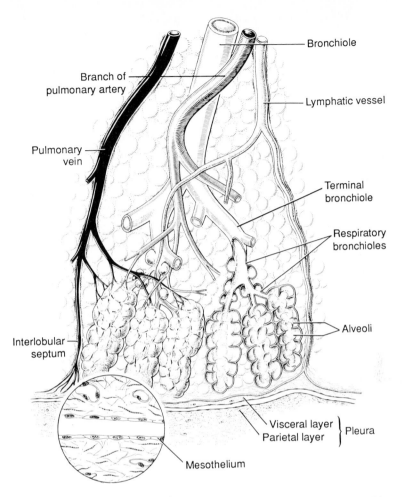

Branch of pulmonary artery

Pulmonary vein

Interlobular septum

Bronchiole

Lymphatic vessel

Terminal bronchiole

Respiratory bronchioles

Alveoli

Visceral layer
Parietal layer } Pleura

Mesothelium

Figure 17–19. Blood and lymph circulation in a pulmonary lobule. Both vessels and bronchi are enlarged out of proportion in this drawing. In the interlobular septum, only the vein is shown (on the left) and the lymphatic vessel (on the right), although both actually coexist in these regions. At lower left, an enlargement of the pleura showing its mesothelial lining. (Based partially on Ham AW: *Histology*, 6th ed. Lippincott, 1969.)

RESPIRATORY MOVEMENTS

During inhalation, contraction of the intercostal muscles elevates the ribs, and contraction of the diaphragm lowers the bottom of the thoracic cavity, increasing its diameter and resulting in pulmonary expansion. The bronchi and bronchioles increase in diameter and length during inhalation. The respiratory portion also enlarges, mainly as a result of expansion of the alveolar ducts; the alveoli enlarge only slightly. The elastic fibers of the pulmonary parenchyma are stretched by this expansion, so that the retraction of the lungs is passive during exhalation caused by muscle relaxation, mainly because of the action of the elastic fibers, which had been under tension.

DEFENSE MECHANISMS

The respiratory system has an exceptionally large area exposed to both blood and the external environment. It is consequently very susceptible to the invasion of airborne infective and noninfective agents. Therefore, it is not surprising that the respiratory system presents an elaborate array of defense mechanisms. Particles larger than 10 μm are retained in the nasal passages, and 2–10-μm particles are trapped by the mucus-coated ciliated epithelium. The cough reflex can eliminate these particles by expectoration or swallowing. Smaller particles are removed by alveolar macrophages. In addition to these nonspecific mechanisms, elaborate immunological processes occur in lymphoid tissues of the bronchus, mainly in nodules containing T and B lymphocytes that interact with lung macrophages.

Tumors of the Lung

Lung tumors, which have historically had their highest incidence in males, are mainly of epithelial origin. Conclusive evidence has been presented that squamous cell carcinoma, the principal lung tumor type, is related to the effects of cigarette smoking on the bronchial and bronchiolar epithelial lining. Chronic smoking induces the transformation of the respiratory epithelium into a stratified squamous epithelium, an initial step in its eventual differentiation into a tumor.

REFERENCES

Bouhuy SA: *Lung Cells in Disease.* Elsevier/North-Holland, 1976.

Breeze RG, Wheeldon EG: The cells of the pulmonary airways. *Am Rev Respir Dis* 1977;**116**:705.

Camner P, Mossberg B, Afzelius BA: Evidence for congenital nonfunctional cilia in the tracheobronchial tract in two subjects. *Am Rev Respir Dis* 1975;**112**:807.

Cummings G (editor): *Cellular Biology of the Lung.* Ettore Majorana International Science Service, 1982.

Evans MJ: Transformation of type II cells to type I cells following exposure to NO_2. *Exp Mol Pathol* 1975; **22**:142.

Gehr P, Bachofen M, Weibel ER: The normal human lung: Ultrastructure and morphometric estimation of diffusion capacity. *Respir Physiol* 1978;**32**:121.

Greenwood M, Holland P: The mammalian respiratory tract surface: A scanning electron microscope study. *Lab Invest* 1972;**27**:296.

Kikkawa Y, Smith F: Cellular and biochemical aspects of pulmonary surfactant in health and disease. *Lab Invest* 1983;**49**:122.

Kuhn C III: The cells of the lung and their organelles. In: *The Biochemical Basis of Pulmonary Function,* Crystal RG (editor). Marcel Dekker, 1976.

Thurlbeck WM, Abell RM (editors): *The Lung: Structure, Function, and Disease.* Williams & Wilkins, 1978.

Skin

18

The skin is the heaviest single organ of the body, accounting for about 16% of total body weight and, in adults, presenting 1.2–2.3 m^2 of surface to the external environment. It is composed of the **epidermis,** an epithelial layer of ectodermal origin, and the **dermis,** a layer of connective tissue of mesodermal origin. The junction of dermis and epidermis is irregular, and projections of the dermis called **papillae** interdigitate with evaginations of the epidermis known as **epidermal ridges** (Fig 18–1). In 3 dimensions, these interdigitations may be of the peg-and-socket variety (thin skin) or formed of ridges and grooves (thick skin). Beneath the dermis lies the **hypodermis** (from Greek, *hypo,* under, + *derma,* skin) or **subcutaneous tissue,** a loose connective tissue that may contain a pad of adipose cells, the **panniculus adiposus.** The hypodermis, which is not considered part of the skin, binds skin loosely to the subjacent tissues and corresponds to the superficial fascia of gross anatomy. Epidermal derivatives include hairs, nails, and sebaceous and sweat glands.

The external layer of the skin is relatively impermeable to water, which prevents extreme water loss by evaporation and allows for terrestrial life. The skin functions as a receptor organ in continuous communication with the environment (see Chapter 24) and protects the organism from impact and friction injuries. **Melanin,** a pigment produced and stored in the cells of the epidermis, provides further protective action against the sun's ultraviolet rays. Glands of the skin, blood vessels, and adipose tissue participate in thermoregulation, body metabolism, and the excretion of various substances. Vitamin D$_3$ is formed, under the action of ultraviolet radiation in sunlight, from precursors synthesized by the skin in the epidermal layer. Because skin is elastic, it can expand to cover large areas in conditions associated with swelling, such as edema and pregnancy.

Upon close observation, certain portions of human skin show ridges and grooves arranged in distinctive patterns. These ridges first appear during intrauterine life—at 13 weeks in the tips of the digits (fingerprints) and later in the volar surfaces of the hands and feet. The patterns assumed by ridges and intervening sulci are known as **dermatoglyphics** (fingerprints). They are unique for each individual, appearing as loops, arches, whorls, or combinations of these

forms. These configurations, which are used for personal identification, are probably determined by multiple genes; the field of dermatoglyphics has come to be of considerable medical and anthropologic as well as legal interest.

EPIDERMIS

The epidermis consists mainly of a stratified squamous keratinized epithelium, but it also contains 3 less abundant cell types: **melanocytes, Langerhans' cells,** and **Merkel's cells.** The keratinizing epidermal cells are called **keratinocytes**. It is customary to distinguish between the **thick skin** (**glabrous,** or smooth and nonhairy) found on the palms and soles and the **thin skin** (hairy) found elsewhere on the body. The designations *thick* and *thin* refer to the thickness of the epidermal layer, which varies between 75 and 150 μm for thin skin (Fig 18–2) and 400 and 600 μm for thick skin (Fig 18–1). Total skin thickness (epidermis plus dermis) also varies according to site. For example, skin on the back is about 4 mm thick, while that of the scalp is about 1.5 mm thick.

From the dermis outward, the epidermis consists of 5 layers of keratin-producing cells (keratinocytes).

A. Stratum Basale (Stratum Germinativum): This consists of a single layer of basophilic columnar or cuboidal cells resting on the basal lamina at the dermal-epidermal junction and separating the dermis from the epidermis. Their long axes are perpendicular to the basal lamina. Desmosomes in great quantity bind the cells of this layer in their lateral and upper surfaces. Hemidesmosomes, found in the basal plasmalemma, help bind these cells to the basal lamina (Fig 4–4B). The stratum basale is characterized by intense mitotic activity and is responsible, in conjunction with the initial portion of the next layer, for constant renewal of epidermal cells. The human epidermis is renewed about every 15–30 days, depending on age, the region of the body, and other factors. All cells in the stratum basale contain filaments about 10 nm in diameter (cytokeratins; see *Intermediate Filaments* in Chapter 3). As the cells progress upward, the number of filaments increases until they represent, in the stratum corneum, half its total protein.

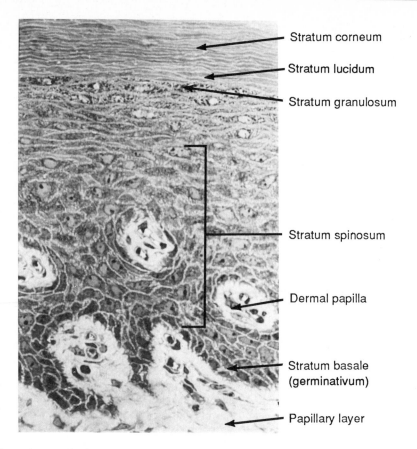

Stratum corneum

Stratum lucidum

Stratum granulosum

Stratum spinosum

Dermal papilla

Stratum basale
(germinativum)

Papillary layer

Figure 18–1. Photomicrograph of a section of human thick skin from the sole of the foot. Observe the papillae of the papillary layer and the thickness of the stratum corneum. H&E stain, × 100.

B. Stratum Spinosum: This layer consists of cuboidal, polygonal, or slightly flattened cells with a central nucleus and a cytoplasm whose processes are filled with bundles of filaments. These bundles converge into many small cellular extensions, terminating with desmosomes located at the tips of these spiny projections (Fig 18–3). The cells of this layer are firmly bound together by the filament-filled cytoplasmic spines and desmosomes that punctuate the cell surface, giving a prickle-studded appearance (Fig 18–4). These tonofilament bundles, visible under the light microscope, are called **tonofibrils;** they end and insert into the cytoplasmic densities of the desmosomes. The filaments play an important role in maintaining cohesion among cells and resisting the effects of abrasion. The epidermis of areas subject to continuous friction and pressure (such as the soles of the feet) has a thicker stratum spinosum with more abundant tonofibrils and desmosomes.

All mitoses are confined to what is termed the **malpighian layer,** which consists of both the stratum basale and stratum spinosum.

C. Stratum Granulosum: This is characterized by 3–5 layers of flattened polygonal cells containing centrally located nuclei and cytoplasm: the latter is filled with coarse basophilic granules called **keratohyalin granules.** Biochemical studies show that these granules contain a phosphorylated histidine-rich protein as well as cystine-containing proteins. The numerous phosphate groups account for the intense basophilia of keratohyalin granules, which are not surrounded by a membrane.

Another characteristic structure found with the electron microscope in the cells of the granular layer of epidermis is the membrane-coated **lamellar granule,** a small (0.1–0.3 μm) ovoid or rodlike structure containing lamellar disks that are formed by lipid bilayers. These granules fuse with the cell membrane and discharge their contents into the intercellular spaces of the stratum granulosum where they are deposited in the form of lipid-containing sheets. The function of this extruded material is similar to that of an intercellular cement in that it acts as a barrier to penetration by foreign materials and provides a very important sealing effect in the skin. Studies made in keratinized and nonkeratinized human oral epithelium

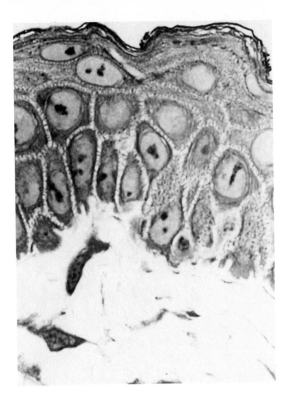

Figure 18–2. Photomicrograph of a section of human abdominal (thin) skin. Compare with Fig 18–1 and note the thinness of the whole epidermis and, specifically, the stratum corneum. The strata are not seen as clearly as in Fig 18–1. H&E stain, × 310.

show that there is no penetration by peroxidase and lanthanum tracers in the regions where this material fills the extracellular space. Formation of this barrier, which appeared first in reptiles, was one of the important evolutionary events that permitted development of terrestrial life.

    D. Stratum Lucidum: More apparent in thick skin this is translucent, thin layer of extremely flattened eosinophilic cells (Fig 18–1). The organelles and nuclei are no longer evident, and the cytoplasm consists primarily of densely packed filaments embedded in an electron-dense matrix. Desmosomes are still evident between adjacent cells.

    E. Stratum corneum: This layer (Figs 18–1 and 18–4) consists of 15–20 layers of flattened nonnucleated keratinized cells whose cytoplasm is filled with a birefringent filamentous scleroprotein, **keratin.** Keratin contains at least 6 different polypeptides with molecular weights ranging from 40,000 to 70,000. Three polypeptide chains coil around one another to form subunits (~ 47 nm long) of the tonofilament. At least one of the polypeptides is different from the others in the subunit, allowing great diversity in composition. Nine of the 3-chain subunits coil around

each other, forming a filament about 10 nm in diameter. End-to-end aggregation of 3-chain subunits increases the length of the tonofilament. The composition of tonofilaments changes as epidermal cells differentiate. Basal cells contain polypeptides of lower molecular weight, while more differentiated cells synthesize the higher-molecular-weight polypeptides. Tonofilaments are packed together in a matrix contributed by the keratohyalin granules.

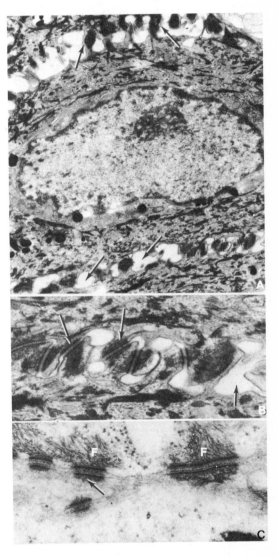

Figure 18–3. Electron micrograph of the stratum spinosum of human skin. **A:** A cell of the stratum spinosum with melanin granules and with its cytoplasm full of tonofibrils. The arrows show the spines, or intercellular bridges, with their desmosomes. × 8400. **B** and **C:** Desmosomes in greater detail. Observe that a dense substance appears between the cell membranes and that bundles of cytoplasmic filaments (tonofilaments; **E**) insert themselves on the desmosomes. × 36,000 and × 45,000. (Courtesy of C Barros.)

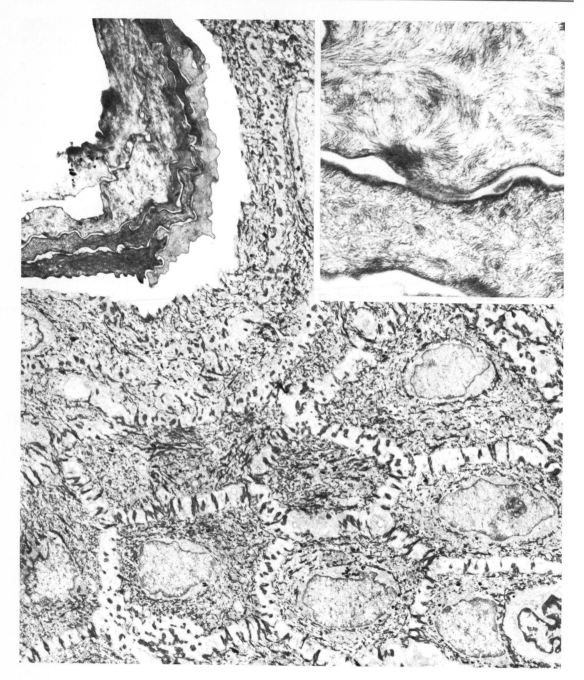

Figure 18–4. Electron micrograph of a section of human skin at the transition between the stratum spinosum and stratum corneum. Observe the cells with their typical cytoplasmic extensions, intercellular bridges, and cytoplasmic tonofibrils. × 5500. At upper left is the stratum corneum, seen in detail in the inset at upper right. × 36,000. Observe that these cells are packed with 10-nm intermediate filaments. (Courtesy of C Barros.)

After keratinization, the cells consist of only fibrillar and amorphous proteins and thickened plasma membranes; they are called **horny cells.** Lysosomal hydrolytic enzymes play a role in the disappearance of the cytoplasmic organelles. These cells are continuously shed at the surface of the stratum corneum.

This description of the epidermis corresponds to its most complex structure in areas where it is very thick, as on the soles of the feet. In thin skin, the stratum granulosum and stratum lucidum are often less well developed, and the stratum corneum may be quite thin.

Renewal of the epidermis under normal conditions occurs every 15–30 days and is due to mitotic activity in the strata germinativum and spinosum.

> In **psoriasis,** a common skin disease, there is an increase in the number of proliferating cells in the stratum basale and stratum spinosum as well as a decrease in the cycle time of these cells. This results in greater epidermal thickness and more rapid renewal of epidermis—7 days instead of 15–30 days.

Melanocytes

The color of the skin results from several factors, but the most important are its content of **melanin** and **carotene,** the number of blood vessels in the dermis, and the color of the blood flowing in them.

Eumelanin is a dark brown pigment produced by the **melanocyte,** a specialized cell of the epidermis found beneath or between the cells of the stratum basale and in the hair follicles. The pigment found in red hair is called **pheomelanin** (from Greek, *phaios,* dusky, + *melas,* black) and contains **cysteine** as part of its structure. Melanocytes are derived from neural crest cells. They have rounded cell bodies from which long irregular extensions branch into the epidermis, running between the cells of the basale and spinosum layers. Tips of these extensions terminate in invaginations of the cells present in the 2 layers. The electron microscope reveals a pale-staining cell containing numerous small mitochondria, a well-developed Golgi complex, and short cisternae of rough endoplasmic reticulum. Intermediate filaments, about 10 nm in diameter, are also present (Figs 18–5 and 18–6). While melanocytes are not attached to the adjacent keratinocytes by desmosomes, hemidesmo-

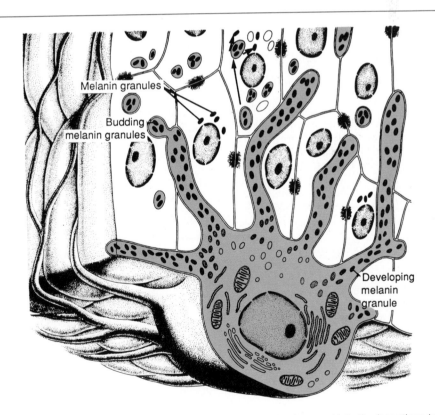

Melanin granules

Budding
melanin granules

Developing
melanin
granule

Figure 18–5. Diagram of a melanocyte (shown in color). Its arms extend upward into the interstices between keratinocytes. The melanin granules are synthesized in the melanocyte, migrate to its arms, and are transferred into the cytoplasm of keratinocytes. Ribosomes, Golgi complex, rough endoplasmic reticulum, and mitochondria are also present. (Based on the work of Fitzpatrick and Szabo, 1959.)

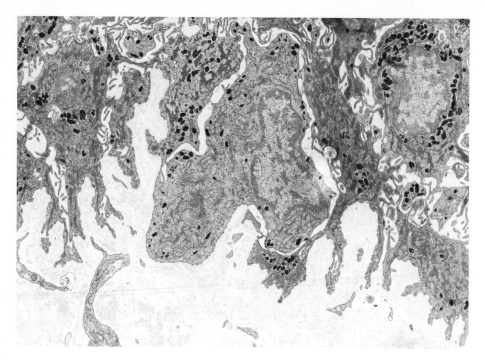

Figure 18–6. Electron micrograph of human skin containing melanocytes and keratinocytes. Note the greater abundance of melanin granules in the keratinocyte at right than in the adjacent melanocyte. The clear material at the bottom is dermal collagen. × 1800.

somes are present that bind melanocytes to the basal lamina.

Synthesis of melanin occurs in the interior of the melanocyte, with tyrosinase playing an important role in the process. As a result of tyrosinase activity, tyrosine is transformed first into **3,4-dihydroxyphenylalanine (dopa)** and then into **dopaquinone,** which is converted, after a series of transformations, into melanin. Tyrosinase is synthesized on ribosomes, transported in the lumen of the rough endoplasmic reticulum of melanocytes, and accumulated in vesicles formed at the Golgi zone (Fig 18–7). Four stages can be distinguished in the development of the mature melanin granule:

A. Stage I: A vesicle is surrounded by a membrane, showing the beginning of tyrosinase activity and formation of fine granular material; at its periphery, electron-dense strands show an orderly arrangement of tyrosinase molecules on a protein matrix.

B. Stage II: The vesicle **(melanosome)** is ovoid now and shows, in its interior, parallel filaments with a periodicity of about 10 nm or cross-striations of about the same periodicity. Melanin is deposited on the protein matrix.

C. Stage III: Increased melanin formation makes the periodic fine structure less visible.

D. Stage IV: The mature melanin granule is visible in the light microscope, and melanin completely

fills the vesicle. No ultrastructure is visible. The mature granules are ellipsoid in shape with a length of 1 μm and a diameter of 0.4 μm.

Once formed, melanin granules migrate within cytoplasmic extensions of the melanocyte and are transferred to cells of the strata germinativum and spinosum of the epidermis. This transferal has been directly observed in tissue cultures of skin.

Melanin granules are essentially injected into keratinocytes in a process called **cytocrine secretion.** Once inside the keratinocyte, melanin granules accumulate in the supranuclear region of the cytoplasm, thus protecting the nuclei of dividing cells from the deleterious effects of solar radiation.

Although melanocytes synthesize melanin, epithelial cells act as a depot and contain more of this pigment than melanocytes. Within the keratinocytes, melanin granules fuse with lysosomes—the reason that melanin disappears in upper epithelial cells. In this interaction between keratinocytes and melanocytes, which causes the pigmentation of the skin, the important factors are the rate of formation of melanin granules within the melanocyte, the transfer of the granules into the keratinocytes, and their ultimate disposition by the keratinocytes. A feedback mechanism may exist between melanocytes and keratinocytes.

Melanocytes can be easily seen by incubating fragments of epidermis in dopa. This compound is con-

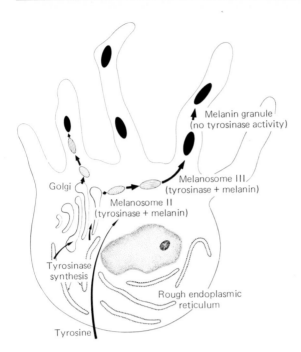

Figure 18–7. Diagram of a melanocyte, illustrating the principal process occurring during melanogenesis. Tyrosinase is synthesized in the rough endoplasmic reticulum and accumulated in vesicles of the Golgi complex. The free vesicles are now called melanosomes. Melanin synthesis begins in the stage II melanosomes, where this compound is accumulated and forms stage III melanosomes. Later, this structure loses its tyrosinase activity and becomes a melanin granule. Melanin granules migrate to the melanocyte's arm tips and are then transferred to the keratinocytes of the malpighian layer.

verted to dark brown deposits of melanin in melanocytes, a reaction catalyzed by the enzyme tyrosinase. Using this method, it is possible to count the number of melanocytes per unit area of the epidermis. Such studies show that these cells are not distributed at random among keratinocytes; rather, there is a pattern, called the epidermal-melanin unit, in their distribution. In humans, the ratio of dopa-positive melanocytes to keratinocytes in the stratum basale is constant within each area of the body but varies from one region to another. For example, there are about 1000 melanocytes/mm^2 in thigh skin and 2000/mm^2 in the skin of the scrotum. The number of melanocytes per unit area is not influenced by sex or race, and differences in skin color are due mainly to differences in the number of melanin granules in the keratinocytes.

Darkening of the skin (tanning) after exposure to ultraviolet rays of sunlight (wavelength = 290–320 nm) is the result of a 2-step process. A physicochemical reaction occurs first, darkening the preexistent melanin and releasing it rapidly into the keratino-

cytes. In the second stage, the rate of melanin synthesis in the melanocytes accelerates, increasing the amount of this pigment.

Lack of cortisol from the adrenal cortex in humans causes overproduction of ACTH, which increases the pigmentation of the skin, as in **Addison's disease,** which is caused by dysfunction of the adrenal glands.

Albinism, a hereditary inability of the melanocytes to synthesize melanin, is caused by the absence of tyrosinase activity or the inability of cells to take up tyrosine. As a result, the skin is not protected from solar radiation by melanin. This leads to a greater incidence of basal and squamous cell carcinomas.

The genetically regulated degeneration and disappearance of entire melanocytes results in a depigmentation disorder called **vitiligo.**

Langerhans' Cells

These star-shaped cells, found mainly in the stratum spinosum of the epidermis, represent 2–8% of the epidermal cells. They are bone-marrow-derived macrophages that are capable of binding and presenting antigens to T lymphocytes, and they participate in the stimulation of these cells. Consequently, they have a significant role in skin immunological reactions.

Merkel's Cells

The Merkel's cells, generally present in the thick skin of palms and soles, somewhat resemble the epidermal epithelial cells but have small dense granules in their cytoplasm. The composition of these granules is not known. Free nerve endings that form an expanded terminal disk are present at the base of the Merkel's cells. These cells may serve as sensory mechanoreceptors, although other evidence suggests that they have functions related to the diffuse neuroendocrine system.

DERMIS

The dermis is composed of the connective tissue that supports the epidermis and binds it to the subjacent layer, the subcutaneous tissue (hypodermis). The thickness of the dermis varies, depending upon the region of the body, and reaches its maximum of 4 mm on the back. The surface of the dermis is very irregular and has many projections (dermal papillae) that interdigitate with projections (epidermal pegs or ridges) of the epidermis (Fig 18–1). These structures are more numerous in skin that is subject to frequent pressure; they are believed to increase and reinforce the dermal-epidermal junction. During embryonic development, the dermis determines the developmental pattern of the overlying epidermis. Dermis obtained from the sole always induces the formation of a heavily keratinized epidermis irrespective of the site of origin of the epithelial cells.

The distinctive dermal-epidermal junction is seen in histologic sections of the human skin; this understructure of the epidermis is unique in each part of the body. A **basal lamina** is always found between the stratum germinativum and the papillary layer of the dermis and follows the contour of the interdigitations between these layers. Underlying the basal lamina is a delicate net of reticular fibers, the **lamina reticularis.** This composite structure is called the **basement membrane,** and can be seen with the light microscope.

> Abnormalities of the dermal-epidermal junction can lead to one type of blistering disorder (**bullous pemphigoid**). An additional type of blistering disease (**pemphigus**) is caused by the loss of intercellular junctions between keratinocytes.

The dermis contains 2 layers with rather indistinct boundaries. They are the outermost papillary layer and the deeper reticular layer. The thin **papillary layer** is composed of loose connective tissue; fibroblasts and other connective tissue cells are present, with the most abundant being mast cells and macrophages. Extravasated leukocytes are also seen. The papillary layer is so called because it constitutes the major part of the dermal papillae. From this layer, special collagen fibrils insert into the basal lamina and extend into the dermis. They bind the dermis to the epidermis and are called **anchoring fibrils (structures);** (Fig 4–4). The **reticular layer** is thicker, composed of irregular dense connective tissue (mainly type I collagen), and therefore has more fibers and fewer cells than does the papillary layer. The glycosaminoglycan content of the dermis varies in different regions. In the skin the principal glycosaminoglycan is dermatan sulfate. The dermis contains a network of elastic fibers (Fig 18–8) in which the thicker fibers are characteristically found in the reticular layer. From this region emerge fibers that become gradually thinner and end by inserting into the basal lamina. As these fibers progress toward the basal lamina, they gradually lose their amorphous elastin component, and only the microfibrillar component inserts into the basal lamina. This elastic network is responsible for the elasticity of the skin.

> Age-related changes in the dermis can be observed histologically and biochemically. Collagen fibers thicken and collagen synthesis decreases with age. Elastic fibers steadily increase in number and thickness, so that the elastin content of human skin increases approximately fivefold from fetal to adult life. In old age, extensive cross-linking of collagen fibers, the loss of elastic fibers, and degeneration of these fibers caused by excessive exposure to the sun (**solar elastosis**) cause the skin to become

more fragile, lose its suppleness, and develop many wrinkles. Several disorders, such as **cutis laxa** and **Ehlers-Danlos syndrome** (Table 5–3), are characterized by a considerable increase in skin and ligament extensibility caused by defective collagen-fibril processing.

The dermis has a rich network of blood and lymph vessels. In certain areas of the skin, blood can pass directly from arteries to veins through arteriovenous anastomoses, or shunts. These play a very important role in temperature and blood pressure regulation, since dermal vessels can accommodate about 4.5% of the blood volume. A rich capillary network in the papillary layer surrounds the epidermal ridges and functions in regulating body core temperature and nourishing the overlying epidermis, which contains no blood vessels of its own.

In addition to these components, the dermis contains such epidermal derivatives as the hair follicles and sweat and sebaceous glands. There is a rich supply of nerves in the dermis, and the effector nerves

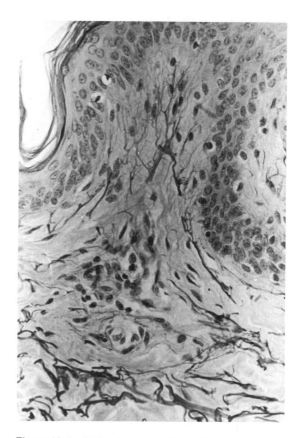

Figure 18–8. Photomicrograph of a section of human abdominal skin stained for elastic fibers. Note the gradual decrease in the diameter of fibers as they approach the epidermis. The very thin superficial fibers are formed only by microfibrils that insert into the basal lamina. × 600.

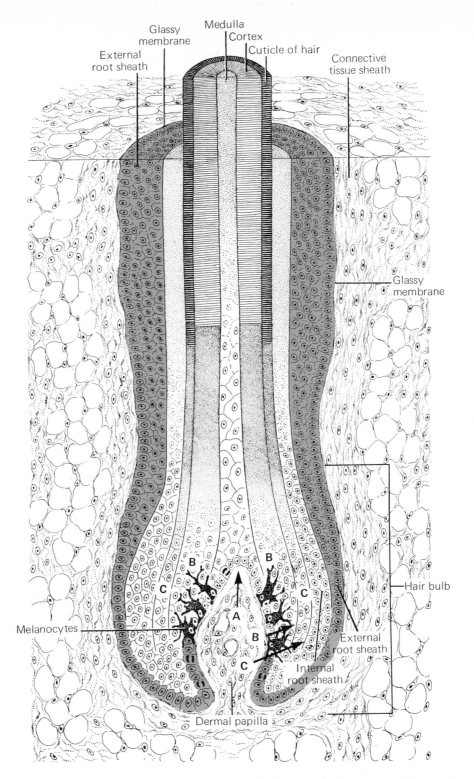

Figure 18–9. Drawing of a hair and its follicle. The follicle has a bulbous terminal expansion with a dermal papilla. The papilla contains capillaries and is covered by cells that form the hair root and develop into the hair shaft. The central cells (A) produce large, vacuolated, moderately keratinized cells (indicated by the arrow) that form the medulla of the hair. The cells that produce the cortex of the hair are located laterally (B). Cells forming the hair cuticle originate in the next layer (C). The peripheral epithelial cells develop into the internal and external root sheaths. The external root sheath (shown in color) is continuous with the epidermis, while the cells of the internal root sheath disappear at the level of the openings of the sebaceous gland ducts (not shown).

to the skin are postganglionic fibers of sympathetic ganglia of the paravertebral chain. No parasympathetic innervation is present. The afferent nerve endings form a superficial dermal network with free nerve endings, a hair follicle network, and the innervation of encapsulated sensory organs (**Meissner's** and **pacinian corpuscles**).

SUBCUTANEOUS TISSUE

This layer consists of loose connective tissue that binds the skin loosely to the subjacent organs, making it possible for the skin to slide over them. The hypodermis often contains fat cells that vary in number according to the area of the body, and in size according to the nutritional status of the individual. This layer is also referred to as the superficial fascia and, where thick enough, the panniculus adiposus.

HAIRS

Hairs are elongated keratinized structures derived from invaginations of epidermal epithelium. Their color, size, and disposition vary according to race, age, sex, and region of the body. Hairs are found everywhere on the body except on the palms, soles, lips, glans penis, clitoris, and labia minora. The face has about 600 hairs/cm^2 while the remainder of the body has about 60/cm^2. Hairs grow discontinuously and have periods of growth followed by periods of rest. This growth does not occur synchronously in all regions of the body or even in the same area; it tends rather to occur in patches. The duration of the growth and rest periods also varies according to the region of the body. Thus, in the scalp, the growth periods (anagen) may last for several years, while the rest periods (catagen and telogen) average 3 months. Hair growth in such regions of the body as the scalp, face, and pubis is strongly influenced not only by sex hormones—especially androgens—but also by adrenal and thyroid hormones.

Each hair arises from an epidermal invagination, the **hair follicle**, which has during its growth period a terminal dilatation called the **hair bulb**. At the base of the hair bulb, a **dermal papilla** can be observed (Figs 18–9 and 18–10) The dermal papilla contains a capillary network that is vital in sustaining the hair follicle. The loss of blood flow or the vitality of the dermal papilla will result in death of the follicle. The epidermal cells covering this dermal papilla form the hair root that produces and is continuous with the hair shaft, which protrudes beyond the skin.

During periods of growth, the epithelial cells that make up the bulb are equivalent to those in the stratum germinativum of the skin. They divide constantly and differentiate into specific cell types. In certain types of thick hairs, the cells of the central region of

the root at the apex of the dermal papilla produce large, vacuolated, and moderately keratinized cells that form the **medulla** of the hair (A in Fig 18–9). The cells located around the central region of the root (B in Fig 18–9) multiply and differentiate into heavily keratinized, compactly grouped fusiform cells that form the **hair cortex.**

Farther toward the periphery are the cells (C in Fig 18–9) that produce the **hair cuticle,** a layer of cells that are cuboidal midway up the bulb, then become tall and columnar. Higher up, they change from horizontal to vertical, at which point they form a layer of flattened, heavily keratinized, shinglelike cells covering the cortex. These cuticle cells are the last cell line in the hair follicle to differentiate.

The outermost cells give rise to the **internal root sheath,** which completely surrounds the initial part of the hair shaft. The internal sheath is a transient structure whose cells degenerate and disappear above the level of the sebaceous glands. The **external root sheath** is continuous with epidermal cells and near

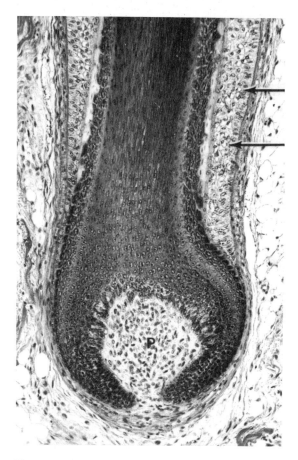

Figure 18–10. Photomicrograph of a section of hair follicle from human skin. Observe the papilla (P) and the outer root sheath (arrows), surrounded by a connective tissue sheath. H&E stain, × 118.

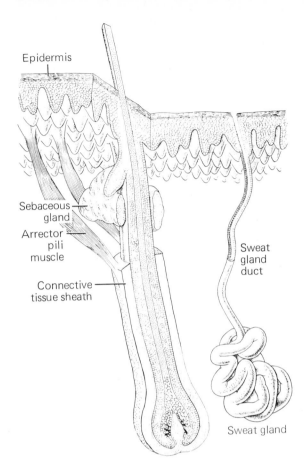

Figure 18–11. Relationships between the skin, hair follicle, arrector pili muscle, and sebaceous and sweat glands. The arrector pili muscle originates in the connective tissue sheath of the hair follicle and inserts into the papillary layer of the dermis, where it ends.

the surface it shows all the layers of epidermis. Near the dermal papilla it is thinner and is composed of cells corresponding to the epidermal stratum germinativum.

Separating the hair follicle from the dermis is a noncellular hyaline layer, the **glassy membrane** (Fig 18–9), which represents a thickening of the basal lamina. The dermis that surrounds the follicle is denser, forming a sheath of connective tissue. Bound to this sheath and connecting it to the papillary layer of the dermis are bundles of smooth muscle cells, the **arrector pili** muscles (Fig 18–11). They are disposed in an oblique direction, and their contraction results in the erection of the hair shaft to a more upright position. Contraction of arrector pili muscles also causes a depression of the skin where the muscles attach to the dermis. This produces the "gooseflesh" of common parlance.

Hair color is caused by the activity of melanocytes

located between the papilla and the epithelial cells of the hair root that produce the pigment present in the medullary and cortical cells of the hair shaft (Fig 18–9). These melanocytes produce and transfer melanin to the epithelial cells by a mechanism similar to that described for the epidermis.

Although the keratinization processes in the epidermis and hair appear to be similar, they differ in several ways:

(1) The epidermis produces relatively soft keratinized outer layers of dead cells that adhere slightly to the skin and desquamate continuously. The opposite occurs in the hair, producing a hard and compact keratinized structure.

(2) Although keratinization in the epidermis occurs continuously and over the entire surface, in the hair it is intermittent and present only in the hair root. The hair papilla has an inductive action on the covering epithelial cells, promoting their proliferation and differentiation. Injuries to the dermal papillae thus result in the loss of hair.

(3) Contrary to what happens in the epidermis, where the differentiation of all cells in the same direction gives rise to the final keratinized layer, cells in the hair root differentiate into various cell types that differ in ultrastructure, histochemistry, and function. Mitotic activity in hair follicles is influenced by androgens.

NAILS

Nails are plates of keratinized epithelial cells on the dorsal surface of each distal phalanx (Fig 18–12). The proximal part of the nail, hidden in the nail groove, is the **nail root.** The epithelium of the fold of skin covering the nail root consists of the usual layers of cells. The stratum corneum of this epithelium forms the **eponychium,** or **cuticle.** The **nail plate,** which corresponds to the stratum corneum of the skin, rests on a bed of epidermis termed the **nail bed.** Only

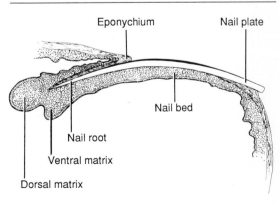

Figure 18–12. The nail and its components.

the stratum basale and the stratum spinosum are present in the nail bed. Nail plate epithelium arises from the **nail matrix.** The proximal end of the matrix extends deep to the nail root. Its distal end extends to the outer edge of the **lunula,** the white, opaque crescent at the proximal end of the nail. Cells of the matrix divide, move distally, and eventually cornify, forming the proximal part of the nail plate. The nail plate then slides forward over the nail bed (which makes no contribution to the formation of the plate). The distal end of the plate becomes free of the nail bed and is worn away or cut off. The nearly transparent nail plate and the thin epithelium of the nail bed provide a useful window on the amount of oxygen in the blood by showing the color of blood in the dermal vessels.

GLANDS OF THE SKIN

Sebaceous Glands

Sebaceous glands are embedded in the dermis over most of the body surface. There are about 100 of these glands per square centimeter over most of the body, but the frequency increases to 400–900/cm² on the face, forehead, and scalp. Sebaceous glands,

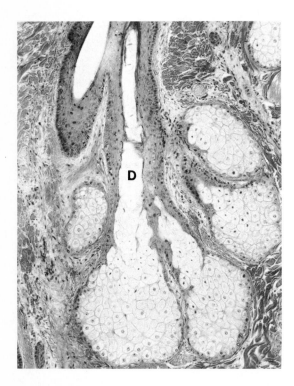

Figure 18–13. Photomicrograph of a sebaceous gland. It consists of several acini, which are limited externally by proliferating, flattened epithelial cells that give rise to the fat-filled cells of the acinar center. D, duct. H&E stain, × 100.

which are not found in the glabrous skin of the palms and soles, are acinar glands that usually have several acini opening into a short duct. This duct usually ends in the upper portion of a hair follicle (Fig 18–11); in certain regions, such as the glans penis, glans clitoridis, and lips, it opens directly onto the epidermal surface. The acini consist of a basal layer of undifferentiated flattened epithelial cells that rest on the basal lamina. These cells proliferate and differentiate, filling the acini with rounded cells containing abundant fat droplets in their cytoplasm (Fig 18–13). Their nuclei gradually shrink, and the cells simultaneously become filled with fat droplets and burst. The product of this process is **sebum,** the secretion of the sebaceous gland, which is gradually moved to the surface of the skin.

This is an example of a holocrine gland, for its product of secretion is released with remnants of dead cells. This product comprises a complex mixture of lipids that includes triglycerides, waxes, squalene, and cholesterol and its esters. Sebaceous glands begin to function at puberty. The primary controlling factor of sebaceous gland secretion in men is testosterone; in women it is a combination of ovarian and adrenal androgens.

> The flow of sebum is continuous, and a disturbance in the normal secretion and flow of sebum is one of the reasons for the development of acne.

The functions of sebum in humans are largely unknown. It may have weak antibacterial and antifungal properties. Sebum does not have any importance in preventing water loss.

Sweat Glands

Sweat glands are widely distributed in the skin. Certain regions, such as the glans penis, are exceptions.

The **eccrine (merocrine)** sweat glands are simple, coiled tubular glands whose ducts open at the skin surface (Fig 18–11). Their ducts do not divide and their diameter is thinner than that of the secretory portion (Fig 18–14). The secretory part of the gland is embedded in the dermis; it measures approximately 0.4 mm in diameter and is surrounded by myoepithelial cells (described in Chapter 4). Contraction of these cells helps discharge the secretion. A fairly thick basal lamina lies outside the secretory portion of the gland. Two types of cells have been described in the secretory portion of eccrine sweat glands. **Dark cells** (mucoid cells) are pyramidal cells that line most of the luminal surface of this portion of the gland. Their basal surface does not touch the basal lamina. The cytoplasm of dark cells contains rod-shaped mitochondria, a well-developed Golgi complex, cisternae of rough endoplasmic reticulum, and numerous free ribosomes. Secretory granules containing glycoproteins are abundant in the apical cytoplasm. **Clear**

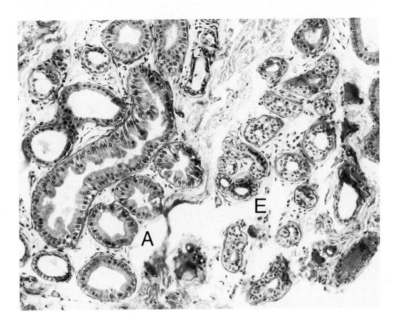

Figure 18–14. Photomicrograph from a region of axillary human skin, showing apocrine (A) and eccrine (E) gland portions. The epidermal side is at the upper border. × 110. (Courtesy of J James).

cells are devoid of secretory granules but contain an abundance of glycogen particles. The basal plasmalemma has the numerous invaginations characteristic of cells involved in transepithelial salt and fluid transport. The ducts are lined by stratified cuboidal epithelium (Fig 18–14).

The fluid secreted by these glands is not viscous and contains little protein. Its main components are water, sodium chloride, urea, ammonia, and uric acid. Its sodium content of 85 meq/L is distinctly below that of blood (144 meq/L), and the cells present in the sweat ducts are responsible for sodium absorption. The fluid in the lumen of the secretory portion of the gland is an ultrafiltrate of the blood plasma. This ultrafiltrate is derived from a network of capillaries that intimately envelop the secretory region of each gland. Following its release on the surface of the skin, sweat evaporates, cooling the surface.

In addition to eccrine sweat glands, another type of sweat gland—the **apocrine** gland—is present in the axillary, areolar, and anal regions. Apocrine glands are much larger (3–5 mm in diameter) than eccrine sweat glands. They are embedded in the subcutaneous tissue, and their ducts open into hair follicles. These glands produce a viscous secretion that is initially odorless—it acquires its distinctive odor as a result of bacterial decomposition. Apocrine glands are innervated by adrenergic nerve endings, while eccrine glands receive cholinergic fibers. The glands of Moll in the margins of the eyelids and the ceruminous glands of the ear are modified sweat glands.

VESSELS & NERVES OF THE SKIN

The arterial vessels that nourish the skin form 2 plexuses. One is located between the papillary and reticular layers, the other between the dermis and the subcutaneous tissue. Thin branches leave these plexuses and vascularize the dermal papillae. Each papilla has only one arterial ascending and one venous descending branch. Veins are disposed in 3 plexuses, 2 in the position described for arterial vessels and the third in the middle of the dermis. Arteriovenous anastomoses with glomera (see Chapter 11) are frequent in the skin. Lymphatic vessels begin as blind sacs in the papillae of the dermis and converge to form 2 plexuses, also as described for the arterial vessels.

One of the most important functions of the skin, with its abundant sensory innervation, is to receive stimuli from the environment. In addition to free nerve endings in the epidermis and cutaneous glands, receptors are present in the dermis and subcutaneous tissue; they are more frequently found in the dermal papillae (see Chapter 24). The hair follicles possess a rich network of nerve endings that are essential in the processing of tactile impressions from the environment.

Tumors of the Skin

One-third of all tumors are of the skin. Most of these derive from the basal cells, the squamous cells of the stratum spinosum, and melanocytes. They produce, respectively, basal cell carcinomas, squamous cell carcinomas, and melanomas. The first two types of tumors can be diagnosed and excised early and consequently are rarely lethal. Skin tumors show an increased incidence in fair-skinned individuals residing in regions with high degrees of solar radiation. **Malignant melanoma** is an invasive tumor of melanocytes. Rapidly dividing, malignantly transformed melanocytes penetrate the basal lamina, enter the dermis, and invade the blood and lymphatic vessels to gain wide distribution through the body. Malignant melanoma represents approximately 1 to 3% of all tumors.

REFERENCES

Edelson RL, Fink JM: The immunologic function of the skin. *Sci Am* (June) 1985;**252**:46.

Green H et al: Differentiated structural components of the keratinocyte. *Cold Spring Harbor Symp Quant Biol,* 1982.

Halprin KM: Epidermal "turnover time": A reexamination. *J Invest Dermatol* 1972;**86**:14.

Hayward AF: Membrane coating granules. *Int Rev Cytol* 1979;**59**:97.

Millington PF, Wilkinson R: *Skin.* Cambridge Univ Press, 1983.

Montagna W: *The Structure and Function of Skin,* 3rd ed. Academic Press, 1974.

Strauss JS, Fochi PE, Downing DT: The sebaceous glands: Twenty-five years of progress. *J Invest Dermatol* 1976;**67**:90.

Winkelmann RK: The Merkel cell system and a comparison between it and the neurosecretory or APUD cell system. *J Invest Dermatol* 1977;**69**:41.

Zelickson AS: *Ultrastructure of Normal and Abnormal Skin.* Lea & Febiger, 1967.

Urinary System

The urinary system consists of the paired kidneys and ureters and the unpaired bladder and urethra. This system contributes to the maintenance of homeostasis by producing urine, in which various metabolic waste products are eliminated. Urine produced in the kidneys passes through the ureters to the bladder, where it is temporarily stored and then released to the exterior through the urethra. The kidneys also regulate the fluid and electrolyte balance of the body and are the site of production of the hormones renin and erythropoietin.

KIDNEYS

1. STRUCTURE

Each kidney has a concave medial border, the **hilum**—where nerves enter, blood and lymph vessels enter and exit, and the ureter exits—and a convex lateral surface (Fig 19–1). The **renal pelvis,** the expanded upper end of the ureter, is divided into 2 or 3 **major calyces.** Several small branches, the **minor calyces,** arise from each major calyx.

The kidney can be divided into an outer **cortex** and an inner **medulla** (Figs 19–1 and 19–2). In humans, the renal medulla consists of 10–18 conical or pyramidal structures, the **medullary pyramids.** From the base of each medullary pyramid, parallel arrays of tubules, the **medullary rays,** penetrate the cortex (Fig 19–1). Each medullary ray consists of one or more collecting tubules together with the straight portions of several **nephrons,** the functional units of the kidney. The mass of cortical tissue surrounding each medullary pyramid is a **renal lobe,** and each medullary ray forms the center of a conical **renal lobule** (Fig 19–20). Cortical tissue is also found between medullary pyramids; these structures are known as the **columns of Bertin** (Fig 19–1).

Nephrons

Each kidney is composed of 1–4 million nephrons (from Greek, *nephros,* kidney). Each nephron consists of a dilated portion, the **renal corpuscle:** the **proximal convoluted tubule:** the thin and thick limbs of the **loop of Henle;** and the **distal convoluted tu-**

bule (Fig 19–1). The **collecting tubules** and **ducts,** which are of different embryologic origin than the nephron, collect the urine produced by nephrons and conduct it to the renal pelvis. The nephron and the collecting duct into which it empties constitute a **uriniferous tubule,** which can be considered the functional unit of the kidney.

Each renal corpuscle is about 200 μm in diameter and consists of a tuff of capillaries, the **glomerulus,** surrounded by a double-walled epithelial capsule called **Bowman's capsule** (Figs 19–1, 19–2, 19–3, and 19–18). The internal layer (the **visceral layer**) of the capsule envelops the capillaries of the glomerulus. The external layer forms the outer limit of the renal corpuscle and is called the **parietal layer** of Bowman's capsule (Figs 19–2 and 19–3). Between the 2 layers of Bowman's capsule is the **urinary space,** which receives the fluid filtered through the capillary wall and the visceral layer. Each renal corpuscle has a **vascular pole,** where the **afferent arteriole** enters and the **efferent arteriole** leaves (Fig 19–3), and a **urinary pole,** where the proximal convoluted tubule begins (Fig 19–3 and 19–4). After entering the renal corpuscle, the afferent arteriole usually divides into 2–5 primary branches, each subdividing into capillaries and forming the renal glomerulus.

The parietal layer of Bowman's capsule consists of a simple squamous epithelium supported by a basal lamina and a thin layer of reticular fibers (Figs 19–3 and 19–5). At the urinary pole, the epithelium changes to the simple columnar epithelium characteristic of the proximal tubule (Figs 19–3 and 19–4).

While the epithelium of the parietal layer remains relatively unchanged, the internal, or visceral, layer is greatly modified during embryonic development. The cells of this internal layer, the **podocytes** (Figs 19–3, 19–6, 19–7, and 19–8), have a cell body from which arise several **primary processes.** Each primary process gives rise to numerous **secondary processes,** called **pedicels** (Figs 19–6, 19–7 and 19–8), that embrace the capillaries of the glomerulus. At a regular distance of 25 nm, the secondary processes are in direct contact with the basal lamina, which is formed jointly by capillary endothelial cells and podocytes. The cell bodies of podocytes and their primary processes do not touch the basal lamina (Figs

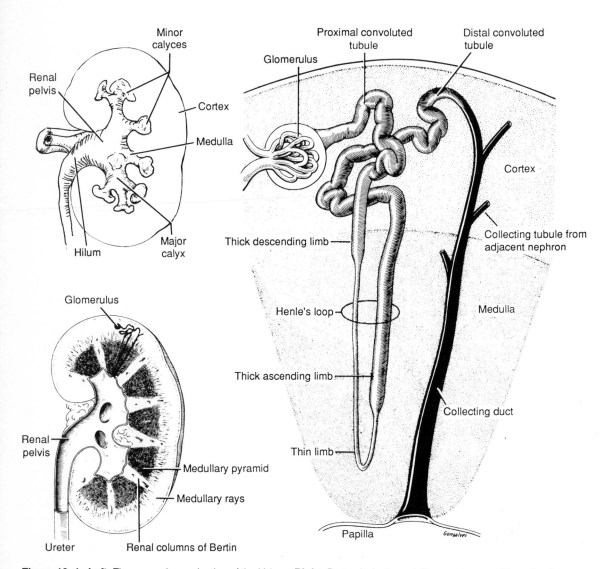

Figure 19–1. Left: The general organization of the kidney. **Right:** Parts of a juxtamedullary nephron and its collecting duct and tubule (shown in black).

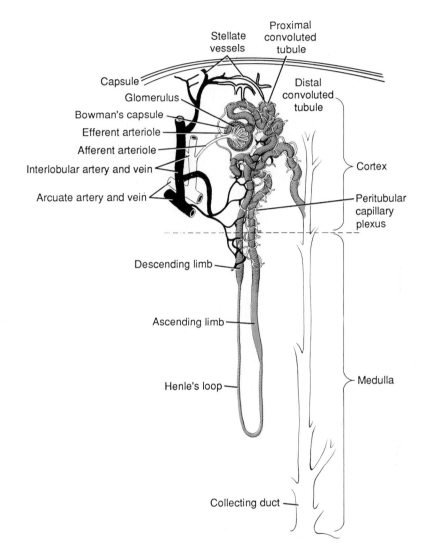

Figure 19–2. Diagram of the vascular supply of a nephron (shown in color) in the outer part of the cortex. Arteries and capillaries are white; veins are black.

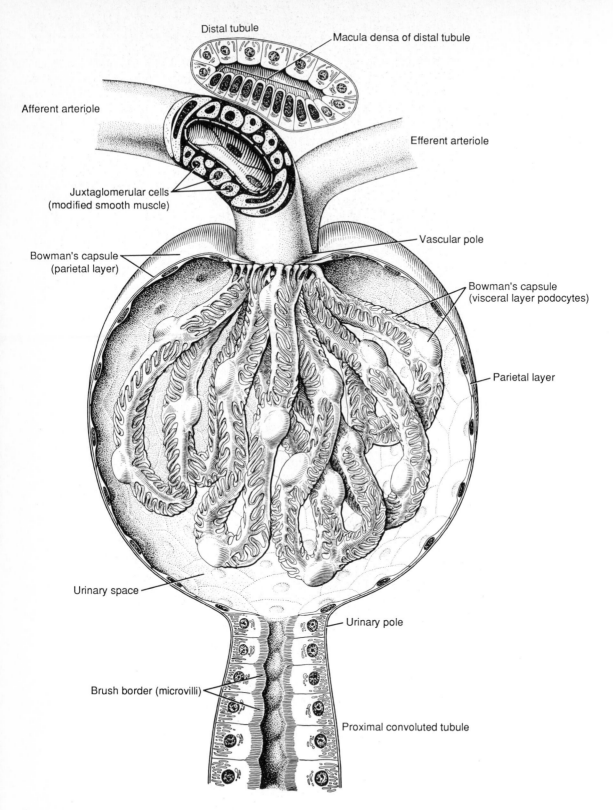

Distal tubule

Macula densa of distal tubule

Afferent arteriole

Efferent arteriole

Juxtaglomerular cells
(modified smooth muscle)

Vascular pole

Bowman's capsule
(parietal layer)

Bowman's capsule
(visceral layer podocytes)

Parietal layer

Urinary space

Urinary pole

Brush border (microvilli)

Proximal convoluted tubule

Figure 19–3. The renal corpuscle. The upper part of the drawing shows the vascular pole, with afferent and efferent arterioles and the macula densa. Note the juxtaglomerular cells in the wall of the afferent arteriole. Podocyte processes cover the outer surfaces of the glomerular capillaries; the part of the podocyte containing the nucleus protrudes into the urinary space. Note the flattened cells of the parietal layer of Bowman's capsule. The lower part of the drawing shows the urinary pole and the proximal convoluted tubule.

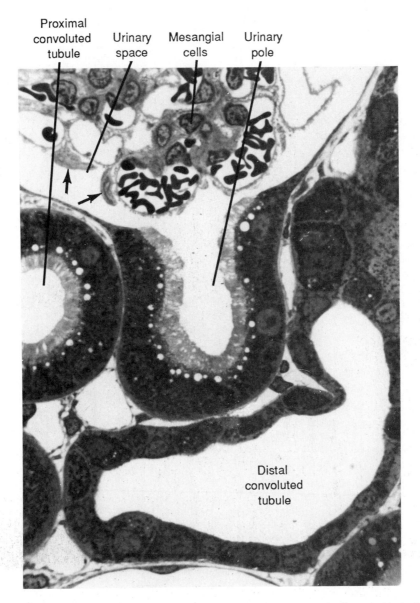

Figure 19–4. Section of rat kidney cortex showing the urinary pole of a renal corpuscle. Arrows point to 2 podocytes that envelop the capillaries of the renal glomerulus. See also the proximal convoluted tubule, distal convoluted tubule, urinary space, and mesangial cells. × 950. (Courtesy of SL Wissig.)

Parietal layer   Peritubular capillary   Visceral layer   Glomerular capillaries   Urinary space   Proximal tubule

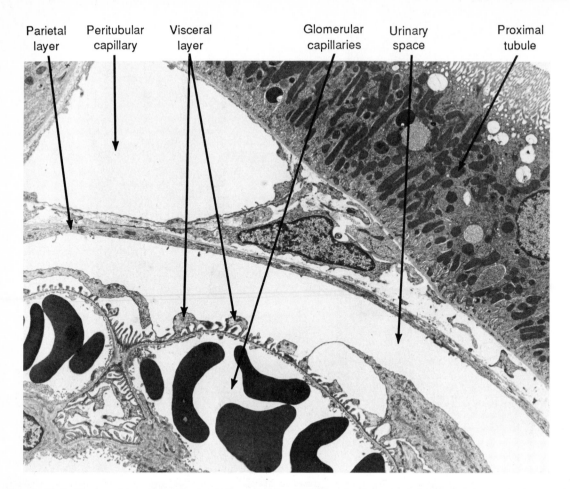

Figure 19–5. Electron micrograph of a rat kidney showing part of a renal corpuscle, including the parietal layer of Bowman's capsule, the urinary space, glomerular capillaries containing erythrocytes, the visceral layer of Bowman's capsule, the peritubular capillary, and the proximal tubule. × 2850. (Courtesy of SL Wissig.)

19–6 and 19–8), however. The pedicels from one podocyte embrace more than one capillary; on a single capillary, the pedicels of 2 podocytes alternate in position next to the basal lamina (Fig 19–8). Although pedicels contain few or no organelles, microfilaments and microtubules are numerous.

The secondary processes of podocytes interdigitate, defining elongated spaces about 25 nm wide—the **filtration slits.** Spanning adjacent processes (and thus bridging the filtration slits), is a diaphragm about 6 nm thick that is comparable to the diaphragm encountered in fenestrated endothelial cells. The cytoplasm of podocytes contains numerous free ribosomes, a few cisternae of rough endoplasmic reticulum, infrequent mitochondria, and a prominent Golgi complex, as well as vesicles and microfilaments (Figs 19–8 and 19–9).

Between the fenestrated endothelial cells of the glomerular capillaries and the podocytes that cover

their external surfaces is a thick (~ 0.1 μm) basal lamina. This layer is believed to be the filtration barrier separating the urinary space and the blood in the capillaries. This basal lamina (or basement membrane) is derived from the fusion of capillary- and podocyte-produced basal laminae. With the aid of the electron microscope, one can distinguish a central electron-dense layer **(lamina densa)** and, on each side, a more electron-lucent layer **(lamina rara;** Fig 19–9). Histochemical methods provide evidence that the 2 electron-lucent zones have biochemical compositions different from those of the denser central zone. Heparan sulfate, a polyanionic molecule, has been detected in the electron-lucent zones, where it could impede the passage of negatively charged proteins across the basal lamina. Thus, the glomerular basal lamina is a selective macromolecular filter in which the type IV collagen present in the lamina densa acts as a physical filter, while the anionic sites in the

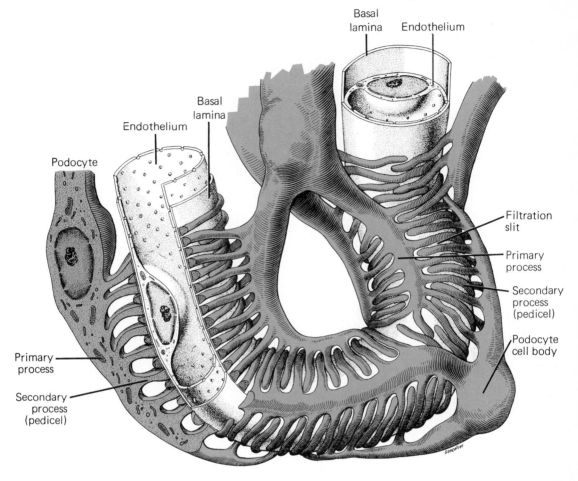

Figure 19–6. Schematic representation of a glomerular capillary with the visceral layer of Bowman's capsule (formed by podocytes; shown in color). In this capillary, endothelial cells are fenestrated, but the basal lamina on which they rest is continuous. At left is a podocyte shown in partial section. As viewed from the outside, the part of the podocyte containing the nucleus protrudes into the urinary space. Each podocyte has many primary processes, from which arise an even greater number of secondary processes that are in contact with the basal lamina. (Redrawn and modified after Gordon. Reproduced, with permission, from Ham AW: *Histology,* 6th ed. Lippincott, 1969.)

laminae rarae act as a charge barrier. Particles greater than 10 nm in diameter do not readily cross the basal lamina, and negatively charged proteins with molecular weights greater than that of albumin (MW 69,000) pass across only sparingly.

In diseases such as diabetes mellitus and glomerulonephritis, the glomerular filter becomes much more permeable to proteins, with the subsequent release of protein into the urine (**proteinuria**).

The endothelial cells of glomerular capillaries have a thin cytoplasm that is thicker around the nucleus, where most of the organelles are clustered. The fenestrae of these cells are larger (70–90 nm in di-

ameter) and more numerous than in the fenestrated capillaries of other organs, and they lack the thin diaphragm commonly observed spanning the openings of other fenestrated capillaries.

Besides endothelial cells and podocytes, the glomerular capillaries have **mesangial** (from Greek, *mesos,* middle, + *angeion*) **cells** adhering to their walls in places where the basal lamina forms a sheath that is shared by 2 or more capillaries (Figs 19–4, 19–10, and 19–11). The cytoplasmic extensions of mesangial cells penetrate between endothelial cells to reach the capillary lumen. The cells synthesize the amorphous matrix that surrounds them and contribute to the support of the capillary walls. Little else is known about their function: they constitute a pericytelike population of cells. After

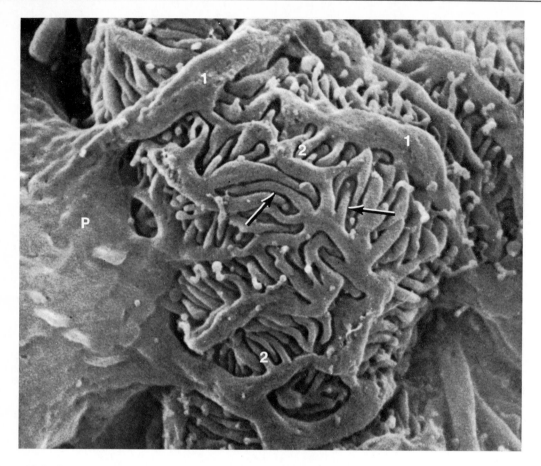

Figure 19–7. Scanning electron micrograph showing Bowman's visceral epithelial cells, or podocytes (P), surrounding capillaries of the renal glomerulus. Two orders of branching of the podocyte processes are apparent: the primary processes (1) and the secondary processes, or pedicels (2). The small spaces between adjacent processes constitute the filtration slits (arrows). × 10,700.

the injection of ferritin (an electron-scattering, iron-containing protein easily identified with the electron microscope), the cytoplasm of mesangial cells appears to be engorged with this protein. These cells may act as macrophages and serve to clean the basal lamina of particulate material that accumulates during the filtration process.

Proximal Convoluted Tubule

At the urinary pole of the renal corpuscle, the squamous epithelium of the parietal layer of Bowman's capsule is continuous with the columnar epithelium of the proximal convoluted tubule (Figs 19–1, 19–2, and 19–4). It is longer than the distal convoluted tubule and is therefore more frequently seen near renal corpuscles in the cortical labyrinth.

The proximal convoluted tubule is lined by simple cuboidal or columnar epithelium (Figs 19–4 and 19–12). The cells of this epithelium have an acidophilic cytoplasm caused by the presence of numerous elon-

gated mitochondria. The cell apex possesses abundant microvilli about 1 μm in length, which form a **brush border** (Figs 19–3, 19–12, and 19–13). Because the cells are large, each transverse section of a proximal tubule contains only 3–5 spherical nuclei, usually located in the center of the cell.

In the living animal, proximal convoluted tubules have a wide lumen and are surrounded by peritubular capillaries. In routine histologic preparations, the brush border is usually disorganized and the peritubular capillary lumens are greatly reduced in size or collapsed.

The apical cytoplasm of these cells has numerous canaliculi between the bases of the microvilli; these have an effect on the capacity of the proximal tubule cells for absorbing macromolecules. Pinocytotic vesicles are formed by evaginations of the apical membranes (Fig 19–14). These vesicles contain macromolecules (mainly proteins with molecular weights of less than 70,000) that have passed across the glom-

Glomerular
capillary   Podocytes   Urinary
space

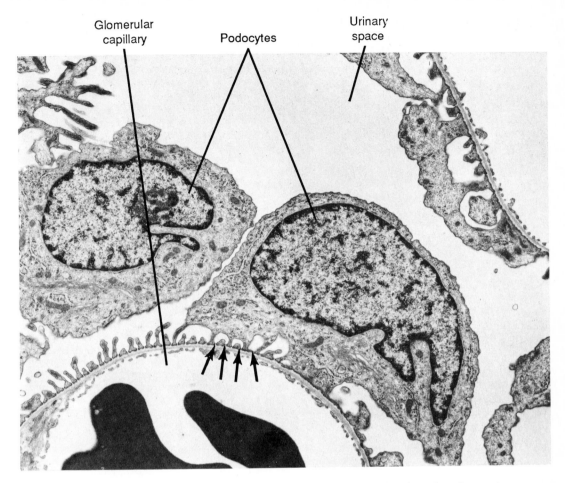

Figure 19–8. Electron micrograph showing the cell bodies of 2 podocytes and the alternation of secondary processes from 2 different cells (arrows). The urinary space and glomerular capillary are indicated. × 9000. (Courtesy of SL Wissig.)

erular filter. The pinocytotic vesicles fuse with lysosomes where degradation of macromolecules occurs, and monomers are returned to the circulation. The basal portions of these cells have abundant membrane invaginations and lateral interdigitations with neighboring cells. The Na^+/K^+-ATPase (sodium pump) responsible for actively transporting sodium ions out of these cells is localized in these basolateral membranes. Mitochondria are concentrated at the base of the cell (Figs 19–12, 19–13, and 19–14) and arranged parallel to the long axis of the cell. This mitochondrial location and the increase in the area of the cell membrane at the base of the cell are characteristic of cells engaged in active ion transport (see Chapter 4). Because of the extensive interdigitation of the lateral membranes, no discrete cell margins can be observed, using the light microscope, between cells of the proximal tubule.

Loop of Henle

The loop of Henle is a U-shaped structure consisting of a **thick descending limb,** very similar in structure to the proximal convoluted tubule; a **thin descending limb;** a **thin ascending limb;** and a **thick ascending limb** that closely resembles the distal convoluted tubule in structure (Fig 19–13). In the outer medulla, the thick descending limb, with an outer diameter of about 60 μm, suddenly narrows to about 12 μm and continues as the thin descending limb. The lumen of this segment of the nephron is wide because the wall consists of squamous epithelial cells whose nuclei protrude only slightly into the lumen (Figs 19–15 and 19–16). A brush border is absent, but short, irregularly spaced microvilli are present. There is some variation in cell structure along the length of the thin limb. The thin ascending limb was at one time believed to actively transport Na^+ from the lumen into the renal interstitium; however, these

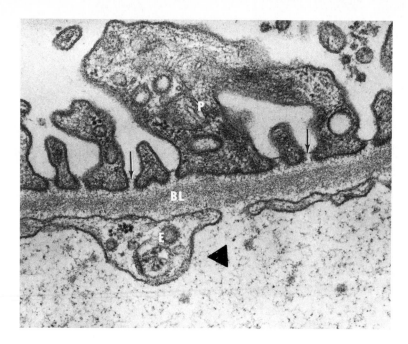

Figure 19–9. Electron micrograph of the filtration barrier in a renal corpuscle. Note the endothelium (E) with open fenestrae (arrowhead), the fused basal laminae (basement membrane) of epithelial and endothelial cells (BL), and the processes of podocytes (P). The basement membrane consists of a central lamina densa bounded on both sides by a light-staining lamina rara. Arrows indicate the thin diaphragms crossing the filtration slits. × 45,750. (Courtesy of SL Wissig.)

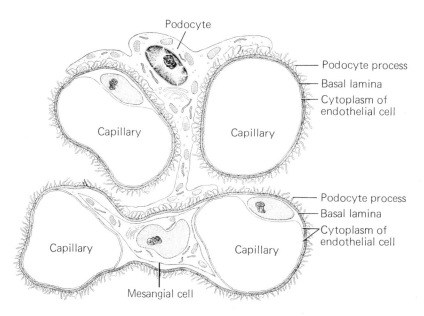

Figure 19–10. Mesangial cells of glomerular capillaries. They are located between 2 capillary lumens that are enveloped by the basal lamina.

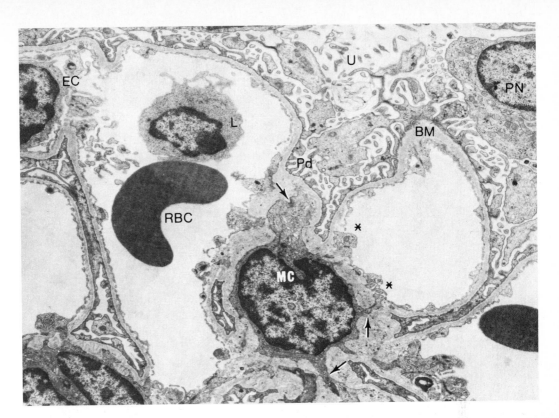

Figure 19–11. Electron micrograph showing a mesangial cell (MC) and the amorphous mesangial matrix surrounding it, aiding the support of capillary loops where a basement membrane is lacking. Some of the mesangial cell's processes (arrows) reach the capillary lumen, passing between endothelial cells (asterisks). The capillary at left contains an erythrocyte and a leukocyte. BM, basement membrane; EC, endothelial cell; L, leukocyte; Pd, pedicels; PN, podocyte nucleus; RBC, red blood cell; U, urinary space.

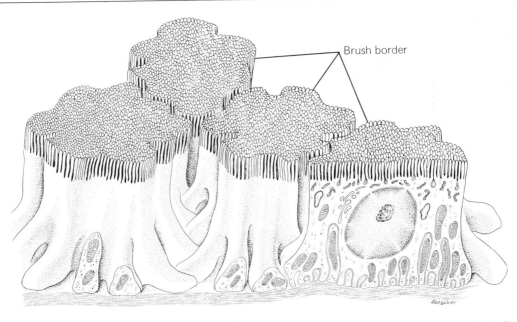

Brush border

Figure 19–12. Schematic drawing of proximal convoluted tubule cells. The apical surfaces of these cuboidal cells have abundant microvilli constituting a brush border. The cells have 2 types of lateral processes, some along the whole side of the cell and others only in its basal half. The latter processes are longer than the former and penetrate deeply among the neighboring cells. Artificial spaces have been shown among the cells to make the drawing more easily understandable. (Modified from a figure by Bulger R: *Amer J Anat* 1965;**116**:237.)

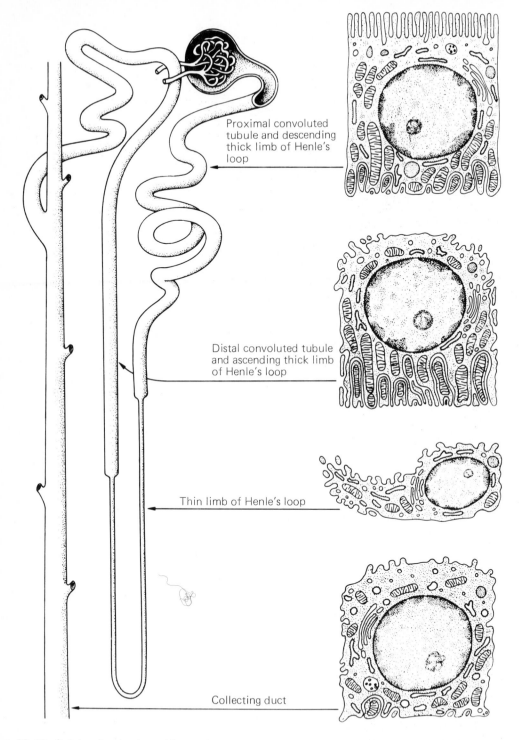

Figure 19–13. Cellular ultrastructure of the nephron, represented schematically. Cells of the ascending thick limb of Henle's loop and the distal tubule are similar in their ultrastructure but different in function.

Microvilli   Pinocytotic vesicles   Lysosome   Mitochondria

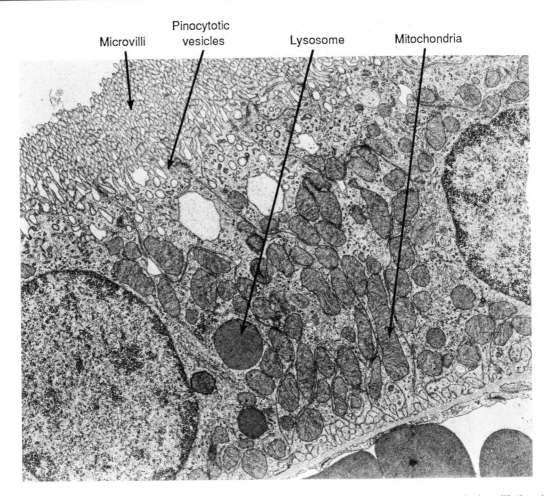

Figure 19–14. Electron micrograph of a proximal convoluted tubule. Note the obliquely sectioned microvilli, the pinocytotic (apical) vesicles, a lysosome, and the mitochondria. A peritubular capillary appears in the lower right corner, × 9500.

cells do not have the ultrastructural characteristics of ion-transporting cells. The thin limbs resemble blood capillaries, with which they may be confused; differences in content, appearance of nuclei, and thickness of the wall are the main criteria used for differentiation.

Approximately one-seventh of all nephrons are located near the corticomedullary junction and are therefore called **juxtamedullary nephrons.** The other nephrons are called **cortical nephrons.** All nephrons participate in the processes of filtration, absorption, and secretion. Juxtamedullary nephrons, however, are of prime importance in establishing the gradient of hypertonicity in the medullary interstitium—the basis of the kidney's ability to produce hypertonic urine. Juxtamedullary nephrons have very long Henle's loops, extending deep into the medulla. These loops consist of a short thick descending limb, long thin descending and ascending limbs, and a thick as-

cending limb (Fig 19–13). Cortical nephrons, on the other hand, have very short descending thin limbs and no thin ascending limbs (Fig 19–2). The thin limbs of juxtamedullary nephrons are responsible for producing the hypertonic environment of the medullary interstitium.

Distal Convoluted Tubule

When the thick ascending limb of Henle's loop penetrates the cortex, it preserves its histologic structure (Fig 19–13) but becomes tortuous and is called the distal convoluted tubule—the last segment of the nephron (Fig 19–1). This tubule is lined by simple cuboidal epithelium.

In histologic sections, the distinction between the proximal and distal convoluted tubules, both found in the cortex, is based on certain characteristics. Cells of proximal tubules are larger than the cells of distal tubules; they have brush borders, which distal tubule

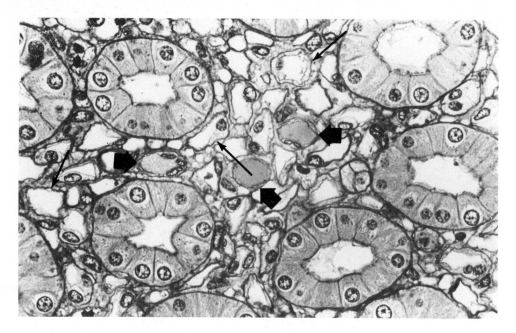

Figure 19–15. Cross section through the medulla of a rat kidney showing collecting tubules, capillary vessels of the vasa recta (arrowheads), and thin limbs of Henle's loop (arrows). × 1100. (Courtesy of SL Wissig.)

cells lack; and they are more acidophilic because of the abundance of mitochondria (Fig 19–14). The lumens of the distal tubules are larger, and because distal tubule cells are flatter and smaller than those of the proximal tubule, more cells and more nuclei are seen in the distal than in the proximal tubule wall in the same histologic section. The apical canaliculi and vesicles that characterize the proximal tubule are absent in distal cells. Lateral boundaries between these cells are not observed with the light microscope because of the interdigitations between adjacent cells. Cells of the distal convoluted tubule have elaborate basal membrane invaginations and associated mitochondria indicative of their ion-transporting function (Fig 19–17).

Along its path in the cortex, the distal convoluted tubule establishes contact with the vascular pole of the renal corpuscle of its parent nephron. At this point of close contact, the distal tubule is modified, as is the afferent arteriole. Cells of the distal convoluted tubule usually become columnar in this juxtaglomerular region, and their nuclei are closely packed together. Most of the cells have a Golgi complex in the basal region. This modified segment of the wall of the distal tubule, which appears darker in microscopic preparations (because of the close proximity of its nuclei), is called the **macula densa** (Figs 19–3 and 19–18). The functional significance of the macula densa, although not certain, may be to transfer data on the osmolarity of the fluid in the distal tubule to the afferent arteriole.

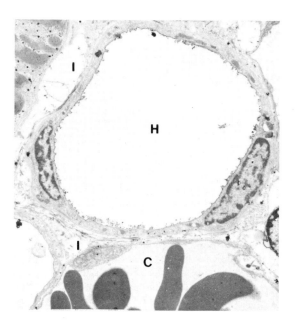

Figure 19–16. Electron micrograph of the thin part of Henle's loop (H) composed entirely of squamous cells. Note fenestrated capillaries with red blood cells (C) and the interstitium (I) with bundles of collagen fibrils. × 3300. (Courtesy of J Rhodin.)

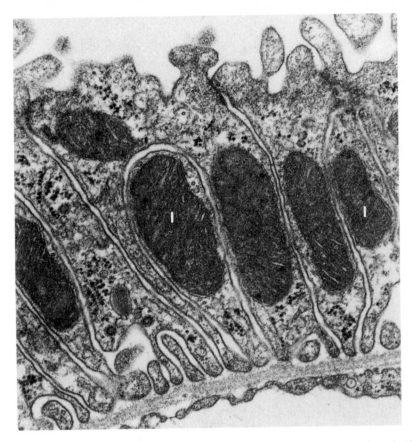

Figure 19–17. Electron micrograph of a distal convoluted tubule showing the numerous invaginations of the basal plasma membrane and associated mitochondria. Regions labeled I are interdigitations of adjacent distal tubule cells. × 30,600. (Courtesy of SL Wissig.)

Collecting Tubules & Ducts

Urine passes from the distal convoluted tubules to collecting tubules that join each other to form larger, straight collecting ducts, the **papillary ducts of Bellini,** which widen gradually as they approach the tips of the pyramids (Fig 19–1).

The smaller collecting tubules are lined with cuboidal epithelium and have a diameter of approximately 40 μm. As they penetrate deeper into the medulla, their cells increase in height (Fig 19–15) until they become columnar. The diameter of the collecting duct reaches 200 μm near the tips of the pyramids.

Along their entire extent, collecting tubules and ducts are composed of cells that stain weakly with the usual stains. They have an electron-lucent cytoplasm with few organelles (Figs 19–13 and 19–19) and almost no invaginations of the basal cell membrane. In collecting tubules and cortical collecting ducts, a dark-staining cell, the intercalated cell, is also seen. Its significance is not understood. The intercellular limits of collecting tubule and duct cells are clearly visible under the light microscope, since there are no interdigitations between the lateral margins of adjacent cells (Fig 19–15). Cortical collecting ducts are joined at right angles by several generations of smaller collecting tubules draining each medullary ray. In the medulla, collecting ducts are a major component of the urine-concentrating mechanism.

Juxtaglomerular Apparatus

Adjacent to the renal corpuscle, the tunica media of the afferent arteriole consists of modified smooth muscle cells. These cells, called **juxtaglomerular (JG) cells** (Fig 19–3), have ellipsoid nuclei and a cytoplasm full of granules that stain with the PAS technique. Secretions of juxtaglomerular cells play a role in the maintenance of blood pressure. The macula densa of the distal convoluted tubule is usually located close to the region of the afferent arteriole containing the juxtaglomerular cells; together, this portion of the arteriole and the macula densa form the juxtaglomerular apparatus (Figs 19–3 and 19–18).

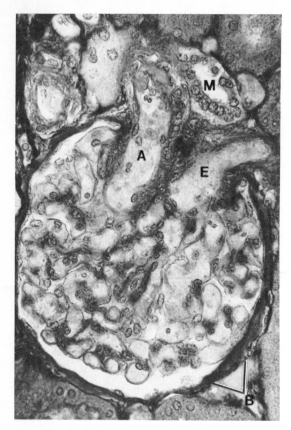

Figure 19–18. Section of a human renal corpuscle, showing the afferent arteriole (A), the efferent arteriole (E), the macula densa (M), and Bowman's capsule (B). × 325.

Also a part of the juxtaglomerular apparatus are some light-staining cells whose functions are not well understood. They are variously called extraglomerular mesangial cells, lacis cells, or polkissen (pole cushions). The internal elastic membrane of the afferent arteriole disappears in the area of the juxtaglomerular cells.

When examined with the electron microscope, juxtaglomerular cells show characteristics of protein-secreting cells, including an abundant rough endoplasmic reticulum, a highly developed Golgi complex, and secretory granules measuring approximately 10–40 nm in diameter. Juxtaglomerular cells produce the hormone **renin,** which acts on a plasma protein called **angiotensinogen,** producing an inactive decapeptide called **angiotensin I.** This substance, as a result of the action of a converting enzyme present in high concentration in lung endothelial cells, loses 2 amino acids and becomes an octapeptide called **angiotensin II.**

There is an increase in renin secretion after a significant hemorrhage. Angiotensin II is pro-

duced, enhancing blood pressure by both constricting arterioles and stimulating the secretion of the adrenocortical hormone **aldosterone** (see Chapter 21). Aldosterone acts on cells of the renal tubules (mostly the distal tubules) to increase the absorption of sodium and chloride ions. This, in turn, expands the fluid volume, leading to an increase in blood pressure.

Decreased blood pressure from other factors (eg. sodium depletion, dehydration) also activates the renin-angiotensin-II-aldosterone mechanism that contributes to the maintenance of blood pressure.

Blood Circulation

Each kidney receives blood from its **renal artery,** which usually divides into 2 branches before entering this organ. One branch goes to the anterior part of the kidney, the other to the posterior part. While still in the hilum, these branches give rise to arteries that branch again to form the **interlobar arteries** located between the renal pyramids (Fig 19–20). At the level of the corticomedullary junction, the interlobar arteries form the **arcuate arteries. Interlobular arteries** branch off at right angles from the arcuate arteries and follow a course in the cortex perpendicular to the renal capsule. Interlobular arteries form the boundaries of renal lobules, which consist of a medullary ray and the adjacent cortical labyrinth (Fig 19–20). From the interlobular arteries arise the **afferent arterioles,** which supply blood to the capillaries of the glomeruli. Blood passes from these capillaries into the **efferent arterioles,** which at once branch again to form a **peritubular capillary network** that will nourish the proximal and distal tubules and carry away absorbed ions and low-molecular-weight materials. The efferent arterioles that are associated with juxtamedullary nephrons form long, thin capillary vessels. These vessels, which follow a straight path into the medulla and then loop back toward the corticomedullary boundary (Fig 19–15), are called **vasa recta,** or straight vessels. The descending vessel is a continuous-type capillary, while the ascending vessel has a fenestrated endothelium. These vessels, containing blood that has been filtered through the glomeruli, provide nourishment and oxygen to the medulla. Because of their looped structure, these vessels do not carry away the high osmotic gradient set up in the interstitium by the thin limbs of Henle's loop (Fig 19–22).

The capillaries of the outer cortex and the capsule of the kidney converge to form the **stellate veins** (so called because of the configuration when seen from the surface of the kidney), which empty into the interlobular veins.

Veins follow the same course as arteries. Blood from interlobular veins flows into arcuate veins and from there to the interlobar veins. Interlobar veins

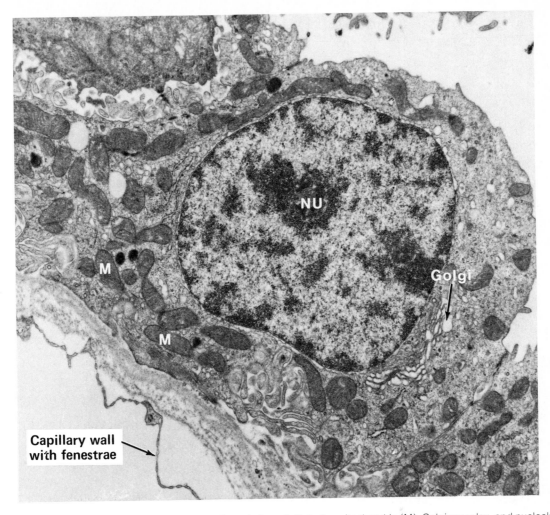

Figure 19–19. Electron micrograph of a collecting tubule wall. Note the mitochondria (M), Golgi complex, and nucleolus (NU). × 15,000.

converge to form the renal vein through which blood leaves the kidney (Fig 19–20).

Renal Interstitium

Both the cortex and the medulla contain specialized cells in the spaces between uriniferous tubules and the blood and lymph vessels. Some of these **interstitial cells** are more frequent in the medulla and are the site of prostaglandin production and the synthesis of ground substance.

2. HISTOPHYSIOLOGY

The kidney regulates the chemical composition of the internal environment by a complex process that involves **filtration, active absorption, passive ab-**

sorption, and **secretion.** Filtration takes place in the glomerulus, where an ultrafiltrate of blood plasma is formed. The tubules of the nephron, primarily the proximal convoluted tubules, absorb from this filtrate the substances that are useful for body metabolism, thus maintaining the homeostasis of the internal environment. They also transfer from blood to the tubular lumen certain waste products that are eliminated with the urine. Under certain circumstance, the collecting ducts are permeable to water, contributing to the concentration of urine—which is usually hypertonic in relation to blood plasma. In this way, the organism controls its water, intercellular fluid, and osmotic balance.

The 2 kidneys produce about 125 mL of filtrate per minute; of this amount, 124 mL is absorbed and only 1 mL is released into the calyces as urine. About 1500 mL of urine are formed every 24 hours.

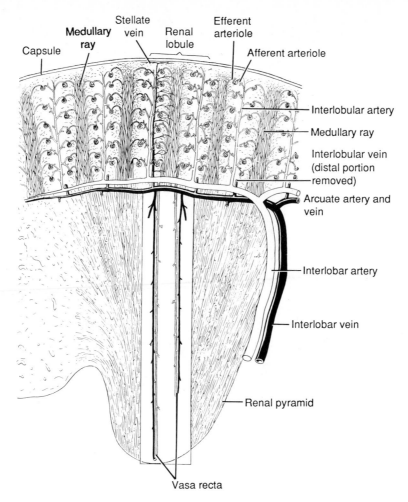

Figure 19–20. Circulation of blood in the kidney. Arcuate arteries are seen in the border between the cortex and medulla.

Filtration

The blood flow in the 2 kidneys of an adult amounts to 1.2–1.3 L of blood per minute. This means that all the circulating blood in the body passes through the kidneys every 4–5 minutes. The glomeruli are composed of arterial capillaries in which the hydrostatic pressure—about 45 mm Hg—is higher than that found in other capillaries.

The glomerular filtrate is formed in response to the hydrostatic pressure of blood, which is opposed by the osmotic (oncotic) pressure of plasma colloids (20 mm Hg), and the hydrostatic pressure of the fluids in Bowman's capsule (10 mm Hg). The net filtration pressure at the afferent end of glomerular capillaries is 15 mm Hg.

The glomerular filtrate has a chemical composition similar to that of blood plasma but contains almost no protein, since macromolecules do not readily cross the glomerular wall. The largest pro-

tein molecules that succeed in crossing the glomerular filter have a molecular weight of about 70,000, and small amounts of plasma albumin appear in the filtrate.

Endothelial cells of glomerular capillaries are fenestrated with numerous openings (70–90-nm in diameter) without diaphragms, so that the endothelium is easily permeated.

Proximal Convoluted Tubule

The glomerular filtrate formed in the renal corpuscle passes into the proximal convoluted tubule, and the processes of absorption and excretion begin here. The site of absorption of diverse substances can be precisely identified since they are absorbed at different points. The proximal convoluted tubule absorbs all the glucose and amino acids and about 85% of the sodium chloride and water contained in the filtrate. Glucose, amino acids, and sodium are absorbed by the tubular cells through an active process involving Na^+/K^+-ATPase located in the basolateral cell membranes. Water diffuses passively, following the osmotic gradient. When the amount of glucose in the filtrate exceeds the absorbing capacity of the proximal tubule, urine becomes more abundant and contains glucose.

Absorption of the small amount of protein present in the filtrate takes place by pinocytosis. The proteins are digested by lysosomes and the amino acids are reused by local cells.

In addition to these activities, the proximal convoluted tubule secretes creatinine and substances foreign to the organism such as para-aminohippuric acid, phenol red, and iodopyracet (an iodinated organic compound used as an x-ray contrast medium) from the interstitial plasma into the filtrate. This is an active process referred to as tubular secretion. Study of the rates of secretion of these substances is useful in the clinical evaluation of kidney function.

Loop of Henle

Henle's loop is involved in water retention; only animals with such loops in their kidneys are capable of producing hypertonic urine and thus maintaining body water. Henle's loop creates a gradient of hypertonicity in the medullary interstitium that influences the concentration of the urine as it flows through the collecting ducts (Fig 19–21).

Although the descending thin limb of the loop is freely permeable to water, the entire ascending limb is impermeable to water. In the thick ascending limb, chloride is actively transported out of the tubule, with sodium following passively, to establish the gradient of hypertonicity in the medullary interstitium necessary for urine concentration. The osmolarity of the interstitium at the tips of the pyramids is about 4 times that of blood (Fig 19–21).

Distal Convoluted Tubule

In the distal convoluted tubule, there is an ion exchange site at which—if aldosterone is present in high enough concentration—sodium is absorbed and potassium ions are secreted. This is the site of the mechanism that controls the total salt and water in the body (mentioned in the discussion of the juxtaglomerular apparatus). The distal tubule also secretes hydrogen and ammonium ions into tubular urine. This activity

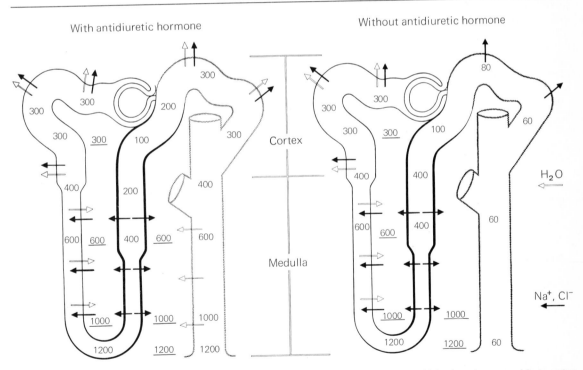

Figure 19–21. Countercurrent multiplier system formed by Henle's loop. The segment of the loop impermeable to water is represented by thick lines. The collecting tubules and ducts, whose cells are impermeable to water but become permeable under the influence of antidiuretic hormone (ADH), are indicated by serrated lines. **Left:** Under the influence of ADH, the urine formed is hypertonic. **Right:** With no or very low levels of ADH, a great quantity of hypotonic urine is formed. The numbers in the tubules and interstitial spaces indicate the local concentration in mosm/L. Solid arrows signify electrolytes; open arrows, water. (Redrawn and reproduced, with permission, from Pitts, RF: *Physiology of the Kidney and Body Fluids,* 2nd ed. Year Book, 1968).

is essential for maintenance of the acid-base balance in the blood.

Collecting Ducts

The epithelium of collecting ducts is responsive to antidiuretic hormone (ADH), secreted by the posterior pituitary. If water intake is limited, ADH is secreted, and the epithelium of the collecting ducts becomes permeable to water. In the presence of ADH, intramembrane particles in the luminal membrane aggregate to form what may be channels for water absorption.

Formation of Hypotonic or Hypertonic Urine

Henle's loop forms a countercurrent multiplier system that generates an osmotic gradient in the medullary interstitium by repetitive transfer of relatively small amounts of sodium and chloride along the length of the loop (Fig 19–21).

Hypotonic or isotonic urine in the collecting ducts of the medulla (the interstitial fluid of the cortex is isotonic) will lose water into the interstitium if there is enough ADH to make the ducts permeable to water, and hypertonic urine will be formed. Without ADH, the walls of the collecting ducts are impermeable to water, so that concentration of urine does not occur and the kidneys produce abundant hypotonic urine (Fig 19–21). In this way, the kidneys participate in the osmotic balance of the internal environment, retaining or eliminating water as needed by the organism.

The vasa recta, or straight vessels, of the medullary region are situated so that blood circulation does not disturb the osmotic gradient created by the ion pump of Henle's loop. This countercurrent exchange system is shown in Fig 19–22. The vasa recta are very thin-walled vessels, similar in structure to capillaries found in other organs. Each straight vessel forms a loop whose branches run side by side (Figs 19–15 and 19–21). While passing through the vasa recta toward the inner medulla, blood loses water and gains sodium because, in the medulla, the interstitial fluid gradually becomes more and more hypertonic. Returning in the opposite direction, blood is exposed to the same—but now decreasing—gradient and therefore loses sodium and gains water. The water lost by the descending vessel is gained by the ascending one, while the sodium that enters the descending vessel is released by the ascending one. These movements of water and sodium are passive, taking place without the use of energy. Thus, while this system produces no net change in interstitial osmolarity, the blood can supply oxygen and nutrients to medullary cells and carry away water that passed out of the collecting ducts under the influence of ADH.

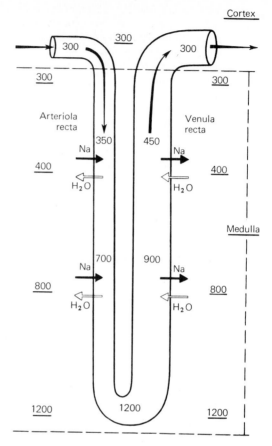

Figure 19–22. The countercurrent exchange system formed by the straight vessels of the kidney. The number 300 in the cortical segment of the arteriole and venule represents blood osmolarity (more accurately, 285–295 mosm/L). The sodium and water exchanges between these straight vessels and the interstitium are passive, depending on the osmotic gradient formed by Henle's loop.

Hormonal Effects

As explained above, water balance is controlled in part by the posterior lobe of the pituitary, which secretes ADH. A high intake of water inhibits production of ADH; the walls of the collecting ducts become impermeable to water, and water is not absorbed. The result is the formation of large amounts of hypotonic urine; water is eliminated, while the ions necessary for osmotic balance are retained. When small amounts of water are ingested or when a great loss of water occurs (eg, from excessive sweating or diarrhea), the walls of collecting ducts become permeable to water, which is absorbed, and the urine is hypertonic.

Steroid hormones of the adrenal cortex, mainly **aldosterone,** increase distal tubular absorption of sodium from the filtrate and thus decrease sodium loss in the urine. Aldosterone also facilitates the elimination of potassium and hydrogen ions. This hormone is critical in maintaining electrolyte balance in the body.

Aldosterone deficiency in adrenalectomized animals and in humans with **Addison's disease** results in an excessive loss of sodium in the urine.

BLADDER & URINARY PASSAGES

The bladder and the urinary passages store the urine formed in the kidneys and conduct it to the exterior. The calyces, pelvis, ureter, and bladder have the same basic histologic structure, with the walls of the ureters becoming gradually thicker as proximity to the bladder increases.

The mucosa of these organs consists of **transitional epithelium** (Fig 19–23) and a lamina propria of loose-to-dense connective tissue. Surrounding the lamina propria of these organs is a dense, woven sheath of smooth muscle.

The transitional epithelium of the bladder in the undistended state is 5–6 cells in thickness; the super-

ficial cells are rounded and bulge into the lumen. These cells are frequently polyploid or binucleate. When the epithelium is stretched, as when the bladder is full of urine, the epithelium is only 3–4 cells in thickness, and the superficial cells become squamous.

More than 90% of urinary bladder tumors originate in the epithelial lining.

The superficial cells of the transitional epithelium have a special membrane of thick plates separated by narrow bands of thinner membrane that are considered to be responsible for the osmotic barrier between urine and tissue fluids. When the bladder contracts, the membrane folds along the thinner regions, and the thicker plates invaginate to form fusiform cytoplasmic vesicles. These vesicles represent a reservoir of these thick plates that can be stored in the cytoplasm of the cells of the empty bladder and used to cover the increased cell surface in the full bladder (Fig 19–24). This luminal membrane is assembled in the Golgi complex and has an unusual chemical composition; cerebroside is the major component of the polar lipid fraction.

The muscular layers in the calyces, renal pelvis, and ureters have a helical arrangement. As the ure-

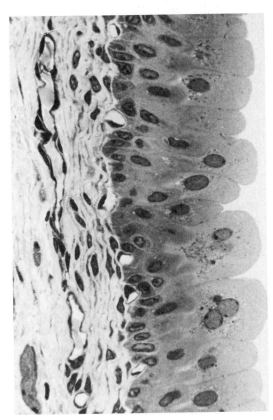
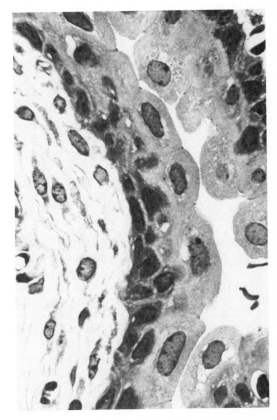

Figure 19–23. Photomicrographs of the urinary bladder wall. **Left:** Empty bladder; **right:** distended bladder. The transitional epithelium lies on a thin lamina propria. H&E stain, reduced from × 320.

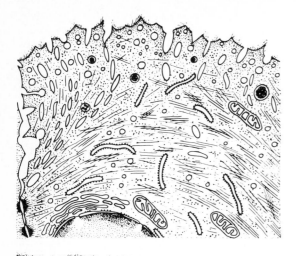

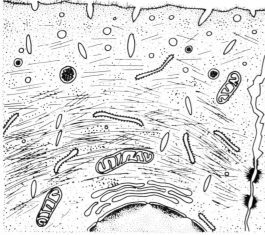

Figure 19–24. Ultrastructure of superficial cells of the bladder's transitional epithelium. **Top:** A contracted bladder. **Bottom:** A bladder distended by a large volume of urine.

teral muscle cells reach the bladder, they become longitudinal. The muscle fibers of the bladder run in every direction (without distinct layers) until they approach the bladder neck, where 3 distinct layers can be identified: The internal longitudinal layer, distal to the bladder neck, becomes circular around the prostatic urethra and the prostatic parenchyma in the male. It extends to the external meatus in the female. Its fibers form the true involuntary urethral sphincter. The middle layer, which ends at the bladder neck. The outer longitudinal layer, which continues to the end of the prostate in the male and to the external urethral meatus in the female.

The ureters pass through the wall of the bladder obliquely, forming a valve that prevents the backflow of urine. The intravesical ureter has only longitudinal muscle fibers.

The urinary passages are covered externally by an adventitial membrane—except for the upper part of the bladder, which is covered by (serous) peritoneum.

Urethra

The urethra is a tube that carries the urine from the bladder to the exterior. In the male, sperm also pass through it during ejaculation. In the female, the urethra is exclusively a urinary organ.

A. Male Urethra: The male urethra consists of 4 parts: **prostatic, membranous, bulbous,** and **pendulous.**

The prostate (see Chapter 22) is situated very close to the bladder, and the initial part of the urethra passes through it. Ducts that transport the secretions of the prostate open into the prostatic urethra.

In the dorsal and distal part of the **prostatic urethra,** there is an elevation, the **verumontanum** (from Latin, mountain ridge), that protrudes into its interior. In the tip of the verumontanum a blind tube called the prostatic utricle opens; this tube has no known function. The ejaculatory ducts open on the sides of the verumontanum. The seminal fluid enters the proximal urethra through these ducts to be stored just prior to ejaculation. The prostatic urethra is lined by transitional epithelium.

The **membranous urethra** extends for only 1 cm and is lined with stratified or pseudostratified columnar epithelium. Surrounding this part of the urethra is a sphincter of striated muscle, the **external sphincter** of the urethra. The voluntary external striated sphincter adds further closing pressure to that exerted by the involuntary urethral sphincter. The latter is formed by the continuation of the internal longitudinal muscle of the bladder.

The **bulbous** and **pendulous** parts of the urethra are located in the **corpus spongiosum** of the penis. The urethral lumen dilates distally, forming the **fossa navicularis.** The epithelium of this portion of the urethra is mostly pseudostratified and columnar, with areas that are stratified and squamous.

Littre's glands are mucous glands found along the entire length of the urethra but mostly in the pendulous part. The secretory portions of some of these glands are directly linked to the epithelial lining of the urethra; others possess excretory ducts.

B. Female Urethra: The female urethra is a tube 4–5 cm long, lined with stratified squamous epithelium with areas of pseudostratified columnar epithelium. The midpart of the female urethra is surrounded by an external striated voluntary sphincter.

REFERENCES

Barger AC, Herd JA: The renal circulation. *N Engl J Med* 1971;**284**:482.

Bulger RE, Dobyan DC: Recent advances in renal morphology. *Annu Rev Physiol* 1982;**44**:147.

Farquhar MG: The glomerular basement membrane: A selective macromolecular filter. In: *Cell Biology of Extracellular Matrix*. Hay E (editor). Plenum Press, 1981.

Ganong WF: Formation and excretion of urine. In: *Review of Medical Physiology*, 14th ed. Appleton & Lange, 1989.

Hicks RM: The mammalian urinary bladder: An accommodating organ. *Biol Rev* 1975;**50**:215.

Maunsbach AB, Olsen TS, Christensen EI (editors): *Functional Ultrastructure of the Kidney*. Academic Press, 1981.

Staehelin LA, Chlapowski FJ, Bonneville MA: Luminal plasma membrane of the urinary bladder. 1. Three-dimensional reconstruction from freeze-etch images. *J Cell Biol* 1972;**53**:73.

20

The Neuroendocrine Hypothalamo-Hypophyseal System (NHS)

In the evolutionary development of the metazoans, multicellularity led to a division of labor in which cells carrying out particular functions assembled into coherent associations known as tissues. The integration and coordination of the activities of various tissues are under the control of the nervous system and of chemical messengers, the **hormones,** synthesized and released by cells of the **endocrine system.** The products of endocrine glands are not secreted through ducts but are released directly into the connective tissue or vascular network.

A hormone is an organic chemical that is liberated—at a specific time and in small amounts—by endocrine cells into the tissue fluids or vascular system. In general, hormones exert their effects at a distance from the site of their secretion. The tissues and organs on which the hormones act are called **target organs.** The endocrine and nervous systems, both of which act to integrate the activities of diverse parts of the organism, are clearly coordinated in function. Hormones of many endocrine glands have an effect on the nervous system, and several endocrine organs are stimulated or inhibited by neural mechanisms. Fig 20–1 illustrates several situations in which endocrine function is controlled by the nervous system. Most biologic phenomena are under the overlapping control of both systems. This interlocking mechanism is so remarkable that its nervous and endocrine elements are regarded as constituting a single **neuroendocrine system.**

COMPONENTS OF THE NHS

The **hypophysis** (*hypo* + Greek, *physis,* growth) or **pituitary gland,** weighs about 0.5 g, and its normal dimensions in humans are about 10 × 13 × 6 mm. It lies in a bony cavity of the sphenoidbone—the

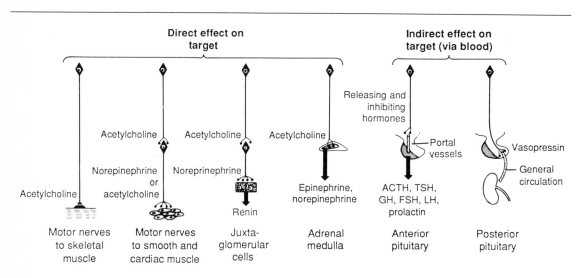

Figure 20–1. Diagrammatic representation of 6 situations in which humoral substances are released by neurons. The last 2 are examples of neurosecretion. (Reproduced, with permission, from Ganong WF. *Review of Medical Physiology.* 14th ed. Appleton & Lange, 1989.)

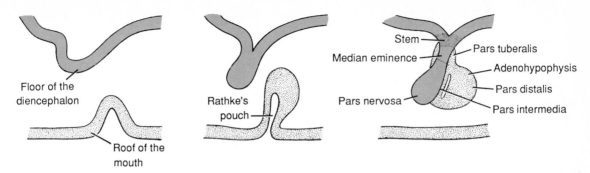

Figure 20–2. Diagram of the development of the adenohypophysis and neurohypophysis. The ectoderm of the roof of the mouth and its derivatives are shown stippled (lower portion). The upper portion shows the neural ectoderm from the floor of the diencephalon (shown in color).

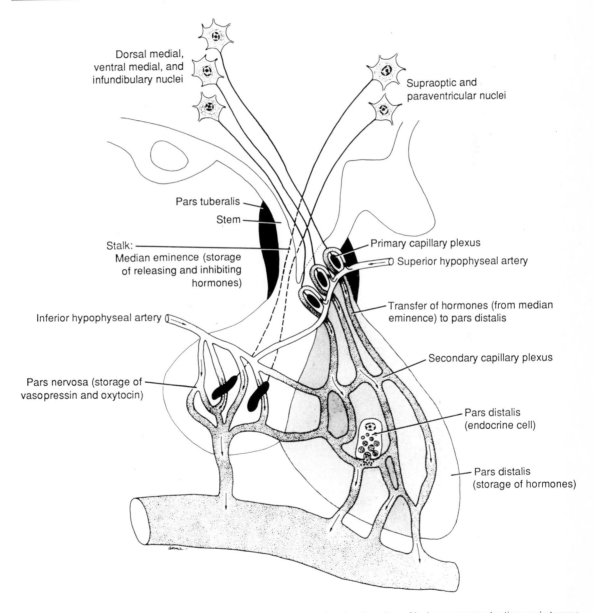

Figure 20–3. Drawing of the hypothalamo-hypophyseal system showing the sites of its hormone production and storage and its vascularization.

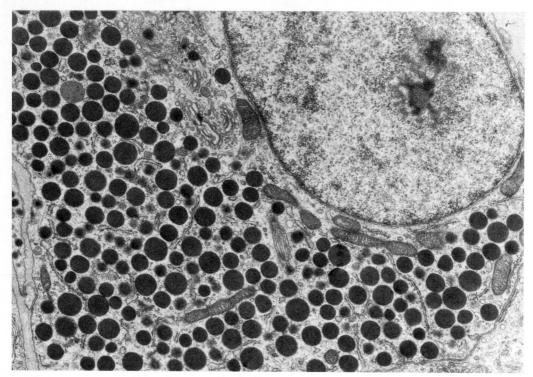

Figure 20–4. Electron micrograph of a somatotrope (growth-hormone-secreting cell) of a cat anterior hypophysis. Note the numerous secretory granules, long mitochondria, cisternae of rough endoplasmic reticulum, and prominent juxta-nuclear Golgi complex. × 10,270.

Table 20–1. Secretory cells of the pars distalis.

Cell Type	Stain Affinity	Hormone Produced	Main Physiologic Activity	Secretory Granules in Humans	Hypothalamic Releasing Hormones	Hypothalamic Inhibiting Hormones
Somatotropic cell	Acidophilic	Somatotropin (growth hormone).	Acts on growth of long bones via somatomedins synthesized in liver.	Numerous, round or oval; 300–400 nm diameter.	Somatotropin-releasing hormone (SRH).	Somatostatin.
Mammotropic cell	Acidophilic	Prolactin.	Promotes milk secretion.	200 nm; increases in size during pregnancy and lactation (600 nm).	Prolactin-releasing hormone (PRH).	Prolactin-inhibiting hormone (PIH).
Gonadotropic cell	Basophilic	Follicle-stimulating hormone (FSH) and luteinizing hormone (LH) in same cell type.	FSH promotes ovarian follicle development and estrogen secretion in female and stimulates spermatogenesis in male. LH promotes ovarian follicle maturation and progesterone secretion in female, Leydig cell stimulation and androgen secretion in male.	250–400 nm.	Gonadotropin-releasing hormone (GnRH). According to some authors there are 2 releasing hormones: FRH and LRH (follicle- and lutein-releasing, respectively).	
Thyrotropic cell	Basophilic	Thyrotropin (TSH).	Stimulates thyroid hormone synthesis, storage, and liberation.	Small granules, 120–200 nm.	Thyrotropin-releasing hormone (TRH).	
Corticotropic cell	Basophilic	Corticotropin (ACTH).	Stimulates secretion of adrenal cortex hormones.	Large granules, 400–550 nm.	Corticotropin-releasing hormone (CRH).	

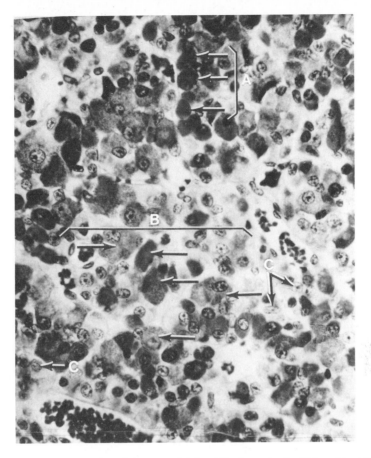

Figure 20–5. Photomicrograph of a section of the pars distalis of the hypophysis. At A, acidophilic cells stain orange-red; at B, basophilic cells (lower arrows) stain blue. At left and right, note unstained chromophobe (C) cells. Mallory's stain. × 185.

sella turcica—an important radiologic landmark. The hypophysis is connected to the hypothalamus at the base of the brain, with which it has important anatomic and functional relationships.

During embryogenesis, the hypophysis develops partly from oral ectoderm and partly from nerve tissue. The neural component arises as an evagination from the floor of the diencephalon and grows caudally as a stalk without detaching itself from the brain. The oral component arises as an outpocketing of ectoderm from the roof of the primitive mouth of the embryo and grows cranially, forming a structure called **Rathke's pouch.** Later, a constriction at the base of this pouch separates it from the oral cavity. Its anterior wall thickens at the same time, reducing the lumen of Rathke's pouch to a small fissure (Fig 20–2).

The **neurohypophysis,** the part of the hypophysis that develops from nerve tissue, consists of a large portion, the **pars nervosa,** and the smaller **infundibulum,** or **neural stalk** (Fig 20–3). The neural stalk is composed of the stem and median

eminence. The part of the hypophysis that arises from oral ectoderm is known as the **adenohypophysis** and is subdivided into 3 portions: a large part, the **pars distalis,** or **anterior lobe;** a cranial part, the **pars tuberalis,** that surrounds the neural stalk; and the **pars intermedia** (Fig 20–3).

Production & Storage of NHS Hormones

The NHS is intimately interconnected by both nerve cells and blood supply; it produces hormones that are active in providing the various levels of both nervous and hormonal control. The hormones can be divided into 2 groups. The first group consists of peptides or small proteins produced by aggregates of secretory neurons (**nuclei**) in the hypothalamus. Some of these hormones are transported via neuronal axons to the median eminence, where they are stored in the dilated blind ends of the axons. Others are stored in the pars nervosa in the dilated ends of axons. Fig 20–3 illustrates the nuclei and the axon

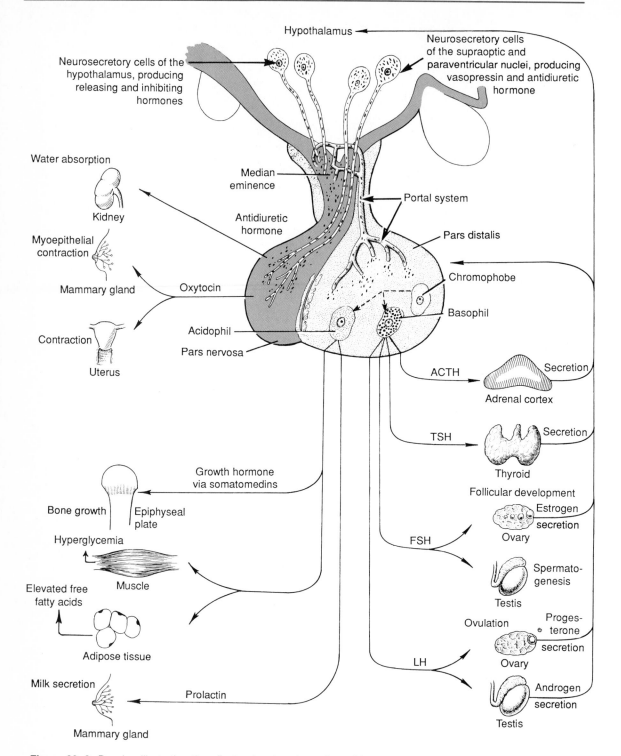

Figure 20–6. Drawing illustrating the effects of various hypophyseal hormones on target organs. Several of the hormones produced by the target organs can act on the hypophysis or hypothalamus to regulate their activity (negative feedback; see Fig 20–7). Neurohypophysis is shown in color; adenohypophysis is stippled.

Table 20–2. Hormones of the neurohypophysis.

Hypothalamus		Pars Nervosa	
Hormone	**Function**	**Hormone**	**Function**
Thyrotropin-releasing hormone (TRH)	Stimulates release of thyroid-stimulating hormone and prolactin	Vasopressin	Increases water permeability of kidney collecting ducts and promotes vascular smooth muscle contraction
Gonadotropin-releasing hormone (GnRH)	Stimulates the release of both follicle-stimulating hormone (FSH) and luteinizing hormone (LH)	Oxytocin	Acts on contraction of uterine smooth muscle and of the myoepithelial cells of the mammary gland
Somatostatin	Inhibits release of both growth hormone (GRH) and thyroid-stimulating hormone (TSH)		
Growth-hormone-releasing hormone (GRH)	Stimulates release of growth hormone		
Prolactin-inhibiting hormone (PIH) Dopamine	Inhibits release of prolactin		
Corticotropin-releasing hormone (CRH)	Stimulates release of both B lipotropin and corticotropin (ACTH)		

bundles (tracts) that produce, transport, and store these hormones.

In the second group of hormones are the secretory products of protein- and glycoprotein-synthesizing and storing cells present in the pars distalis. These hormones are stored in these endocrine epithelial cells as secretory granules (Fig 20–4). Both groups of hormones are released according to external stimuli; they constitute a delicately balanced system of neuroendocrine regulation for the organism.

Blood Supply & Innervation

The blood supply of the hypophysis derives from 2 groups of blood vessels that come from the internal carotid artery. From above, the right and left **superior hypophyseal arteries** supply the median eminence and the neural stalk; from below, the right and left **inferior hypophyseal arteries** provide mainly for the neurohypophysis, with a small supply to the stalk. The superior hypophyseal arteries form a **primary capillary plexus** of fenestrated capillaries that irrigate the stalk and median eminence. They then rejoin to form veins that develop a **secondary plexus** in the adenohypophysis (Fig 20–3). This **hypophyseal portal system** is of utmost importance in regulating hypophyseal function: it carries neurohormones from the median eminence to the neurohypophysis.

The nerve supply of the anterior lobe is derived from the carotid plexus, which accompanies the arteriolar branches. These nerves appear to have a vasomotor function and do not directly affect the cells of the anterior lobe. Blood from both hypophyseal lobes drains into the cavernous sinuses through a number of venous channels.

ADENOHYPOPHYSIS

Pars Distalis

This portion of the NHS is formed by cords of aggregated cells interspersed with capillaries. The few fibroblasts present produce reticular fibers that support the cords of hormone-secreting cells. The pars distalis accounts for 75% of the mass of the hypophysis. Cells of the pars distalis have been described as **chromophobes** (*chroma* + Greek, *phobos*, fear) and **chromophils,** based on their staining affinities. The chromophobes do not stain intensely, and when observed with an electron microscope, show 2 populations of cells. One has few secretory granules, and the other has none. The latter group probably contains undifferentiated cells and follicular cells. The long branching processes of follicular cells form a supporting network for the other cells. Chromophils, which can be stained with basic or acid dyes, are called basophilic or acidophilic according to their affinity (Table 20–1; Figs 20–5 and 20–6). The 5 types of endocrine secretory cells of the pars distalis secrete 6 protein and glycoprotein hormones and exhibit the general characteristics of cells that synthesize, segregate, store, and export proteins (see Chapters 3 and 4 and Figs 3–18 and 20–5). As shown in Table 20–1, these secretory cells are named according to the hormones they produce. Most cells produce only a single hormone each, with the exception of the gonadotropic cell, which produces 2 hormones. These hormones have widespread physiologic activity (Fig 20–6); they regulate almost all endocrine glands, the secretion of milk, and the metabolism of muscle, bone, and adipose tissue.

Many dyes have been used in an attempt to distinguish the 5 types of hormone-secreting cells, but with little success. Immunocytochemistry and electron microscopy are currently the only reliable techniques to distinguish these cell types.

Control of the Pars Distalis

The activities of the cells of the pars distalis are controlled by more than one mechanism. The main mechanism uses the peptide hormones (Table 20–2) produced in the hypothalamic aggregates of neurosecretory cells and stored in the median eminence. Most of these hormones are called **hypothalamic releasing hormones;** when liberated, they go to the pars distalis through the primary and secondary capillary plexuses (see Fig 20–3). Two of these hormones, which act on specific cells of the par distalis, inhibit hormone release **(hypothalamic inhibiting hormones;** see Table 20–1).

A second general control mechanism is the direct effect of hormones from stimulated endocrine cells on the release of peptides from the median eminence and the pars distalis. Fig 20–7 illustrates both these mechanisms, using the thyroid as an example. The figure also illustrates the complex chain of events that begins with the action of neurons on neurosecretory cells of the hypothalamic nuclei and ends on the effector cells with the action of the last hormone in the sequence. This mechanism participates in fine tuning the coordination of these events and may offer insights into the effects of psychic stimulation and depression.

Pars Tuberalis

This funnel-shaped region surrounds the infundibulum of the neurohypophysis (Fig 20–3). Most of the cells of the pars tuberalis secrete gonadotropins (FSH and LH) and are arranged in cords alongside the blood vessels.

Pars Intermedia

The pars intermedia, which develops from the dorsal portion of Rathke's pouch (Fig 20–2), is, in humans, a rudimentary region made up of cords of weakly basophilic cells that contain small secretory granules. The function of these cells is not known (Fig 20–3).

NEUROHYPOPHYSIS

The neurohypophysis consists of the pars nervosa and the neural stalk. The pars nervosa, which contains no secretory cells, is composed of some 100,000 unmyelinated axons of secretory neurons from the supraoptic and paraventricular nuclei (Fig 20–3). The secretory neurons have all the characteristics of typical neurons, including the ability to conduct an action potential, but have more developed Nissl bodies

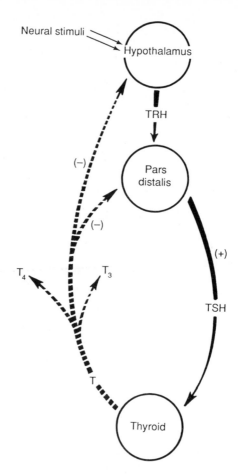

Figure 20–7. Relationship between the hypothalamus, the hypophysis, and the thyroid. Thyrotropin-releasing hormone (TRH) promotes secretion of thyrotropin (TSH), which regulates the synthesis and secretion of the hormones T_3 and T_4. In addition to their effect on peripheral tissues, these hormones regulate TSH and TRH secretion from the pars distalis and the hypothalamus by a negative feedback mechanism. T, thyroglobulin. Solid arrows indicate stimulation; dashed arrows, inhibition.

related to the production of the neurosecretory material. In addition, the axons and the cell bodies contain granular inclusions that can be studied by specific techniques such as staining with Gomori's chrome hematoxylin stain.

The electron microscope reveals that these neurosecretory granules have a diameter of 100–200 nm, are surrounded by a membrane, and are more numerous in the dilated terminal parts of the axons that are apposed to fenestrated blood capillaries. Here they form accumulations, known as **Herring bodies,** that are visible with the light microscope. The hormones contained in these stored granules are released as needed by the organism.

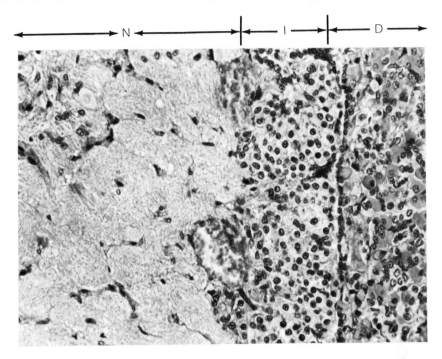

Figure 20–8. Section of the hypophysis of a rat showing (from left to right) the neurohypophysis (N), the pars intermedia (I), and the pars distalis (D). Chromophilic and chromophobic cells are apparent in the pars distalis. The pars intermedia consists of cords of one cell type. Nuclei of pituicytes are clearly visible in the neurohypophysis. × 340.

The **neurosecretory material** consists of hormones (either **oxytocin** or **vasopressin**), a binding protein (**neurophysin**) specific for each hormone, and **ATP**. The hormones are 9-amino-acid peptides with a ring structure formed by a disulfide bridge. Each has a slightly different composition, which results in greatly different functions. The hormone-neurophysin complex is synthesized as a single long peptide on ribosomes of rough endoplasmic reticulum. The peptide is partly glycosylated in the lumen of the endoplasmic reticulum and then passed on to the Golgi complex, where further glycosylation and packaging in secretory granules occur. As the granules pass down axons of the hypothalamo-hypophyseal tract, proteolysis of the precursor yields the hormone and its specific binding protein. Vasopressin and oxytocin are stored in the posterior pituitary and released into the blood by impulses in the nerve fibers from the hypothalamus. Although there is some overlap, the fibers from supraoptic nuclei are mainly concerned with vasopressin secretion, while most of those from the paraventricular nuclei are concerned with oxytocin secretion.

Neurohypophyseal Cells

Although the neurohypophysis consists mainly of axons from hypothalamic neurons, about 25% of the volume of this structure consists of a specific type of highly branched glial cell called a **pituicyte** (Fig 20–8). Endothelial cells of capillaries are also present.

Histophysiology

The neurohypophysis of all mammals except members of the pig family secretes 2 hormones, both cyclic peptides made up of 9 amino acids. These hormones are **arginine vasopressin**—also called **antidiuretic hormone (ADH)**—and **oxytocin.** These hormones are present in different secretory granules and in different neurons. In large doses, vasopressin promotes the contraction of smooth muscle of blood vessels, raising the blood pressure. It acts mainly on the muscle layers of small arteries and arterioles. It is doubtful if the amount of endogenous vasopressin secreted is sufficient to exert any appreciable effect on blood pressure homeostasis.

Vasopressin is secreted whenever the osmotic pressure of the blood increases. The blood then acts on osmoreceptor cells in the anterior hypothalamus, stimulating the secretion of the hormone from supraoptic neurons. Its main effect is to increase the permeability to water of the collecting tubules of the kidney. As a result, water is absorbed by these tubules and urine becomes hypertonic. Thus, vasopressin helps to regulate the osmotic balance of the internal milieu. Sections of the neurohypophysis of animals previously given injections of hypertonic solutions do not contain the neurosecretory material usually present in control animals.

Oxytocin stimulates contraction of the smooth muscle of the uterine wall during copulation and childbirth and contraction of myoepithelial cells that surround the alveoli and ducts of the mammary glands. The secretion of oxytocin is stimulated by distention of the vagina or of the uterine cervix and by nursing. This occurs via nerve tracts that act on the hypothalamus. The neurohormonal reflex triggered by nursing is called the **milk-ejection reflex** (Fig 20–6).

Lesions of the hypothalamus, which destroy the neurosecretory cells, cause **diabetes insipidus,** a disease characterized by loss of renal capacity to concentrate urine. As a result, an individual suffering from this disease may excrete up to 20 liters of urine per day (polyuria) and will drink enormous quantities of liquids.

Tumors of the Hypophysis

Tumors of the hypophysis are usually benign. About two-thirds of them have been shown to produce hormones that cause clinical symptoms. These tumors can produce growth hormone, prolactin, adrenocorticotropin and, less frequently, thyroid-stimulating hormone. Clinical diagnosis of these tumors can be confirmed by immunocytochemistry after their surgical removal.

REFERENCES

Bhatnagar AS (editor): *The Anterior Pituitary Gland.* Raven Press, 1983.

Brownstein MJ, Russell JT, Gainer H: Synthesis, transport, and release of posterior pituitary hormones. *Science* 1980;**207**:373.

Cross BA, Leng G (editors): The neurohypophysis; Structure, function and control. *Prog Brain Res* 1982;**60**:3.

Daniel PM: The blood supply of the hypothalamus and pituitary gland. *Br Med Bull* 1966;**22**:202.

Girod C: Immunocytochemistry of the vertebrate adenohypophysis. In: *Handbook of Histochemistry.* Vol 8, Suppl 5. Graumann W, Neumann K (editors). Gustav Fischer, 1983.

Pantic VR: The specificity of pituitary cells and regulation of their activities. *Int Rev Cytol* 1975;**40**:153.

Pelletier G, Robert F, Hardy J: Identification of human anterior pituitary cells by immunoelectron microscopy. *J Clin Endocrinol Metab* 1978;**46**:534.

Phifer RF, Midgley AR, Spicer SS: Immunohistologic and histologic evidence that follicle-stimulating hormone and luteinizing hormone are present in the same cell type in the human pars distalis. *J Clin Endocrinol Metab* 1973;**36**:125.

Phifer RF, Spicer SS, Orth DN: Specific demonstration of the human hypophyseal cells which produce adrenocorticotropic hormone. *J Clin Endocrinol* 1970;**31**:347.

Reichlin S (editor): *The Neurohypophysis: Physiological and Clinical Aspects.* Plenum, 1984.

Seyama S, Pearl GS, Takei Y: Ultrastructural study of the human neurohypophysis. 1. Neurosecretory axons and their dilatations in the pars nervosa. *Cell Tissue Res* 1980;**205**:253.

Seyama S, Pearl GS, Takei Y: Ultrastructural study of the human neurohypophysis. 3. Vascular and perivascular structures. *Cell Tissue Res* 1980;**206**:291.

Takei Y et al: Ultrastructural study of the human neurohypophysis. 2. Cellular elements of neural parenchyma, the pituicytes. *Cell Tissue Res* 1980;**205**:273.

Adrenals, Islets of Langerhans, Thyroid, Parathyroids, & Pineal Gland

21

ADRENAL (SUPRARENAL) GLANDS

The adrenal glands are paired organs that lie near the superior poles of the kidneys, embedded in adipose tissue (Fig 21–1). They are flattened structures with a half-moon shape; in the human, they are about 4–6 cm long, 1–2 cm wide, and 4–6 mm thick. Together they weigh about 8 g, but their weight and size vary depending upon the age and physiologic condition of the individual. Examination of a fresh section of adrenal gland shows it to be covered by a capsule of dense collagenous connective tissue. The gland consists of 2 concentric layers: a yellow peripheral layer, the **adrenal cortex;** and a reddish-brown central layer, the **adrenal medulla** (Figs 21–2 and 21–7). Cortical and medullary tissues sometimes occur at other sites, as shown in Fig 21–1.

These 2 layers can be considered as 2 organs with distinct functions and morphologic characteristics that become united during embryonic development. They arise from different germ layers. The cortex arises from coelomic intermediate mesoderm; the medulla consists of cells derived from the neural crest, from which sympathetic ganglion cells also originate. The medulla might, in fact, be considered a modified sympathetic ganglion whose postganglionic neurons lost their processes during development and became secretory cells. The general histologic appearance is typical of an endocrine gland in which cells of both cortex and medulla are grouped in cords along capillaries (see Chapter 4).

The collagenous connective tissue capsule that covers the gland sends thin septa to the interior of the gland as trabeculae. The stroma consists mainly of a rich network of reticular fibers that support the secretory cells.

Blood Supply

The adrenals are supplied by a number of arteries that enter at various points around their periphery (Fig 21–2). The 3 main groups are the **superior suprarenal artery,** arising from the inferior phrenic

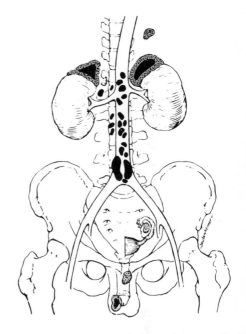

Figure 21–1. Human adrenal glands. Adrenocortical tissue is shown stippled; adrenal medullary tissue is shown black. Note the location of adrenals at the superior pole of each kidney. Also shown are extra-adrenal sites where cortical and medullary tissues are sometimes found. (Reproduced, with permission, from Forsham in: *Textbook of Endocrinology,* 4th ed. Williams RH [editor]. Saunders, 1968).

artery; the **middle suprarenal artery,** arising from the aorta; and the **inferior suprarenal artery,** arising from the renal artery. The several arterial branches form a subcapsular plexus from which arise 3 groups of vessels: arteries of the capsule; arteries of the cortex, which branch repeatedly to form the capillary bed between the parenchymal cells (these capillaries drain into medullary capillaries); and arteries of the medulla, which pass through the cortex before breaking up to form part of the extensive capillary network of the medulla (Fig 21–2).

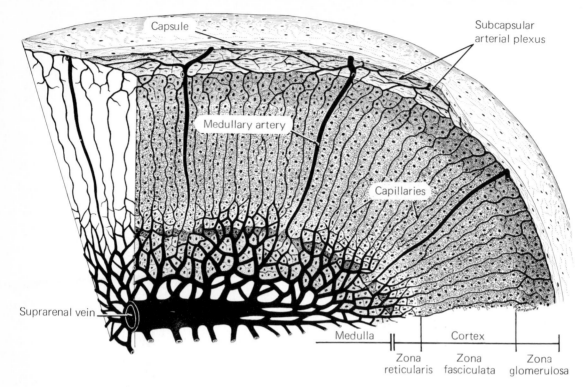

Figure 21–2. Diagram of the general architecture and blood circulation of the adrenal gland.

This dual vascular supply provides the medulla with both arterial (via **medullary arteries**) and venous (via **cortical arteries**) blood. The endothelium of these capillaries is extremely attenuated and interrupted by small fenestrae that are closed by thin diaphragms. A continuous basal lamina is present beneath the endothelium. Capillaries of the medulla, together with those that supply the cortex, form the medullary veins, which join to constitute the **adrenal** or **suprarenal vein** (Fig 21–2).

Adrenal Cortex

Because of the differences in disposition and appearance of its cells, the adrenal cortex can be subdivided into 3 concentric layers that are usually not sharply defined in humans (Figs 21–2 and 21–3): the **zona glomerulosa,** the **zona fasciculata,** and the **zona reticularis.** The cells of the adrenal cortex have the characteristics of steroid-synthesizing cells described in Chapter 4. The glomerulosa, fasciculata, and reticularis zones occupy, respectively, 15%, 65%, and 7% of the total volume of the adrenals.

The layer immediately beneath the connective tissue capsule is the zona glomerulosa, in which the columnar or pyramidal cells are arranged in closely packed, rounded, or arched clusters surrounded by capillaries (Fig 21–3A, B).

The next layer of cells is known as the zona fas-

ciculata because of the arrangement of the cells in straight cords, one or two cells thick (Fig 21–3C), that run at right angles to the surface of the organ and have capillaries between them. The cells of the zona fasciculata are polyhedral, with a great number of lipid droplets in their cytoplasm. As a result of the dissolution of the lipids during tissue preparation, the fasciculata cells appear vacuolated in common histologic preparations (Fig 21–3C). The smooth endoplasmic reticulum is even more highly developed in the zona fasciculata than in the zona glomerulosa.

The zona reticularis (Fig 21–3D), the innermost layer of the cortex, lies between the zona fasciculata and the medulla; it contains cells disposed in irregular cords that form an anastomosing network. These cells are smaller than those of the other 2 layers. Lipofuscin pigment granules in these cells are large and quite numerous. Irregularly shaped cells with pyknotic nuclei—suggesting cellular degradation—are often found in this layer (Fig 21–3D).

Cells of the adrenal cortex do not store their secretory products in granules; rather, they synthesize and secrete steroid hormones only upon demand. Steroids, being low-molecular-weight lipid-soluble molecules, can freely diffuse through the plasma membrane and do not require the specialized process of exocytosis for their release. These cells (Fig 21–4) have the typical ultrastructure of steroid-secreting cells detailed in Chapter 4.

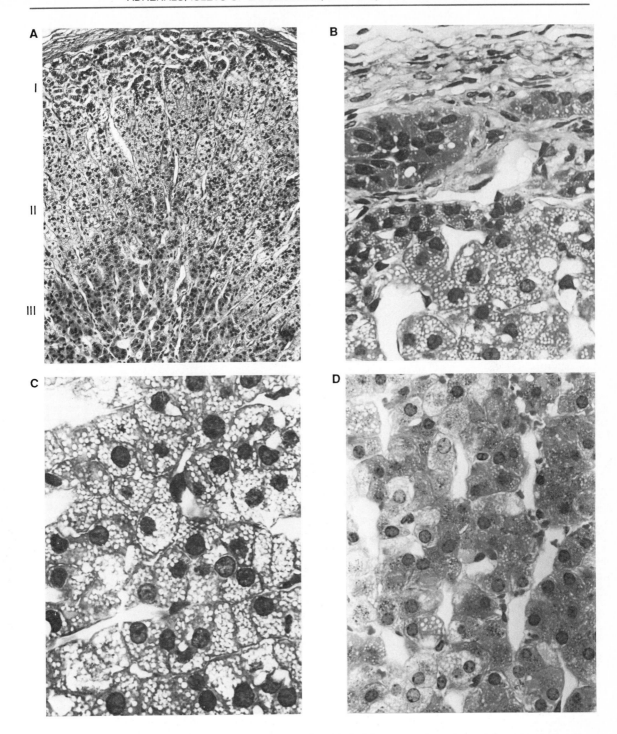

Figure 21–3. Photomicrographs of the adrenal cortex (H&E stain). **A:** A low-power general view. I, the zona glomerulosa; II, the zona fasciculata; III, the zona reticularis. × 80. **B:** The capsule and the zona glomerulosa. × 330. **C:** The zona fasciculata. × 330. **D:** The zona reticularis. × 330.

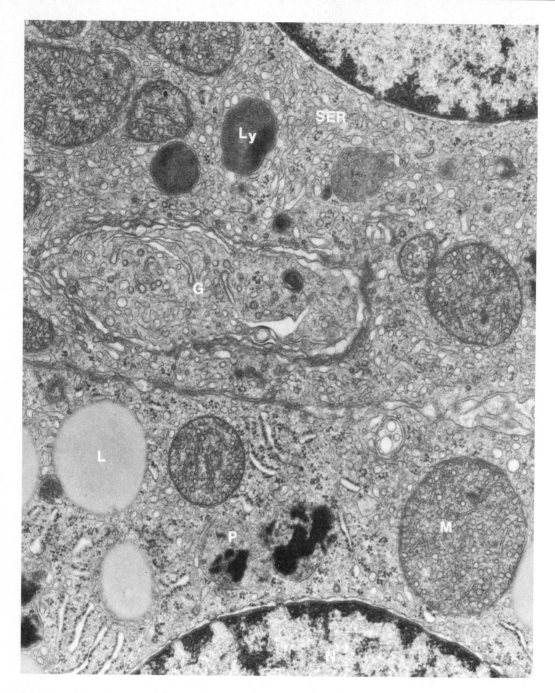

Figure 21–4. Fine structure of 2 steroid-secreting cells from the zona fasciculata of the human adrenal cortex. The lipid droplets (L) contain cholesterol esters. M, mitochondria with characteristic tubular and vesicular cristae; SER, smooth endoplasmic reticulum; N, nucleus; G, Golgi complex; Ly, lysosomes; P, lipofuscin pigment granules. × 25,700.

Histophysiology

The steroids secreted by the cortex can be divided into 3 groups, according to their main physiologic actions: **glucocorticoids, mineralocorticoids,** and **androgens** (Fig 21–5). The zona glomerulosa secretes mineralocorticoids, primarily aldosterone, that are involved with the maintenance of electrolyte (eg, sodium and potassium) and water balance. The zona fasciculata and probably the zona reticularis secrete the glucocorticoids cortisone and cortisol or, in some animals, corticosterone; these are concerned with the regulation of carbohydrate, protein, and fat metabolism. Androgens and perhaps estrogens are produced in small amounts in these 2 zones.

The localization of the enzymes participating in aldosterone synthesis has been determined through differential centrifugation. The synthesis of cholesterol from acetate takes place in smooth endoplasmic reticulum, and the conversion of cholesterol to pregnenolone takes place in the mitochondria. The enzymes associated with the synthesis of progesterone and deoxycorticosterone from pregnenolone are found in smooth endoplasmic reticulum; those enzymes that convert deoxycorticosterone → corticosterone → 18-hydroxycorticosterone → aldosterone are located in mitochondria. This is a clear example of collaboration between 2 cell organelles.

The **glucocorticoids,** mainly cortisol and corticosterone, exert a profound effect upon the metabolism of carbohydrates, as well as on that of proteins and lipids. In the liver, glucocorticoids promote the uptake and use of fatty acids (energy source), amino acids (enzyme synthesis), and carbohydrates (glucose synthesis) that are used in gluconeogenesis and glycogenesis (glycogen assembly). In fact, these hormones can stimulate the synthesis of so much glucose that the resulting high levels in the blood produce a condition similar to diabetes mellitus. Outside the liver, however, glucocorticoids induce an opposite, or catabolic, effect on peripheral organs (eg, skin, muscle, adipose tissue). In these structures, these steroid hormones not only decrease synthetic activity, but they also promote protein and lipid degradation. The by-products of degradation, amino and fatty acids, are removed from the blood and used by the synthetically active hepatocytes.

Glucocorticoids also suppress the immune response by decreasing the number of circulating lymphocytes. This reduction is a result of both their increased destruction and inhibition of mitotic activity in lymphocyte-forming organs.

The **mineralocorticoids** act mainly on the distal renal tubules as well as on the gastric mucosa and the salivary and sweat glands, stimulating the absorption of sodium. They may increase the concentration of potassium and decrease that of sodium in muscle and brain cells.

Dehydroepiandrosterone is the only sex hormone secreted in significant physiologic quantities by the adrenal cortex. It has masculinizing and anabolic effects, but it is less than one-fifth as potent as testicular androgens. For this reason, and because it is secreted in small quantities, it produces a negligible physiologic effect under normal conditions.

As in other endocrine glands, control of the adrenal cortex occurs initially through the release of its corresponding releasing hormone stored in the median eminence. This is followed by secretion of ACTH, which stimulates the synthesis and secretion of cortical hormones (eg, glucocorticoids). Free glucocorticoids may then inhibit ACTH secretion. The degree of pituitary inhibition is proportionate to the circulating glucocorticoid level and is exerted at both the pituitary and hypothalamic levels (Figs 21–6 and 21–7).

Fetal, or Provisional, Cortex

In humans and some other animals, the adrenal gland of the newborn is proportionately larger than that of the adult. At this early age, a layer known as the **fetal,** or **provisional, cortex** is present between the medulla and the thin permanent cortex. This layer is fairly thick, and its cells are disposed in cords. After birth, the provisional cortex undergoes involution, while the permanent cortex—the initially thin layer—develops, differentiating into the 3 layers described above. A major function of the fetal cortex is the secretion of sulfate conjugates of androgens, which are converted in the placenta to active androgens and estrogens that enter the maternal circulation.

Adrenal Medulla

The adrenal medulla is composed of polyhedral parenchymal cells arranged in cords or clumps and supported by a reticular fiber network (Fig 21–8). A profuse capillary supply intervenes between adjacent cords, and there are a few parasympathetic ganglion cells. Medullary parenchymal cells arise from neural crest cells, as do the postganglionic neurons of sympathetic and parasympathetic ganglia. Parenchymal cells of the adrenal medulla can be regarded as modified sympathetic postganglionic neurons that have lost their axons and dendrites.

Medullary parenchymal cells have abundant membrane-limited electron-dense secretory granules, 150–350 nm in diameter. These granules contain one or the other of the catecholamines, epinephrine or norepinephrine. (Fig 21–9). These granules also contain ATP, proteins called **chromogranins** (which may serve as binding proteins for catecholamines), dopamine β-hydroxylase (which converts dopamine to norepinephrine), and opiatelike peptides (enkephalins). Fig 21–10 shows the participation of cell organelles in the synthetic processes that lead to the formation of medullary-cell secretory granules.

A large body of evidence shows that epinephrine

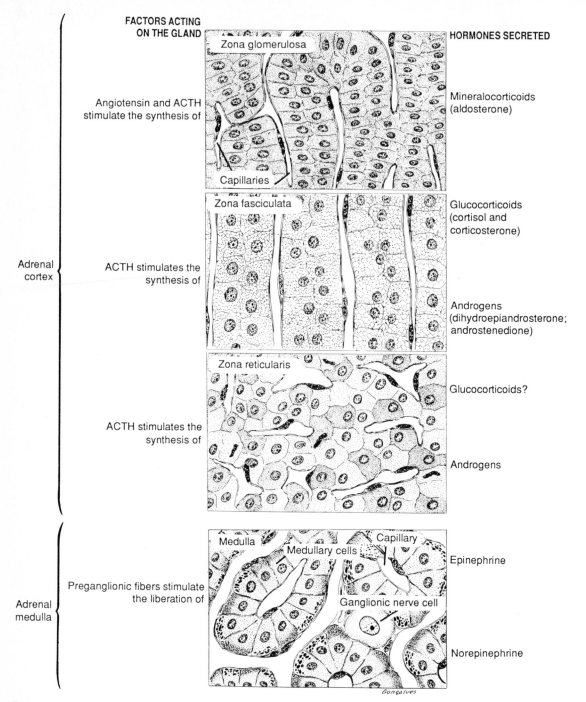

FACTORS ACTING ON THE GLAND

Zona glomerulosa

Angiotensin and ACTH stimulate the synthesis of

Capillaries

Zona fasciculata

ACTH stimulates the synthesis of

Zona reticularis

ACTH stimulates the synthesis of

Adrenal cortex

Preganglionic fibers stimulate the liberation of

Adrenal medulla

Medulla   Capillary
Medullary cells

Ganglionic nerve cell

HORMONES SECRETED

Mineralocorticoids (aldosterone)

Glucocorticoids (cortisol and corticosterone)

Androgens (dihydroepiandrosterone; androstenedione)

Glucocorticoids?

Androgens

Epinephrine

Norepinephrine

Gonçalves

Figure 21–5. Structure and histophysiology of the adrenal gland. **Left:** Factors acting on the gland. **Right:** The hormones secreted.

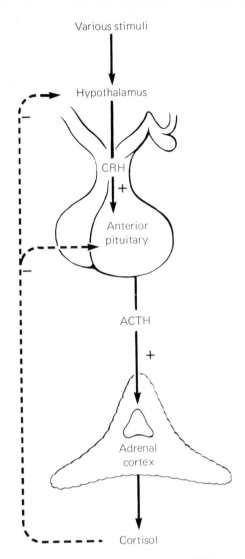

Figure 21–6. Feedback mechanism of ACTH-glucocorticoid secretion. Solid arrows indicate stimulation; dashed arrows, inhibition.

oids, cells of the medulla accumulate and store their hormones in granules.

Epinephrine and norepinephrine are secreted in large quantities in response to intense emotional reactions (eg, fright). Secretion of these substances is mediated by the preganglionic fibers that innervate medullary cells. Vasoconstriction, hypertension, changes in heart rate, and metabolic effects such as blood glucose elevation result from the secretion and release of catecholamines into the bloodstream. These effects are part of the organism's defense reaction to stress (the fight-or-flight response). In contrast, during normal activity, the medulla secretes (continuously) only small quantities of these hormones.

Medullary cells are also found in the paraganglia (collections of catecholamine-secreting cells adjacent to autonomic ganglia) as well as in various viscera. Paraganglia are a diffuse source of catecholamines.

Adrenal Dysfunction

A common disorder of the adrenal medulla is **pheochromocytoma,** a tumor of its cells that causes hyperglycemia and transient elevations of blood pressure. These tumors can also develop in extramedullary sites (Fig 21–1).

Disorders of the adrenal cortex can be classified as **hyperfunction** or **hypofunction.** Tumors of the adrenal cortex can result in excessive production of glucocorticoids **(Cushing's syndrome)** or aldosterone **(Conn's syndrome).** Cushing's syndrome is most often (90%) due to a pituitary adenoma that results in excessive production of ACTH; it is rarely caused by adrenal hyperplasia or an adrenal tumor. Excessive production of adrenal androgens has little effect in mature males. Hirsutism (abnormal hair growth) is seen in females, and precocious puberty (males) and virilization (females) are encountered in prepubertal children. These adrenogenital syndromes are the result of several enzymatic defects in steroid metabolism that cause increased biosynthesis of androgens by the adrenal cortex.

Adrenocortical insufficiency **(Addison's disease)** is mainly caused by autoimmune destruction of the adrenal cortex (80%), or it can be a complication of tuberculosis (20%). The signs and symptoms suggest failure of secretion of both glucocorticoids and mineralocorticoids by the adrenal cortex.

Carcinomas of the adrenal cortex are rare, but most are highly malignant. About 90% of these tumors produce steroids associated with endocrine symptoms.

and norepinephrine are secreted by 2 different types of cells in the medulla. Epinephrine-secreting cells have smaller, less-electron-dense granules, and their contents fill the granule. On the other hand, norepinephrine-secreting cells have larger, more-electron-dense granules. Their contents are irregular in shape, and there is an electron-lucent layer beneath the surrounding membrane. About 80% of the catecholamine output of the adrenal vein is epinephrine.

All adrenal medullary cells are innervated by cholinergic endings of preganglionic sympathetic neurons. Unlike the cortex, which does not store ster-

FACTORS ACTING
ON THE GLAND

GLAND REACTION

Hypophysectomy causes

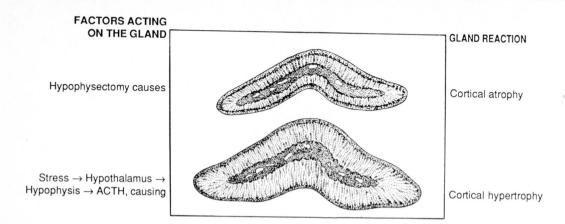

Cortical atrophy

Stress → Hypothalamus →
Hypophysis → ACTH, causing

Cortical hypertrophy

Figure 21–7. Effects of decreased and increased stimulation of the structure of the adrenal gland.

ISLETS OF LANGERHANS

The islets of Langerhans are multihormonal endocrine microorgans of the pancreas; they appear as rounded clusters of cells embedded within exocrine pancreatic tissue.

While most islets are 100–200 μm in diameter and contain several hundred cells, small islets of endocrine cells can also be found interspersed among pancreatic exocrine cells. There may be more than 1 million islets in the human pancreas, with a slight tendency for islets to be more abundant in the tail region.

Each islet consists of lightly stained polygonal or rounded cells arranged in cords separated by a net-work of fenestrated blood capillaries (Figs 21–11 and 21–12). Both the parenchymal cells and the blood vessels are innervated by autonomic nerve fibers. A fine capsule of reticular fibers surrounds each islet, separating it from the adjacent exocrine pancreatic tissue.

Using immunocytochemical methods (Figs 21–13, 21–14, and 21–15), 4 types of cells—A, B, D, and F—have been located in the islets. The secretory granules of these cells vary according to the species studied. In humans, the A cells have regular granules with a dense core surrounded by a clear region bounded by a membrane. The B cells have irregular granules with a core formed by irregular crystals of insulin complexed with zinc (Fig 21–13). Insulin syn-

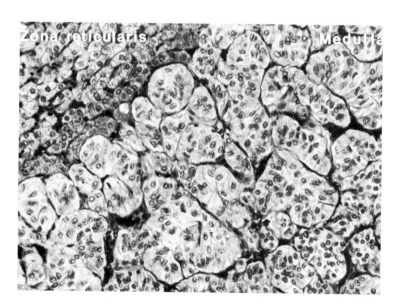

Figure 21–8. Photomicrograph of a section of the corticomedullary transition in the adrenal gland, showing cords of medullary cells. H&E stain. × 200.

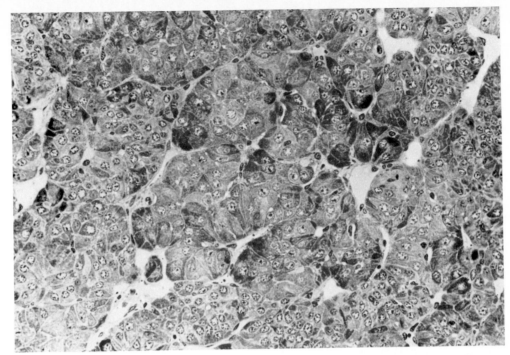

Figure 21–9. Photomicrograph of adrenal medulla showing cords of cells and interspersed capillaries. The majority are epinephrine-producing cells; a smaller number of darker norepinephrine-producing cells are also present.

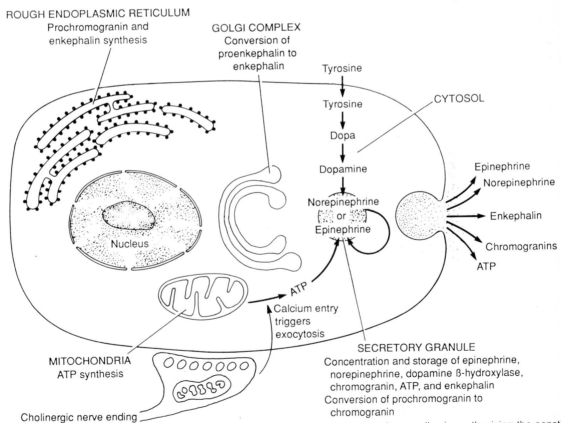

Figure 21–10. Diagram of an adrenal medullary cell showing the role of several organelles in synthesizing the constituents of secretory granules. Norepinephrine synthesis and conversion to epinephrine take place in the cytosol, as indicated.

411

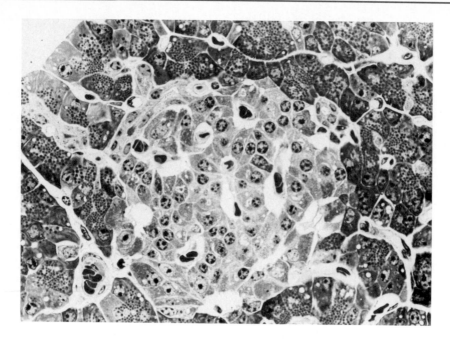

Figure 21–11. Photomicrograph of a section of the pancreas. Observe the islet of Langerhans, where the A cells appear mainly in the periphery as large cells with a dark cytoplasm. The remaining cells are mostly B cells. The islet is formed of cell cords and capillaries and is surrounded by pancreatic acinar cells.

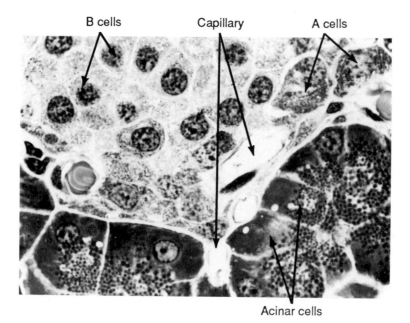

Figure 21–12. Photomicrograph of a pancreatic islet of Langerhans. The A cells exhibit larger, darker granules than do the B cells.

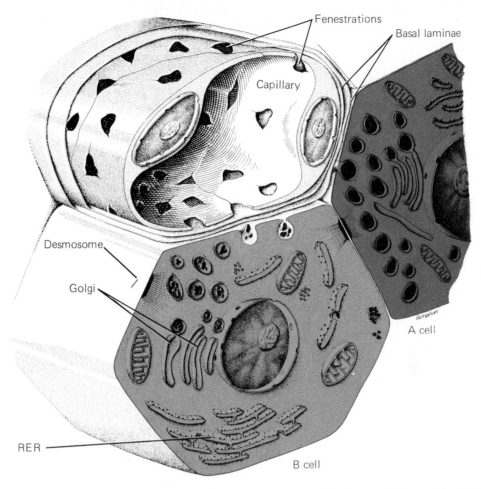

Figure 21–13. Schematic drawing of the A and B cells, showing the morphologic features of the secretory granules and their relation to blood vessels. The B cell's granules are irregular, while the granules are round and uniform in the A cells. RER, rough endoplasmic reticulum.

thesis has been well studied; its main steps are shown in Fig 21–16.

The relative quantities of the 4 cell types found in islets are not uniform but vary considerably with their location in the pancreas. Table 21–1 summarizes the types, quantities, and functions of the hormones produced by the islet cells. The ultrastructure of these cells (Fig 21–13) resembles that of cells synthesizing polypeptides (see Chapter 4).

Terminations of nerve fibers on islet cells can be observed by light or electron microscopy. Both sympathetic and parasympathetic nerve endings have been found in close association with about 10% of the A, B, and D cells. Gap junctions presumably serve to transfer the ionic changes associated with autonomic discharge to the other cells. These nerves function as part of the insulin and glucagon control system.

Several tumor types arise from islet cells that produce such hormones as insulin, glucagon, so-

matostatin, and pancreatic polypeptide. Some pancreatic tumors have been described that produce 2 or more of these hormones simultaneously, generating complex clinical symptoms.

It is currently known that one of the principal types of diabetes (type I) is an autoimmune disease in which antibodies against B cells depress their activity.

THYROID

In early embryonic life, the thyroid is derived from the cephalic portion of the alimentary canal endoderm. Its function is to synthesize the hormones thyroxine (T_4) and triiodothyronine (T_3), which stimulate the rate of metabolism.

The thyroid gland, located in the cervical region anterior to the larynx, consists of 2 lobes united by an isthmus (Fig 21–17). Thyroid tissue is composed of

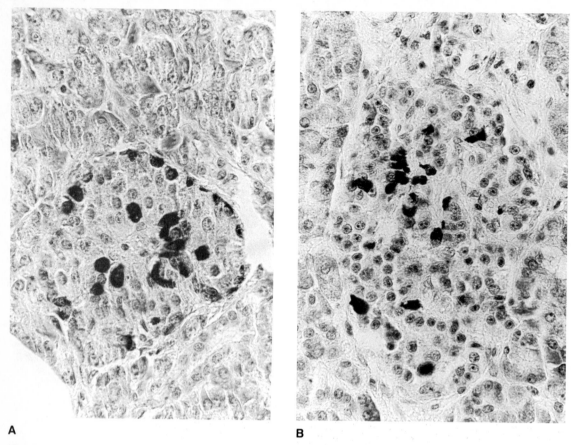

A   **B**

Figure 21–14. Photomicrographs of human pancreatic islets of Langerhans treated by immunohistochemical methods to demonstrate glucagon-secreting **(A)** and somatostatin-secreting **(B)** cells. × 250. (Courtesy of V Alberti.)

follicles consisting of a simple epithelial sphere whose lumen contains **colloid,** a gelatinous substance (Fig 21–18). In typical sections, follicular cells range from squamous to low columnar; the follicles have a variable diameter. The gland is covered by a loose connective tissue capsule that sends septa into the parenchyma. These septa gradually become thinner; they reach all the follicles, separating one from another by fine irregular connective tissue composed mainly of reticular fibers. The thyroid is an extremely vascularized organ, having an extensive blood and lymphatic capillary network surrounding the follicles. Endothelial cells of these capillaries are fenestrated, as in other endocrine glands. This configuration facilitates the passage of the hormones into the blood capillaries.

Innervation of the thyroid, via the sympathetic and parasympathetic systems, serves an essentially vasomotor function. Ultrastructural and radioautographic studies have shown a network of adrenergic fibers terminating near the basal lamina of the follicular cells. These findings, together with evidence that adrenergic and other amines influence thyroid iodine metabolism in isolated thyroid cells and in vivo, indicate that neurogenic stimuli can influence thyroid function through a direct effect on the epithelial cells. The major regulator of the anatomic and functional state of the thyroid gland, however, is thyroid-stimulating hormone (TSH, or thyrotropin), which is secreted by the anterior pituitary.

The morphologic appearance of thyroid follicles varies according to the region of the gland and its functional activity. In the same gland, larger follicles that are full of colloid and have a cuboidal or squamous epithelium are found alongside follicles that are lined by columnar epithelium. In spite of this variation, the gland is considered hypoactive when the average composition of these follicles is squamous. When drugs capable of stimulating the synthesis of thyroid hormone are administered, a marked increase in the height of the follicular epithelium is observed. This phenomenon is accompanied by a decrease in the quantity of the colloid and the size of the follicles.

The thyroid epithelium always rests on a basal lamina. The ultrastructure of the follicular epithelium

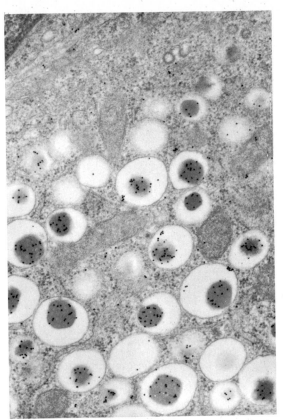

Figure 21–15. Immunocytochemical localization of insulin in a B cell of a Langerhans islet. The black granules are gold particles used to label anti-insulin. They indicate the sites where this antibody was attached to the insulin in the secretory granules. Observe also the clear zone between the secretory material and the granule membrane. × 35,000. (Courtesy of M Bendayan.)

exhibits all the characteristics of a cell that simultaneously synthesizes, secretes, absorbs, and digests proteins (Fig 21–21). The basal part of these cells is rich in rough endoplasmic reticulum. The nucleus is generally round and situated in the center of the cell. The apical pole has a discrete Golgi complex and small secretory granules with the morphologic characteristics of follicular colloid. Abundant lysosomes, 0.5–0.6 μm in diameter, and some large phagosomes are found in this region. The cell membrane of the apical pole has a moderate number of microvilli. Mitochondria, distended cisternae of rough endoplasmic reticulum, and ribosomes are dispersed throughout the cytoplasm.

Another type of cell, the **parafollicular,** or **C, cell,** is found as part of the follicular epithelium or as isolated clusters between thyroid follicles (Fig 21–19). Parafollicular cells are somewhat larger and stain less intensely than thyroid follicular cells. They present a small amount of rough endoplasmic reticulum, long mitochondria, and a large Golgi complex.

The most striking feature of these cells is their numerous small (100–180 nm in diameter) hormone-containing granules (Fig 21–20). These cells are responsible for the synthesis and secretion of **calcitonin,** a hormone whose main effect is to lower blood calcium levels by inhibiting bone resorption. Secretion of calcitonin is triggered by an elevation in blood calcium concentration.

Histophysiology

The thyroid is the only endocrine gland whose secretory product is stored in great quantity. This accumulation is also unusual in that it occurs in the extracellular colloid. In humans, there is sufficient hormone within the follicles to supply the organism for up to 3 months. Thyroid colloid is composed of a glycoprotein (thyroglobulin) of high molecular weight (660,000).

Control of the activity of thyroid follicular cells was discussed in Chapter 20 and summarized in Fig 20–7. This mechanism maintains an adequate quantity of thyroxin. (T_4) and triiodothyronine (T_3) within the organism. TSH secretion is also increased by exposure to cold and depressed by heat and stressful stimuli.

Synthesis & Accumulation of Hormones by Follicular Cells

This process takes place in 4 stages: synthesis of thyroglobulin, uptake of iodide from the blood, activation of the iodide, and iodination of the tyrosine residues of thyroglobulin.

These stages, diagrammed in Fig 21–21, take place in the following manner:

(1) The **synthesis of thyroglobulin** occurs in a manner typical of other protein-exporting cells (described in Chapter 4). Briefly, the secretory pathway consists of the synthesis of protein in the rough endoplasmic reticulum, addition of carbohydrate in the endoplasmic reticulum and the Golgi complex, and release from formed vesicles at the apical surface of the cell into the lumen of the follicle.

(2) The **uptake of circulating iodide** is accomplished in the thyroid by a mechanism of active transport, using the iodide pump. This pump, located within the cytoplasmic membrane of the basal region of the follicular cells, is readily stimulated by thyrotropin. The uptake of iodide can be inhibited by such drugs as perchlorate and thiocyanate, which act by competing with iodide.

(3) During the **activation of iodide,** it is oxidized by thyroid peroxidase to an intermediate, which in turn combines in the colloid with the tyrosine residues of thyroglobulin.

(4) In contrast to the processes described above, **iodination of tyrosine residues** bound to thyroglobulin takes place not inside the follicular cells but in the colloid in contact with the membrane of the apical region of the cells.

Table 21–1. Cell types in human islets of Langerhans.

Cell Type	Quantity	Position	Hormone Produced	Hormonal Function
A	~20%	Usually in periphery.	Glucagon.	Acts on several tissues to make energy stored in glycogen and fat available through glycogenolysis and lipolysis. Increases blood glucose content.
B	~70%	Central region.	Insulin.	Acts on several tissues to cause storage of energy from excess nutrients. Promotes decrease of blood glucose content.
D	<5%	Variable.	Somatostatin.	Inhibits release of other islet cell hormones through local paracrine action.
F	Rare	Variable.	Pancreatic polypeptide.	Not well established.

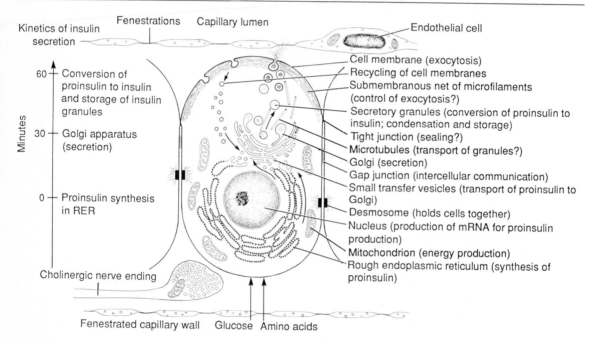

Figure 21–16. The physiology of the B cell of the pancreatic islet. Note the complex secretory process (simplified elsewhere in this book for teaching purposes). The process begins with the entrance of blood-borne amino acids into the cell, probably aided by an active amino acid pump in the cell membrane. The amino acids are polymerized to preproinsulin by the polyribosomes on the surface of the rough endoplasmic reticulum, and the polypeptide chain is injected through the membrane of the RER into the lumen. The preproinsulin undergoes a limited proteolysis and becomes proinsulin. The latter is then transferred into small vesicles by a process of budding that occurs in the cisternae close to the Golgi complex. (No polyribosomes cover the endoplasmic reticulum in this region.) The small vesicles are transported to the Golgi cisternae. Their contents are then packed into immature secretory granules by the Golgi complex; the granules gradually condense to form the mature secretory granule. In the secretory granules, proinsulin is cleaved enzymatically to yield insulin; microtubules play a role in the transport of these granules to the cell surface. Granule extrusion occurs when the cell membrane fuses with the membrane of the granule. The contents of the granule spill into the extracellular space and diffuse into a blood vessel. Evidence has been presented suggesting that a submembranous net of microfilaments participates in mechanical inhibition of the extrusion process until the appropriate stimulus has been received.

The granule membrane is incorporated into the cell membrane and is probably recycled by the cell by means of small endocytotic vesicles (shown at upper left). The secretory processes of the B cell are regulated mainly by the blood glucose level and by autonomic nerve endings. (Based on data presented by Orci L: A portrait of the pancreatic B cell. *Diabetologia* 1974;**10**:163.)

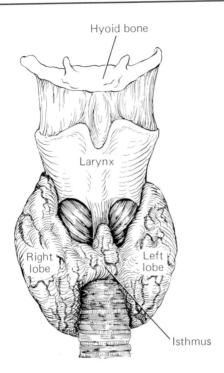

Figure 21–17. Anatomy of the human thyroid. (Reproduced, with permission, from Ganong, WF: *Review of Medical Physiology,* 15th ed. Lange, 1991.)

It is postulated that the union of the iodinated tyrosines is catalyzed by an enzymatic mechanism. Thyroglobulin must have the correct spatial configuration for this process to occur normally. When disease causes the production of abnormal thyroglobulin, this process is blocked, resulting in deficient synthesis of thyroid hormone. The process can also be blocked by drugs (eg, propylthiouracil, carbimazole) that inhibit the peroxidase-catalyzed iodination of thyroglobulin. Some forms of thyroid dysfunction are related to a genetic deficiency of peroxidase or the iodide pump.

Liberation of T_3 & T_4

When stimulated by TSH, thyroid follicular cells take up colloid by a form of pinocytosis. Folds of apical cytoplasm (lamellipodia) encircle a portion of colloid and bring it into the follicular cell. The pinocytotic vesicles then fuse with lysosomes. The peptide bonds between the iodinated residues and the thyroglobulin molecule are broken by proteases in lysosomes, and T_4, T_3, diiodotyrosine (DIT), and monoiodotyrosine (MIT) (Fig 21–22) are liberated into the cytoplasm. The free T_4 and T_3 then cross the cell membrane and are discharged into the capillaries. MIT and DIT are not secreted into the blood since their iodine is removed as a result of the intracellular action of **iodotyrosine dehalogenase.** The products of this enzymatic reaction, iodine and tyrosine, are reused by the follicular cells. T_4 is the more abundant of these compounds, constituting 90% of the circu-

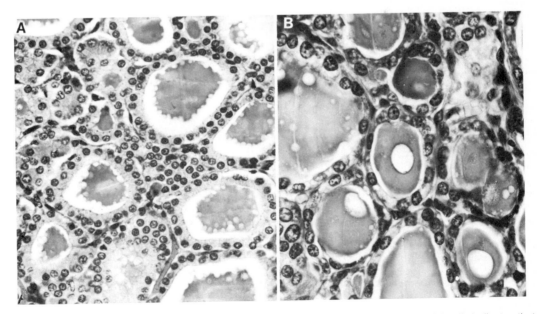

Figure 21–18. Photomicrographs of sections of thyroid glands. The presence of taller epithelial cells indicates that the section on the left is from a more active gland. H&E stain. × 200 **(A)** and × 400 **(B).**

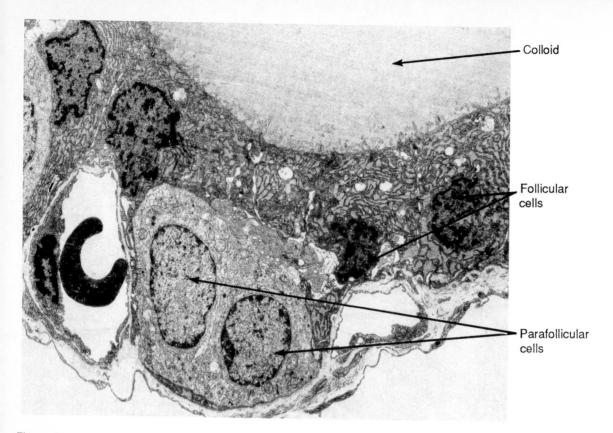

— Colloid

— Follicular
cells

— Parafollicular
cells

Figure 21–19. Electron micrograph of thyroid showing 2 calcitonin-producing parafollicular cells and part of a thyroid follicle. Observe 2 capillaries at both sides of the parafollicular cells.

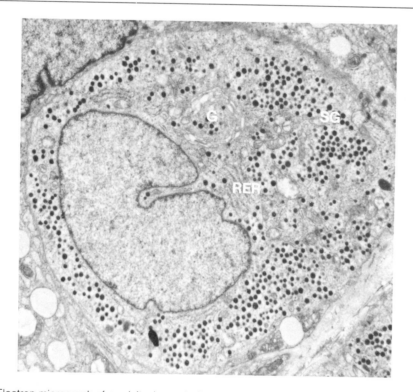

Figure 21–20. Electron micrograph of a calcitonin-producing cell. Observe the small secretory granules (SG) and the scarcity of rough endoplasmic reticulum (RER). G. Golgi region. × 5000.

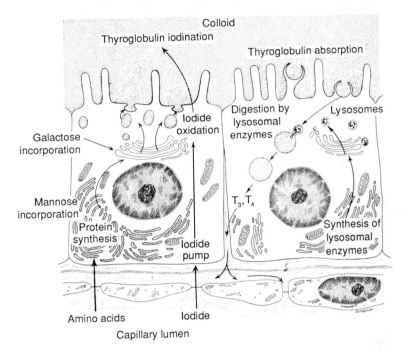

Figure 21–21. Diagram showing the processes of synthesis and iodination of thyroglobulin **(left)** and its absorption and digestion **(right).** These events occur in the same cell.

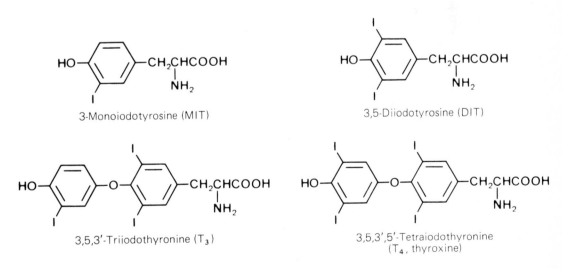

Figure 21–22. Formulas of 3-monoiodotyrosine (MIT) and 3, 5–diiodotyrosine (DIT). The condensation of 2 molecules of DIT with the elimination of an alanine residue results in the formation of tetraiodothyronine (T_4 [thyroxine]). The condensation of one molecule of MIT and one molecule of DIT with the elimination of one alanine residue results in the formation of triiodothyronine (T_3).

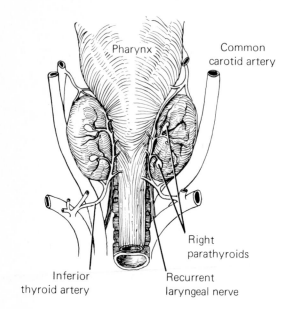

Figure 21–23. The human parathyroid glands, viewed from behind. (Redrawn and reproduced, with permission, from Nordland in: *Surg Gynecol Obstet* 130;**51**:449; and from *Gray's Anatomy of the Human Body*, 29th ed. Goss CM [editor]. Lea & Febiger, 1973.)

lating thyroid hormone, although T_3 acts more rapidly and is more potent than T_4.

Thyroxine stimulates mitochondrial respiration and oxidative phosphorylation. Since this effect is blocked by dactinomycin, it is dependent on mRNA synthesis. T_3 and T_4 increase the numbers of both mitochondria and their cristae. Mitochondrial protein synthesis is increased and degradation of their proteins is decreased.

Most of the effects of thyroid hormones are secondary to their effects on the basal metabolic rate; they increase the absorption of carbohydrates from the intestine and regulate lipid metabolism. Thyroid hormones also influence body growth and the development of the nervous system during fetal life.

Factors Affecting the Synthesis of Thyroid Hormones

A diet that contains less that 10 μg/d of iodine hinders the synthesis of thyroid hormones. Thyroid hypertrophy as a result of increased TSH secretion causes the disorder known as **iodine deficiency goiter,** which occurs widely in some regions of the world.

The syndrome of adult hypothyroidism, **myxedema,** may be the result of a number of diseases of the thyroid gland, or it may be secondary to pituitary or hypothalamic failure. Children who are hypothyroid from birth are called **cretins;** they are characterized by dwarfing and mental retardation.

Hyperthyroidism or thyrotoxicosis may be caused by a variety of thyroid diseases, but the most common form is **Graves' disease,** or **exophthalmic goiter.** The levels of TSH are subnormal in this disease, and the thyroid hyperfunction is due to an immunologic dysfunction with production of a circulating immunoglobulin whose effects resemble those of TSH.

Autoimmune disease of this gland promotes its destruction by lymphocytes with consequent hypothyroidism (Hashimoto's disease).

PARATHYROID GLANDS

The parathyroids are 4 small glands—3 × 6 mm— with a total weight of about 0.4 g. They are situated behind the thyroid gland, one at each end of the upper and lower poles, usually in the capsule that covers the lobes of the thyroid (Fig 21–23). Sometimes they are found embedded in the thyroid gland. The parathyroid glands are derived from pharyngeal pouches— the superior glands from the fourth pouch and the inferior glands from the third. They can be found in the mediastinum, lying beside the thymus; the parathyroid glands and the thymus originate from the same pharyngeal pouches.

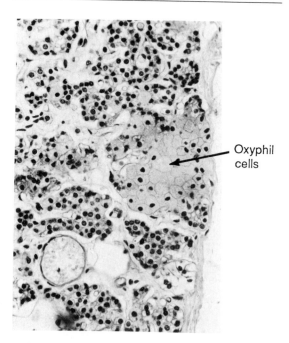

Figure 21–24. Photomicrograph of a section of the parathyroid gland. Observe a group of large, acidophilic oxyphil cells at the middle right. × 220. (Courtesy of J James.)

Histology

Each parathyroid gland is contained within a connective tissue capsule. These capsules send septa into the gland, where they merge with the reticular fibers supporting elongated cordlike clusters of secretory cells.

The parenchyma of the parathyroid glands consists of 2 types of cells: the chief, or principal, cells and the oxyphil cells (Fig 21–24).

The **chief cells** are small polygonal cells with a vesicular nucleus and a pale-staining, slightly acidophilic cytoplasm. Electron microscopy shows irregularly shaped granules 200–400 nm in diameter in their cytoplasm. They are the secretory granules containing **parathyroid hormone (PTH),** which in its active form is a polypeptide. **Oxyphil cells** are polygonal in shape and larger than chief cells; their nuclei are smaller and stain many densely, and their cytoplasm contains many acidophilic granules that consist of mitochondria with abundant cristae. The function of the oxyphil cell is unknown.

Cells with structural characteristics intermediate between chief and oxyphil cells are also seen, suggesting that they are transitions of a single cell type. With increasing age, secretory cells are replaced by adipocytes. Adipose cells can constitute over 50% of the gland in older individuals.

Histophysiology

Parathyroid hormone acts on the cells of bone tissue, increasing the number and activity of osteoclasts, thus promoting the absorption of the calcified bone matrix and the release of calcium into the blood. An increase in the concentration of calcium in the blood suppresses the production of parathyroid hormone. Calcitonin from the thyroid gland also influences osteoclasts by inhibiting both their resorptive action on bone and the liberation of calcium. Calcitonin thus lowers blood calcium and increases osteogenesis; its effect is opposite to that of parathyroid hormone. These hormones constitute a dual mechanism regulating blood levels of calcium, an important factor in homeostasis.

In addition to increasing the concentration of calcium, parathyroid hormone reduces the concentration of phosphate in the blood. This effect is a consequence of the activity of parathyroid hormone on kidney tubule cells, diminishing the absorption of phosphate and causing an increase of phosphate excretion in urine. There is also strong evidence that parathyroid hormone increases the absorption of calcium from the gastrointestinal tract and that vitamin D is necessary for this effect.

In **hyperparathyroidism,** blood phosphate is low and blood calcium is increased. This frequently produces pathologic deposits of calcium in several organs, such as the kidneys and arteries. Bones are decalcified and become subject to fracture. The bone disease caused by hyperparathyroidism, which is characterized by multiple bone cysts, is known as **osteitis fibrosa cystica.**

Hypoparathyroidism causes an increase in the concentration of phosphate and a decrease in

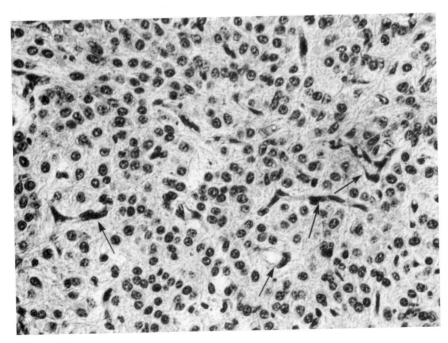

Figure 21–25. Section of a pineal gland. The arrows indicate blood vessels that surround the cellular cords. × 350.

the concentration of calcium in the blood. The bones become denser and more mineralized. This condition causes spastic contractions of the skeletal muscles and generalized convulsions called **tetany.** These symptoms are caused by the exaggerated excitability of the nervous system, which is due to the lack of calcium ions in the blood. The administration of calcium or of parathyroid hormone terminates the convulsions —the former much more rapidly than the latter.

The secretion of the parathyroid cells is regulated by the blood calcium level and is apparently not directly affected by other endocrine glands or the nervous system.

PINEAL GLAND

The pineal gland is also known as the **epiphysis cerebri,** or **pineal body.** In the adult, it is a flattened conical organ measuring approximately 5–8 mm in length and 3–5 mm at its greatest width, weighing about 120 mg. It is found in the posterior extremity of the third ventricle, above the roof of the diencephalon, to which it is connected by a short stalk.

The pineal gland is covered by pia mater. Connective tissue septa (containing blood vessels and unmyelinated nerve fibers) originate in the pia mater and penetrate the pineal tissue. Along with the capillaries, they surround the cellular cords and follicles, forming irregular lobules (Fig 21–25).

The pineal gland consists of several types of cells, principally pinealocytes and astroglial (*astron +*

glia) cells. **Pinealocytes** have a slightly basophilic cytoplasm with large irregular or lobate nuclei and sharply defined nucleoli. When impregnated with silver salts, the pinealocytes appear to have long and tortuous branches reaching out to the vascular connective tissue septa, where they end as flattened dilatations. These cells produce **melatonin,** serotonin, and some ill-defined pineal peptides.

The **astroglial cells** of the pineal gland are a specific type of cell characterized by elongated nuclei that stain more heavily than do those of parenchymal cells. They are observed between the cords of pinealocytes and in perivascular areas. These cells have long cytoplasmic processes containing a large number of intermediate filaments 10 nm in diameter.

Innervation

Nerve fibers lose their myelin sheaths when they penetrate the pineal gland; the unmyelinated axons end among pinealocytes, with some forming synapses. A great number of small vesicles containing norepinephrine are observed in these nerve endings. Serotonin is also present, in both the pinealocytes and the sympathetic nerve terminals.

Histophysiology

The pineal gland responds mainly to external visual stimuli relayed by the sympathetic nerves. Melatonin, serotonin, and specific methylindols are released upon stimulation. These in turn promote rhythmic changes in the secretory activity of the gonads and hypophysis. The pineal gland is therefore considered a neuroendocrine transducer that modifies the functions of different endocrine organs.

REFERENCES

Adrenal Glands
Christy NP (editor): *The Human Adrenal Cortex.* Harper & Row, 1971.
James VHT (editor): *The Adrenal Gland.* Raven Press, 1979.
Neville AM, O'Hare MJ: *The Human Adrenal Cortex.* Springer-Verlag, 1982.

Islets of Langerhans
Cooperstein SJ, Watkins D (editors): *The Islets of Langerhans.* Academic Press, 1981.
Ganong WF: *Review of Medical Physiology,* 15th ed. Appleton & Lange, 1991.
Orci L, Vassali JD, Perrelet A: The insulin factory. *Sci Am* (Sept) 1988;**259**:85.

Thyroid Gland
Nunez EA, Gershon MD: Cytophysiology of thyroid parafollicular cells. *Int Rev Cytol* 1978;**52**:1.

Parathyroid Glands
Gaillard PJ, Talmage RV, Budy AM (editors): *The Parathyroid Glands.* Univ of Chicago Press, 1965.

Pineal Gland
Tapp E, Huxley M: The histological appearance of the human pineal gland from puberty to old age. *J Pathol* 1972;**108**:137.

The Male Reproductive System

22

The male reproductive system is composed of the testes, genital ducts, accessory glands, and penis. The dual function of the **testis** is to produce hormones and spermatozoa. It is surrounded by a thick capsule of collagenous connective tissue, the **tunica albuginea.** The tunica albuginea is thickened on the posterior surface of the testis to form the **mediastinum testis,** from which fibrous septa penetrate the gland, dividing it into about 250 pyramidal compartments called the **testicular lobules** (Fig 22–1). These septa are incomplete, and there is frequently intercommunication between the lobules. Each lobule is occupied by 1–4 seminiferous tubules enmeshed in a web of loose connective tissue rich in blood and lymphatic vessels, nerves, and interstitial (Leydig) cells. Seminiferous tubules produce male reproductive cells, the sperma-

tozoa. Interstitial cells secrete testicular androgens (Fig 22–2).

The genital ducts and accessory glands produce secretions that, aided by smooth muscle contractions, propel spermatozoa toward the exterior. These secretions also provide nutrients for spermatozoa while they are confined to the male reproductive tract. Spermatozoa plus the secretions of the genital ducts and accessory glands make up the **semen** (from Latin, seed), which is introduced into the female reproductive tract through the penis.

The testes develop retroperitoneally in the dorsal wall of the abdominal cavity. They are later suspended within the scrotum at the ends of the spermatic cords. Each carries with it a serous sac, the **tunica vaginalis** (Fig 22–1), derived from the peri-

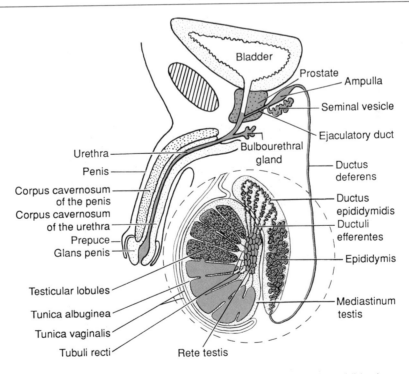

Figure 22–1. Diagram of the male genital system (shown in color). The testis and the epididymis are shown in different scales than the other parts of the reproductive system. Observe the communication between the testicular lobules.

Seminiferous tubule
produces spermatazoa

Interstitial cell
secretes androgen

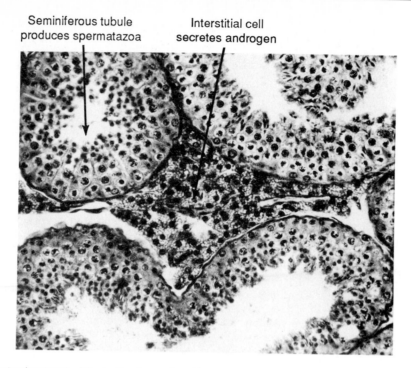

Figure 22–2. Photomicrograph of the testis of a monkey. The interstitial cells in the middle of the field contain vacuoles resulting from the dissolution of lipid droplets during preparation. H&E stain, × 400.

toneum. The tunic consists of an outer parietal and an inner visceral layer, covering the tunica albuginea on the anterior and lateral sides of the testis. The scrotum has an important role in maintaining the testes at a temperature lower than the intra-abdominal temperature.

TESTIS

Seminiferous Tubules

Each seminiferous tubule is lined with a complex stratified epithelium; it is about 150–250 μm in diameter and 30–70 cm long. The combined length of the tubules of one testis is about 250 m. The convoluted tubules form a network in which individual tubules are either blind-ended or branched. At the termination of each tubule, the lumen narrows and continues in short segments, known as **straight tubules,** or **tubuli recti,** that connect the seminiferous tubules to an anastomosing labyrinth of epithelium-lined channels, the **rete testis.** The rete, present in the connective tissue of the mediastinum, is connected to the cephalic portion of the **epididymis** by 10–20 **ductuli efferentes** (Fig 22–1).

The seminiferous tubules consist of a tunic of fibrous connective tissue, a well-defined basal lamina,

and a complex **germinal,** or **seminiferous, epithelium** (Figs 22–2 and 22–3).

The fibrous **tunica propria** enveloping the seminiferous tubule consists of several layers of fibroblasts. The innermost layer adhering to the basal lamina consists of flattened **myoid cells,** which exhibit smooth muscle characteristics.

The epithelium consists of 2 types of cells: **Sertoli,** or **supporting, cells** and cells that constitute the **spermatogenic lineage.** The cells of spermatogenic lineage are stacked in 4–8 layers that occupy the space between the basal lamina and the lumen of the tubule. These cells divide several times and finally differentiate, producing spermatozoa. They represent various stages in the continuous process of differentiation of the male germ cells. This phenomenon, from start to finish, is called **spermatogenesis** and can be divided into 3 phases: **spermatocytogenesis** (from Greek, *sperma,* seed, + *kytos* + *genesis*), during which spermatogonia divide, producing successive generations of cells that finally give rise to **spermatocytes; meiosis,** during which the spermatocyte goes through 2 successive divisions, with reduction by half of the number of chromosomes and amount of DNA per cell, producing **spermatids;** and **spermiogenesis,** during which the spermatids go through an elaborate process of cytodifferentiation, producing **spermatozoa.**

The process begins with a primitive germ cell, the **spermatogonium,** situated next to the basal lamina. It is a relatively small cell, about 12 μm in diameter, and its nucleus contains pale-staining chromatin (Fig 22–3). At sexual maturity, this cell undergoes a series of mitoses, and the newly formed cells can follow one of 2 paths: they can continue, after one or more mitotic divisions, as undifferentiated stem cells (**type A spermatogonia** [*sperma* + Greek, *gone,* generation]), or they can differentiate during progressive mitotic cycles to become **type B spermatogonia.**

Type B spermatogonia give rise to the **primary spermatocytes** (Fig 22–7). Soon after their formation, these cells enter the prophase of the first meiotic division. At this point, the primary spermatocyte has 46 (44 + XY) chromosomes and 4N of DNA. (N denotes either the haploid set of chromosomes [23 chromosomes in humans] or the amount of DNA in this set.) In this prophase, the cell passes through 4 stages—leptotene, zygotene, pachytene, and diplotene—and reaches the stage of diakinesis, resulting in the separation of the chromosomes. The crossing over of genes of the chromosomes occurs during these stages of meiosis. The cell then enters the metaphase, and the chromosomes move toward each pole in the following anaphase. Since the prophase of this division takes

about 22 days, the majority of cells seen in sections will be in this phase. The primary spermatocytes are the largest cells of the spermatogenic lineage and are characterized by the presence of chromosomes in different stages of the coiling process within their nuclei.

From this first meiotic division come smaller cells called **secondary spermatocytes** (Fig 22–3) with only 23 chromosomes (22 + X or 22 + Y). This decrease in number (from 46 to 23) is accompanied by a reduction in the amount of DNA per cell (from 4N to 2N). Secondary spermatocytes are difficult to observe in sections of the testis because they are short-lived cells that remain in interphase very briefly and quickly enter into the second meiotic division. Division of the secondary spermatocytes results in spermatids, cells that contain 23 chromosomes. Because no S phase (DNA synthesis) occurs between the first and second meiotic divisions of the spermatocytes, the amount of DNA per cell is reduced by half in this second division, forming haploid (1N) cells. The meiotic process therefore results in the formation of cells with a haploid number of chromosomes. With fertilization, they return to the normal diploid number. It is the meiotic process that, because of the reductional process of cell division, guarantees a constant (fixed) number of chromosomes for the species.

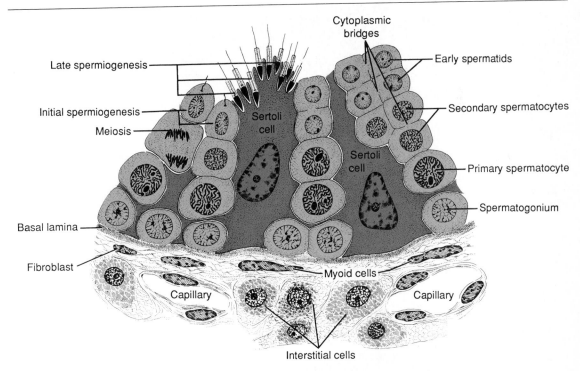

Figure 22–3. Diagram of the structure of part of a seminiferous tubule and interstitial tissue. This figure does not show the lymphatic vessels found in the connective tissue.

Spermiogenesis

Spermatids are the cells that result from the division of secondary spermatocytes. They can be distinguished by their small size (7–8 μm in diameter), nuclei with areas of condensed chromatin, and juxtaluminal location within the seminiferous tubules (Fig 22–3). Spermatids undergo **spermiogenesis,** a complex process of differentiation that includes formation of the acrosome (from Greek, *akron,* extremity, + *soma*), condensation and elongation of the nucleus, development of the flagellum, and the loss of much of the cytoplasm. The end result is the mature spermatozoon, which is then released into the lumen of the seminiferous tubule.

Spermiogenesis can be divided into 3 phases (Figs 22–4 and 22–5).

A. The Golgi Phase: The cytoplasm of spermatids contains a prominent Golgi complex near the nucleus, mitochondria, a pair of centrioles, free ribosomes, and tubules of smooth endoplasmic reticulum. Small PAS-positive proacrosomal granules accumulate in the Golgi complex and subsequently coalesce to form a single **acrosomal granule** contained within a membrane-limited **acrosomal vesicle.** The centrioles migrate to a position near the cell surface and opposite the location of the forming acrosome. Formation of the flagellar axoneme is initiated, and the centrioles migrate back toward the nucleus, spinning out the axonemal components as they move.

B. The Acrosomal Phase: The acrosomal vesicle and granule spread to cover the anterior half of the condensing nucleus and are now known as the **acrosome.** The acrosome contains several hydrolytic enzymes, such as hyaluronidase, neuraminidase, acid phosphatase, and a protease that has trypsinlike activity. The acrosome thus serves as a specialized type of lysosome. These enzymes are known to dissociate cells of the corona radiata and to digest the zona pellucida, structures that surround recently ovulated eggs (Fig 23–3). When spermatozoa encounter ova, the outer membrane of the acrosome fuses with the plasma membrane at multiple sites, liberating the acrosomal enzymes. This process, the **acrosomal reaction,** is one of the first steps in fertilization.

During this phase the anterior pole of the cell, containing the acrosome, becomes oriented toward the base of the seminiferous tubule. In addition, the nucleus becomes more elongated and condensed. This process may be facilitated by a cylinder of microtubules, the **manchette,** that surrounds the nucleus (Fig 22–5). One of the centrioles grows concomitantly, forming the **flagellum.** The mitochondria aggregate around the proximal part of the flagellum, forming a thickened region known as the **middle piece,** the region where the movements of the spermatozoa are generated.

This disposition of mitochondria is another example of a concentration of these organelles in sites

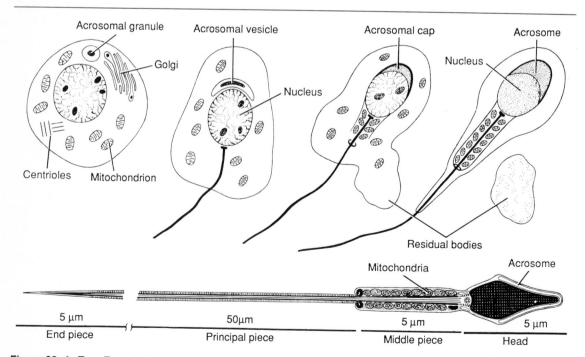

Figure 22–4. Top: The principal changes occurring in spermatids during spermiogenesis. The basic structural feature of the spermatozoon is the head, which consists primarily of condensed nuclear chromatin. The reduced volume of the nucleus permits the sperm greater mobility and may protect the genome from damage while in transit to the egg. The rest of the spermatozoon is structurally arranged to provide motility. **Bottom:** The structure of a spermatozoon.

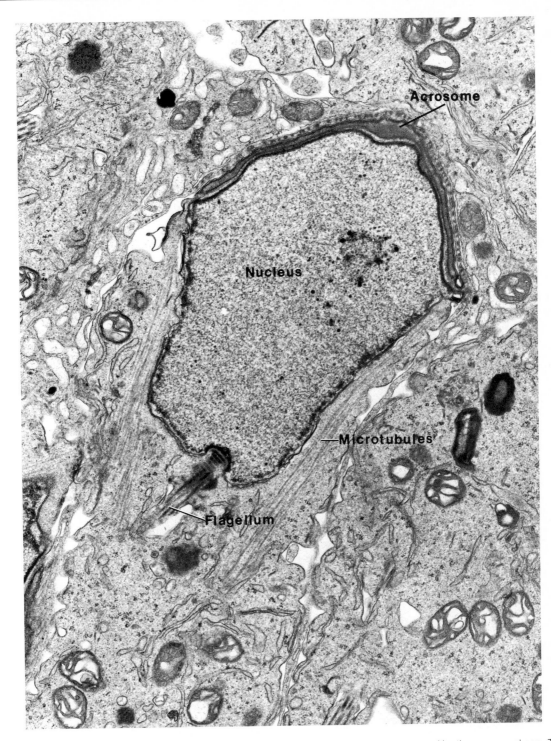

Figure 22–5. Electron micrograph of a mouse spermatid. In the center is its nucleus, covered by the acrosomal cap. The flagellum can be seen emerging in the lower region below the nucleus. A cylindrical bundle of microtubules, the manchette, limits the nucleus laterally. × 15,000. (Courtesy of KR Porter.)

related to cell movement and high energy consumption. (Flagellar structure and function are described in Chapter 3.) Movement of the flagellum is a result of the interaction among microtubules, ATP, and **dynein,** a protein with ATPase activity.

> **Immotile spermatozoa syndrome** is characterized by immotile spermatozoa and consequent infertility. It is due to a lack of dynein or other proteins required for flagellar motility in the patient's spermatozoa. This disorder is usually coincident with chronic respiratory infections, since a similar deficiency exists in the ciliary axonemes of respiratory epithelial cells.

C. The Maturation Phase: Residual cytoplasm is shed and phagocytized by Sertoli cells (Figs 22–4 and 22–9), and the spermatozoa are released into the lumen of the tubule. Mature spermatozoa are shown in Figs 22–4 and 22–6.

During division of the spermatogonia, the resulting cells do not separate completely but remain attached by cytoplasmic bridges. This concept is illustrated in Fig 22–7. The intercellular bridges provide communication between every primary and secondary spermatocyte and spermatid derived from a single spermatogonium. By permitting the interchange of information from cell to cell, these bridges play an important role in coordinating the sequence of events in spermatogenesis. This detail may be of importance in understanding the cycle of the seminiferous epithelium (described below). When the process of spermatogenesis is completed, the sloughing of the cytoplasm and cytoplasmic bridges as residual bodies leads to a separation of the spermatids.

Experimental injection of ^{3}H-thymidine into the testes of volunteers shows that, in men, the changes that occur between the spermatogonia stage and the formation of the spermatozoa take about 64 days. Aside from the slowness of the process, spermatogenesis occurs neither simultaneously nor synchronously in all the seminiferous tubules, but occurs instead in wavelike fashion. This explains the irregular appearance of the tubules, where each region exhibits a different phase of spermatogenesis. It also explains why spermatozoa are encountered in some regions of the seminiferous tubules while only spermatids are found in others. The **cycle of the seminiferous epithelium** refers to the sequence of maturation changes occurring in a given area of the germinal epithelium between 2 successive appearances of a given cell stage. In the human, each cycle lasts 16 ± 1 days, and spermatogenesis ends about 4 cycles (64 ± 4.5 days) later. The seminiferous cycle

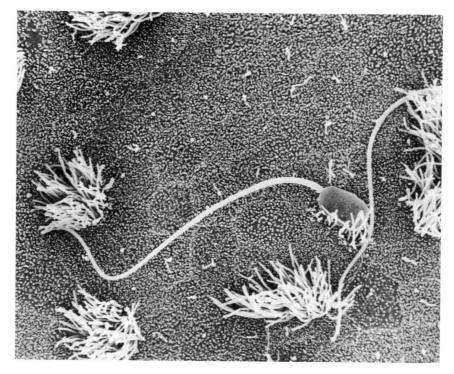

Figure 22–6. Spermatozoon in the uterine cavity of a rodent seen using scanning electron microscopy. The tufts are ciliated cells. × 2000. (Reproduced with permission, from Motta P, Andrews PM, Porter KR. *Microanatomy of Cell and Tissue Surfaces: An Atlas of Scanning Electron Microscopy.* Lea & Febiger, 1977. Copyright © Societa Editrice Libraria [Milan].)

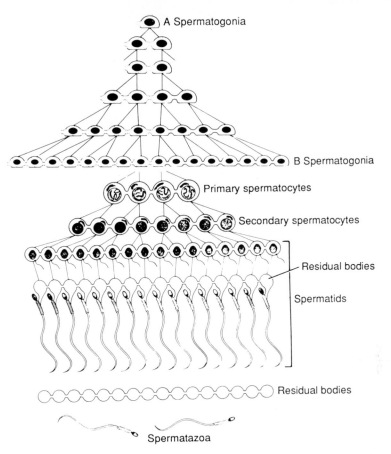

Figure 22–7. Diagram showing the clonal nature of the germ cells. Only the initial spermatogonia divide and produce separate daughter cells. Once committed to differentiation, the cells of all subsequent divisions are connected by intercellular cytoplasmic bridges. Only after they are separated from the residual bodies can the spermatozoa be considered isolated individuals. The actual number of cells is greater than shown in this figure. See the text for the function of the intercellular bridges. (Reproduced, with permission, from Bloom W, Fawcett DW. *A Textbook of Histology,* 10th ed. Saunders, 1975.)

is clearly seen in rodents, in which 12 stages have been described. In men, 6 stages are known to occur, but their occurrence is not as easily visualized. Fig 22–8 shows the sequence of stages in the human testis.

Sertoli Cells

The **Sertoli cells** are elongated pyramidal cells that partially envelop cells of the spermatogenic lineage. The bases of the Sertoli cells adhere to the basal lamina, while their apical ends frequently extend into the lumen of the seminiferous tubule. In the light microscope, Sertoli cell outlines appear poorly defined because of the numerous lateral processes that surround spermatogenic cells (Figs 22–3 and 22–9). Studies with the electron microscope reveal that these cells contain abundant smooth endoplasmic reticulum, some rough endoplasmic reticulum, a

well-developed Golgi complex, and numerous mitochondria and lysosomes. The elongated nucleus, which is often triangular in outline, possesses numerous infoldings and a prominent nucleolus; it exhibits little heterochromatin (Figs 22–8 and 22–9).

Adjacent Sertoli cells are bound together by occluding junctions at the level of the spermatogonia, which lie in a **basal compartment** that has free access to materials found in blood. During spermatogenesis, progeny of spermatogonia somehow traverse these junctions and come to lie in the **adluminal compartment.** Here, the more advanced stages of spermatogenesis are protected from blood-borne products by a **blood-testis barrier** formed by the occluding junctions between Sertoli cells. Spermatocytes and spermatids lie within deep invaginations of the lateral and apical margins of the Sertoli cells. As the flagellar tails of the spermatids develop, they ap-

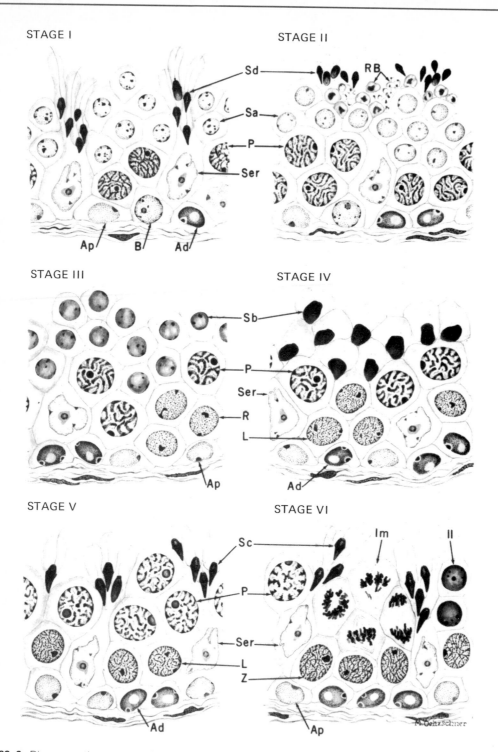

Figure 22–8. Diagrammatic representation showing the 6 recognizable cell associations corresponding to the stages of the cycle of the human seminiferous epithelium. Ser, Sertoli cell; Ad and Ap, dark and pale type A spermatogonia; B, type B spermatogonia; R, resting primary spermatocyte; L, leptotene spermatocyte; Z, zygotene spermatocyte; P, pachytene spermatocyte; Im, primary spermatocyte in division; II, secondary spermatocyte in interphase; Sa, Sb, and Sd, spermatids in various stages of differentiation; RB, residual bodies of Regnaud. (Reproduced, with permission, from Clermont Y: *Am J Anat* 1963;**112**:35.)

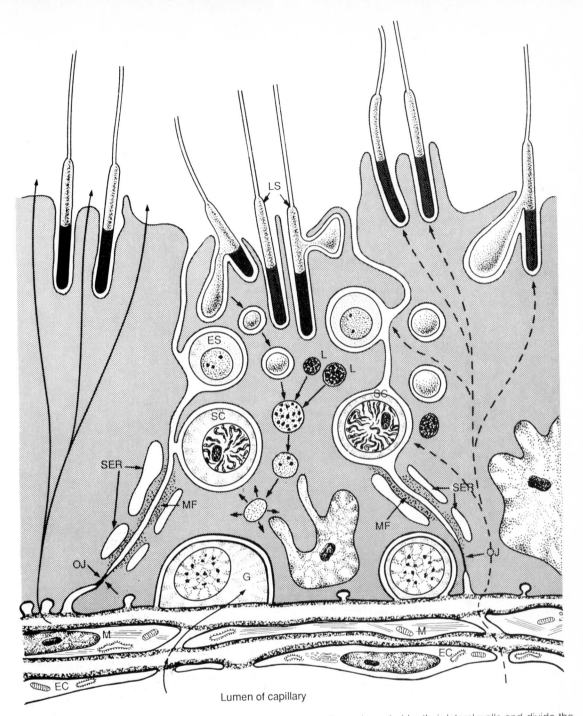

Figure 22–9. The position and functions of Sertoli cells. These cells are bounded by their lateral walls and divide the seminiferous tubules into 2 compartments. The lower part is the basal compartment and comprises the lumen of the blood vessels, the interstitial space, and the regions occupied by the spermatogonia (G). The second (upper) part represents the adluminal compartment of the seminiferous tubules, down to the level of the occluding junctions (OJ). The arrows pointing to the occluding junctions show the zones where the membranes converge and impede the passage of substances from the first to the second compartment. Above the junctional membrane, specialized regions are characterized by the presence of circularly disposed microfilaments (MF) and of cisternae of the smooth endoplasmic reticulum (SER). Some functions of Sertoli cells are also portrayed. In the cell at left, the arrows indicate the secretion of testicular fluid. In the middle cell, cytoplasmic residual bodies from the forming spermatids undergo phagocytosis and are digested by lysosomes (L). In the cell at right, the dotted arrows indicate the transport of metabolites from the extracellular space to the spermatocytes (SC) and the early (ES) and late (LS) spermatids and spermatozoa. Observe that the transport of material from the basal compartment to the lumen and spermatogenic cells passes through the Sertoli cells. Note also the myoid cells (M) and the endothelial cells (EC).

pear as tufts extending from the apical ends of the Sertoli cells. Sertoli cells are also connected by gap junctions that provide ionic and chemical coupling of the cells; this may be important in coordinating the cycle of the seminiferous epithelium described above.

Sertoli cells have at least 4 main functions:

(1) Support, protection, and nutritional regulation of the developing spermatozoa. As mentioned above, the cells of the spermatogenic series are interconnected via cytoplasmic bridges. This network of cells is physically supported by extensive cytoplasmic ramifications of the Sertoli cells. Because spermatocytes, spermatids, and spermatozoa are isolated from the blood supply by the blood-testis barrier, these spermatogenic cells depend upon the Sertoli cells to mediate the exchange of nutrients and metabolites. The Sertoli cell barrier also protects the developing sperm cells from immunologic attack (discussed below).

(2) Phagocytosis. During spermiogenesis, excess spermatid cytoplasm is shed as residual bodies. These cytoplasmic fragments are phagocytized and broken down by Sertoli cell lysosomes.

(3) Secretion. Sertoli cells continuously secrete into the seminiferous tubules a fluid that flows in the direction of the genital ducts and is utilized for sperm transport. Secretion of an androgen-binding protein by Sertoli cells is under the control of FSH and tes-

tosterone and serves to concentrate testosterone in the seminiferous tubule, where it is necessary for spermatogenesis. Sertoli cells can convert testosterone to estradiol. They also secrete a peptide called **inhibin,** which suppresses FSH synthesis and release in the anterior pituitary gland.

(4) Production of the anti-Müllerian hormone. This hormone is a glycoprotein that acts during embryonic development to promote regression of the Müllerian ducts in the male fetus. Immunocytochemistry has revealed its presence in immature Sertoli cells of various mammals, including humans.

Sertoli cells in humans and other animals do not divide during the reproductive period. They are extremely resistant to such adverse conditions as infection, malnutrition, and x-ray irradiation and survive these insults much better than do cells of the spermatogenic lineage.

In mammals, the release of spermatozoa probably occurs as a result of cellular movements, with the participation of microtubules and microfilaments present in the Sertoli cell apex.

Interstitial Tissue

The spaces between the seminiferous tubules in the testis are filled with accumulations of connective tissue, nerves, blood, and lymphatic vessels. Testicular capillaries are fenestrated and permit the free passage of macromolecules such as the blood pro-

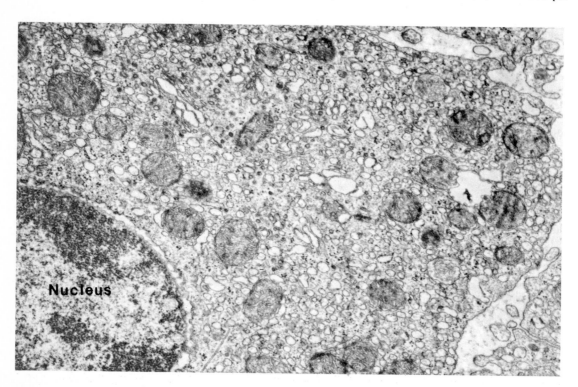

Figure 22–10. Electron micrograph of a section of an interstitial cell from the testis of a rat. There are abundant mitochondria and vesicles of smooth endoplasmic reticulum. × 12,000.

teins. The extensive network of lymphatic vessels present in the interstitial space explains the similarity of composition between the interstitial fluid and lymph collected from this organ. The connective tissue consists of various cell types, including fibroblasts, undifferentiated connective cells, mast cells, and macrophages. During puberty, an additional cell type becomes apparent that is either rounded or polygonal in shape and which has a central nucleus and an eosinophilic cytoplasm rich in small lipid droplets (Figs 22–3 and 22–10). These are the **interstitial,** or **Leydig, cells** of the testis, which have the characteristics of steroid-secreting cells (described in Chapter 4). These cells produce the male hormone **testosterone,** responsible for the development of the secondary male sex characteristics. A direct correlation is thus observed between the presence of interstitial cells and the production of androgen by the testis. The presence in the interstitial cells of enzymes necessary for the synthesis of testosterone has been demonstrated with histochemical and biochemical methods. Cholesterol, stored in lipid droplets or newly synthesized from acetate, is the substrate for side-chain cleaving enzymes located in interstitial cell mitochondria. The product of this reaction is pregnenolone, which is subjected to a series of reactions—culminating in testosterone synthesis—that are mediated by enzymes located in the smooth endoplasmic reticulum (Fig 22–11).

Both the activity and the quantity of the interstitial cells depend on hormonal stimuli. During human pregnancy, placental gonadotropic hormone passes from the maternal blood to the fetus, stimulating the abundant fetal testicular interstitial cells that produce androgenic hormones. The presence of these hormones is required for the embryonic differentiation of the male genitalia. The embryonic interstitial cells remain fully differentiated up to 4½ months of gestation; they then regress, with an associated decrease in testosterone synthesis. They remain quiescent throughout the rest of the pregnancy and up to the prepubertal period, when they resume testosterone synthesis in response to the stimulus of luteinizing hormone from the hypophysis.

Histophysiology

Temperature is very important in the regulation of spermatogenesis, which occurs only at temperatures below the core body temperature of 37 °C. Testicular temperature is about 35 °C and is controlled by several mechanisms. A rich venous plexus (the **pampiniform plexus**) surrounds each testicular artery and forms a countercurrent heat-exchange system that is important in maintaining the testicular temperature. Other factors are evaporation of sweat from the scrotum, which contributes to heat loss, and contraction of cremaster muscles of the spermatic cords, which pull the testes into the inguinal canals, where their temperature can be increased.

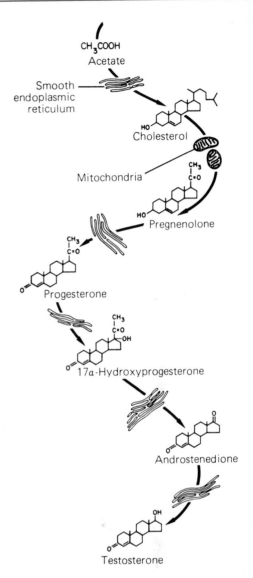

Figure 22–11. A schematic representation of the steps in the conversion of acetate to testosterone. All the enzymes are present in the microsomal fraction (smooth endoplasmic reticulum) except the cholesterol side-chain cleaving enzymes, which are found in the mitochondria. (Reproduced, with permission, from Dym M: The male reproductive system. In: *Histology: Cell and Tissue Biology,* 5th ed. Weiss L [editor]. Elsevier, 1983.)

Failure of descent of the testis (**cryptorchidism** [from Greek, *kryptos*, hidden, + *orchis*, testis]) maintains the testes at the core temperature of 37 °C, which inhibits spermatogenesis. In cases that are not too far advanced, spermatogenesis can occur normally if the testes are moved surgically to the scrotum. Although germ cell proliferation is inhibited by abdominal tempera-

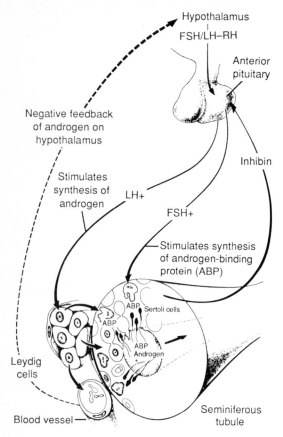

Hypothalamus
FSH/LH–RH

Anterior
pituitary

Negative feedback
of androgen on
hypothalamus

Inhibin

Stimulates
synthesis of
androgen

LH+

FSH+

Stimulates synthesis
of androgen-binding
protein (ABP)

ABP Sertoli cells

ABP

ABP
Androgen

Leydig
cells

Blood vessel

Seminiferous
tubule

Figure 22–12. Diagram of the hypophyseal control of male reproduction. Luteinizing hormone (LH) acts upon the Leydig cells, and follicle-stimulating hormone (FSH) acts upon the seminiferous tubules. A testicular hormone called inhibin inhibits FSH secretion in the pituitary. (Modified and reproduced, with permission, from Bloom W, Fawcett DW: *A Textbook of Histology,* 10th ed. Saunders, 1975.)

Without doubt, however, endocrine factors have the most important effect on spermatogenesis. Spermatogenesis depends on the action of the follicle-stimulating (FSH) and luteinizing (LH) hormones of the hypophysis on the testicular cells. LH acts on the interstitial cells, stimulating the production of testosterone necessary for the normal development of cells of the spermatogenic lineage. FSH is known to act on the Sertoli cells, stimulating adenylate cyclase and consequently increasing the presence of cAMP; it also promotes the synthesis and secretion of **androgen-binding protein (ABP).** This protein combines with testosterone and transports it into the lumen of the seminiferous tubules (Fig 22–12). Spermatogenesis is stimulated by testosterone and inhibited by estrogens and progestogens. The mechanisms of endocrine control are shown in Fig 22–12.

Spermatozoa are transported to the epididymis in an appropriate medium, **testicular fluid,** produced by the Sertoli cells and rete testis. This fluid contains steroids, proteins, ions, and androgen-binding protein associated with testosterone.

Blood-Testis Barrier

The existence of a barrier between the blood and the interior of the seminiferous tubules accounts for the observation of few substances from the blood in the testicular fluid. (The testicular capillaries are of the fenestrated type and permit free passage of large molecules.) The occluding junctions between Sertoli cells are responsible for this barrier, which is of importance in protecting male germ cells against blood-borne noxious agents.

> Differentiation of spermatogonial cells leads to the appearance of sperm-specific proteins. Since sexual maturity occurs long after the development of immunocompetence, differentiating sperm cells could be recognized as foreign and provoke an immune response that would destroy the germ cells. The blood-testis barrier would eliminate any interaction between developing sperm and the immune system. This barrier prevents the passage of immunoglobulins into the seminiferous tubule and would account for the absence of any impairment of fertility in patients whose serum possesses high levels of sperm antibodies. The Sertoli cell barrier thus functions in protecting the seminiferous epithelium against an autoimmune reaction.

INTRATESTICULAR GENITAL DUCTS

The intratesticular genital ducts are the **tubuli recti** (straight tubules), the **rete testis,** and the **ductuli efferentes** (Fig 22–1). Most seminiferous tubules are in the form of loops, both ends of which join the rete testis by structures known as **tubuli recti.** These tu-

ture, testosterone synthesis is not. This explains why individuals with cryptorchidism can be sterile but still develop secondary male characteristics and achieve erection.

Malnutrition, alcoholism, and the action of certain drugs lead to alterations in spermatogonia, with a consequent decreased production of spermatozoa. X-ray irradiation and cadmium salts are quite toxic to the cells of spermatogenic lineage, causing the death of those cells and sterility in animals. The drug busulfan acts on the germinal cells; when administered to pregnant female rats, it promotes the death of the germinal cells of their male offspring. The offspring are therefore sterile, and their seminiferous tubules contain only Sertoli cells. Androgen-producing interstitial cell tumors can cause precocious puberty in males.

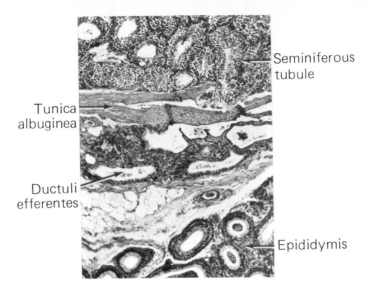

Figure 22–13. Photomicrograph of a section of testis showing the ductuli efferentes, the thick tunica albuginea, and the epididymis. H&E stain, × 80.

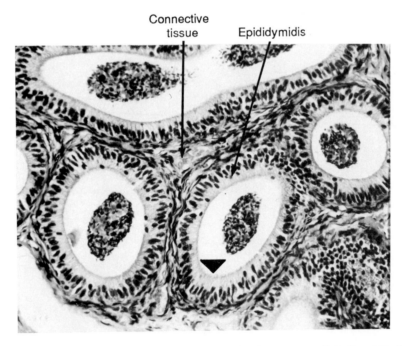

Figure 22–14. Photomicrograph of a section of epididymis showing its structure. Note the epithelium of the ductus epididymidis, the connective tissue, and the stereocilia (arrow head). Note aggregates of spermatozoa in the lumen of the duct. H&E stain, × 200.

bules are recognized by the gradual loss of spermatogenic cells, with an initial part in which only Sertoli cells remain to form their walls, followed by a main segment consisting of cuboidal epithelium supported by a dense connective tissue sheath.

Tubuli recti empty into the **rete testis,** contained within the mediastinum, a thickening of the tunica albuginea. The rete testis is a highly anastomotic network of channels lined with cuboidal epithelium.

From the rete testis extend 10–20 **ductuli efferentes** (Figs 22–1 and 22–13). They have an epithelium composed of groups of nonciliated cuboidal cells alternating with ciliated cells that beat in the direction of the epididymis. This gives the epithelium a characteristic scalloped appearance. The nonciliated cells absorb much of the fluid secreted by the seminiferous tubules. Ciliated cell activity and fluid absorption create a fluid flow that sweeps spermatozoa toward the epididymis. A thin layer of circularly oriented smooth muscle cells is seen outside the basal lamina of the epithelium. The ductuli efferentes gradually fuse to form the **ductus epididymidis** of the epididymis (Fig 22–1).

EXCRETORY GENITAL DUCTS

The ducts that transport the spermatozoa produced in the testis toward the penile meatus are the ductus epididymidis, the ductus deferens (vas deferens), and the urethra.

The **ductus epididymidis** is a single highly coiled tube about 4–6 m in length. This long canal forms, with surrounding connective tissue and blood vessels, the body and tail of the **epididymis.** It is lined by pseudostratified columnar epithelium composed of rounded basal cells and columnar cells. These cells are supported on a basal lamina surrounded by smooth muscle cells whose peristaltic contractions help to move the sperm along the duct and by loose connective tissue rich in blood capillaries (Fig 22–14). Their surface is covered by long, branched, irregular microvilli called **stereocilia.** These cells secrete glycerophosphocholine, which may inhibit **capacitation,** a process that prepares spermatozoa for fertilization. The epithelium of the ductus epididymidis participates in the uptake and digestion of residual bodies that are eliminated during spermatogenesis.

From the epididymis the **ductus (vas) deferens,** a straight tube with a thick, muscular wall, continues toward the prostatic urethra and empties into it (Fig 22–1). It is characterized by a narrow lumen and a thick layer of smooth muscle (Fig 22–15). Its mucosa forms longitudinal folds and is covered along most of its extent by pseudostratified columnar epithelium with stereocilia. The lamina propria is a layer of connective tissue rich in elastic fibers, and the thick muscular layer consists of longitudinal inner and outer layers separated by a circular layer. The ductus deferens forms part of the spermatic cord, which includes the testicular artery, the pampiniform plexus, and nerves. The spermatic cord is surrounded by lon-

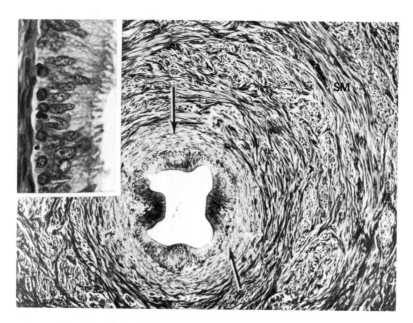

Figure 22–15. Photomicrograph of a section of ductus deferens. The ductus has a thick wall formed by smooth muscle cells (SM). The arrows point to the thin lamina propria. × 16. Observe in the inset the details of the pseudostratified columnar epithelium with aggregated stereocilia. × 400.

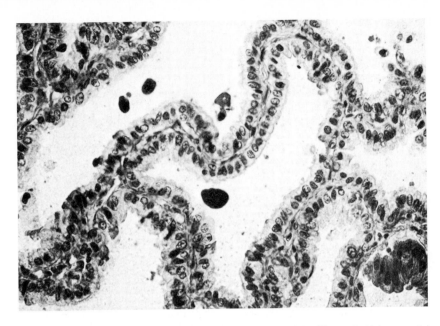

Figure 22–16. Photomicrograph of a section of human seminal vesicle. Masson's trichrome stain, × 300.

gitudinally oriented fibers of skeletal cremaster muscle. Before it enters the prostate, the ductus deferens dilates, forming a region called the **ampulla.** In this area, the epithelium becomes thicker and extensively folded. At the final portion of the ampulla, the seminal vesicles join the duct. From there on, the ductus deferens enters the prostate, opening into the prostatic urethra. The segment entering the prostate is called the **ejaculatory duct.** While the mucous layer of the ductus deferens continues through the ampulla into the ejaculatory duct, the muscle layer ends after the ampulla.

ACCESSORY GENITAL GLANDS

The accessory genital glands are the seminal vesicles, the prostate gland, and the bulbourethral glands.

The **seminal vesicles** consist of 2 highly tortuous tubes 15 cm in length; they are not reservoirs for spermatozoa. When the organ is sectioned, the same tube is observed in different orientations. It has a folded mucosa lined with pseudostratified columnar epithelium rich in secretory granules. They have ultrastructural characteristics of protein-synthesizing cells (see Chapter 4). The lamina propria of the seminal vesicles is rich in elastic fibers and surrounded by a thin layer of smooth muscle (Fig 22–16). The viscid, yellowish secretion of the seminal vesicles contains spermatozoa-activating substances such as fructose, citrate, inositol, prostaglandins, and several proteins. Carbohydrates produced by the glands as-

sociated with the male reproductive system and secreted in the seminal fluid are the source of energy for sperm motility. The monosaccharide **fructose** is the most abundant of these carbohydrates. Seventy percent of human ejaculate originates from the seminal vesicles. The height of the epithelial cells of the seminal vesicles and the degree of activity of the secretory processes are testosterone-dependent.

The **prostate** is a collection of 30–50 branched tubuloalveolar glands whose ducts empty into the prostatic urethra. The prostate produces prostatic fluid and stores it in its interior for expulsion during ejaculation. The prostate is surrounded by a fibroelastic capsule rich in smooth muscle. Septa from this capsule penetrate the gland and divide it into lobes that

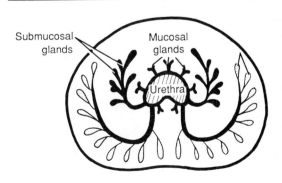

Figure 22–17. Diagram illustrating the position of the prostatic glands.

are indistinct in the adult male. An exceptionally rich fibromuscular stroma surrounds the glands.

From the biomedical point of view, the prostate has two distinct groups of glands. One group is localized more in the anterior and lateral portion of the urethra just below its lining epithelium (the **mucosal glands**). The other portion (**submucosal** and **main glands**) occupies the rest of the gland (Fig 22–17). The main glands contribute most to the volume of the prostatic secretion.

> **Benign prostatic hypertrophy,** which is present in 50% of men more than 50 years of age, progresses gradually to 95% who are older than 70. It leads to obstruction of the urethra with clinical symptoms in only 5–10% of the cases and is caused by hyperplasia of the mucosal glands. The submucosal and main glands are the source of malignant cells which cause carcinoma of the prostate. This is the second most common form of cancer in males and the third leading cause of cancer-related mortality.

Small spherical bodies of glycoprotein composition, 0.2–2 mm in diameter, are frequently observed in the lumen of prostatic glands. They are called **prostatic concretions,** or **corpora amylacea** (Fig 22–18). These bodies are often calcified. Their significance is not understood, but their number increases with age.

The **bulbourethral glands (Cowper's glands),** 3–5 mm in diameter, are located proximal to the membranous portion of the urethra and empty into it. They are tubuloalveolar glands lined with mucus-secreting simple cuboidal epithelium. Skeletal and smooth muscle cells are present in the septa that divide each gland into lobes. The secretion is a clear mucus that acts as a lubricant.

PENIS

The penis consists mainly of 3 cylindrical masses of erectile tissue, plus the urethra, surrounded externally by skin. Two of these cylinders—the **corpora**

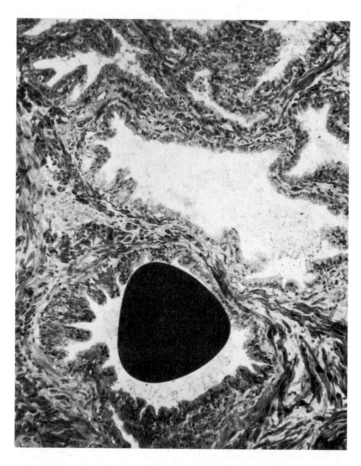

Figure 22–18. Section of a prostate, showing its epithelium, smooth muscle fibers, and a typical prostatic concretion (corpus amylaceum). H&E stain, × 300.

cavernosa of the penis—are placed dorsally. The other, ventrally located, is called the **corpus cavernosum of the urethra,** or **corpus spongiosum,** and surrounds the urethra. At its end it dilates, forming the **glans penis** (Fig 22–1). The corpora cavernosa are covered by a resistant layer of dense connective tissue, the **tunica albuginea** (Fig 22–19). The corpora cavernosa of the penis and urethra are composed of erectile tissue—venous spaces lined by unfenestrated endothelial cells and separated by trabeculae that consist of connective tissue fibers and smooth muscle cells.

The prepuce is a retractile fold of skin that contains connective tissue with smooth muscle in its interior. Sebaceous glands are present in the internal fold and in the skin that covers the glans.

Most of the penile urethra is lined with pseudostratified columnar epithelium; in the glans penis, it becomes stratified squamous epithelium. Mucus-secreting **glands of Littre** are found throughout the length of the penile urethra.

The arterial supply of the penis derives from the internal pudendal arteries, which give rise to the deep arteries and the dorsal arteries of the penis. The deep arteries branch to form nutritive and helicine arteries. The former supply oxygen and nutrients to the trabeculae, while the latter empty directly into the cavernous spaces (erectile tissue). There are arteriovenous shunts between helicine arteries and the deep dorsal vein.

Penile erection is a hemodynamic event that is controlled by neural input to both arterial muscle and smooth muscle in the walls of the vascular spaces in the penis; in the flaccid state, there is minimal blood flow in the penis. The nonerect state is maintained by both the intrinsic tone of penile smooth muscle and the tone induced by continuous sympathetic input. Erection occurs when vasodilator impulses of parasympathetic origin effect relaxation of the penile vessels and cavernous smooth muscle. Vasodilation also involves the concomitant inhibition of sympathetic vasoconstrictor impulses to penile tissues. Opening of the penile arteries and cavernous spaces accounts for the increase in blood flow, filling of the cavernous spaces, and the resultant rigidity of the penis.

After ejaculation and orgasm have been achieved, parasympathetic activity declines, allowing the penis to return to its flaccid state.

Tumors of the Male Reproductive System

Testicular tumors are derived mainly from germ cells, Leydig (interstitial) cells, or Sertoli cells. Interstitial cell tumors can secrete steroid hormone (androgens and estrogens), producing characteristic endocrine symptoms.

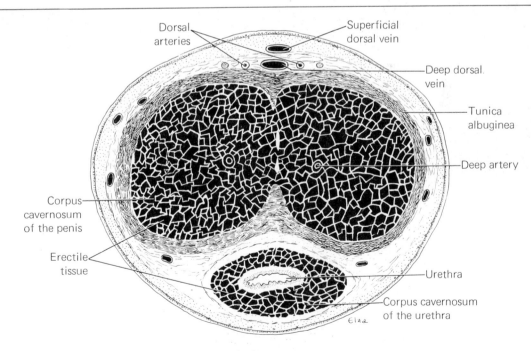

Figure 22–19. Drawing of a transverse section of the penis. (Redrawn and reproduced, with permission, from Leeson TS, Leeson CR: *Histology,* 2nd ed. Saunders, 1970.)

REFERENCES

Afzelius BA et al: Lack of dynein arms in immotile human spermatozoa. *J Cell Biol* 1975;**66**:225.

Dail WG: Autonomic control of penile erectile tissue. Pages 340–344 in: *Experimental Brain Research.* Series 16. Springer-Verlag, 1987.

Fawcett DW: The mammalian spermatozoon. *Dev Biol* 1975;**44**:394.

Hafez ESE, Spring-Mills E (editors): *Accessory Glands of the Male Reproductive Tract.* Ann Arbor Science Publishers, 1979.

Johnson AD, Gomes WR (editors): *The Testis.* Vols 1–4. Academic Press, 1970–1977.

Stambough R, Buckley J: Identification and subcellular localization of the enzymes affecting penetration of the zona pellucida of rabbit spermatozoa. *J. Reprod Fertil* 1969;**19**:423.

Tindall DJ et al: Structure and biochemistry of the Sertoli cell. *Int Rev Cytol* 1985;**94**:127.

Trainer TD: Histology of the normal testis. *Am J Surg Pathol* 1987;**11**:797.

The Female Reproductive System

The female reproductive system (Fig 23–1) consists of 2 ovaries, 2 oviducts (uterine tubes), the uterus, the vagina, and the external genitalia. Between menarche and menopause, the system undergoes cyclic changes in structure and functional activity. These modifications are controlled by neurohumoral mechanisms. **Menarche** is the time when the first menses occurs; **menopause** is a variable period during which the cyclic changes become irregular and eventually disappear altogether. In the postmenopausal period there is a slow involution of the reproductive system. Although the mammary glands do not belong to the genital system, we shall study them also, because they undergo changes directly connected with the functional state of the reproductive system.

OVARY

The ovary is an almond-shaped body approximately 3 cm long, 1.5 cm wide, and 1 cm thick. It consists of a **medullary region,** containing a rich vascular bed within a cellular loose connective tissue; and a **cortical region,** where ovarian follicles, containing the oocytes, predominate. There are no sharp limits between the cortical and medullary regions (Fig 23–2). After about the first month of embryonic life, primordial germ cells **(oogonia)** can be identified in the endodermal yolk sac. They divide mitotically several times while migrating to the genital ridges. Oogonia populate the cortex of the future ovary, and mitotic divisions continue until about the fifth month of fetal life. At this time, each ovary contains more than 3 million oogonia. Beginning in the third fetal month, some oogonia enter the prophase of the first meiotic division and become **primary oocytes** (from Greek, *oon,* egg, + *kytos*). In the human, this process is completed by the end of the seventh month of gestation. During this time, many primary oocytes are lost as a result of a degenerative process called **atresia.**

The stroma of the cortical region is composed of characteristic spindle-shaped fibroblasts that respond in a different way to hormonal stimuli than do fibroblasts of other organs. The surface of the ovary is covered by a simple squamous or cuboidal epithelium, the **germinal epithelium.** Under the germinal epithelium, the stroma forms the **tunica albuginea,** a poorly delineated layer of dense connective tissue. The tunica albuginea is responsible for the whitish color of the ovary (Fig 23–2).

Ovarian Follicles

Ovarian follicles are embedded in the stroma of the cortex. A follicle consists of an oocyte surrounded by one or more layers of follicular cells, the **granulosa cells.** There are several stages of follicular development (described below). The total number of follicles in the 2 ovaries of a normal young adult woman is estimated to be 400,000, but most of them will disappear through atresia during the reproductive years. This follicular regression begins before birth and continues over the entire span of reproductive life. After menopause, only a small number of follicles remain. Atresia can affect any type of follicle, from the primordial to those that are nearly mature. Since generally only one ovum is liberated by the ovaries in each menstrual cycle (average duration: 28 days) and the reproductive life of a woman lasts about 30–40 years, only about 450 ova are liberated. All the other follicles, with their oocytes, fail to mature; they become atretic and degenerate.

A. Primordial Follicles: The primordial follicles are most numerous before birth. Each consists of a primary oocyte enveloped by a single layer of flattened follicular cells (Fig 23–3).

The oocyte in the primordial follicle is a spherical cell about 25 μm in diameter. Its slightly eccentrically situated nucleus is large and has a large nucleolus. The chromosomes have become mostly uncoiled and do not stain intensely. The organelles in the cytoplasm tend to form a clump adjacent to the nucleus. There are numerous mitochondria, several Golgi complexes, and cisternae of endoplasmic reticulum. The squamous follicular cells contain endoplasmic reticulum, mitochondria, and lipid droplets. They are joined to one another by desmosomes. A basal lamina underlies the follicular cells and marks the boundary between the avascular follicle and the surrounding stroma.

B. Growing Follicles: Follicular growth involves mainly the follicular cells but also the primary oocyte and the stroma surrounding the follicle (Figs 23–2,

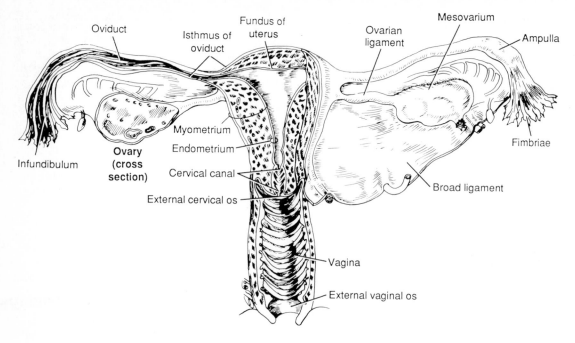

Figure 23–1. Internal organs of the female reproductive system.

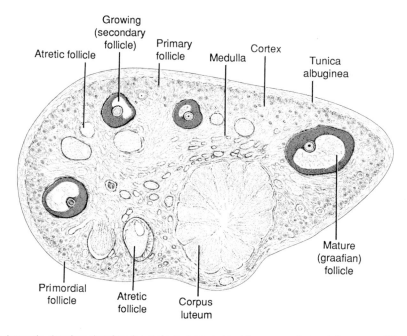

Figure 23–2. Schematic drawing showing the main components of the ovary of an adult woman. (Redrawn and reproduced, with permission, from Copenhaver WM, Bunge RP, Bunge MTS: *Bailey's Textbook of Histology,* 16th ed. Williams & Wilkins, 1972.)

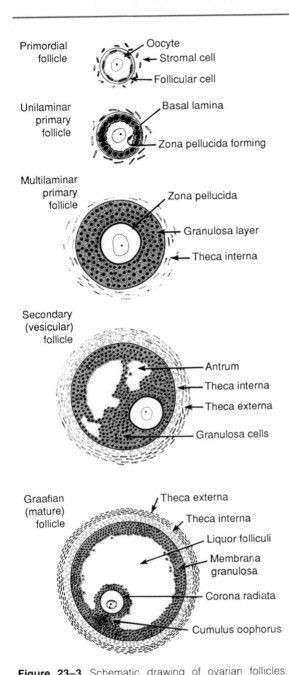

Primordial follicle — Oocyte, Stromal cell, Follicular cell

Unilaminar primary follicle — Basal lamina, Zona pellucida forming

Multilaminar primary follicle — Zona pellucida, Granulosa layer, Theca interna

Secondary (vesicular) follicle — Antrum, Theca interna, Theca externa, Granulosa cells

Graafian (mature) follicle — Theca externa, Theca interna, Liquor folliculi, Membrana granulosa, Corona radiata, Cumulus oophorus

Figure 23–3. Schematic drawing of ovarian follicles, starting with the primordial follicle and ending with mature follicles.

Follicular cells form a single layer of cuboidal cells, and the follicle is now called a **unilaminar primary follicle** (Fig 23–3). Follicular cells proliferate by mitosis and form a stratified follicular epithelium or **granulosa layer.** The follicle is now called a **multilaminar primary follicle** (Fig 23–3), and gap junctions are found between follicular cells. A thick coat, the **zona pellucida,** composed of at least 3 different glycoproteins, surrounds the oocyte (Figs 23–4, 23–5, and 23–6). It is thought that both the oocyte and follicular cells contribute to the synthesis of the zona pellucida. Filopodia of follicular cells and microvilli of the oocyte penetrate the zona pellucida and make contact with one another via gap junctions (Fig 23–5).

While these modifications are taking place, the stroma immediately around the follicle differentiates to form the **theca folliculi.** This layer subsequently differentiates into the **theca interna** and the **theca externa** (Figs 23–3 and 23–7). The cells of the theca (from Greek, *theke,* box) interna, when completely differentiated, have the same ultrastructural characteristics as cells that produce steroids. These characteristics include abundant profiles of smooth endoplasmic reticulum, mitochondria with tubular cristae, and numerous lipid droplets. Evidence suggests that these cells synthesize **androstenedione,** which is converted into estradiol by cells of the granulosa. Like all organs of endocrine function, the theca interna is richly vascularized. The theca externa consists mainly of connective tissue. Small vessels penetrate it and supply a rich capillary plexus around the secretory cells of the theca interna. There are no blood vessels in the granulosa cell layer during the stage of follicular growth. The boundary between the 2 thecas is not clear; neither is the boundary between the theca externa and the ovarian stroma. The boundary between the theca interna and the granulosa layer is well defined, since their cells are morphologically different and there is a thick basement membrane between them (Fig 23–7).

As the follicle grows—owing mainly to the increase in size and number of granulosa cells—accumulations of follicular fluid (**liquor folliculi**) appear between the cells. The cavities that contain this fluid coalesce and form a cavity, the **antrum** (Figs 23–3 and 23–4). These follicles are termed **secondary (vesicular) follicles** (Fig 23–3). Follicular fluid contains transudates of plasma and products secreted by follicular cells. Most inorganic ions are present in concentrations similar to those found in plasma. Glycosaminoglycans, several proteins (including steroid-binding proteins), and high concentrations of steroids (progesterone, androgens, and estrogens) are also present. The cells of the granulosa layer are more numerous at a certain point on the follicular wall, forming a small hillock of cells, the **cumulus oophorus,** which contains the oocyte. The cumulus oophorus protrudes toward the interior

23–3, and 23–4). Oocyte growth is most rapid during the first part of follicular growth, with this cell reaching a maximum diameter of 125–150 μm. The nucleus enlarges and is now called a **germinal vesicle.** Mitochondria increase in number and become uniformly distributed throughout the cytoplasm; the endoplasmic reticulum hypertrophies, and the Golgi complexes migrate to just beneath the cell surface.

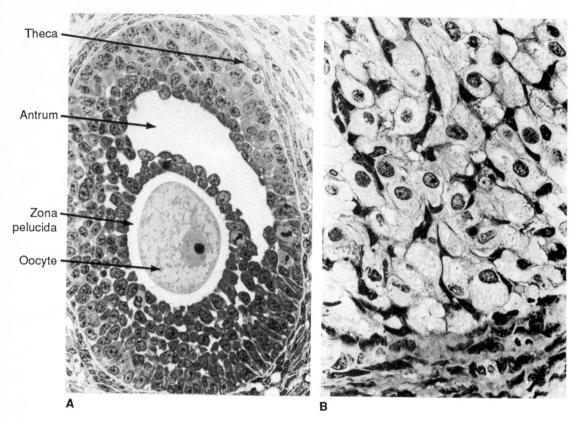

Figure 23–4. A: Developing ovarian follicle, showing the oocyte, zona pellucida, surrounding granulosa cells, theca cells and the antrum of the follicle. **B:** Corpus luteum contains lutein cells interspersed with capillaries. A portion of ovarian stroma is seen in the lower right of the micrograph.

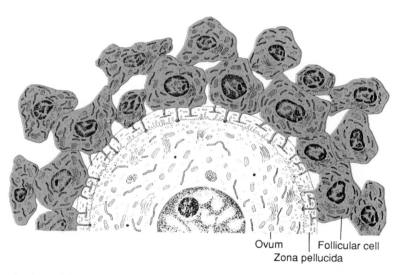

Figure 23–5. Ultrastructure of the ovum, zona pellucida, and follicular cells. The zona pellucida is composed of glycoproteins penetrated by oocyte microvilli and by longer processes from follicular cells (shown in color). In the cytoplasm of the ovum are annulate lamellae, arrays of parallel layers of membranes perforated by pores that resemble the nuclear envelope. The nucleus is in prophase of the first meiotic division.

Oocyte   Follicular cells

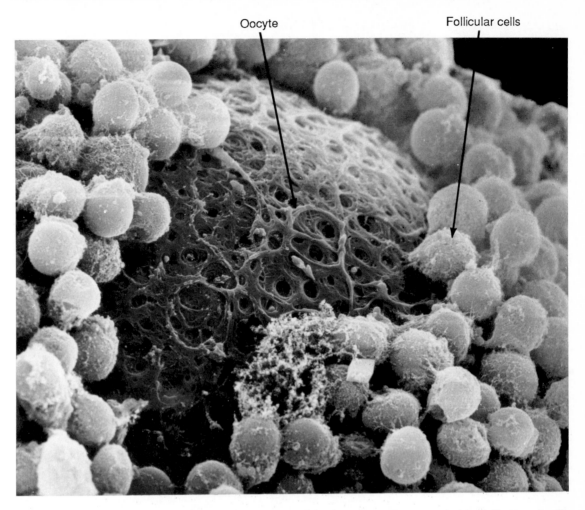

Figure 23–6. Scanning electron micrograph of dog ovary, showing an oocyte surrounded by follicular cells. The structure covering the oocyte is the zona pellucida, which appears as an irregular meshwork. × 2950.

of the antrum (Fig 23–3). The oocyte grows no more thereafter.

C. Mature Follicles: The **mature (graafian) follicle** is about 2.5 cm in diameter and can be seen as a transparent vesicle that bulges from the surface of the ovary. As a result of the accumulation of liquid, the follicular cavity increases in size, and the oocyte adheres to the wall of the follicle through a pedicle formed by granulosa cells. Since the granulosa cells do not multiply in proportion to the accumulation of liquid, the granulosa layer becomes thinner.

The granulosa cells that form the first layer around the ovum—and are, therefore, in close contact with the zona pellucida—become elongated and form the **corona radiata,** which accompanies the ovum when it leaves the ovary. The corona radiata is still present when the spermatozoon fertilizes the ovum; it is retained for some time during the passage of the ovum through the oviduct.

Follicular Atresia

Most ovarian follicles undergo follicular atresia, in which follicular cells and oocytes die and are disposed of by phagocytic cells. This process is characterized by cessation of mitosis in the granulosa cells, detachment of granulosa cells from the basal lamina, and death of the oocyte. Although follicular atresia takes place from before birth until a few years after the menopause, there are times at which it is particularly intense. It is greatly accentuated just after birth, when the effect of maternal hormones ceases, and during puberty and pregnancy, when marked qualitative and quantitative hormonal modifications take place. The process of atresia can take place during any stage in the development of a follicle.

Interstitial Glands

Although granulosa cells and the oocytes undergo degeneration during follicular atresia, the theca in-

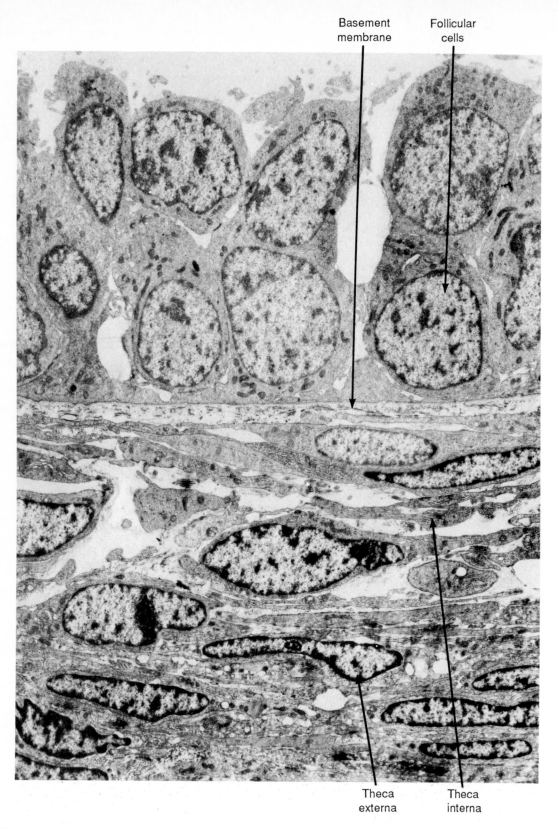

Basement
membrane

Follicular
cells

Theca
externa

Theca
interna

Figure 23–7. Electron micrograph of the wall of a growing ovarian follicle. In the upper part of the figure are several cuboidal follicular cells. A basement membrane separates these cells from the flattened cells of the theca interna. × 6400.

terna cells frequently persist and become active steroid secretors. These active thecal cells are called **interstitial cells.** Present from childhood through menopause, these cells are the source of ovarian androgens.

Ovulation

The process of ovulation consists of rupture of the mature follicle and liberation of the ovum, which will be caught by the dilated end of the oviduct. In the human female, usually only one ovum is liberated by the ovary at a time, but 2 or more can be expelled at the same time. In the latter case, if 2 or more of the liberated ova are fertilized, there may be more than one fetus (fraternal twins).

Ovulation takes place in approximately the middle of the menstrual cycle, ie, around the 14th day of a 28-day cycle. The mechanism of ovulation is still being investigated. Careful measurements have shown that there is no increase in intrafollicular pressure that could account for follicular rupture. Smooth muscle cells, which are present in the ovarian stroma, are probably not an important factor in ovulation. A current hypothesis invokes increased activity of proteases, such as collagenase and plasmin, which could cause dissolution of connective tissues around the follicle that will ovulate. In any case, a midcycle surge of luteinizing hormone (LH) concentration appears to be indispensable for ovulation.

Before ovulation, the ovum—together with the cells of the corona radiata—detaches itself from the wall of the follicle and floats in the follicular fluid. An indication of impending ovulation is the appearance on the surface of the follicle of the **stigma,** in which the flow of blood ceases, resulting in a local change in color and translucence of the follicular wall. The germinal epithelium in this area becomes discontinuous, and the stroma becomes thinner. The wall then ruptures and the ovum is released from the ovary together with the follicular liquid and blood.

The extremity of the oviduct that faces the ovary is funnel-shaped and fringed with numerous fingerlike processes called **fimbriae.** At the moment of ovulation, this end is very close to the surface of the ovary and receives the ovum. Promoted by muscle contraction and activity of ciliated cells, the ovum enters the infundibulum of the oviduct, where it may be fertilized. Once fertilized, the ovum, now called the **zygote** (from Greek, *zygotos,* yolked), begins to undergo cleavage and is transported to the uterus, a trip that lasts about 5 days. If the ovum is not fertilized within the first 24 hours after ovulation, it begins to degenerate.

Origin & Maturation of Oocytes

Oocytes are formed during intrauterine life, and their number does not increase after birth. The cells that are precursors of the oocytes, the **primordial germ cells,** originate in the endoderm of the yolk sac.

They migrate to the genital ridge and then into the developing ovary.

Primordial as well as growing follicles contain primary oocytes equivalent to primary spermatocytes of the seminiferous tubules (see Chapter 22). These oocytes are in the prophase of the first meiotic division.

The first meiotic division is completed just before ovulation. The chromosomes are equally divided between the daughter cells, but one of the secondary oocytes retains almost all of the cytoplasm. The other becomes the **first polar body,** a very small cell containing the nucleus and a minimal amount of cytoplasm.

Immediately after expulsion of the first polar body and while it is still in the cortical region of the ovary, the nucleus of the ovum starts the second meiotic division, which stops in metaphase and will be completed only when fertilization has taken place. Fertilization consists of penetration of the ovum by the spermatozoon (the fertilized ovum is called a zygote).

The ovum remains viable for an estimated maximum of 24 hours. Penetration by the sperm cell reconstitutes the diploid number of chromosomes typical of the species and serves as a stimulus for the ovum to complete the second meiotic division and

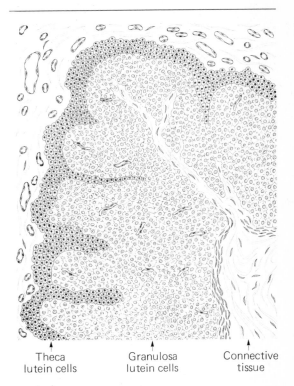

| Theca lutein cells | Granulosa lutein cells | Connective tissue |

Figure 23–8. Drawing of a small portion from a corpus luteum. Granulosa lutein cells derived from the granulosa layer are larger and less darkly stained than the theca lutein cells, which derive from the theca interna.

cast off the second polar body. When fertilization does not take place, the ovum undergoes autolysis in the oviduct without completing the second maturation division.

Corpus Luteum

After ovulation, the granulosa cells and those of the theca interna (Fig 23–7) that remain in the ovary form a temporary endocrine gland called the corpus luteum (yellow body) (Fig 23–8). The corpus luteum, which is localized in the cortical region of the ovary, secretes progesterone and estrogens. Progesterone prevents the development of new ovarian follicles and thus prevents ovulation.

Release of the follicular fluid results in collapse of the follicle's wall so that it becomes folded. Some blood flows into the follicular cavity, where it coagulates and is later invaded by connective tissue. This connective tissue, with remnants of blood clots that are gradually removed, remains as the most central part of the corpus luteum.

Although the granulosa cells do not divide after ovulation, they increase greatly in size (20–35 μm in diameter). They comprise about 80% of the parenchyma of the corpus luteum and are now called **granulosa lutein cells** (Fig 23–8), with the characteristics of steroid-secreting cells (Fig 23–4). This is in contrast to their structure in the preovulatory follicle, where they appear to be protein-secreting cells (Fig 23–7).

Cells of the theca interna also contribute to the formation of the corpus luteum by giving rise to **theca lutein cells** (Fig 23–8). These cells are similar in structure to granulosa lutein cells but are smaller (about 15 μm in diameter) and stain more intensely. They are located in the folds of the wall of the corpus luteum.

The blood capillaries and lymphatics of the theca interna grow into the interior of the corpus luteum and form the rich vascular network of this structure.

The corpus luteum is formed as a result of the stimulus provided by luteinizing hormone synthesized by the pars distalis of the pituitary under hypothalamic control. Since the progesterone produced by the corpus luteum has an inhibitory effect on the production of LH, the corpus luteum will soon degenerate unless it receives a stimulus from another source. This inhibitory effect of progesterone on luteinizing hormone production is indirect; it is mediated through the hypothalamus (Fig 23–9).

When pregnancy does not occur, the corpus luteum lasts only 10–14 days; ie, it persists only during the second half of the menstrual cycle. After this period, the lack of luteinizing hormone causes it to degenerate and disappear. This is the **corpus luteum of menstruation.**

When pregnancy occurs, **chorionic gonadotropin** produced by the placenta will stimulate the corpus luteum, which is maintained for about 6 months and

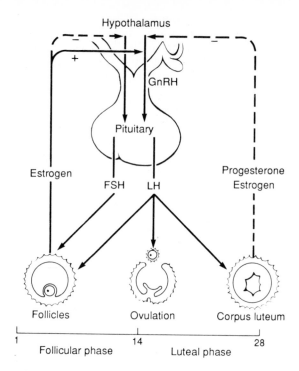

Figure 23–9. Diagram showing the relationships of the hypothalamus, hypophysis, and ovaries. This feedback mechanism regulates the secretion of hormones produced during the menstrual cycle. GnRH, gonadotropin-releasing hormone; solid arrows, stimulation; broken arrows, inhibition.

then gradually declines. It does not disappear completely, however, and continues to secrete progesterone until the end of pregnancy. This is the **corpus luteum of pregnancy.** It has been shown by immunohistochemistry that the corpus luteum of pregnancy also secretes **relaxin,** a polypeptide hormone that softens the connective tissue of the symphysis pubica, facilitating parturition. The corpus luteum of pregnancy is larger than the corpus luteum of menstruation, sometimes reaching a diameter of 5 cm.

The cells of the corpus luteum of menstruation or pregnancy undergo degeneration by autolysis, and their cellular remnants are phagocytized by macrophages. The site is occupied by a scar of dense connective tissue, forming a **corpus albicans.** The corpus albicans remains for a variable period and is gradually absorbed by macrophages of the stroma.

OVIDUCT

The oviduct is a muscular tube (Fig 23–1) of great mobility, measuring about 12 cm in length. One of its extremities opens into the peritoneal cavity next to the ovary; the other passes through the wall of the

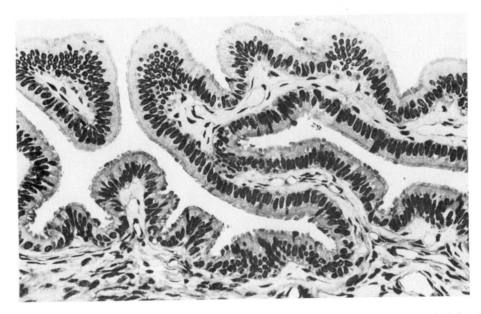

Figure 23–10. Photomicrograph of a cross section through the oviduct. The mucosa projects many folds into the lumen.

uterus and opens into the interior of this organ. The free extremity of the oviduct has a fringe of fingerlike extensions called **fimbriae** (Fig 23–1).

Histologic Structure

The wall of the oviduct is composed of 3 layers: a mucosa, a muscularis, and a serosa composed of visceral peritoneum (Fig 23–10).

The mucosa has longitudinal folds that are most numerous in the ampulla. In cross sections, the lumen of the ampulla resembles a labyrinth (Fig 23–10). These folds become smaller in the segments of the tube that are closer to the uterus. In the intramural portion, the folds are reduced to small bulges in the lumen, so that its internal surface is almost smooth.

The epithelium lining the mucosa is simple columnar and contains 2 types of cells. One is provided with cilia, the other is secretory (Figs 23–11 and 23–12). Most of the cilia beat toward the uterus, causing movement of the viscous liquid film that covers its surface. This liquid consists mainly of products of the secretory cells interspersed between ciliated cells. This secretion has nutrient and protective functions for the ovum and promotes activation (**capacitation**) of spermatozoa. Movement of the film that covers the mucosa of the tube, in conjunction with contractions of the muscle layer, helps to transport the ovum or the conceptus toward the uterus. It also hampers the passage of microorganisms from the uterus to the peritoneal cavity. Microcinematographic films of the uterine tube lining, however, reveal that some cilia beat toward the ovary. It is believed that

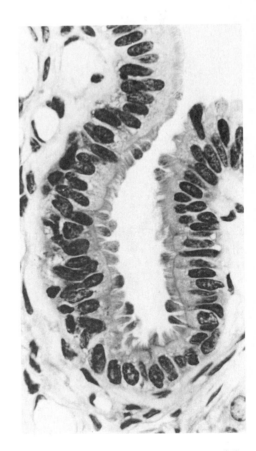

Figure 23–11. Photomicrograph of mucosa of the oviduct. The section was made at the level of the ampulla. Observe ciliated cells.

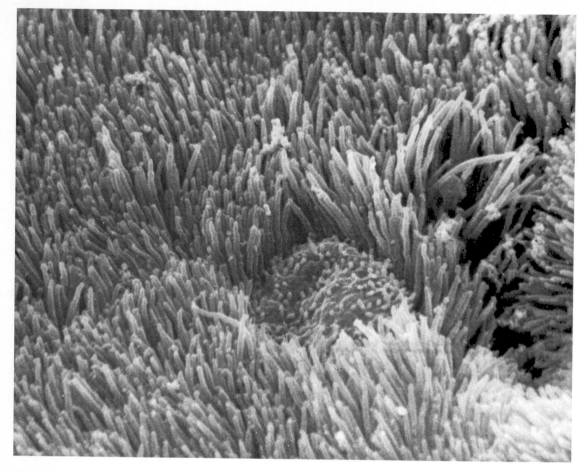

Figure 23–12. Scanning electron micrograph of the lining of an oviduct. Observe the abundant cilia. In the middle is the apex of a secretory cell covered by short microvilli. × 8000. (Courtesy of KR Porter.)

these cilia facilitate the movement of the sperm toward the unfertilized egg.

The lamina propria of the mucosa is composed of loose connective tissue. The muscularis is composed of smooth muscle fibers disposed as an inner circular or spiral layer and an outer longitudinal layer.

Histophysiology

The oviduct receives the ovum expelled by the ovary and carries it toward the uterus. Its lumen represents an environment adequate for fertilization, and its secretions contribute to the nutrition of the embryo during the early phases of development.

At the time of ovulation, the oviduct exhibits active movement. The fimbriae of the infundibulum move closer to the surface of the ovary, and the funnel shape of the infundibulum facilitates the recovery of the liberated ovum.

The wall of the oviduct is richly vascularized, and its vessels become dilated at the time of ovulation. This gives rigidity and distention to the organ, facilitating its approximation to the ovary. Fertilization usually takes place in the lateral third of the oviduct.

In cases of abnormal nidation, in which the embryo implants itself in the tube (**ectopic pregnancy**), the lamina propria reacts like the endometrium, forming numerous decidual cells. Because of its small diameter, the oviduct cannot contain this increase and bursts during ectopic pregnancy, causing extensive hemorrhage that can be fatal if not treated immediately.

UTERUS

The uterus is a pear-shaped organ that consists of a **body (corpus),** which lies above a narrowing of the uterine cavity (the **internal os**), and a lower cylindrical structure, the **cervix,** which lies below the internal os. The part of the body of the uterus lying above the points of entrance of the uterine tubes is called the **fundus** (Fig 23–1).

The wall of the uterus is relatively thick and is formed of 3 layers. Depending on the part of the uterus, there is either an outer **serosa** (connective tissue and mesothelium) or **adventitia** (connective tissue). The other uterine layers are the **myometrium,** a thick tunic of smooth muscle, and the **endometrium,** or mucosa of the uterus.

Myometrium

The myometrium (*mys* + Greek, *metra*, uterus), the thickest tunic of the uterus, is composed of bundles of smooth muscle fibers separated by connective tissue. The bundles of smooth muscle form 4 layers that are not well defined. The first and the fourth are composed mainly of fibers disposed longitudinally, ie, parallel to the long axis of the organ. The middle layers contain the larger blood vessels.

During pregnancy, the myometrium goes through a period of great growth. The growth is due to both **hypertrophy** and an increase in the number of smooth muscle cells (**hyperplasia**). During pregnancy, many smooth muscle cells have ultrastructural characteristics of protein-secreting cells and actively synthesize collagen, promoting a significant increase in uterine collagen content.

After pregnancy, there is destruction of some smooth muscle cells, reduction in the size of others, and an enzymatic degradation of the collagen. The uterus is reduced in size almost to its prepregnancy dimensions.

Endometrium

The endometrium consists of epithelium and lamina propria containing simple tubular glands that sometimes branch in their deeper portions (near the myometrium). Its epithelial cells are simple columnar and are a mixture of ciliated and secretory cells. The epithelium of the uterine glands is similar to the superficial epithelium, but ciliated cells are rare within the glands.

The connective tissue of the lamina propria is rich in fibroblasts and contains abundant amorphous ground substance. Connective tissue fibers are mostly reticular.

The endometrial layer can be subdivided into 2 zones: the **functionalis,** which constitutes the portions sloughed off at menstruation and replaced during each menstrual cycle; and the **basalis,** the portion retained after menstruation that subsequently proliferates and provides a new epithelium and lamina propria for the renewal of the endometrium. The bases of the uterine glands, which lie deep within the basalis, are the source of the cells that divide and migrate over the exposed connective tissue of the menstrual-phase endometrium, thereby providing for the new epithelial lining of the uterus after menstruation.

The blood vessels supplying the endometrium are of special significance in the periodic sloughing of most of this layer. **Arcuate arteries** are circumferentially oriented in the middle layers of the myometrium. From these vessels, 2 sets of arteries arise to supply blood to the endometrium: **straight arteries,** which supply the basalis; and **coiled arteries,** which bring blood to the functionalis.

Uterine Cervix

As previously noted, the **cervix** is the lower, cylindrical part of the uterus (see Figs 23–1 and 23–18). This portion differs in histologic structure from the rest of the uterus. The lining consists of a mucus-secreting simple columnar epithelium. The cervix has few smooth muscle fibers and consists mainly (85%) of dense connective tissue. The external aspect of the cervix that bulges into the lumen of the vagina (Latin, *sheath*) is covered by stratified squamous epithelium.

The mucosa of the cervix contains the mucous **cervical glands,** which are extensively branched. This mucosa does not desquamate during menstruation, although its glands undergo small variations in their structure during the menstrual cycle. When the ducts of these glands are blocked, the retained secretion causes a dilatation that gives rise to **nabothian cysts.** During pregnancy, the cervical mucous glands proliferate and secrete a more viscous and abundant mucus.

Cervical secretions play a significant role in fertilization of the ovum. At the time of ovulation, the mucous secretions are watery and allow penetration of the uterus by sperm. In the luteal phase or in pregnancy, the progesterone levels alter the mucous secretions so that they become more viscous and prevent the passage of the microorganisms, as well as sperm, into the body of the uterus (cervical mucous plug; see Fig 23–18). The dilation of the cervix that precedes parturition is due to intense collagenolysis, which promotes its softening.

> Cancer of the cervix (**cervical carcinoma**) is derived from its stratified squamous epithelium. Although it is frequently observed, the mortality rate is low (8 per 100,000). This low rate is due to the usual discovery of the carcinoma in its early stages, made possible by yearly physical observation of the cervix and by cytological analysis of smears of the cervical epithelium (Papanicolaou's stain test).

1. THE MENSTRUAL CYCLE

The action of ovarian hormones (estrogens and progesterone) under the stimulus of the anterior lobe of the pituitary causes the endometrium to undergo cyclic structural modifications during the menstrual cycle. The duration of the menstrual cycle is variable but averages 28 days (Fig 23–22).

Menstrual cycles usually start between 12 and 15 years of age and continue until about age 45–50. Since menstrual cycles are a consequence of ovarian modifications related to the production of ova, the female is fertile only during the years when she is having menstrual cycles. This does not mean that sexual activity is terminated by menopause—only that fertility ceases.

For practical purposes, the beginning of the menstrual cycle is taken as the day when menstrual bleeding appears. The menstrual discharge consists of degenerating endometrium mixed with blood from the ruptured blood vessels. The **menstrual phase** is defined as the first to the fourth days of the cycle; the **proliferative phase** is the fifth to the fourteenth days; and the **secretory phase** is the fifteenth to the twenty-eighth days. The duration of each phase is variable, and the intervals given are only averages.

Although the menstrual cycle can be described as having a proliferative phase, a secretory or luteal phase, and a menstrual phase, the structural changes that occur during the cycle are gradual; the clear division of the phases implied in the text has mainly teaching value.

A. The Proliferative Phase: After the menstrual phase, the uterine mucosa is reduced to a small band of connective tissue (lamina propria) containing the basal portions of the glands. The proliferative phase is also known as the **follicular phase** because it coincides with the development of ovarian follicles and the production of estrogens.

Cellular proliferation continues during the entire proliferative phase, and reconstitute both the glands and the surface epithelium lining the endometrium (Fig 23–13). Proliferation of the connective cells and deposition of the ground substance in the lamina propria also occur, causing growth of the endometrium as a whole.

At the end of the proliferative phase, the endometrium is 2–3 mm thick, and the glands, which consist of simple columnar epithelial cells, are straight tubules with narrow lumens. During this phase, these cells gradually accumulate more cisternae of rough endoplasmic reticulum, and the Golgi complex increases in size in preparation for secretory activity. Coiled arteries grow into the regenerating stroma.

B. The Secretory, or Luteal, Phase: This phase starts after ovulation and depends upon progesterone secreted by the corpus luteum. Acting upon glands already developed by the action of estrogen, progesterone stimulates the gland cells to secrete glycoproteins that will be the major source of embryonic nutrition before implantation occurs.

The glands become highly coiled (Fig 23–14) and the epithelial cells begin to accumulate glycogen below their nuclei. Later, the amount of glycogen diminishes, and glycoprotein secretory products dilate the lumens of the glands. In this phase, the endometrium reaches its maximum thickness (5 mm) as a result of the accumulation of secretions and edema of the stroma. Mitoses are rare during the secretory phase. The elongation and convolution of the coiled arteries continue, and they extend into the superficial portion of the endometrium. Progesterone inhibits the contractions of smooth muscle cells of the myo-

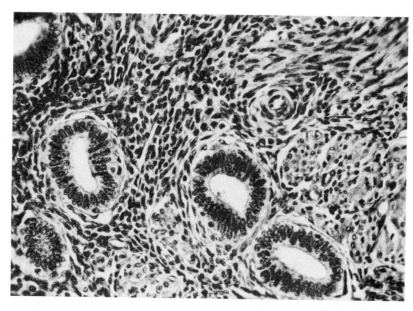

Figure 23–13. Endometrium in the proliferative phase. The epithelial cells of the uterine gland are usually organized as a simple columnar lining, although during the active proliferation phase, the close proximity of nuclei may assume a pseudostratified appearance. H&E stain, × 320.

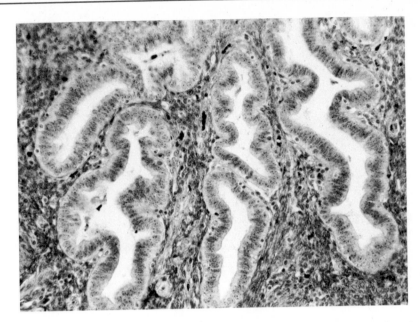

Figure 23–14. Endometrium in the secretory phase (21st day of the menstrual cycle). The uterine glands have broad lumens with an irregular outline; the lumens are dilated by accumulation of secretory material. H&E stain, × 224.

metrium that might otherwise interfere with the implantation of the embryo.

C. The Menstrual Phase: When fertilization and implantation of the ovum released by the ovary fail to occur, the corpus luteum spontaneously ceases functioning after about 14 days. The levels of progesterone and estrogens in the blood drop rapidly, and the endometrium developed in response to these hormones undergoes involution and is partially shed. If implantation occurs, **human chorionic gonadotropin (hCG)** begins to be synthesized by the developing embryo. This sustains the life of the corpus luteum, and menstruation does not occur.

At the end of the secretory phase, the walls of the coiled arteries contract, closing off blood flow and producing ischemia, which leads to death (necrosis) of their walls and of the functionalis layer of the endometrium. At this time, blood vessels above the constrictions rupture, and bleeding begins.

The endometrium becomes partially detached. The amount lost is variable in different women and even in the same woman at different times. At the end of the menstrual phase, the endometrium is almost always reduced to nothing but the basal layer, containing the basal ends of the endometrial glands. Proliferation of the gland cells and their migration to the surface initiate the proliferative phase, restarting the cycle.

2. PREGNANCY & IMPLANTATION

The human ovum is fertilized at the ampullar-isthmic junction of the oviduct, and cleavage of the zygote occurs as it moves passively toward the uterus. Through successive mitoses, a compact collection of cells, the **morula,** is formed. The morula, covered by the zona pellucida, is about the same size as the fertilized ovum (Fig 23–15). The cells that result from segmentation of the zygote are called **blastomeres** (*blastos + meros*). They do not grow in size at this time but divide the zygote into smaller cells that will subsequently differentiate along several pathways.

A cavity at the center of the morula appears as a result of the gradual accumulation of liquid transferred from the lumen of the oviduct; the cells form a fluid-filled sphere, the **blastocyst.** The blastomeres arrange themselves in a peripheral layer (**trophoblast**) that is thickened at the point where a collection of cells (**inner cell mass**) remains and bulges into the cavity. This stage of development corresponds approximately to the fourth or fifth day after ovulation. At this time, the embryo reaches the uterus. The blastocyst remains in the lumen of the uterus for 2 or 3 days and comes into contact with the surface of the endometrium, immersed in the secretion of the endometrial glands.

In the blastocyst stage, the zona pellucida becomes thinner and disappears, allowing cells of the trophoblast, which have the capacity to invade the mucosa, to come into direct contact with the endometrium. Immediately thereafter, the cells of the trophoblast begin to multiply, ensuring, with the help of the endometrium, the nourishment of the embryo. The inner cell mass, from which the body of the embryo will originate, grows slightly during this phase.

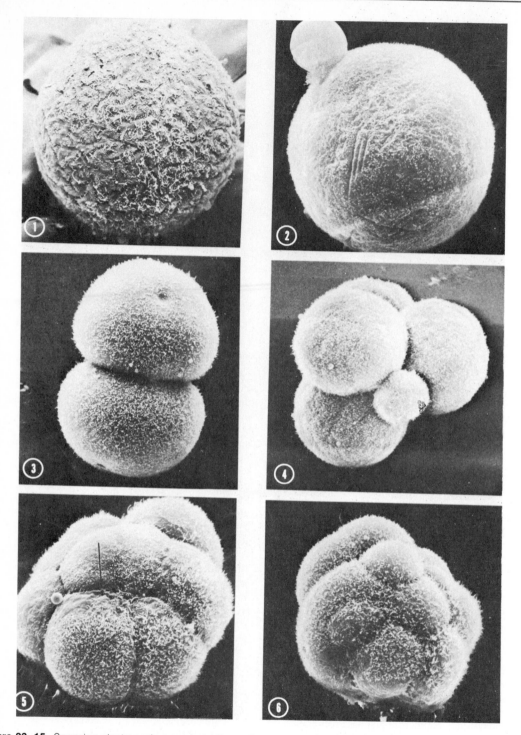

Figure 23–15. Scanning electron micrographs of the surface of a mouse ovum after fertilization and up to the morula stage. The zona pellucida has been digested with pronase. **1:** The ovum shortly after its release from an ovarian follicle. The ovum's germinal vesicle is intact at this stage. × 1380. **2:** Fertilized egg. Note the microvillous surface of the egg and the smooth surface of the first polar body. × 1300. **3:** Two-cell stage, evenly covered with microvilli. × 1320. **4:** Four-cell stage with second polar body. × 1870. **5:** Eight-cell stage. Note smoother regions of membrane where cells come into contact (arrow). × 1400. **6:** Morula. Microvilli are quite numerous, particularly adjacent to the area of cell contact. × 1540. (Reproduced, with permission, from Calarco P: Mammalian preimplantation development. In: *Scanning Electron Microscopy Atlas of Mammalian Reproduction.* Hafez ESE [editor]. Igaku Shoin Ltd, 1975.

Implantation, or nidation (Fig 23–16), involves penetration through the uterine epithelium, with little sign of necrosis. This type of **interstitial** implantation occurs in humans and a few other mammals. The process starts around the seventh day, and on about the ninth day after ovulation the embryo is totally submerged in the endometrium, from which it will receive protection and nourishment during pregnancy.

Implantation takes place when the endometrium is in the secretory phase. The uterine glands secrete glycoproteins, the vessels dilate, and the lamina propria swells slightly.

During implantation, the trophoblast differentiates into 2 layers, the **syncytiotrophoblast** and the **cytotrophoblast** (Figs 23–16, 23–17, and 23–20). The former, a multinucleated syncytial external layer arises from the fusion of mononucleated cytotropho-

blasts. The cytotrophoblast (*kytos* + *trophe* + *blastos*) consists of an irregular layer of mononucleated ovoid cells immediately under the syncytiotrophoblast.

The surface of the syncytiotrophoblast has irregular microvilli, and the superficial cytoplasm contains vesicles covered by smooth membranes. This suggests an intense pinocytotic process in the syncytiotrophoblast, possibly related to the transfer of material from the maternal circulation to the fetus. Below that level, the cytoplasm of the syncytiotrophoblast shows an abundance of both rough and smooth endoplasmic reticulum, a well-developed Golgi complex, and numerous mitochondria. These ultrastructural characteristics are consistent with the role attributed to the syncytiotrophoblast in the secretion of chorionic gonadotropin (a glycoprotein hormone), placental

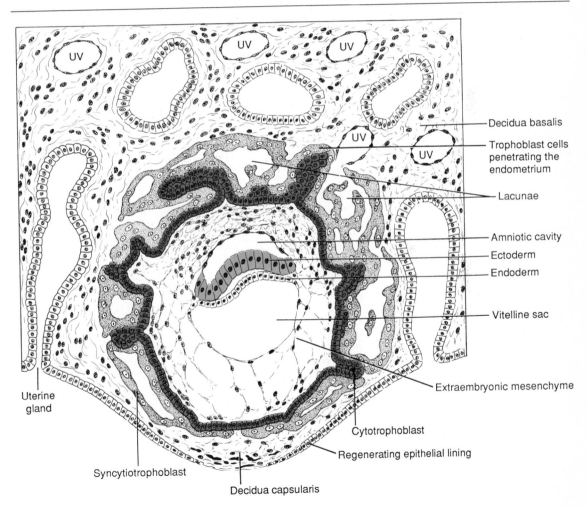

Figure 23–16. Schematic drawing of a human embryo at the end of implantation (12 days), showing the relationships between the embryo and the endometrium (called the decidua) after implantation. UV, uterine vessels, one of which opens into a lacuna, filling its spaces with blood. Darker color shows the cytotrophoblast; lighter color highlights the ectoderm and amnion.

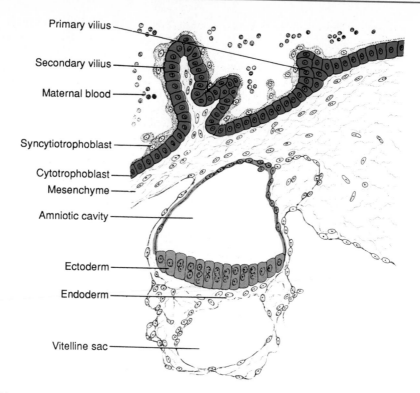

Primary vilius

Secondary vilius

Maternal blood

Syncytiotrophoblast

Cytotrophoblast

Mesenchyme

Amniotic cavity

Ectoderm

Endoderm

Vitelline sac

Figure 23–17. Human embryo at 15 days. Primary and secondary chorionic villi are shown at upper left, protruding into a lacuna that contains maternal blood.

lactogen (a protein hormone), and estrogen and progesterone (steroids). The syncytiotrophoblast contains lipid droplets whose composition (as determined by cytochemical methods) is compatible with the presence of cholesterol, the immediate precursor of steroid hormones.

The syncytiotrophoblasts delineate extracytoplasmic cavities. These cavities increase in size and communicate with one another, resulting in a spongy structure (Fig 23–16). Thus, lacunae are formed, lined with syncytiotrophoblast. The lytic activity of the syncytiotrophoblast causes the rupture of both arterial and venous maternal blood vessels, with overflow of blood into these lacunar spaces. Blood flows from the arterial vessels to the lacunae and from there to the veins.

After implantation of the embryo, the endometrium goes through profound changes and is called the **decidua.** Cells of the stroma become enlarged and polygonal and are called decidual cells. The decidua can be divided into the **decidua basalis,** situated between the embryo and the myometrium; **decidua capsularis,** between the embryo and the lumen of the uterus; and **decidua parietalis,** the remainder of the decidua (Fig 23–18).

The trophoblast in contact with the decidua capsularis develops only to a slight extent, since its nutri-

tion is deficient. Growth of the trophoblast in the part of the embryo facing the myometrium is ensured by the maternal blood, and its growth is rapid. From this part of the trophoblast, elongated projections, **primary villi,** are formed (Fig 23–17). Their main characteristic is their composition of only cytotrophoblasts and an external syncytiotrophoblastic covering. During this stage of embryonic development, an extraembryonic mesenchyme appears before the intraembryonic mesenchyme and contributes to the formation of the placenta and the fetal membranes. The extraembryonic mesenchyme and the trophoblast form the **chorion** (from Greek, *choreon,* fetal membrane). On the side of the **decidua capsularis,** the chorion develops very slightly (**smooth chorion, or chorion laeve**); on the side of the decidua basalis, the chorion grows extensively and forms the **chorion frondosum.** The layers of the chorion (beginning at the surface) are the syncytiotrophoblast, cytotrophoblast, and extraembryonic mesenchyme.

When the mesenchyme invades the primary villi, it transforms them into **secondary villi** (Figs 23–17 and 23–19). Within the villi, vessels are formed gradually and later will join those formed in the body of the embryo, establishing a circulation and thus allowing exchange of substances and gases between the fetal and maternal blood (Fig 23–19).

Placenta

The placenta is a temporary organ found only in eutherian mammals; it is the site of physiologic exchanges between the mother and the fetus. It consists of a fetal part (chorion) and a maternal part (decidua basalis).

The placenta is the only organ composed of cells derived from 2 different individuals. The boundary between maternal and fetal tissues is marked by extracellular—**fibrinoid**—products of necrosis. Since the embryo and mother are of different genetic constitution, there should be an immunologic attack by the maternal organism against the foreign implanting embryo. Why this does not occur remains an active area of investigation.

A. Fetal Part: The fetal part of the placenta, the chorion, has a **chorionic plate** at the point where the **chorionic villi** arise—the secondary villi already described. These villi consist of a connective tissue core derived from the extraembryonic mesenchyme surrounded by the syncytiotrophoblast and the cytotrophoblast (Fig 23–20). The syncytiotrophoblast remains until the end of pregnancy, but the cytotrophoblast disappears gradually during the second half. Although the cytotrophoblast undergoes extensive proliferation and concomitant cell fusion during early placentation, in the second half of pregnancy, proliferation slows while the fusion continues. This results in a loss of the cytotrophoblast cells, which become incorporated into the growing **syncytium.**

The chorionic villi may be either free or anchored to the decidua basalis. Both villi have the same struc-

ture, but the free ones do not reach the decidua, while the anchored chorionic villi become embedded within the decidua basalis. The surfaces of the villi are bathed with blood from the lacunae of the basal decidua; it is here that the exchange of substances between fetal and maternal blood occurs.

B. Maternal Part: The maternal part of the placenta—the decidua basalis—supplies arterial blood to and receives venous blood from the lacunae situated between the secondary villi. Although the maternal blood vessels are open during implantation, the fetal vessels contained in the secondary villi remain intact. Fetal blood and maternal blood do not mix except, on rare occasions, at the end of pregnancy. During this period, the cytotrophoblast is no longer continuous, and the capillaries of the villi are close to the surface; a very slight exchange of blood cells may occur. At that time, the walls of the fetal capillaries are separated from the maternal blood only by the syncytiotrophoblast.

During pregnancy, cells from the connective tissue stroma of the decidua basalis and a lesser number of cells from the decidua parietalis and decidua capsularis form the **decidual cells.** These cells are large and exhibit the characteristics of protein-synthesizing cells; they produce prolactin and other biologically active substances.

At the end of a full-term pregnancy, the placenta has the shape of a disk. The umbilical cord usually arises at the center of the placenta and forms a connection between the fetal and placental circulations.

C. Histophysiology: Fetal venous blood reaches

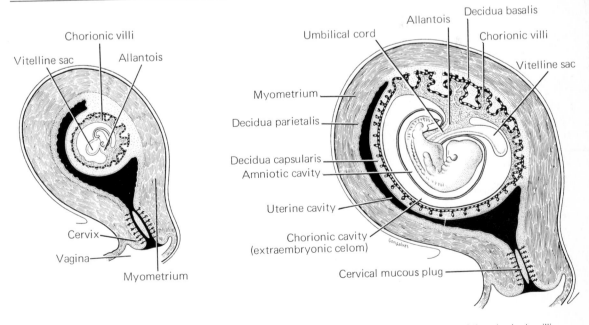

Figure 23–18. Schematic drawings showing formation of the 3 regions of the decidua and the chorionic villi.

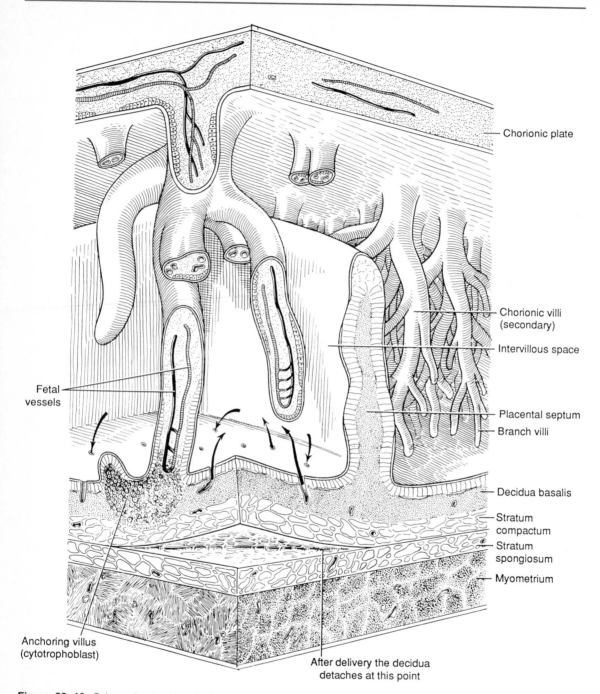

Chorionic plate

Chorionic villi (secondary)

Intervillous space

Placental septum

Branch villi

Fetal vessels

Decidua basalis

Stratum compactum

Stratum spongiosum

Myometrium

Anchoring villus (cytotrophoblast)

After delivery the decidua detaches at this point

Figure 23–19. Schematic drawing of placental structure. Arrows indicate the blood flow from decidual arteries to intervillous space and back to decidual veins. This direction is determined by the difference in pressure between arterial and venous blood. Observe free and anchored chorionic villi. (Redrawn and reproduced, with permission, from Duplessis GDT, Haegel P: *Embryologie.* Masson, 1971 [English edition, Springer-Verlag, 1972; Chapman & Hall, 1972; Masson, 1972].)

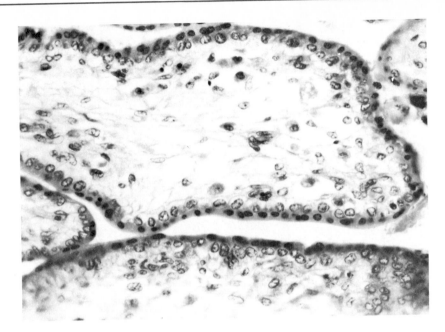

Figure 23–20. Photomicrograph of a chorionic villus in the second half of pregnancy. The syncytiotrophoblast is a continuous layer at the surface with dark nuclei. Cytotrophoblast cells form a discontinuous layer of cells with lighter and larger nuclei just beneath the syncytiotrophoblast. H&E stain, × 320.

the placenta through the 2 umbilical arteries, which branch and ultimately give rise to the vessels of the chorionic villi. In these villi, the fetal blood receives oxygen, loses its CO_2, and returns to the fetus through the umbilical vein.

Since the chorionic villi are submerged in maternal blood, the fetal blood remains isolated by the structures that form the **placental barrier:** the endothelium of the fetal capillaries and the basal lamina of these capillaries; the mesenchyme in the interior of the villus; the basal lamina of the trophoblast; the cytotrophoblast (during the first half of pregnancy); and the syncytiotrophoblast.

The placenta is permeable to several substances; it normally transfers oxygen, water, electrolytes, carbohydrates, lipids, proteins, vitamins, hormones, some antibodies, and some drugs from maternal blood to fetal blood. CO_2, water, hormones, and residual products of metabolism are transferred from fetal blood to the maternal blood.

The placenta is also an endocrine organ, producing such hormones as chorionic gonadotropin, chorionic thyrotropin, chorionic corticotropin, estrogens, and progesterone. It also secretes a protein hormone called human placental lactogen, which has lactogenic and growth-stimulating activity. All these hormones are synthesized by the syncytiotrophoblast.

Radioautographic studies after injection of radioactive thymidine show that the cells of the cytotrophoblast multiply actively and incorporate themselves into the syncytiotrophoblast. This indicates that the syncytiotrophoblast grows as a result of the growth and mitotic activity of the cytotrophoblast.

VAGINA

The wall of the vagina is devoid of glands and consists of 3 layers: a **mucosa,** a **muscular layer,** and an **adventitia.** The mucus found in the lumen of the vagina comes from the glands of the uterine cervix.

The epithelium of the mucosa is stratified squamous and has a thickness of 150–200 μm. Its cells may contain a small amount of keratohyalin. Intense keratinization, however, with the cells changing into keratin plates, as in typical keratinized epithelia, does not occur (Fig 23–21). Under the stimulus of estrogen, the vaginal epithelium synthesizes and accumulates a large quantity of glycogen, which is deposited in the lumen of the vagina when the vaginal cells desquamate. Bacteria in the vagina metabolize glycogen and form lactic acid, which is responsible for the usually low pH of the vagina.

The lamina propria of the vaginal mucosa is composed of loose connective tissue that is very rich in elastic fibers. Among the cells present are lymphocytes and neutrophils in relatively large quantities. During certain phases of the menstrual cycle, these 2 types of leukocytes invade the epithelium and pass into the lumen of the vagina. Although the lamina propria lacks glands, it exhibits a rich vascularization

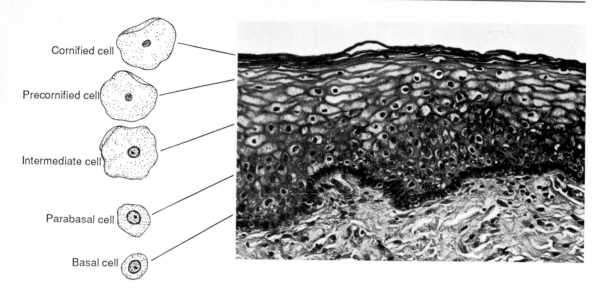

Figure 23–21. Photomicrograph of a section of vaginal mucosa and drawings of the cells found in various epithelial layers. Masson's stain, × 250.

that is the source of the fluid exudate that seeps through the squamous epithelium during sexual stimulation. The vaginal mucosa is virtually devoid of sensory nerve endings, and the few naked nerve endings that do exist are probably pain fibers.

The muscular layer of the vagina is composed mainly of longitudinal bundles of smooth muscle fibers. There are some circular bundles, especially in the innermost part (next to the mucosa).

Outside the muscular layer, a coat of dense connective tissue, the adventitia, rich in thick elastic fibers, unites the vagina with the surrounding tissues. The great elasticity of the vagina is related to the large number of elastic fibers in the connective tissues of its wall. In this connective tissue are an extensive venous plexus, nerve bundles, and groups of nerve cells.

EXTERNAL GENITALIA

The female external genitalia, or vulva, consists of the **clitoris, labia minora, labia majora,** and some glands that open into the vestibulum, a space enclosed by the labia minora.

The urethra and the ducts of the vestibular glands open into the vestibulum. The 2 **glandulae vestibulares majores,** or **glands of Bartholin,** are situated with one on each side of the vestibulum. These glands are homologous to the bulbourethral glands in the male. The more numerous **glandulae vestibulares minores** are scattered, occurring with greater frequency around the urethra and clitoris. All the glandulae vestibulares secrete mucus.

The clitoris and the penis are of homologous em-

bryonic origin and histologic structure. The clitoris is formed by 2 erectile bodies ending in a rudimentary **glans clitoridis** and a prepuce. The clitoris is covered with stratified squamous epithelium.

The labia minora are folds of skin with a core of spongy connective tissue permeated by elastic fibers. The stratified squamous epithelium that covers them has a thin layer of keratinized cells on the surface. Sebaceous and sweat glands are present on the inner and outer surfaces of the labia minora.

The labia majora are folds of skin that contain a large quantity of adipose tissue and a thin layer of smooth muscle. Their inner surface has a histologic structure similar to that of the labia minora. The external surface is covered by skin and coarse, curly hair. Sebaceous and sweat glands are numerous on both surfaces.

The external genitalia are abundantly supplied with sensory tactile nerve endings including Meissner's and Pacini's corpuscles, which contribute to the physiology of sexual arousal.

ENDOCRINE INTERRELATIONSHIPS

Female reproductive function is regulated through certain nuclei of the hypothalamus. Nerve cells in the hypothalamus produce and introduce into the portal blood vessels specific polypeptides that act on the pars distalis of the hypophysis to liberate gonadotropins; these gonadotropins in turn stimulate the secretion of ovarian hormones (estrogens and progesterone; Fig 23–22). The hypothalamic localization of the ovarian hormone control mechanism might ex-

THE FEMALE REPRODUCTIVE SYSTEM / 461

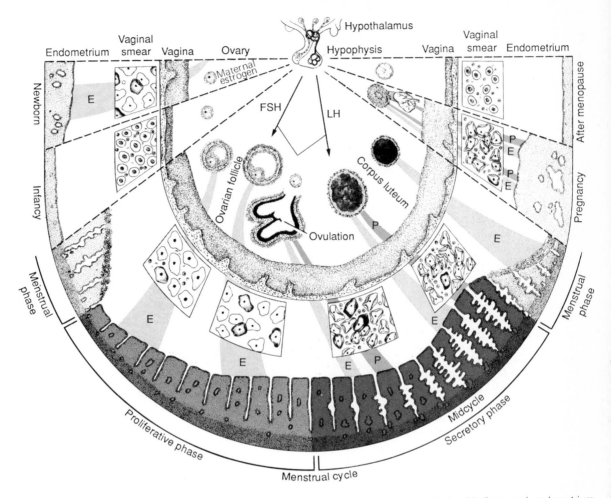

Figure 23–22. Functional changes relating to the hypothalamus, pituitary, ovary, vaginal epithelium, and endometrium. E, estrogen (grey); P, progesterone (dark grey). (Modified and redrawn from FH Netter.)

plain why strong, nonspecific cerebral stimuli occasionally affect reproductive function, resulting in **false pregnancy (pseudocyesis)** or the phenomenon of women who live or work together menstruating at virtually the same time.

The developing ovarian follicle synthesizes **estrogens,** and the corpus luteum synthesizes estrogens and **progesterone.** The main source of estrogens in the human ovarian follicle seems to be granulosa cells that have all the enzymes necessary to convert cholesterol to **estradiol-17β.** Estradiol found in blood is produced mainly by the theca interna cells of the follicle. Estradiol is rapidly converted to **estrone,** which is further metabolized to **estriol,** probably in the liver. Estradiol is the most potent of the 3 estrogen compounds.

The hypophyseal gonadotropins, follicle-stimulating hormone (FSH) and luteinizing hormone (LH), are produced under the control of a single releasing hormone (GnRH) liberated by the hypothalamus.

FSH stimulates the growth of the ovarian follicles and the formation of estrogens. It is important to note that at any particular time in the cycle, the ovary possesses follicles in all stages of growth. The release of FSH does not promote the formation of a graafian follicle from a primordial follicle during one cycle. The most immediate effect of FSH is probably the maturation of existing late primary or secondary follicles. LH promotes ovulation and the formation of the corpus luteum (Fig 23–22).

The ovary also acts on the hypophysis, both directly and through the hypothalamus. Estrogen inhibits the secretion of FSH and stimulates the secretion of LH, whose production is inhibited by progesterone. Just prior to midcycle, estrogen secretion reaches a peak and causes a brief surge of LH secretion. Luteinizing hormone promotes ovulation, maturation of the oocyte, and formation of the corpus luteum. As the secretion of LH is inhibited by progesterone produced by the corpus luteum, this structure is soon deprived of the hypophyseal stimulus (LH) necessary for its functioning, and it consequently degenerates.

When fertilization and implantation occur, syncytiotrophoblast cells synthesize the chorionic gonadotropins that stimulate and maintain the function of the corpus luteum during pregnancy.

There is no evidence that prolactin, which stimulates the corpus luteum in rats and mice, has any influence on the human corpus luteum. In humans, prolactin initiates and maintains milk secretion by mammary glands already stimulated by estrogens and progesterone.

EXFOLIATIVE CYTOLOGY

Exfoliative cytology is the study of the characteristics of cells that normally desquamate from various surfaces of the body. Cytologic examination of cells collected from the vagina gives information of clinical importance.

In fully mature vaginal mucosa, 5 types of cells are easily identifiable: cells of the internal portion of the basal layer (basal cells), cells of the external portion of the basal layer (called parabasal cells), cells of the intermediate layers, precornified cells, and cornified cells (Fig 23–21). Based on the numbers of cell types that appear in a vaginal smear, valuable information can be obtained on the hormonal status of the patient (action of estrogen and progesterone). It is also useful in the early detection of cervical cancer.

MAMMARY GLANDS

Each mammary gland consists of 15–25 lobes of the compound tubuloalveolar type whose function is to secrete milk to nourish newborns (Fig 23–23). Each lobe, separated from the others by dense connective tissue and much adipose tissue, is really a gland in itself with its own **excretory lactiferous duct.** These ducts, 2–4.5 cm long, emerge independently in the **nipple,** which has 15–25 openings, each about 0.5 mm in diameter. The histologic structure of the mammary glands varies according to sex, age, and physiologic status.

Embryonic Breast Development

The mammary glands appear in a 6-week-old human embryo as a pair of thickenings of the epidermis, the **milk lines.** They extend from the forelimb to the hindlimb on the ventral side of the fetus. The caudal parts of the milk lines regress early in development. In the thoracic region of a second-trimester fetus, 15–25 ingrowths of the epithelium penetrate the underlying connective tissue and give rise to the future lactiferous ducts. Most of the remainder of each milk line degenerates.

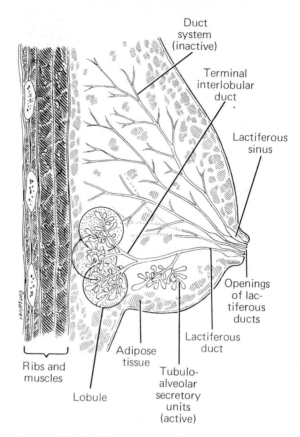

Figure 23–23. Schematic drawing of female breast showing the mammary glands with ducts that open in the nipple. The outlines of the lobules do not exist in vivo but are shown for instructional purposes. The stippling indicates the loose intralobular connective tissue.

In newborns of both sexes, the glands have a diameter of 3.5–9 mm and consist of ducts that may be swollen with secretory material. Secretion of a fluid by neonates is not unusual, since these glands are affected by placental and maternal hormones.

Breast Structure During Puberty & in the Adult

Before puberty, the mammary glands are composed of **lactiferous sinuses** and several branches of these sinuses, the **lactiferous ducts** (Fig 23–23).

The development of mammary glands in females during puberty constitutes one of the secondary sex characteristics. During this period, the breasts increase in size and develop a prominent nipple. In males, the breasts normally remain flattened.

Breast enlargement during puberty is the result of the accumulation of adipose tissue and collagenous connective tissue, with increased growth and branching of lactiferous ducts. The proliferation of the lactiferous ducts and accumulation of fat are due to an increase in the amount of ovarian estrogens during puberty.

The characteristic structure of the adult female gland—the **lobule**—is developed at the tips of the smallest ducts (**terminal interlobular ducts,** Fig 23–23). A lobule consists of several **intralobular** ducts that empty into one terminal interlobular duct. Each lobule is embedded in loose, cellular, intralobular connective tissue. A denser, less cellular interlobular connective tissue separates the lobules.

Near the opening of the nipple, the lactiferous ducts dilate to form the lactiferous sinuses (Fig 23–23). The lactiferous sinuses are lined by stratified squamous epithelium at their external openings. This epithelium very quickly changes to stratified columnar or cuboidal epithelium. Examination of the lactiferous ducts with the electron microscope reveals that the cells adjacent to the lumen are ductal epithelial cells, while the cells lying on the basal lamina are closely packed myoepithelial cells. The epithelial cells are joined by tight junctions and desmosomes. The terminal interlobular ducts (Fig 23–

23) consist of simple cuboidal epithelium resting on basal lamina and a discontinuous layer of myoepithelial cells.

In the intralobular connective tissue surrounding the alveoli are lymphocytes and plasma cells. The plasma cell population increases significantly toward the end of pregnancy; it is responsible for the secretion of immunoglobulins (secretory IgA) that confer passive immunity on the newborn.

Small alterations in the histologic structure of these glands occur during the menstrual cycle, eg, proliferation of cells of the ducts at about the time of ovulation. These changes coincide with the time at which circulating estrogen is at its peak. Greater hydration of connective tissue in the premenstrual phase produces breast enlargement.

The **nipple** has a conical shape and may be pink, light brown, or dark brown in color. Externally, it is covered by keratinized stratified squamous epithelium continuous with that of the adjacent skin. The skin around the nipple constitutes the **areola.** The color of the areola darkens during pregnancy, owing to the

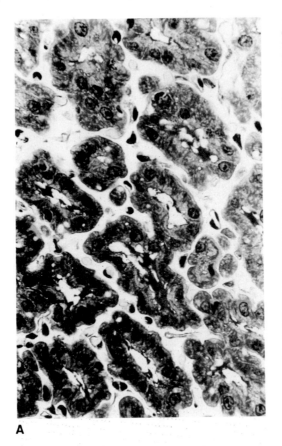

A

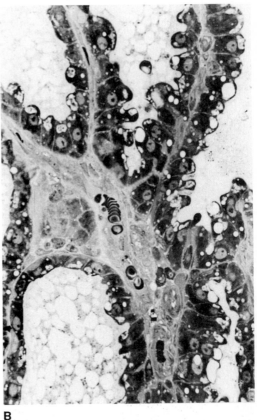

B

Figure 23–24. A. Photomicrograph of a mammary gland during pregnancy. There is intense proliferation of the alveoli. No secretion is seen. **B.** Photomicrograph of lactating mammary gland. The alveoli are distended by the secretion (milk) accumulated in their lumens. Observe the presence of lipid droplets and protein granules in the lumen of the alveolus.

local accumulation of melanin. After delivery, the areola may become lighter in color but rarely returns to its original shade. The epithelium of the nipple rests on a layer of connective tissue rich in smooth muscle fibers. These fibers are disposed in circles around the deeper lactiferous ducts and parallel to them where they enter the nipple. The nipple is abundantly supplied with sensory nerve endings.

The Breasts During Pregnancy & Lactation

The mammary glands undergo intense growth during pregnancy as a result of the proliferation of **alveoli** at the ends of the terminal interlobular ducts. Alveoli are spherical collections of epithelial cells that become the active milk-secreting structures in lactation. A few fat droplets, not surrounded by a membrane, can be seen in the apical cytoplasm of alveolar cells. Also present are a few membrane-limited secretory vacuoles containing from one to several dense aggregates of milk proteins. The number of secretory vacuoles and fat droplets greatly increases in lactation (see below). Four to six stellate myoepithelial cells encompass each alveolus; they are found between the alveolar epithelial cells and the basal lamina. The amounts of connective tissue stroma and adipose tissue, relative to the parenchyma, decrease considerably. Despite this growth process, there are few signs of secretion until late in pregnancy (Fig 23–24A).

Growth of the mammary glands during pregnancy is the result of the synergistic action of several hormones, mainly estrogen, progesterone, prolactin, and human placental lactogen. These hormones stimulate the growth of the secretory parts (alveoli) of the mammary glands. The mammary gland is the only structure in the body that undergoes such a striking structural and physiologic change during the hormonal cycles of pregnancy (Fig 23–25).

During lactation, milk is produced by the epithelial cells of the alveoli and accumulates in their lumens and inside the lactiferous ducts. The secretory cells become small and low cuboidal, and their cytoplasm contains spherical droplets of various sizes containing mainly neutral triglycerides. These lipid droplets pass out of the cells into the lumen and in the process are enveloped with a portion of the apical cell membrane (Fig 23–24B). Lipids constitute 4% of human milk.

In addition to the lipid droplets, which are at the apical pole of the secretory cell, there are a large number of membrane-limited vacuoles that contain granules composed of caseins and other milk proteins. Milk proteins include several caseins, α-lactalbumin, and immunoglobulin A, which are released by exocytosis (Fig 23–26). Proteins constitute approximately 1.5% of human milk. Lactose, the sugar of milk, is synthesized from glucose and galactose and constitutes about 7% of human milk.

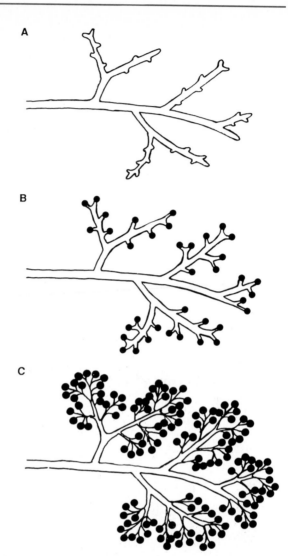

Figure 23–25. Diagram illustrating changes in the mammary gland. **A:** In nonpregnant women, the gland has an inactive duct system. **B:** During pregnancy, alveoli proliferate at the end of the ducts and prepare for the secretion of milk. **C:** During lactation, alveoli are fully differentiated and milk secretion is abundant. Once lactation is completed, the gland reverts to the nonpregnant condition. The gland is normally quiescent and undifferentiated, undergoing this differentiation and secretion only during each cycle of pregnancy and lactation.

The first secretion to appear after birth is called **colostrum.** It contains less fat and more protein than regular milk and is rich in antibodies (predominantly secretory IgA) that provide some degree of passive immunity to the newborn, especially within the gut lumen.

When a woman is breast-feeding, the nursing action of the child stimulates tactile receptors in

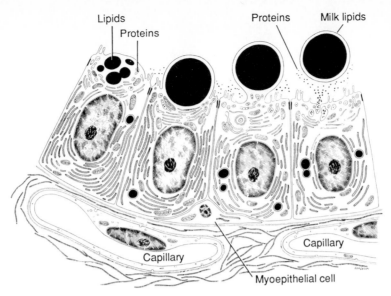

Figure 23–26. Schematic drawing of alveolar cells from the mammary gland. Observe (from left to right) the accumulation and extrusion of milk lipids and proteins. The proteins are released through exocytosis.

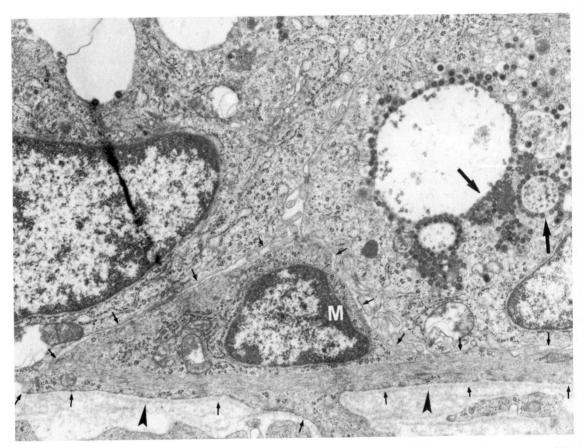

Figure 23–27. Electron micrograph of a mouse mammary gland. A myoepithelial cell (M) is seen in the lower part of the picture, outlined by small arrows. The myoepithelial cell is contained within the basal lamina that surrounds the secretory cells (arrowheads). In this species, but not in humans, the secretory cells may contain numerous virus particles (large arrows) that may eventually induce cancer in this gland. × 17,500. (Reproduced, with permission, from Junqueira LCU, Salles LMM: *Ultra-Estrutura e Função Celular.* Edgard Blücher, 1975.)

the nipple, resulting in liberation of the posterior pituitary hormone **oxytocin.** This hormone causes contraction of myoepithelial cells (Fig 23–27) in alveoli and ducts, resulting in ejection of milk (**milk-ejection reflex**). Negative emotional stimuli, such as frustration, anxiety, or anger, can inhibit the liberation of oxytocin, thus preventing the reflex.

Postlactational Regression of the Breasts

With cessation of breast-feeding (weaning), most alveoli that develop during pregnancy undergo degeneration. This includes sloughing of whole cells as well as autophagic absorption of cellular components. Dead cells and debris are removed by macrophages. Myoepithelial cells and the basal lamina persist and are reused in the next pregnancy.

Senile Involution of the Breasts

After menopause, involution of the mammary glands is characterized by a reduction in size and the atrophy of their secretory portions and, to a certain extent, the ducts. Atrophic changes also occur in the interlobular connective tissue.

Cancer of the Breast

About 9% of all women born in the USA will develop breast cancer at some time during their lives. Most of these cancers arise from epithelial cells of the lactiferous ducts (carcinomas). If these cells metastasize to the lungs, brain, or bone, breast carcinoma becomes a major cause of death. Early detection (eg, through self-examination, mammography, ultrasound, and other techniques) and consequent early treatment have significantly reduced the mortality rate from breast cancer.

REFERENCES

Beaconsfield P. Birdwood G, Beaconsfield R: The placenta. *Sci Am* (Aug) 1980;**243**:94.

Gulyas BJ: Fine structure of the luteal tissue. Pages 238–254 in: *Ultrastructure of Endocrine Cells and Tissues.* Motta PM (editor). Martinus Nijhoff, 1984.

Guraya SS: Recent advances in the morphology, histochemistry and biochemistry of the developing mammalian ovary. *Int Rev Cytol* 1977;**51**:49.

Mathieu P, Rahier J, Thomas K: Localization of relaxin in human gestational corpus luteum. *Cell Tissue Res* 1981;**219**:213.

Motta PM, Hafez ESE (editors): *Biology of the Ovary.* Martinus Nijhoff, 1980.

Peters H, McNatty KP: *The Ovary: A Correlation of Structure and Function in Mammals.* Granada Publishing, 1980.

Pitelka DR, Hamamoto ST: Ultrastructure of the mammary secretory cell. In: *Biochemistry of Lactation.* Mepham TB (editor). Elsevier, 1983.

Segal SJ: The physiology of human reproduction. *Sci Am* (Sept) 1974;**231**:52.

Tersakis J: The ultrastructure of normal human first trimester placenta. *J Ultrastruct Res* 1963;**9**:268.

Vorherr H: *The Breast: Morphology, Physiology and Lactation.* Academic Press, 1974.

Wynn RM (editor): *Biology of the Uterus.* Plenum Press, 1977.

Yoshida Y: Ultrastructure and secretory function of the syncytial trophoblast of human placenta in early pregnancy. *Exp Cell Res* 1964;**34**:305.

Zuckerman S, Weir BJ (editors): *The Ovary,* 2nd ed. Vol. 1. General Aspects. Academic Press, 1977.

The Sense Organs

24

Information about the external world is conveyed to the central nervous system by sensory units called **receptors**. These structures transduce stimuli (heat, pressure, light, sound, etc) into signals that are capable of triggering action potentials in sensory nerves. These receptors are grouped into somatic and visceral receptor, proprioceptor, chemoreceptor, photoreceptor, and audioreceptor systems.

SUPERFICIAL & DEEP SENSATION: THE SOMATIC & VISCERAL RECEPTOR SYSTEM

These receptors can be divided into free and encapsulated nerve terminals, according to the absence or presence of a connective tissue capsule. The receptors consist of dendritic nerve endings or specialized nonneuronal cells and are responsible for the senses discussed below.

Touch & Pressure

The sense of touch and pressure is detected by Meissner's corpuscles, Ruffini's endings, Merkel's touch corpuscles, sensory endings around hairs, and perhaps by free nerve endings. The best-studied mechanoreceptor is the **pacinian corpuscle**. Consisting of 20–70 layers of fibroblasts alternating with thin collagen fibers, it resembles a sliced onion in histologic sections (Figs 24–1 and 24–2). These corpuscles are found in the dermis and are especially numerous in the dermis of the digits; they are also present in mesenteries and periosteum. Pacinian corpuscles have been associated mainly with the detection of vibration.

Meissner's corpuscles are composed of fibroblasts and thick collagen fibers surrounding an inner core of Schwann cells and nerve terminals. In histologic sections, the horizontal arrangement of groups of Schwann cells forms layers that enfold the nerve terminals as they wind their way upward. They respond to tactile stimuli and are present mainly in the hairless skin of the palms, soles, nipples, and lips (Fig 24–1).

Ruffini's endings are spindle-shaped encapsulated nerve endings found in joints and in the dermis of both hairless and hairy skin (Fig 24–1).

Hair follicles have both circumferential and longitudinal arrays of unmyelinated fibers around most of the length of the follicle. When a hair is bent, the sensation of touch is elicited.

Heat, Cold, & Pain

These sensations are mainly mediated by free nerve endings that branch in the dermis, penetrate the basement membrane, and extend into the lower cell layers of the epidermis (Fig 24–1).

DETECTION OF BODY POSITION IN SPACE: THE PROPRIOCEPTOR SYSTEM

All human striated muscles contain encapsulated proprioceptors (from Latin, *proprius*, one's own, + *capio*, to take) known as **muscle spindles** (Fig 24–1). These structures consist of a connective tissue capsule surrounding a fluid-filled space that contains a few long, thick muscle fibers and some short, thinner fibers (collectively called **intrafusal fibers**). Several sensory nerve fibers penetrate the muscle spindles, where they detect changes in the length of extrafusal muscle fibers and relay this information to the spinal cord. Here reflexes of varying complexity are activated to maintain posture and to regulate the activity of opposing muscle groups involved in motor activities such as walking.

In tendons, near the insertion sites of muscle fibers, a connective tissue sheath encapsulates a number of large bundles of collagen fibers that are continuous with the collagen fibers that make up the myotendinous junction. Sensory nerves penetrate the connective tissue capsule. These structures, known as **Golgi tendon organs**, contribute to proprioception by detecting tensional differences in tendons (Fig 24–1).

Because these structures are sensitive to increases in tension, they permit blind persons to know the exact position of their limbs and thereby regulate the amount of effort required to perform movements that call for variable amounts of muscular force.

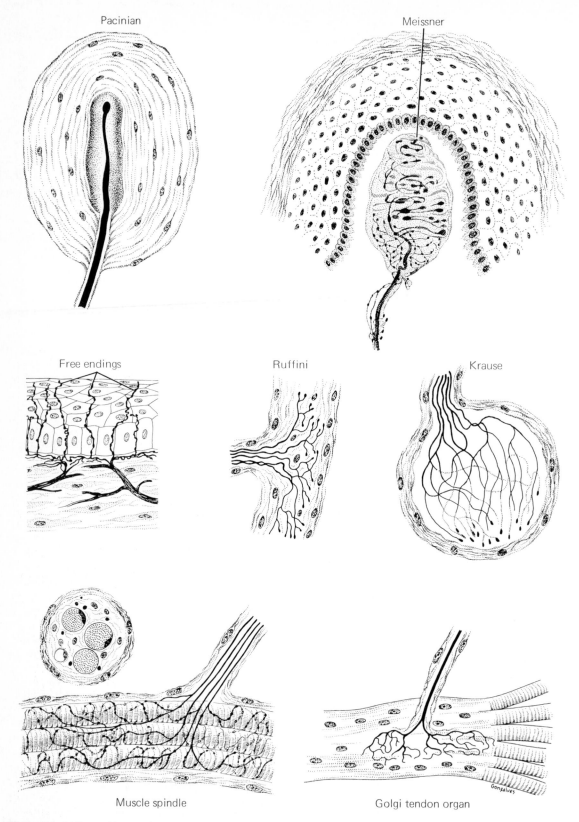

Pacinian

Meissner

Free endings

Ruffini

Krause

Muscle spindle

Golgi tendon organ

Figure 24–1. Several types of sensory endings of nerves (not drawn to the same scale). (Based partially on a drawing in Ham AW: *Histology*, 6th ed. Lippincott, 1969.)

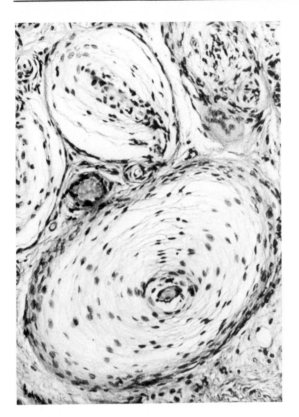

Figure 24–2. Photomicrograph of transverse and oblique sections of human pacinian corpuscles. Observe the concentric layers of connective tissue surrounding the centrally disposed unmyelinated nerve. H&E stain, × 320.

TASTE & SMELL: THE CHEMORECEPTOR SYSTEM

Taste

Taste is a sensation perceived by **taste buds,** receptors located principally on the tongue (there are about 2000 taste buds on the human tongue) and in smaller numbers on the soft palate and laryngeal surface of the epiglottis. Lingual taste buds are embedded within the stratified epithelium of the **circumvallate, foliate,** and **fungiform papillae.** Chemicals enter through the **taste pore,** a small aperture providing access to the receptor cells (Figs 24–3 and 24–4).

Taste buds are composed of at least 4 types of cells, which can be distinguished with the electron microscope. **Type I** and **type II** cells are tall, with microvilli at their surface. Although their function is uncertain, they may support the activity of type III cells. The **type III** cell is also a long cell, characterized by the presence of numerous vesicles that resemble synaptic vesicles. A fourth cell type is a relatively undifferentiated basal cell that may be the precursor of more specialized cells in the taste buds. Dendritic processes of sensory nerves are found in close prox-

imity to these accumulations of synaptic vesicles (Fig 24–4). This is the basis for assigning taste reception to the type III cell.

Smell (Olfaction)

The olfactory chemoreceptors are located in the **olfactory epithelium,** a specialized area of the mucous membrane in the roof of the nasal cavity. In humans, it is about 10 cm^2 in area and up to 100 μm in thickness. This is a pseudostratified columnar epithelium composed of 3 types of cells.

The **supporting cells** have broad, cylindrical apexes and narrower bases. On their free surface are microvilli submerged in a fluid layer consisting of both serous and mucous secretions and covering the entire epithelial surface. Well-developed junctional complexes bind the supporting cells to the adjacent olfactory cells. The cells contain a light yellow pigment that is responsible for the color of the olfactory mucosa (Fig 24–5).

The **basal cells** are small; they are spherical or cone-shaped and form a single layer at the base of the epithelium.

Between the basal cells and the supporting cells are the **olfactory cells,** bipolar neurons distinguished from the supporting cells by the position of their nu-

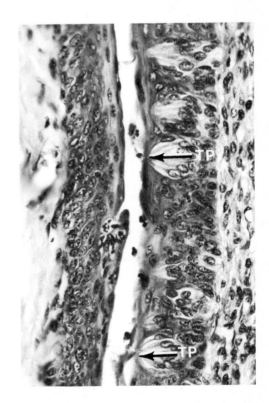

Figure 24–3. Photomicrograph of a section of a circumvallate papilla of the tongue, showing the taste buds embedded in the epithelial layer. TP, taste pore. H&E stain, × 400.

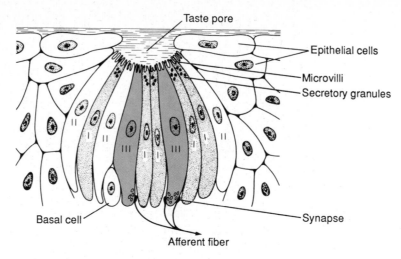

Figure 24–4. Structure and innervation of a taste bud. Four types of cells are shown. Type I cells are dark and possess apical secretory granules. The function of the light type II cells is not known. The sensory cell is type III (shown in color), with basally located synaptic vesicles and associated afferent nerve endings. Basal cells proliferate and give rise to the other cells. Although only one afferent fiber is shown, in reality, about 50 fibers innervate a single taste bud.

clei, which lie below the nuclei of the supporting cells. Their apexes possess dilated areas from which arise 6–20 cilia (Fig 24–6). These cilia are long and nonmotile and are considered to be receptors, ie, the structures that respond to odoriferous substances by generating a receptor potential. They considerably increase the receptor surface (Fig 24–7). The afferent axons of these bipolar neurons unite in small bundles directed toward the central nervous system.

VISION: THE PHOTORECEPTOR SYSTEM

1. THE EYE

The eye is a complex and highly developed photosensitive organ that permits an accurate analysis of the form, light intensity, and color reflected from objects. The eyes are located in protective bony structures of the skull—the **orbits.** Each eye includes a tough, fibrous globe to maintain its shape, a lens system to focus the image, a layer of photosensitive cells, and a system of cells and nerves whose function it is to collect, process, and transmit visual information to the central nervous system. Each eye is composed of 3 concentric layers: an external layer that consists of the **sclera** and the **cornea;** a middle layer—also called the **vascular layer,** or **uveal tract**—consisting of the **choroid, ciliary body,** and **iris;** and an inner layer of nerve tissue, the **retina,** which consists of an outer pigment epithelium (Fig 24–9) and an inner retina proper. The photosensitive retina proper communicates with the cerebrum through the **optic nerve** (Figs 24–8 and 24–9) and extends forward to the **ora serrata.**

The **lens** of the eye is a biconvex transparent structure held in place by a circular system of fibers, the **zonule,** which extends from the lens into a thickening

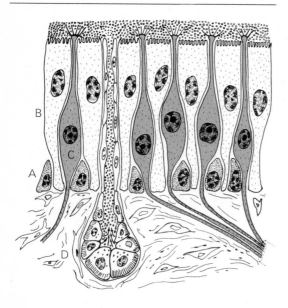

Figure 24–5. Olfactory mucosa showing the 3 cell types and Bowman's gland. **A:** Basal cells; **B:** supporting cells; **C:** olfactory cells (shown in color); **D:** Bowman's gland.

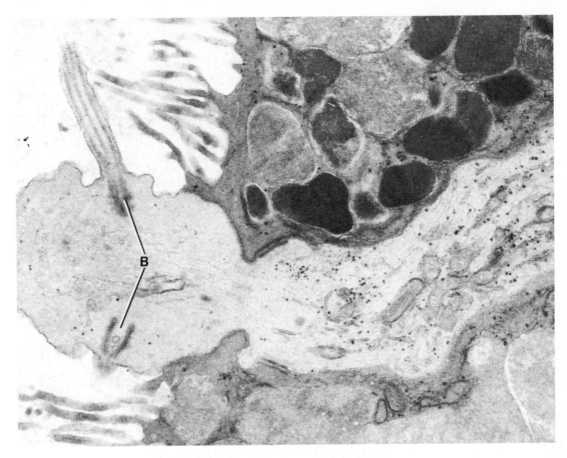

Figure 24–6. Electron micrograph of a section of olfactory mucosa from a frog. In the center is a pale olfactory cell and its terminal dilation with 2 basal bodies (B), from which cilia emerge. × 28,000. (Courtesy of KR Porter.)

of the middle layer, the **ciliary body,** and by close apposition, to the vitreous on its posterior side (Figs 24–8 and 24–9). Partly covering the anterior surface of the lens is an opaque pigmented expansion of the middle layer called the **iris.** The round hole in the middle of the iris is the **pupil** (Fig 24–8).

The eye contains 3 compartments: the **anterior chamber,** which occupies the space between the cornea and the iris and lens; the **posterior chamber,** between the iris, ciliary process, zonular attachments, and the lens; and the **vitreous space,** which lies behind the lens and zonular attachments and is surrounded by the retina (Figs 24–8 and 24–9). Both the anterior and posterior chambers contain a protein-poor fluid called **aqueous humor.** The vitreous space is filled by a gelatinous substance called the **vitreous body.**

Note that the terms **outer** (**external**) and **inner** (**internal**) refer to the gross structure of the eye. Inner denotes a structure closer to the center of the globe, while outer means closer to the surface of the eyeball.

External Layer, or Tunica Fibrosa

The opaque white posterior five-sixths of the external layer of the eye is the **sclera,** forming in the human a segment of a sphere roughly 22 mm in diameter (Figs 24–8 and 24–9). The sclera consists of tough, dense connective tissue made up mainly of flat collagen bundles intersecting in various directions while remaining parallel to the surface of the organ, a moderate amount of ground substance, and a few fibroblasts. The external surface of the sclera—the **episclera**—is connected by a loose system of thin collagen fibers to a dense layer of connective tissue called **Tenon's capsule.** It comes into contact with the loose conjunctival stroma at the junction of the cornea with the sclera. Between Tenon's capsule and the sclera is **Tenon's space.** It is because of this loose space that the eyeball can make rotating movements in all directions. Between the sclera and the choroid is the **suprachoroidal lamina,** a thin layer of loose connective tissue rich in melanocytes, fibroblasts, and elastic fibers. The sclera is relatively avascular.

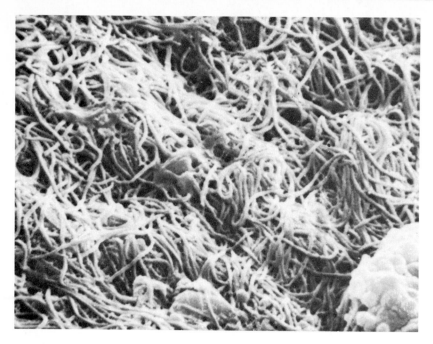

Figure 24–7. Scanning electron micrograph of the surface of the olfactory mucosa of a turtle. Observe the dense net of cilia covering its surface. × 6600. (Courtesy of PP Graziadei.)

In contrast to the posterior five-sixths of the eye, the anterior one-sixth—the **cornea**—is colorless and transparent (Figs 24–8 and 24–9). A transverse section of the cornea shows that it consists of 5 layers: epithelium, Bowman's membrane, stroma, Descemet's membrane, and endothelium (Fig 24–10). The corneal epithelium is stratified, squamous, and nonkeratinized and consists of 5 or 6 layers of cells. In the basal part of the epithelium are numerous mitotic figures that are responsible for the cornea's remarkable regenerative capacity: the turnover time for these cells is approximately 7 days. The surface corneal cells show microvilli protruding into the space filled by the precorneal tear film, a protective layer of lipid and glycoprotein, about 7 μm in thickness. The cornea has one of the richest sensory nerve supplies of any eye tissue.

Beneath the corneal epithelium lies a thick homogeneous layer 7–12 μm in thickness. It consists of collagen fibers crossing at random, a condensation of the intercellular substance, and no cells (Fig 24–11). This is **Bowman's membrane,** which contributes greatly to the stability and strength of the cornea.

The **stroma** is formed by many layers of parallel collagen bundles that cross at approximately right angles to each other. The collagen fibrils within each lamella are parallel to each other and run the full width of the cornea. Between the several layers, the cytoplasmic extensions of fibroblasts are flattened like the wings of a butterfly. Both cells and

fibers of the stroma are immersed in an amorphous metachromatic glycoprotein substance rich in chondroitin sulfate. Although the stroma is avascular, migrating lymphoid cells are normally present in the cornea.

Descemet's membrane is a thick (5–10 μm) homogeneous structure composed of fine collagenous filaments organized in a 3-dimensional network (Fig 24–10B).

The **endothelium** of the cornea is a simple squamous epithelium. These cells possess organelles characteristic of cells engaged in active transport and protein synthesis for secretion, which may relate to the synthesis and maintenance of Descemet's membrane. The corneal endothelium and epithelium are responsible for maintaining the transparency of the cornea. Both layers are capable of transporting sodium ions toward their apical surfaces. Chloride ions and water follow passively, maintaining the corneal stroma in a relatively dehydrated state. This, along with the regular orientation of the very thin collagen fibrils of the stroma, accounts for the transparency of the cornea.

The **corneoscleral junction,** or **limbus,** is an area of transition from the transparent collagen bundles of the cornea to the white opaque fibers of the sclera. It is highly vascularized, and its blood vessels assume an important role in corneal inflammatory processes. The cornea—an avascular structure—receives its metabolites by diffusion from adjacent vessels and from

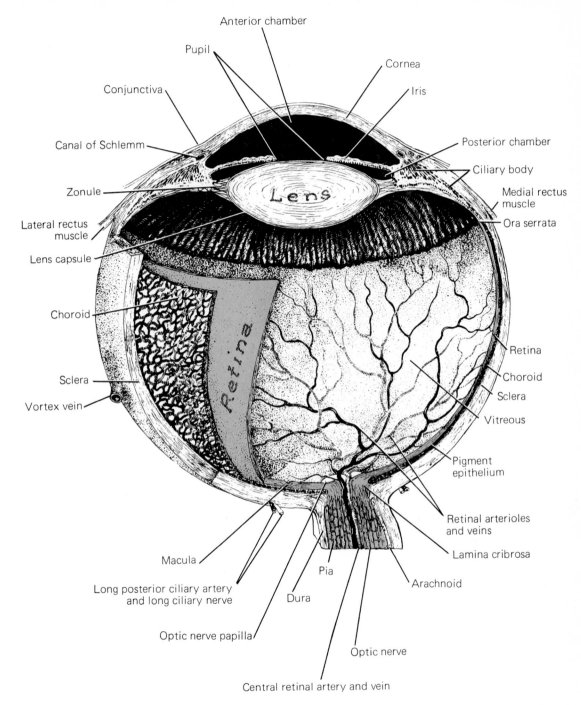

Figure 24–8. Internal structures of the human eye. The retina and optic nerve are shown in color. (Redrawn from an original drawing by Paul Peck and reproduced, with permission, from *The Anatomy of the Eye*. [Courtesy of Lederle Laboratories.])

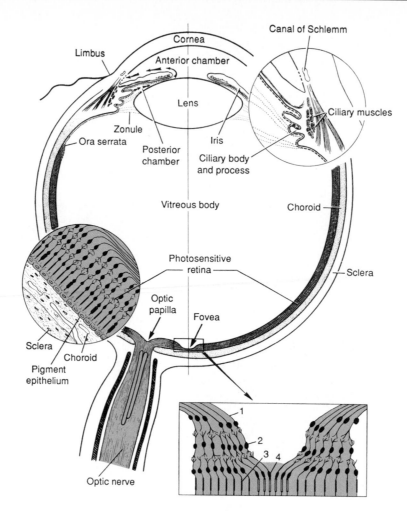

Figure 24–9. Diagram of the right eye, seen from above, showing the structure of the eye, retina, fovea, and ciliary body. Arrows in the anterior chamber show the direction of flow of aqueous humor. An enlarged diagram of the fovea is shown at lower right. 1, axons of ganglion cells; 2, bipolar cells; 3, rods; 4, cones. (Modified and reproduced, with permission, from Ham AW: *Histology*, 6th ed. Lippincott, 1969.)

the fluid of the anterior chamber of the eye. In the region of the limbus in the stromal layer, irregular endothelium-lined channels, the trabecular meshwork, merge to form the **canal of Schlemm** (Figs 24–8 and 24–9), which drains fluid from the anterior chamber of the eye. The canal of Schlemm communicates externally with the venous system.

Middle, or Vascular, Layer

The middle (vascular) layer of the eye consists of 3 parts: choroid, ciliary body, and iris (Fig 24–8). These 3 parts are known collectively as the uveal tract.

A. Choroid: The choroid is a highly vascularized coat, with loose connective tissue rich in fibroblasts, macrophages, lymphocytes, mast cells, plasma cells, collagen fibers, and elastic fibers between its blood vessels. Melanocytes are abundant in this

layer and give it its characteristic black color. The inner layer of the choroid is richer than the outer layer in small vessels and is called the **choriocapillary layer.** It has an important function in nutrition of the retina, and damage to this tissue causes serious damage to the retina. A thin (3–4 μm) amorphous hyaline membrane separates the choriocapillary layer from the retina. This is known as **Bruch's membrane** and extends from the **optic disk** to the ora serrata. The optic disk, also called **optic papilla,** is the region where the optic nerve enters the eyeball (Fig 24–9).

Bruch's membrane is formed of 5 different layers. The central layer is composed of a network of elastic fibers. This network is lined on its 2 surfaces by layers of collagen fibers that are covered by the basal lamina of the capillaries of the choriocapillary layer

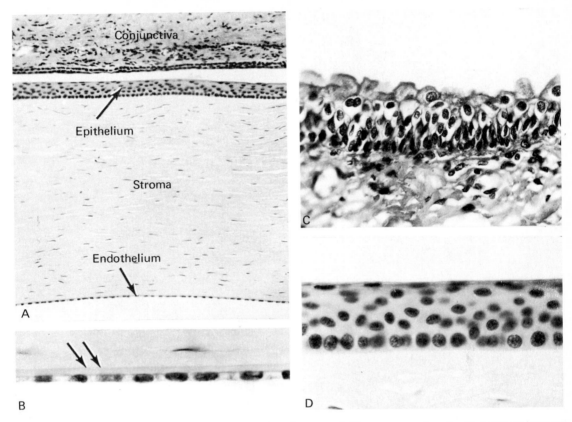

Figure 24–10. Photomicrographs of a transverse section of cornea. **A:** The cornea and conjunctiva seen at low magnification. × 80. **B:** The posterior corneal epithelium—also called endothelium (arrows indicate Descemet's membrane). × 400. **C:** Conjunctival epithelium. × 300. **D:** Anterior corneal epithelium. Note the smooth contour of the surface of this epithelium. × 400.

on one side and the basal lamina of the pigment epithelium on the other side (Fig 24–12). (See page 479, under *Retina,* for a description of the pigment epithelium.) The choroid is bound to the sclera by the **suprachoroidal lamina,** a loose layer of connective tissue rich in melanocytes.

B. Ciliary Body: The ciliary body, an anterior expansion of the choroid at the level of the lens (Figs 24–8 and 24–9), is a continuous thickened ring that lies at the inner surface of the anterior portion of the sclera; it forms a triangle in transverse section. One of its faces is in contact with the vitreous body, one with the sclera, and the third with the lens and the posterior chamber of the eye. The histologic structure of the ciliary body is basically loose connective tissue (rich in elastic fibers, vessels, and melanocytes) surrounding the **ciliary muscle** (Fig 24–9). This structure consists of 2 bundles of smooth muscle fibers that insert on the sclera anteriorly and on different regions of the ciliary body posteriorly. One of these bundles has the function of stretching the choroid; another bundle, when contracted, relaxes the tension on the lens.

These muscular movements are important in visual accommodation (see the discussion on the lens). The surfaces of the ciliary body that face the vitreous, posterior chamber, and lens are covered by the anterior extension of the retina (Fig 24–9). In this region, the retina consists of only 2 cell layers. The layer directly adjacent to the ciliary body consists of simple columnar cells rich in melanin and corresponds to the forward projection of the pigment layer of the retina. The second layer, which covers the first, is derived from the sensory layer of the retina and consists of simple nonpigmented columnar epithelium (Fig 24–13A).

C. Ciliary Processes: The ciliary processes are ridgelike extensions of the ciliary body. They have a loose connective tissue core and numerous fenestrated capillaries (see Chapter 11) and are covered by the 2 simple epithelial layers described above (Fig 24–13B). From the ciliary processes emerge fibers **(zonule fibers)** that insert into the capsule of the lens and anchor it in place. The apical ends of the epithelial cells are found at the junction between pigmented

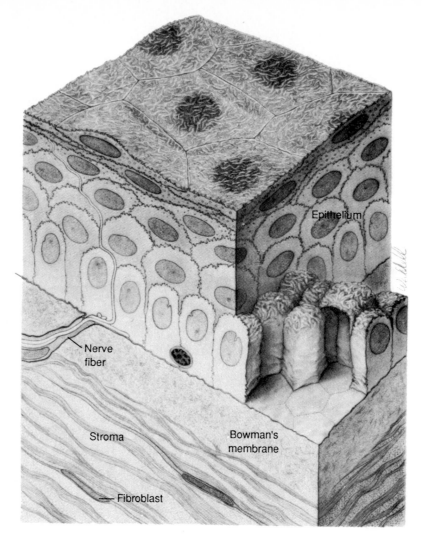

Figure 24–11. Three-dimensional drawing of the cornea. (Reproduced, with permission, from Hogan MJ, Alvarado JA, Weddell JE: *Histology of the Human Eye.* Saunders, 1971.)

and nonpigmented cells, and the cells thus meet each other head-to-head. The basement membrane of the outer, pigmented cells is adjacent to the main mass of the ciliary body, while the basement membrane of the inner, nonpigmented cells is adjacent to the posterior chamber. It is in this basement membrane that the zonular fibers have their origin. The apical ends of the epithelial cells are joined by desmosomes, and elaborate tight junctions are found around the apical surfaces of epithelial cells of both layers. The unpigmented inner layer of cells has extensive basal infoldings and interdigitations characteristic of ion-transporting cells (see Chapter 4). These cells actively transport certain constituents of plasma into the posterior chamber, thus forming the **aqueous humor.** This fluid has an inorganic ion composition similar to plasma but contains less than 0.1% protein (plasma has about 7% protein). Aqueous humor flows toward the lens and passes between it and the iris, reaching the anterior chamber of the eye (see arrows in Fig 24–9). Once in the anterior chamber, it proceeds to the angle formed by the cornea with the basal part of the iris. It penetrates the tissue of the limbus in a series of labyrinthine spaces (the trabecular meshwork) and finally reaches the irregular canal of Schlemm, lined by endothelial cells (Figs 24–8 and 24–9). This structure communicates with small veins of the sclera, through which the aqueous humor escapes.

Any impediment to the drainage of aqueous humor caused by an obstruction in the outflow

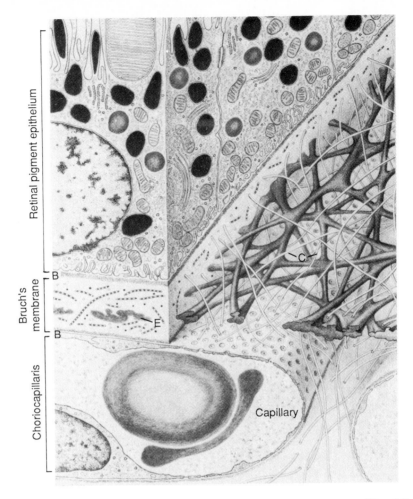

Figure 24–12. Three dimensional drawing showing the constitution of Bruch's membrane and its relation to the pigment cell layer and choriocapillary layer. B, basal lamina; observe the anastomosing network of dark elastic fibers interspersed with thin, light, nonanastomosing collagen fibers. (Slightly modified and reproduced, with permission, from Hogan MJ, Alvarado JA, Weddell JE: *Histology of the Human Eye.* Saunders, 1971.)

channels results in an increase in intraocular pressure, causing **glaucoma.**

D. Iris: The iris is an extension of the choroid that partially covers the lens, leaving a round opening in the center called the **pupil** (Fig 24–8). The anterior surface of the iris is irregular and rough, with grooves and ridges. It is formed by a discontinuous layer of pigment cells and fibroblasts. Beneath this layer is a poorly vascularized connective tissue with few fibers and many fibroblasts and melanocytes. The next layer is rich in blood vessels embedded in loose connective tissue. The smooth posterior surface of the iris is covered by 2 layers of epithelium, which also cover the ciliary body and its processes. The inner epithelium, in contact with the posterior chamber, is heavily pigmented with melanin granules. The outer epithe-

lial cells have radially directed tonguelike extensions of their basal region; they are filled with overlapping myofilaments, creating the **dilator pupillae muscle** of the iris. The heavy pigmentation prevents the passage of light into the interior of the eye except through the pupil.

The function of the abundant melanocytes or melanin-containing pigment cells in several regions of the eye is to keep stray light rays from interfering with image formation. The melanocytes of the stroma of the iris are responsible for the color of the eyes. If the layer of pigment in the interior region of the iris consists of only a few cells, the light reflected from the black pigment epithelium present in the posterior surface of the iris will be blue. As the amount of pigment increases, the iris assumes various shades of greenish-blue, gray, and finally brown. Albinos have

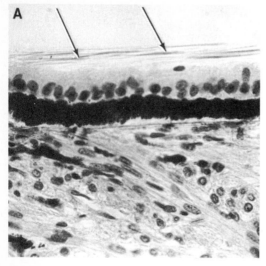

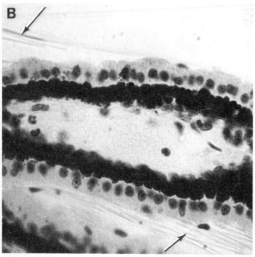

Figure 24–13. Photomicrographs of a ciliary body. **A:** Note the double layer, one of which consists of pigmented cells. **B:** The ciliary process is covered by epithelium on both sides. Arrows indicate zonular fibers. H&E stain, × 400.

A. Lens Capsule: The lens is enveloped by a thick (10–20 μm), homogeneous, refractile, carbohydrate-rich capsule coating the outer surface of the epithelial cells. It is elastic and consists mainly of collagen type IV and amorphous glycoprotein.

B. Subcapsular Epithelium: This consists of a single layer of cuboidal epithelial cells that are present only on the anterior surface of the lens. The lens increases in size and grows throughout life as new lens fibers develop from cells located at the equator of the lens. The cells of this epithelium exhibit many interdigitations with the lens fibers. Their cytoplasm has few organelles and stains lightly. The cells are bound together by gap junctions.

C. Lens Fibers: These are elongated and appear as thin flattened structures. They are highly differentiated cells derived from cells of the subcapsular epithelium. They eventually lose their nuclei and other organelles and become greatly elongated, attaining dimensions of 7–10 mm in length, 8–10 μm in width, and 2 μm in thickness. These cells are filled with a group of proteins called **crystallins.** Although lens fiber production continues throughout life, it is at an ever-decreasing rate.

The lens is held in place by a radially oriented group of fibers, the **zonule,** that inserts on one side on the lens capsule and on the other on the ciliary body (Fig 24–14). Zonular fibers are similar to the microfibrils of elastic fibers. This system is important in the process known as **accommodation,** which permits focusing on near and far objects by changing the curvature of the lens. When the eye is at rest or gazing at distant objects, the lens is kept stretched by the zonule in a plane perpendicular to the optical axis. To focus on a near object, the ciliary muscles contract, causing forward displacement of the choroid and ciliary body. The tension exerted by the zonule is relieved, and the lens becomes thicker, keeping the object in focus.

Advancing age reduces the elasticity of the lens, making accommodation for near objects difficult. This is a normal aging process (presbyopia), which can be corrected by wearing glasses with convex lenses. In older individuals, a brownish pigment accumulates in lens fibers, making them less transparent. When the lens becomes opaque, the condition is termed **cataract.** Cataract may also be caused by excessive exposure to ultraviolet radiation. In diabetes mellitus, the high levels of glucose are thought to produce cataract.

Vitreous Body

The vitreous body occupies the region of the eye behind the lens. It is a transparent gel that consists of water (about 99%), collagen, and heavily hydrated glycosaminoglycans whose principal component is hyaluronic acid.

almost no pigment, and the pink color of their irises is due to the reflection of incident light from the blood vessels of the iris.

The iris contains smooth muscle bundles disposed in circles concentric with the pupillary margin, forming the **sphincter pupillae muscle** of the iris. The dilator and sphincter muscles have sympathetic and parasympathetic innervation, respectively.

Lens

This biconvex structure is characterized by great elasticity, a feature that is lost with age as the lens hardens. The lens has 3 principal components.

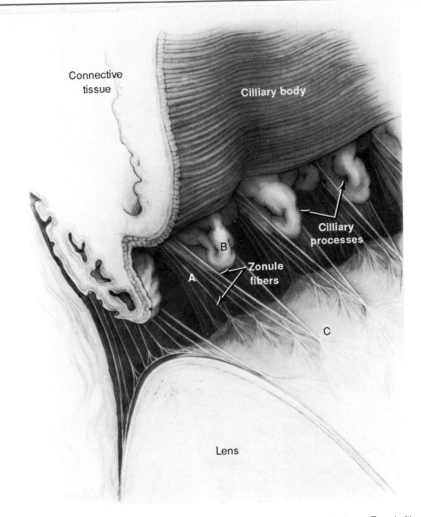

Figure 24–14. Anterior view of the ciliary processes showing the zonules attaching to the lens. Zonule fibers are bundles of microfilaments (oxytalan fibers) from the elastic fiber system. The zonules form columns (A) on either side of the ciliary processes (B), which meet on a single site (C) as they attach to the lens. (Reproduced, with permission, from Hogan MJ, Alvarado JA, Weddell JE: *Histology of the Human Eye.* Saunders, 1971.)

Retina

The retina, the inner layer of the globe, consists of 2 portions. The posterior portion is photosensitive; the anterior part, which is not photosensitive, constitutes the inner lining of the ciliary body and the posterior part of the iris (Figs 24–9 and 24–15). The retina derives from an evagination of the anterior cephalic vesicle or prosencephalon. As this so-called **optic vesicle** comes into contact with the surface ectoderm, it gradually invaginates in its central region, forming a double-walled **optic cup.** In the adult, the outer wall gives rise to a thin membrane called the **pigment epithelium;** the optical or functioning part of the retina—the **neural retina**—is derived from the inner layer.

The pigment epithelium consists of columnar cells with a basal nucleus. The basal regions of the cells adhere firmly to Bruch's membrane, and the cell membranes have numerous basal invaginations (Fig 24–21). Mitochondria are more abundant in the region of the cytoplasm near these invaginations. These characteristics suggest an ion-transporting activity for this region.

The lateral cell membranes show cell junctions with conspicuous zonulae occludentes and adherentes at their apexes; there are also desmosomes and gap junctions. These morphologic details indicate that the apical and basal regions of this epithelial sheet are sealed off and that intercellular communication exists. The existence of an electrical potential difference resulting from ion transport between the 2 surfaces of this epithelium can be accounted for by these junctional specializations.

The cell apex has abundant extensions of 2 types:

Epithelium   Choroid   Sclera

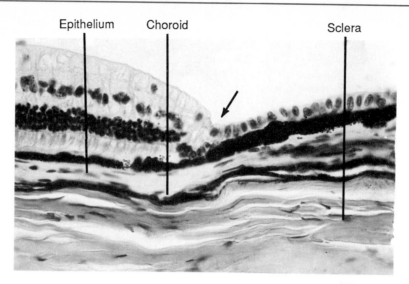

Figure 24–15. Photomicrograph of a section of retina in the transition (arrow) between the photosensitive (at left) and blind (at right) parts. This transition is called the ora serrata. Note the pigment epithelium, the choroid, and the sclera. H&E stain, × 200.

Internal
limiting membrane   External
limiting membrane

Ganglion cell

Internal plexiform

Internal nuclear

External plexiform

External nuclear

Inner segments

Outer segments

Retinal pigment
epithelium

Choroid

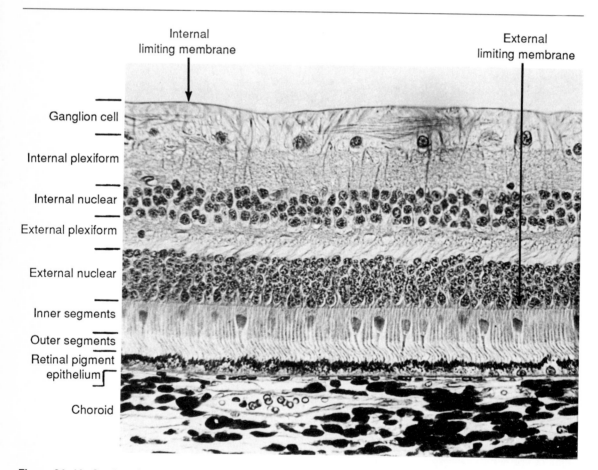

Figure 24–16. Section of the retina of a monkey. It is basically composed of 3 layers of cells: photoreceptors, bipolar neurons, and ganglion cells. Light enters from the top and traverses the layers shown in the figure. The internal nuclear layer contains bipolar neurons, and the external nuclear layer contains the nuclei of rods and cones. Note the inner segments of rods (narrow lines) and cones (triangular dark structures). × 655.

slender microvilli and cylindrical sheaths that invest the tips of the photoreceptors.

> Because neither type of extension is anatomically joined to the photoreceptors, these regions can become separated, as in a **detachment of the retina.** This common and serious disorder in humans is currently being treated effectively by laser surgery.

The cytoplasm of pigment epithelial cells has abundant smooth endoplasmic reticulum, believed to be a site of vitamin A esterification and transport to the photoreceptors. Melanin granules are numerous in the apical cytoplasm and microvilli. Melanin is synthesized in these cells by a mechanism similar to that described for the melanocytes in the skin (see Chapter 18). This dark pigment has the function of absorbing light after the photoreceptors have been stimulated.

The cell apex has numerous dense vesicles of variable shape that represent various stages in the phago-cytosis and digestion of the tips of photoreceptor outer segments. The structure of these cells and the shedding of their tips are discussed below (Fig 24–21).

The optical part of the retina—the posterior or photosensitive part—is a complex structure containing at least 15 types of neurons, and these cells form at least 38 distinct kinds of synapses with one another. The optical retina consists of an outer layer of photosensitive cells, the **rods** and **cones** (Figs 24–9, 24–16, and 24–17); an intermediate layer of **bipolar neurons,** which connects the rods and cones to the ganglion cells; and an internal layer of **ganglion cells,** which establishes contact with the bipolar cells through its dendrites and sends axons to the central nervous system. These axons converge at the optic papilla, forming the **optic nerve.**

Between the layer of rods and cones and the bipolar cells is a region called the **external plexiform,** or **synaptic, layer** where synapses between these 2 types of cells occur. The region where the synapses between the bipolar and ganglion cells are established is

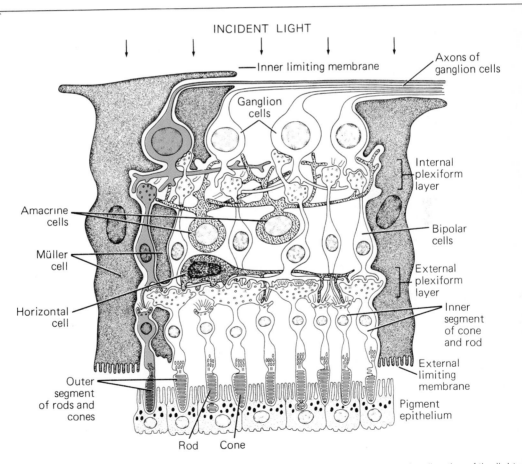

Figure 24–17. Schematic drawing of the 3 layers of retinal neurons. The arrows represent the direction of the light path. The stimulation generated by the incident light on rods and cones proceeds in the opposite direction. (Redrawn and reproduced, with permission, from Boycott and Dowling: *Proc R Soc Lond [Biol]* 1966;**166**:80.)

called the **internal plexiform layer** (Fig 24–17). The retina has an inverted structure, for the light will first cross the ganglion layer and then the bipolar layer to reach the rods and cones.

The following paragraphs examine the structure of the retina in greater detail. The rods and cones, named for the forms they assume, are polarized neurons; at one pole is a single photosensitive dendrite, and at the other are synapses with cells of the bipolar layer (Figs 24–17 and 24–18). The rod and cone cells can be divided into outer and inner segments, a nuclear region, and a synaptic region. The outer segments are modified cilia and contain stacks of flattened membrane-limited saccules with a flattened disklike shape. The photosensitive pigment of the retina is in the membranes of these saccules. Both rod and cone cells pass through a thin layer, the **external limiting membrane,** that is a series of junctional complexes between the photoreceptors and glial cells of the ret-

ina (Müller cells) (Fig 24–22). The nuclei of the cones are generally disposed near the limiting membrane, while rod nuclei lie near the center of the inner segment.

The **rod cells** are thin, elongated cells (50 x 3 μm) composed of 2 portions as shown in Figs 24–17 and 24–18. The external photosensitive rod-shaped portion is composed mainly of numerous (600–1000) flattened membranous disks piled up like a stack of coins. The disks in rods are not continuous with the plasma membrane; the **outer segment** is separated from the **inner segment** by a constriction. Just below this constriction is a basal segment from which a cilium arises and passes to the outer segment. The inner segment is rich in glycogen and has a remarkable accumulation of mitochondria, most of which lie near the constriction (Figs 24–18 and 24–19). This local accumulation of mitochondria is related to the production of energy necessary for the visual process and protein synthesis. Polyribosomes, present in large numbers below the mitochondrial region of the inner segment, are involved in protein synthesis. Some of these proteins migrate to the outer segment of the rod cells, where they are incorporated into membranous disks. The flattened disks of the rod cells contain the pigment **visual purple,** or **rhodopsin,** which is bleached by light and initiates the visual stimulus. This substance is globular in form and is located in the outer surface of the lipid bilayer of the flattened membranous disks.

It has been estimated that the human retina has approximately 120 million rods. They are extremely sensitive to light and are considered the receptors used when low levels of light are encountered, such as dusk or nighttime. The outer segment is the site of photosensitivity; the inner segment contains the metabolic machinery necessary for the biosynthetic and energy-producing processes of these cells.

Radioautographic studies show that proteins of the rod vesicles are synthesized in the polyribosome-rich inner segments of these cells. From there, they migrate to the outer segment and aggregate at its basal region, where they are incorporated into membranes formed by a double layer of phospholipids, producing flattened disks (Figs 24–18 and 24–19). These structures gradually migrate to the cell apex, where they are shed, phagocytized, and digested by the cells of the pigment epithelium (Figs 24–20 and 24–21). It has been calculated that, in the monkey, approximately 90 vesicles per cell are produced daily. The whole process of migration, from assembly at the basal cell region to apical shedding, takes 9–13 days.

In **hereditary retinal dystrophy** in the rat, the vesicles shed from the rods are not phagocytized, probably as a result of a dysfunction of the pigment epithelium. They are instead deposited at the surface of the pigment layer.

The **cone cells** are also elongated (60 × 1.5 μm)

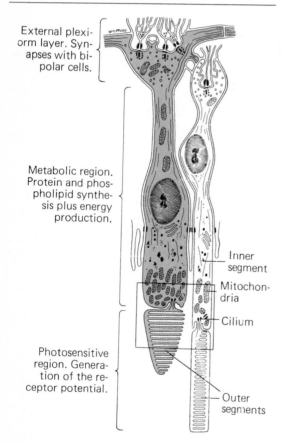

External plexiform layer. Synapses with bipolar cells.

Metabolic region. Protein and phospholipid synthesis plus energy production.

Inner segment

Mitochondria

Cilium

Photosensitive region. Generation of the receptor potential.

Outer segments

Figure 24–18. The ultrastructure of the rods is shown at right and the cones at left. The outlined region is illustrated in the electron micrograph in Fig 24–19. (Redrawn and reproduced, with permission, from Chevremont M: *Notions de Cytologie et Histologie.* S.A. Desoer Editions [Liege], 1966.)

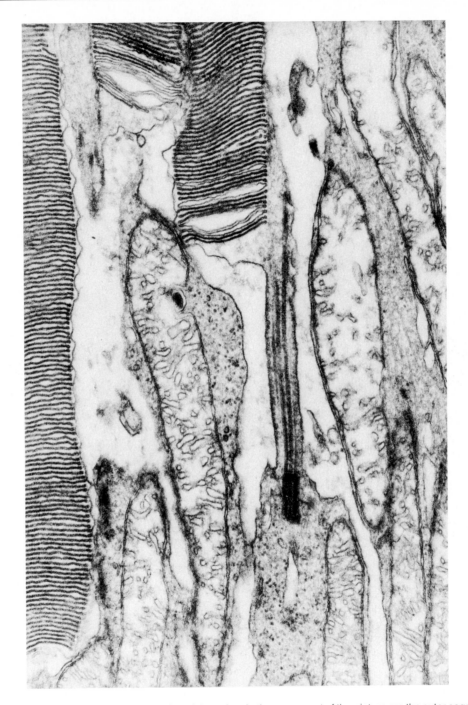

Figure 24–19. Electron micrograph of a section of the retina. In the upper part of the picture are the outer segments. This photosensitive region consists of parallel membranous flat disks. Mitochondrial accumulation occurs in the inner segment (see Fig 24–18). In the middle of the figure is a basal body giving rise to a cilium that is further modified into an outer segment.

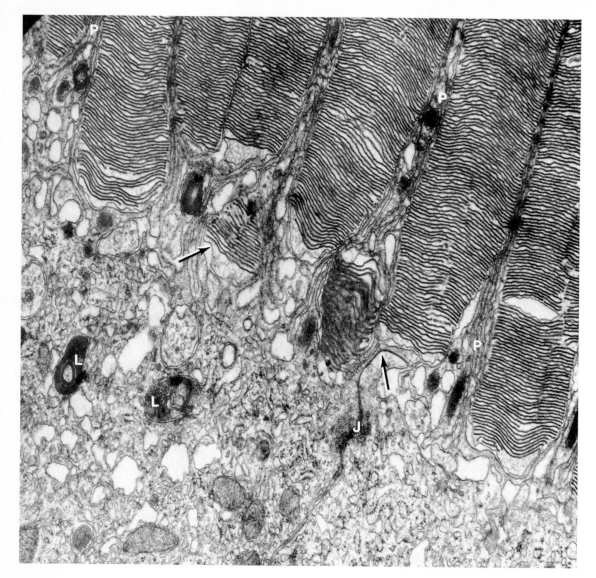

Figure 24–20. Electron micrograph of the interface between the photosensitive and pigmented layers in a rat retina. In the lower portion are parts of 2 pigment epithelial cells, revealing specialized junctions (J) between their lateral plasmalemmas. Above the pigment cells are the tips of several outer segments of rod cells that interdigitate with apical processes of the pigment epithelium (P). The large vacuoles containing flattened membranes (arrows) have been shed from the tips of the rods. Lysosomal vesicles are indicated by L.

neurons. Each human retina has about 6 million cone cells. The structure is similar to that of the rods, with outer and inner segments, basal body with cilium, and an accumulation of mitochondria and polyribosomes (Fig 24–18). The cones differ from the rods in their conical form and the structure of their outer segments. This region is also composed of stacked membranous disks; however, they are not independent of the outer plasma membrane but arises as invaginations of this structure (Fig 24–18). In cones, newly synthesized protein is not concentrated in re-

cently assembled disks (as it is in rods) but is distributed uniformly throughout the outer segment. There are at least 3 functional types of cones that cannot be distinguished by their morphologic characteristics. Each type contains a variety of the cone photopigment called **iodopsin,** and its maximum sensitivity is in the red, green, or blue region of the visible spectrum. The cones, sensitive only to light of a higher intensity than that required to stimulate the rods, are believed to permit better visual acuity than do the rods.

FOUR FUNCTIONS OF A RETINAL PIGMENT CELL

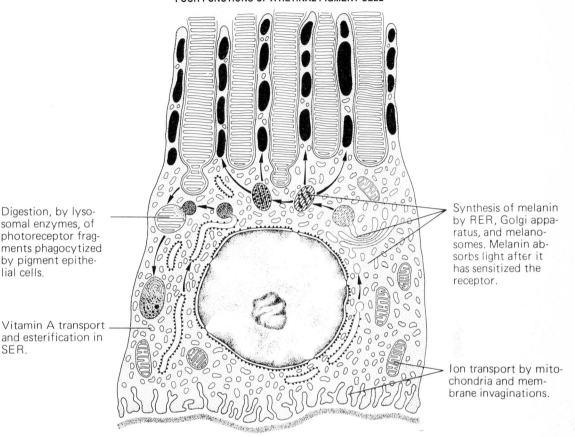

Digestion, by lyso-
somal enzymes, of
photoreceptor frag-
ments phagocytized
by pigment epithe-
lial cells.

Vitamin A transport
and esterification in
SER.

Synthesis of melanin
by RER, Golgi appa-
ratus, and melano-
somes. Melanin ab-
sorbs light after it
has sensitized the
receptor.

Ion transport by mito-
chondria and mem-
brane invaginations.

Figure 24–21. Drawing of a pigment epithelial cell. Observe that the apical portion has abundant cell processes that fill the spaces between the outer segments of the photosensitive cells and the membrane of the basal region has invaginations into the cytoplasm. This is a cell type with several functions, including the synthesis of melanin granules (by a process described in Chapter 18) that absorb stray light in the eye chamber. This is depicted on the right side of the figure, which shows the organelles that participate in melanin synthesis. On the left side of the figure, lysosomes containing enzymes synthesized in the rough endoplasmic reticulum coalesce with the phagocytized apical parts of the photoreceptors, digesting them. In addition to these activities, these cells are probably active in ion transport, since they maintain an electrical potential between the 2 surfaces of the epithelial membrane. The relatively well developed smooth endoplasmic reticulum participates in the processes of vitamin A esterification. SER, smooth endoplasmic reticulum; RER, rough endoplasmic reticulum.

The layer of bipolar cells consists of 2 types of cells (Fig 24–17): **diffuse bipolar cells,** which have synapses with 2 or more photoreceptors; and **monosynaptic bipolar cells,** which establish contact with the axon of only one cone photoreceptor and only one ganglion cell. There are, therefore, a certain number of cones that transmit their impulses directly to the central nervous system.

The cells of the ganglion layer, in addition to establishing contact with the bipolar cells, project their axons to a specific region of the retina, where they come together to form the **optic nerve** (Fig 24–17). This region, which is devoid of receptors, is known as **the blind spot** of the retina, the **papilla of the optic nerve,** or the **optic nerve head** (Fig 24–9). The **ganglion cells** are typical nerve cells, containing a large euchromatic nucleus, basophilic Nissl substance, etc. These cells, like the bipolar cells, are also classified as diffuse or monosynaptic types in their connections with other cells.

In addition to these 3 main types of cells (photoreceptor, bipolar, and ganglion cells), there are other types of cells distributed more diffusely in the layers of the retina.

(1) Horizontal cells (Fig 24–17) establish contact between different photoreceptors. Their exact function is not known, but it is possible that they act to integrate stimuli.

(2) Amacrine cells are various types of neurons that establish contact between the ganglion cells. Their function is also obscure.

(3) Supporting cells are neuroglia that possess, in addition to the astrocyte and microglial cell types, some large, extensively ramified cells called **Müller cells.** The processes of these cells bind together the neural cells of the retina and extend from the inner to the outer limiting membranes of the retina (Fig 24–17). They contain abundant microfilaments and glycogen in their cytoplasm and are known to have a high metabolic rate. The outer limiting membrane is a zone of adhesion (tight junctions) between photoreceptors and Müller cells. These latter cells are functionally analogous to neuroglia in that they support, nourish, and insulate the retinal neurons and fibers (Fig 24–22).

Retinal Histophysiology

Light passes through the layers of the retina to the rods and cones, where it is absorbed, initiating a series of reactions that result in what we call vision—an extraordinarily sensitive process. There is experimental evidence to suggest that a single photon is enough to trigger the production of a receptor potential in a rod. Light acts to bleach the visual pigments, a photochemical process amplified by mechanisms that cause the local production of responses which are subsequently transmitted to the central nervous system.

The visual pigment of rods, **rhodopsin,** is composed of an aldehyde of vitamin A (retinal) bound to specific proteins called **opsins.** Because the rods (the receptors used for low levels of illumination) have a low resolution they form images without clear details; they are not sensitive to colors. Cones, on the other hand, have a higher threshold and are responsible for sharp images and color vision. They contain 3 not yet completely characterized pigments (iodopsins) in humans, which may provide a possible chemical basis for the classic tricolor theory of color vision.

When light strikes rhodopsin molecules, retinal undergoes isomerization from the 11-*cis* form to the all-*trans* form. This change results in the dissociation of retinal from opsin, a reaction termed **bleaching.** Bleaching of the visual pigment incorporated in the membrane disks increases the calcium conductance of the disk membranes and promotes a diffusion of calcium to the intracellular space of the outer segment of the photoreceptor. This calcium acts on the cell membrane, reducing its permeability to sodium ions and promoting cell hyperpolarization. The electrical signals produced by closing these sodium channels spreads to the inner segment and through gap junctions to neighboring cells.

In a second step, the visual pigment is reassembled, and the calcium ions are transported back into the disks by an energy-consuming process. The high energy requirement would seem to account for the abundance of mitochondria near the photosensitive

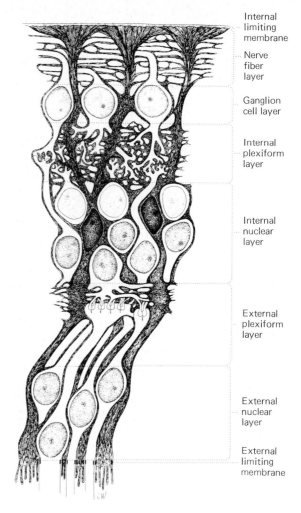

Figure 24–22. Illustration showing the close association of Müller cells with neural elements in the sensory retina. Müller cells (dark fibrous cells) appear to be structurally and functionally equivalent to the astrocytes of the central nervous system in that they envelop and support the neurons and nerve processes of the retina. (Reproduced, with permission, from Hogan MJ, Alvarado JA, Weddell JE: *Histology of the Human Eye.* Saunders, 1971.)

Labels on figure:
- Internal limiting membrane
- Nerve fiber layer
- Ganglion cell layer
- Internal plexiform layer
- Internal nuclear layer
- External plexiform layer
- External nuclear layer
- External limiting membrane

site of rods and cones. Contrary to what happens in other receptors where action potentials are generated through cell depolarization, the rods and cones are hyperpolarized by light. This signal is transmitted to the bipolar, amacrine, and horizontal cells and then to the ganglion cells. Only the ganglion cells generate action potentials along their axons, which relay the information to the central nervous system.

The clinical observation that the retina is damaged when it becomes detached suggests that the photosensitive cells derive their metabolites from the choriocapillary layer. The superficial localization of the vessels of the retina provides for their easy observation with an ophthalmoscope. This examination is of great value in the diagnosis and evaluation of disorders that affect blood vessels, such as diabetes mellitus and hypertension.

At the posterior pole of the optical axis lies the **fovea,** a shallow depression in whose center the retina is very thin. This is because the bipolar and ganglion cells accumulate in the periphery of this depression, so that its center consists only of cone cells (Fig 24–9). Cone cells in the fovea are long and narrow, resembling rod cells in shape. This is an adaptation to permit closer packing of cones and thereby increase visual acuity. In this area, blood vessels do not cross over the photosensitive cells. Light falls directly on the cones in the central part of the fovea, which helps account for the extremely precise visual acuity of this region. Light not absorbed by the photoreceptors is absorbed by the pigment cells of the retinal pigment epithelium and the choroid.

The structure of the retina varies according to the region. The fovea has only cones, and the blind spot, or papilla, has no receptors (Fig 24–9). Other structural variations of physiologic significance are also observed in the retina. The number of ganglion cells per unit area is one such example. In the periphery of the retina, these cells are relatively few in number—hundreds of cells per square millimeter—in sharp contrast to the fovea, where the cells are counted in hundreds of thousands per square millimeter. Therefore, vision at or near the fovea is much sharper than at the peripheral part of the retina.

2. ACCESSORY STRUCTURES OF THE EYE

Conjunctiva

The conjunctiva (Fig 24–10A) is a thin, transparent mucous membrane that covers the anterior portion of the eye up to the cornea and the internal surface of the eyelids. It has a stratified columnar epithelium with numerous goblet cells, and its lamina propria is composed of loose connective tissue.

Eyelids

Eyelids (Fig 24–23) are movable folds of tissue that protect the eye. The skin of the lids is loose and elastic, permitting extreme swelling and subsequent return to normal shape and size.

The three types of glands in the lid are the meibomian glands and the glands of Moll and Zeis. The meibomian glands are long sebaceous glands in the tarsal plate. They do not communicate with the hair follicles. There are about 25 in the upper lid and 20 in the lower lid, appearing as yellow vertical streaks deep into the conjunctiva. The meibomian glands pro-

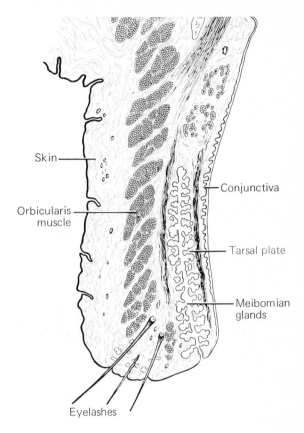

Figure 24–23. Diagram illustrating the structure of the eyelid.

duce a sebaceous substance that creates an oily layer on the surface of the tear film, helping to prevent rapid evaporation of the normal tear layer. The glands of Zeis are smaller, modified sebaceous glands connected with the follicles of the eyelashes. The sweat glands of Moll are unbranched sinuous tubules that begin in a simple spiral and not in a glomerulus like ordinary sweat glands. They empty their secretion into the follicles of the eyelashes.

Lacrimal Apparatus

The lacrimal apparatus (Figs 24–24 and 24–25) consists of the lacrimal gland, canaliculi, lacrimal sac, and nasolacrimal duct. The **lacrimal gland** is a tear-secreting gland located in the anterior superior temporal portion of the orbit. It consists of several separate glandular lobes with 6–12 excretory ducts that connect the gland to the superior conjunctival fornix. (Fornices are the conjunctiva-lined recesses between the lids and the eyeball.) A tubuloalveolar gland that usually has distended lumens, it is composed of column-shaped cells of the serous type, resembling the parotid acinar cells. They show lightly stained secretory granules, and a basal lamina sepa-

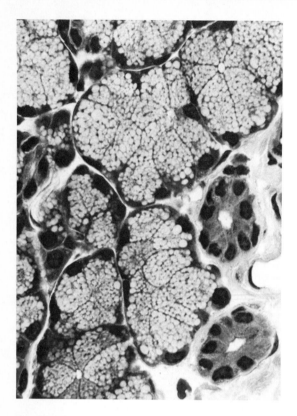

Figure 24–24. Photomicrograph of a section of a lacrimal gland. Ducts are shown on the right, the secretory portion in the center. H&E stain, × 350.

rates them from the surrounding connective tissue.

Well-developed myoepithelial cells surround the secretory portions of this gland. The secretion of the gland passes down over the cornea and the bulbar and palpebral conjunctiva, moistening the surfaces of these structures. It drains into the **lacrimal canaliculi** through the **lacrimal puncta,** round apertures about 0.5 mm in diameter on the medial aspect of both the upper and lower lid margins (Fig 24–25). The canaliculi are about 1 mm in diameter and 8 mm long and join to form a common canaliculus just before opening into the lacrimal sac. The canaliculi are lined by a thick stratified squamous epithelium. Diverticuli of the common caniliculus, which may be part of the normal structure, are frequently susceptible to fungal infections.

The **lacrimal sac** is the dilated portion of the lacrimal drainage system that lies in the bony lacrimal fossa. The **nasolacrimal duct** is the downward continuation of the lacrimal sac. It opens into the inferior meatus lateral to the inferior turbinate. Both the lacrimal sac and the nasolacrimal duct are lined with ciliated pseudostratified epithelium. The lacrimal glands produce a fluid secretion rich in the enzyme lysozyme, whose main functions are to moisten the surface of the eye and to hydrolyze the cell walls of certain species of bacteria.

HEARING: THE AUDIORECEPTOR SYSTEM

The Ear (Vestibulocochlear Apparatus)

The functions of the vestibulocochlear apparatus (Fig 24–26) are related to equilibrium and hearing. The organ consists of 3 parts: the **external ear,** which receives the sound waves; the **middle ear,** where these waves are transmitted from air to bone and by bone to the internal ear; and the **internal ear,** where these vibrations are transduced to specific nerve impulses that pass via the acoustic nerve to the central nervous system. The internal ear also contains the vestibular organ, which maintains equilibrium.

External Ear

The **auricle (pinna)** consists of an irregularly shaped plate of elastic cartilage covered by tightly adherent skin on all sides.

The **external auditory meatus** is a somewhat flattened canal extending from the surface into the temporal bone. Its internal limit is the tympanic membrane. A stratified squamous epithelium continuous with the skin lines the canal. Hair follicles, sebaceous glands, and a type of modified sweat gland—the **ceruminous glands**—are found in the submucosa. Ceruminous glands are coiled tubular glands that produce the cerumen—or earwax—a brownish, semisolid mixture of fats and waxes. Hairs and cerumen probably have a protective function. The wall of the external auditory meatus is supported by elastic cartilage in its outer third, while the temporal bone provides support for the inner part of the canal.

Across the deep end of the external auditory meatus lies an oval membrane, the **tympanic membrane** (eardrum). Its external surface is covered by a thin layer of epidermis and its inner surface by simple cuboidal epithelium continuous with the lining of the tympanic cavity (see below). Between the 2 epithelial coverings is a tough connective tissue layer composed of collagen and elastic fibers and fibroblasts. The anterior upper quadrant of the tympanic membrane is flaccid and more transparent, since the connective tissue layer is much thinner here. This region is known as **Schrapnell's membrane.** The tympanic membrane is the structure that transmits sound vibrations to the ossicles of the middle ear (Fig 24–26).

Middle Ear

The middle ear, or tympanic cavity, is an irregular space that lies in the interior of the temporal bone between the tympanic membrane and the bony surface of the internal ear. It communicates anteriorly with the pharynx by the **auditory tube (eustachian**

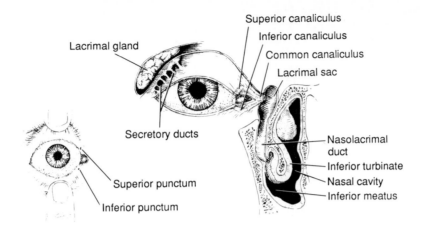

Figure 24–25. The lacrimal drainage system. (Redrawn with modifications and reproduced, with permission, from Thompson: Radiography of the nasolacrimal passageways. *Med Radiogr Photogr* 1949;**25**:66.)

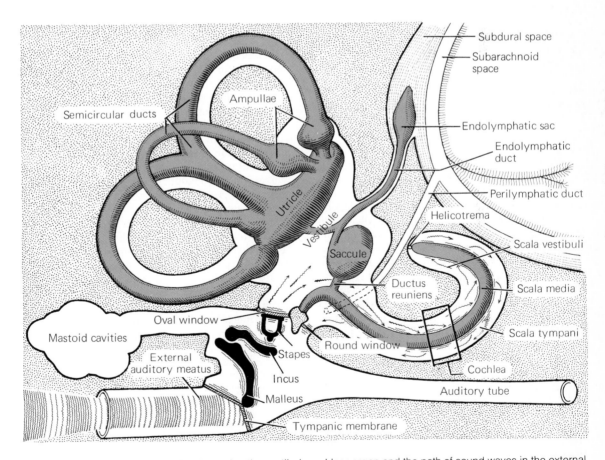

Figure 24–26. Schematic drawing illustrating the vestibulocochlear organ and the path of sound waves in the external, middle, and internal ear. Components of the internal ear are shown in color. A cross section of the cochlea, as outlined, is illustrated in Fig 24–30. (Redrawn and reproduced, with permission, from Best CH, Taylor NB: *The Physiological Basis of Medical Practice,* 8th ed. Williams & Wilkins, 1966.)

tube) and posteriorly with the air-filled cavities of the mastoid process of the temporal bone. The middle ear is lined by simple squamous epithelium resting on a thin lamina propria that is strongly adherent to the subjacent periosteum. Near the auditory tube and in its interior, the simple epithelium that lines the middle ear is gradually transformed into ciliated pseudostratified columnar epithelium. Although the walls of the tube are usually collapsed, the tube opens during the process of swallowing, balancing the pressure of the air in the middle ear with atmospheric pressure. In the medial bony wall of the middle ear are 2 membrane-covered oblong regions devoid of bone; these are the **oval** and **round windows** (Fig 24–26), which will be described later.

The tympanic membrane is connected to the oval window by a series of 3 small bones—the **auditory ossicles:** the **malleus, incus,** and **stapes** (Fig 24–26)—that transmit the mechanical vibrations generated in the tympanic membrane to the inner ear. The malleus inserts itself into the tympanic membrane and the stapes into the membrane of the oval window. These bones are articulated by synovial joints and, like all structures of this cavity, they are covered by simple squamous epithelium. In the middle ear, 2 small muscles are present that insert themselves into the malleus and stapes. They too have a function in sound conduction.

Internal Ear

The internal ear is composed of 2 **labyrinths.** The **bony labyrinth** consists of a series of spaces within the petrous portion of the temporal bone that house the **membranous labyrinth** (Fig 24–26). The membranous labyrinth is a continuous epithelium-lined series of cavities of ectodermal origin. It derives from the auditory vesicle that is developed from the ectoderm of the lateral part of the embryo's head. During embryonic development, this vesicle invaginates into the subjacent connective tissue, loses contact with the cephalic ectoderm, and moves deeply into the rudiments of the future temporal bone. During this process, it undergoes a complex series of form changes, giving rise to 2 specialized regions of the membranous labyrinth: the **utricle** and the **saccule.** The **semicircular ducts** take their origin from the utricle, while the elaborate **cochlear duct** is formed from the saccule. In each of these areas, the epithelial lining becomes specialized to form such sensory structures as the **maculae** of the utricle and saccule, the **cristae** of the semicircular ducts, and the **organ of Corti** of the cochlear duct.

The **bony labyrinth** consists of spaces in the temporal bone. There is an irregular central cavity, the **vestibule,** housing the saccule and the utricle. Posteriorly, 3 **semicircular canals** enclose the semicircular ducts, while the anterolaterally directed **cochlea** contains the cochlear duct (Fig 24–26).

The cochlea, about 35 mm in total length, makes 2.5 turns around a bony core known as the **modiolus.** The modiolus has spaces within it containing blood vessels and the cell bodies and processes of the acoustic branch of the eighth cranial nerve (spiral ganglion). Extending laterally from the modiolus is a thin bony ridge, the **osseous spiral lamina.** This structure extends farther across the cochlea in the basal than it does at the apex (Fig 24–30).

The bony walls of the vestibule and semicircular canals are lined by several layers of flattened connective tissue cells that form a mesothelium. From this layer, thin trabeculae, consisting of fine fibrils and fibroblasts, extend to the outer walls of the utricle, saccule, and semicircular ducts and support these parts of the membranous labyrinth. Blood vessels are also found in this connective tissue.

The bony labyrinth is filled with **perilymph,** which is similar in ionic composition to extracellular fluids elsewhere but has a very low protein content. The membranous labyrinth contains **endolymph,** which is characterized by its low sodium and high potassium content. The protein concentration in endolymph is low.

Histology of the Membranous Labyrinth

A. Saccule and Utricle: These structures are composed of a thin sheath of connective tissue lined by simple squamous epithelium. The membranous labyrinth is bound to the periosteum of the osseous labyrinth by thin strands of connective tissue that also contain blood vessels supplying the epithelia of the membranous labyrinth. In the wall of the saccule and utricle, one can observe small regions, called **maculae,** of differentiated neuroepithelial cells innervated by branches of the vestibular nerve (Fig 24–27). The macula of the saccule lies in its floor, while that of the utricle occupies the lateral wall so that the maculae are perpendicular to one another. Maculae in both locations have basically the same histologic structure. They consist of a thickening of the wall and possess 2 types of receptor cells, some supporting cells, and the afferent and efferent nerve endings.

Receptor cells (**hair cells**) are characterized by the presence of 40–80 long, rigid stereocilia, which are actually highly specialized microvilli, and one cilium (Fig 24–27). Stereocilia are arranged in rows of increasing length, with the longest—about 100 μm in length—located adjacent to a cilium. The cilium has a basal body and the usual 9 + 2 arrangement of microtubules in its proximal portion, but the central 2 microtubules soon disappear. This cilium is usually called a kinocilium, but it probably is immotile. Hair cells have a dense terminal web, numerous mitochondria, a well-developed Golgi complex, and an abundance of smooth endoplasmic reticulum. There are 2 types of hair cells distinguished by the form of their afferent innervation. Type I cells have a large, cup-shaped ending surrounding most of the base of the

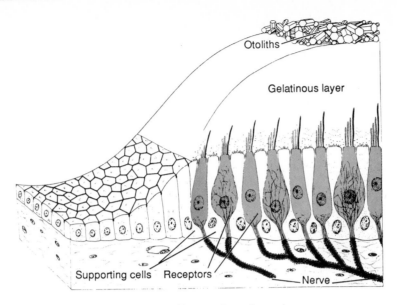

Figure 24–27. The structure of maculae.

cell, while type II receptors have many small afferent endings. Both types have efferent nerve endings that are probably inhibitory.

The supporting cells disposed between the receptors are columnar in shape with the nucleus at the base of the cell and microvilli on the apical surface (Fig 24–27). Covering this neuroepithelium is a thick, gelatinous glycoprotein layer, probably secreted by the supporting cells, with surface deposits of crystals composed mainly of calcium carbonate and called **otoliths (otoconia)** (Figs 24–27 and 24–28).

B. Semicircular Ducts: These structures have the same general form as the corresponding parts of the bony labyrinth. The receptor areas present in their **ampullae** (Fig 24–26) have an elongated ridgelike form; they are called **cristae ampullares.** The ridge is oriented perpendicular to the long axis of the duct. Cristae are structurally similar to maculae, but their glycoprotein layer is thicker; it has a conical form called a **cupula** and is not covered by otoliths. The cupula extends across the ampullae, establishing contact with its opposite wall (Fig 24–29).

C. Endolymphatic Duct and Sac: The endolymphatic duct initially has a simple squamous epithelial lining. As it nears the endolymphatic sac, it gradually changes to tall columnar epithelium composed of 2 cell types, one of which has microvilli on its apical surface and abundant pinocytotic vesicles and vacuoles. It has been suggested that these cells are responsible for the absorption of endolymph and the endocytosis of foreign material and cellular remnants that may be present in endolymph.

D. Cochlear Duct: This structure, a diverticulum of the saccule, is highly specialized as a sound recep-

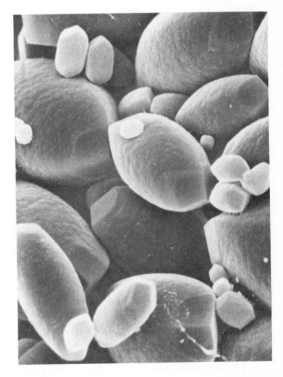

Figure 24–28. Scanning electron micrograph of the surface of a pigeon's macula showing the otoliths. (Courtesy of DJ Lim.)

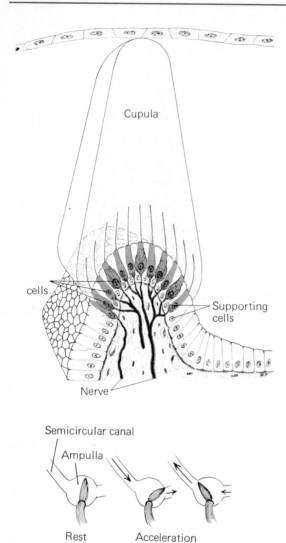

Cupula

cells

Supporting
cells

Nerve

Semicircular canal

Ampulla

Rest   Acceleration

Figure 24–29. Crista ampullaris. **Top:** Schematic drawing of the structure of the crista ampullaris. **Bottom:**
Movements of the cupula in an ampullary crista during
rotational acceleration. Arrows indicate the direction of
fluid movement. (Redrawn and reproduced, with permission, from Wersall J: Studies on the structure and innervation of the sensory epithelium of the cristae ampullares
in the guinea pig. *Acta Otolaryngol [Stockh] Suppl*
1956;**126**:1.)

tor. It is about 35 mm long and is surrounded by
specialized perilymphatic spaces. When observed in
histologic sections, the cochlea (in the bony labyrinth) appears to be divided into 3 spaces: the **scala
vestibuli** above the **scala media** (cochlear duct) and
the **scala tympani** below (Fig 24–30). The cochlear
duct, which contains endolymph, ends blindly at the
apex of the cochlea. The other 2 scalae contain perilymph and are in reality one long tube, beginning at
the **oval window** and terminating at the **round win-**

dow (Fig 24–26). They communicate at the apex of
the cochlea via an opening known as the **helicotrema.**

The cochlear duct has the following histologic
structure (Fig 24–30). The **vestibular (Reissner's)
membrane** consists of 2 layers of squamous epithelium, one derived from the cochlear duct and the
other from the lining of the scala vestibuli. Cells of
both layers are joined by extensive tight junctions that
help preserve the very high ionic gradients across this
membrane. The **stria vascularis** is an unusual vascularized epithelium located in the lateral wall of the
cochlear duct. It consists of 3 types of cells: marginal,
intermediate, and basal. Marginal cells have many
deep infoldings of their basal plasma membranes, and
numerous mitochondria are found here. These characteristics indicate that marginal cells are ion- and
water-transporting cells, and it is generally believed
that these cells are responsible for the characteristic
ionic composition of endolymph.

The **organ of Corti** contains hair cells that can
respond to different sound frequencies. It rests on a
thick layer of amorphous ground substance—the
basilar membrane—containing fibrils related to keratin that is formed by cells of the organ of Corti as
well as by mesothelial cells lining the scala tympani.
The basilar membrane is about 100 μm wide in the
basal turn of the cochlea and 500 μm wide in the
apical turn. Supporting and hair (receptor) cells of
the organ of Corti rest on this membrane. Many different types of supporting cells and 2 types of hair
cells can be distinguished. Three to five rows of **outer
hair cells** can be seen, depending on the distance
from the base of the organ, and a single row of **inner
hair cells** is present. Both types of hair cells are
columnar, with basally located nuclei, numerous mitochondria, and distinctive cisternae of smooth endoplasmic reticulum aligned beneath the lateral plasma
membranes. The most characteristic feature of these
cells is the W-shaped (outer hair cells) or linear (inner hair cells) array of stereocilia (Fig 24–31), which
increases in height from one side of the array to the
other. A basal body is found in the cytoplasm adjacent to the tallest stereocilia. In contrast to vestibular
receptors, no kinocilium is present. This absence imparts a symmetry to the hair cell that is important in
sensory transduction. In addition, the apical cytoplasm contains numerous fine filaments that impart
stiffness to this part of the cell, the **reticular lamina.**

The tips of the tallest stereocilia of the outer hair
cells are embedded in the **tectorial membrane,** a
glycoprotein-rich secretion of certain cells of the spiral limbus (Fig 24–30).

Of the supporting cells, the **pillar cells** should be
singled out for special mention. Pillar cells contain a
large number of microtubules that seem to impart
stiffness to these cells. They outline a triangular space
between the outer and inner hair cells—the **inner
tunnel** (Fig 24–30). This structure is of importance
in sound transduction, as discussed below.

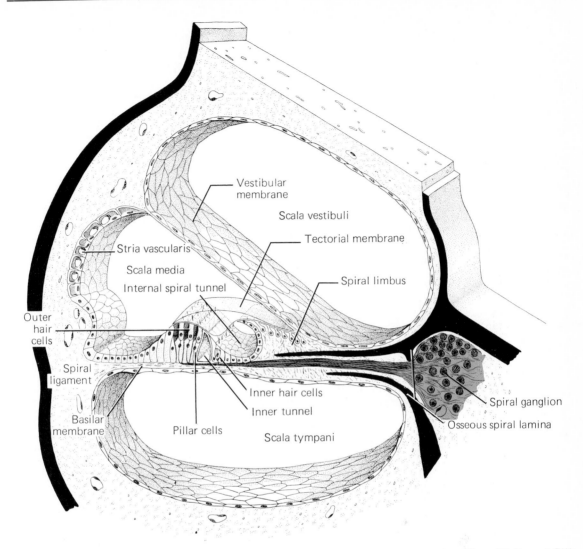

Figure 24–30. The structure of the cochlea. (Redrawn and reproduced, with permission, from Bloom W, Fawcett DW: *A Textbook of Histology*, 9th ed. Saunders, 1968.)

Both outer and inner hair cells have afferent and efferent nerve endings, and although the inner hair cells have by far the greater afferent innervation, the functional significance of this difference is not understood. The cell bodies of the bipolar afferent neurons of the organ of Corti are located in the modiolus and constitute the spiral ganglion (Fig 24–30).

Histophysiology of the Inner Ear

A. Vestibular Functions: Increase or decrease in the velocity of circular movement—angular acceleration or deceleration—causes a flow of fluid in the semicircular ducts as a consequence of the inertia of the endolymph. This induces a corresponding movement of the cupula over the crista ampullaris and results in the bending of the sterocilia on the sensory cells. Measurement of electrical impulses along vestibular nerve fibers indicates that movement of the cupula in the direction of the kinocilium results in excitation of the receptors, accompanied by the action potentials in the vestibular nerve fibers. Movement in the opposite direction inhibits neuronal activity. When uniform movement returns, acceleration ceases, the cupula returns to its normal position, and excitation or inhibition of the receptors no longer occurs (Fig 24–29).

The semicircular ducts respond to fluid displacement and therefore body position following angular acceleration. The maculae of the saccules and the utricles respond to linear acceleration. Because of their greater density, the otoliths are displaced when there is a change in the position of the head. This

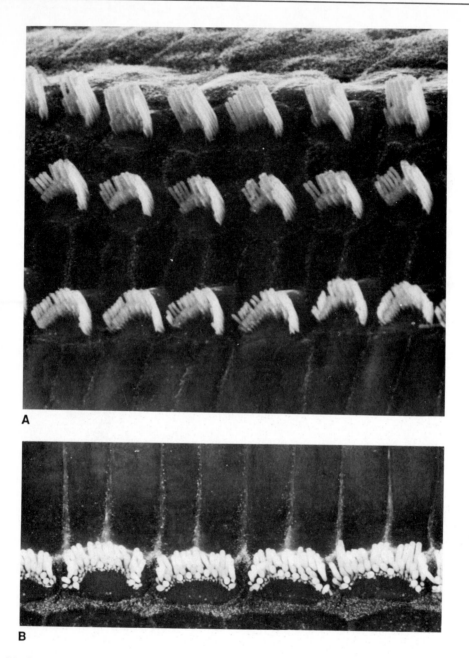

Figure 24–31. Scanning electron micrograph of 3 rows of outer hair cells **(A)** and a single row of inner hair cells **(B)** in the middle turn of a cat cochlear duct. × 2700. (Courtesy of P Leake.)

displacement is transferred to the underlying hair cells via the gelatinous otolithic membrane. Deformation of stereocilia of the hair cells results in action potentials that are carried to the central nervous system by the vestibular branch of the eighth cranial nerve. Maculae are thus sensitive to the force of gravity on the otoliths. The vestibular apparatus is important for the perception of movement and orientation in space and for the maintenance of equilibrium or balance.

B. Auditory Functions: Sound waves impinging on the tympanic membrane set the auditory ossicles into motion. The large difference in area of the tympanic membrane and the footplate of the stapes ensures the efficient transmission of mechanical motion from air to the fluids of the inner ear. Two striated skeletal muscles are found in the middle ear—the **tensor tympani** muscle (attached to the malleus) and the **stapedius** muscle (attached to the stapes). Loud sounds result in reflex contractions of these muscles, which limit excursions of the tympanic membrane and the stapes; this helps prevent damage to the inner ear. These reflexes are too slow to guard against sudden loud sounds, such as gunshots.

The following is a step-by-step explanation of how sound waves are converted to electrical impulses in the inner ear (Fig 24–26). Sound waves are longitudinal waves with **compression** and **rarefaction** phases. The compression phase causes the stapes to move inward. Since the fluids of the inner ear are almost incompressible, the pressure change is transmitted across the vestibular membrane and the basilar membrane, causing them to be deflected downward toward the scala tympani. This pressure change also causes the covering of the round window to bulge outward, thereby relieving the pressure. Because the tips of the pillar cells form a pivot, downward deflection of the basilar membrane is converted into lateral shearing of stereocilia of hair cells against the tectorial membrane. The tips of stereocilia are deflected toward the modiolus and away from the position of the basal body.

During the rarefaction phase of the sound wave, everything is reversed—the stapes moves outward, the basilar membrane moves upward toward the scala vestibuli, and stereocilia of the hair cells are bent toward the stria vascularis and the position of the basal body. Deflection in this direction sets up depolarizing generator potentials in the hair cells that result in release of a neurotransmitter (chemical nature unknown) that causes the production of action potentials in bipolar neurons of the spiral ganglion (**excitation**).

Frequency discrimination is based on the response of the basilar membrane to the frequency of sound. The membrane responds with maximal displacement at different points along its length, depending on the frequency. High frequencies are detected at the basal end of the membrane, while low frequencies result in maximal movement of the basilar membrane in the apex of the organ of Corti. This **tonotopic** localization can be correlated with the width and stiffness of the basilar membrane—the narrow basilar membrane, with greater stiffness at the base, responds best to high-frequency sounds. Maximal displacement of the basilar membrane at the threshold of hearing is very small; 0.1 nm is a commonly quoted figure for a 3000-Hz tone.

REFERENCES

Cutaneous & Other Sensory Mechanisms

Beidler LM (editor): Olfaction. In: *Handbook of Sensory Physiology*. Vol 4. Springer, 1971.

Beidler LM (editor): Taste. In: *Handbook of Sensory Physiology*, Vol 4. Springer, 1971.

Graziadei PPC: The olfactory mucosa of vertebrates. In: *Handbook of Sensory Physiology*. Vol 4. Beidler LM (editor). Springer, 1971.

Iggo A, Andres KH: Morphology of cutaneous receptors. *Annu Rev Neurosci* 1985;**5**:1.

Keverne EB: Chemical senses: Smell. In: *The Senses*. Barlow HB, Mollon JD (editors). Cambridge Univ Press, 1982.

Moulton DG: Dynamics of cell populations in the olfactory epithelium. *Trans NY Acad Sci* 1974;**237**:52.

Schmidt RF (editor): *Fundamentals of Sensory Physiology*. Springer-Verlag, 1978.

The Eye

Bok D, Hall MO: The role of the retinal pigment epithelium in the etiology of inherited retinal dystrophy in the rat. *J Cell Biol* 1971;**49**:664.

Botelho SY: Tears and the lacrimal gland. *Sci Am* (Oct) 1964;**211**:78.

Dowling JE: Organization of vertebrate retinas. *Invest Ophthalmol*. 1970;**9**:665.

Hogan MJ et al: *Histology of the Human Eye*. Saunders, 1971.

McDevitt D (editor): *Cell Biology of the Eye*. Academic Press, 1982.

Schwartz EA: First events in vision: The generation of responses in vertebrate rods. *J Cell Biol* 1982;**90**:271.

Young RW: Visual cells and the concept of renewal. *Invest Ophthalmol* 1976;**15**:700.

The Ear

Hudspeth AJ: The hair cells of the inner ear. *Sci Am* (Jan) 1983;**248**:54.

Kimura RS: The ultrastructure of the organ of Corti. *Int Rev Cytol* 1975;**42**:173.

Lim DJ: Functional structure of the organ of Corti: A review. *Hear Res* 1986;**22**:117.

Index

NOTE: Page numbers in **boldface** type indicate a major discussion. A *t* following a page number indicates tabular material and an *i* following a page number indicates an illustration.

Corticotropic cells, 396*t*
Corticotropin (adrenocorticotropic hormone; ACTH)
connective tissue metabolism affected by, 124–125
corticotropic cells producing, 396*t*
hypersecretion of, 409
target organs affected by, 398*i*
thymic lymphocytes affected by, 268
Corticotropin-releasing hormone, 399*t*
Corti's organ, 490, 492–493
histology of, 492–493
Cortisol (hydrocortisone)
adrenal cortex secreting, 408*i*
connective tissue metabolism affected by, 124
Countercurrent exchange system, of straight vessels of kidney, 390*i*
Countercurrent multiplier system, of Henle's loop, 389*i*
Covering epithelium, 74–77
Cowper's glands, 438
Cranial flat bones
formation of, 150
growth of, 154
Creatine kinase, in M line, 198
Cretins, 420
CRH. *See* Corticotropin-releasing hormone
Cricoid cartilage, 343
Cristae
ampullaris, 491, 492*i*
mitochondrial, 31*i*, 32
of semicircular ducts, 490
Cross-bridges, in muscle contraction, 201, 202, 202*i*
Crown, of tooth, 284*i*, 285
Cryofracture, 7, 9*i*
Cryptorchidism, 433–434
Crypts
intestinal (intestinal glands, glands of Lieberkühn)
in large intestine, 306–308
in small intestine, 299, 300*i*
of palatine tonsils, 280
Crystallins, in lens fibers, 478
CSF. *See* Colony-stimulating factors
Cuboidal epithelium, 66, 76
simple, 66*i*, 75*t*, 76
stratified, 75*t*, 76
Cultures, living cells examined by
cell, **11–13**
tissue, **11–13**
Cumulus oophorus, 443–445
Cuneiform cartilage, 343
Cupula, 491, 492*i*
Cushing's syndrome, 409
Cutaneous basophil hypersensitivity, 241
Cuticle
hair, 365*i*, 366
nail, 367
Cutis laxa, 364
Cycle of seminiferous epithelium, 428–429, 430*i*
Cyclic AMP, in smooth muscle contraction, 213
Cysteine, in pheomelanin, 361
Cystic ducts, 333
Cytocenter, 47
Cytochemistry, **15–24**
basic principles of, 15
Cytocrine secretion, of melanin, 362
Cytogenetics, 57
Cytokeratins, 50, 48*t*, 93
in stratum basale, 357
Cytology, exfoliative, **462**
Cytomatrix, **51**
Cytopathy, mitochondrial, 64*t*

Cytoplasm, **25**
autophagosomes in digestion of, 41
Cytoplasmic deposits, 48*i*, **51**
Cytoskeleton, **44–51**. *See also specific component*
Cytosol, 51
Cytotoxic T cells (killer T cells), 242*t*, 243, 263
differentiation of, 263, 264*i*
in graft rejection, 268, 269*i*
Cytotrophoblast, 455, 456*i*, 459*i*

D cells, 297
in gastrointestinal tract, 304*t*
in islets of Langerhans, 410, 426*t*
nerve fiber terminations and, 413
D₁ cells, in gastrointestinal tract, 304*t*
DAB method, peroxidase identified by, 18–19
Dark cells (mucoid cells), in sweat glands, 368
Decidua, 456, 457*i*
basalis, 455*i*, 456, 457, 457*i*
capsularis, 455*i*, 456, 457*i*
parietalis, 456, 457*i*
Decidual cells, 457
Deciduous teeth (baby teeth), 285
Deep sensation, **467**
Defense
connective tissue in, 123–124
respiratory system in, 355–356
spleen in, 278
Degeneration
of nerve tissue, **185–188**
transneuronal, 185
Dehydration, for embedding, 2, 3*t*
Dehydroepiandrosterone, adrenal cortex secreting, 407
Dehydrogenases, histochemical methods for identification of, 18
Delta granules (dense bodies), in platelets, 246
Demarcation membranes, of megakaryocytes, 260
Demilunes, serous, in salivary glands, 312, 313*i*, 315*i*
Dendrites, 163–164, **168**
Dendritic cells (follicular cells), in lymph node, 272
Dendrodendritic synapse, 169
Dense bodies
in platelets (delta granules), 246
in smooth muscle, 213
Dense connective tissue
irregular, 120–122, 120*i*, 121*i*
regular, 120–122, 120*i*, 122*i*, 123*i*
Dense tubular system, in platelets, 245
Dense undercoating, 169
Density gradient centrifugation, in cell fractionation, 13
Dental lamina, in tooth development, 287, 288*i*
Dental papilla, in tooth development, 287
Dental pulp, 284*i*, 285, 286, 287*i*
Dentin, 284*i*, 285, 286*i*
formation of, 288
Dentinal tubules, 285, 286*i*, 288
Deoxyribonuclease
lysosomal, 40
pancreas secreting, 318
Deoxyribonucleic acid. *See* DNA
Dermal papillae, 358*i*, 363, 365*i*, 366
Dermal-epidermal junction, 364
abnormalities of, 364
Dermatan sulfate, 95
composition of, 96*t*
distribution of, 95, 96*t*
Dermatoglyphics (fingerprints), 357

Dermis, 357, **363–366**
age-related changes in, 364
blood vessels of, 364
nerves of, 364–366
Descemet's membrane, 472
Desmin (skeletin), 48*t*, 50
in skeletal muscle, 200
in smooth muscle, 213
Desmosine, in elastin, 107
Desmosomes (maculae adherentes), 69*i*, 70*i*, 73
in cardiac muscle, 209, 210*i*
of stratum basale, 357
of stratum spinosum, 358
Detachment, of retina, 481
Diabetes
insipidus, hypothalamic lesions causing, 402
mouse (*Acomys*), 64*t*
proinsulin, 64*t*
Diads, in cardiac muscle, 210
3,3-Diaminoazobenzidine (DAB), peroxidase identified by, 18–19
Diapedesis, 116, 124, 237, 256
and capillary permeability, 222
Diaphyseal funnels, 155
Diaphyseal shaft, 155
Diaphysis, bone, 146
growth of, 154–155
Diarthroses, 159, **159–162**
Diastole, arteries during, 224
Differential centrifugation, in cell fractionation, 12*i*, 13
Differential interference (Nomarski) optics, in phase contrast microscopy, 4, 5*i*
Differentiation, cell, **25**
of erythrocytes, 253
in hematopoiesis, **248–251**
Diffuse bipolar cells, 485
Diffuse neuroendocrine system, **87–88**
gastrointestinal tract and, 302, 303*i*, 304*t*
DiGeorge's syndrome, 168
Digestion, in small intestine, 305–306
Digestive system, **281–311**. *See also specific organ or structure*
cancer of, 310
cell renewal in, 308–310
glands associated with, **312–335**. *See also specific type*
tumors of, 333
structure of, 281–282
Dihydroepiandrosterone, adrenal cortex secreting, 407, 408*i*
3,4-Dihydroxyphenylalanine (dopa), in melanin synthesis, 362
Diiodotyrosine, 417
structure of, 419*i*
Dilator pupillae muscle, 477
Dipalmitoyl lecithin, in pulmonary surfactant, 350
Diploë, 147
Disks, intervertebral, **140**
herniation of, 140
Disse's space, 320
Distal convoluted tubules
histophysiology of, 389–390
structure of, 371, 372*i*, 373*i*, 374*i*, 375*i*, **383–384**, 385*i*
Distributing arteries, 224
Distributing veins, in liver, 321
DIT. *See* Diiodotyrosine
DNA
chromatin, 54, 55, 55*i*
histochemical methods for demonstration of, 15–16
in mitochondrial matrix, 33
nucleolar-organizer, 57, 58*i*